Advanced Procedures for Pain Management

Sudhir Diwan • Timothy R. Deer
Editors

Advanced Procedures for Pain Management

A Step-by-Step Atlas

Springer

Editors
Sudhir Diwan, MD, FIPP, DABIPP
Lenox Hill Hospital
New York, NY, USA

Manhattan Spine and Pain Medicine
New York, NY, USA

Timothy R. Deer, MD
The Center for Pain Relief
Charleston, WV, USA

ISBN 978-3-030-09854-4 ISBN 978-3-319-68841-1 (eBook)
https://doi.org/10.1007/978-3-319-68841-1

Printed on acid-free paper

This Springer imprint is published by the registered company Springer International Publishing AG part of Springer Nature.
The registered company address is: Gewerbestrasse 11, 6330 Cham, Switzerland

This atlas is dedicated to my mother, late Raniba Diwan, for teaching me the true meaning of life; to my wife Indira for her unconditional love and support; to our children Kaushal, Shira, Sneh, and Christian; and to our most wonderful grandchildren, Belen and Jonathon, for bringing joy and happiness to our lives. I am a better person because of my family.

I dedicate this book to the internationally renowned expert in neuromodulation for his dedication, research, and education, my dear friend and esteemed colleague, Timothy Deer. His contribution to the specialty of interventional pain medicine is unparalleled.

This atlas is also dedicated to the hard work of the section editors (Leonardo Kapural, Jason Pope, Steven Falowski, Ken Aló, Timothy Davis, and Corey Hunter) and all authors. Lastly, I dedicate this atlas to all my former fellows who made me an educator and mentor.

Sudhir Diwan, MD, FIPP, DABIPP

This book is a creation based on many people. My gratitude to my friend and colleague, Sudhir Diwan, for all of his vision and for shaping our field with his training of many young minds. He is a truly wonderful person and has a very kind heart. Greatest appreciation to our fellow authors and friends who led to this excellent piece of work.

The book is dedicated to my wife, Melissa, and to my children, Morgan, Taylor, Reed, and Bailie, for all the support over the years to build my career; to Jane, Jim, and Joe for guidance; to my Korean brother, Christopher Kim; to my family of physicians, nurses, physician assistants, and staff at the practice who make my work achievable; and to Jeff and Michelle for keeping my daily life functioning and successful.

Most of all, this book is dedicated to my patients who give me so much purpose in trying to make things better and reduce suffering, improve function, and reduce the need for opioids. Lastly, and most importantly, all praise and thanks go to my God, to whom I owe all blessings.

Timothy R. Deer, MD

Preface

The spine is a complicated structure that has led to great suffering and medical intrigue since antiquity. The process of being debilitated by spinal disease and subsequently reborn after a spinal intervention is a familiar story in our culture and in many cultures around the world. The ability for patients to continue in pain is unacceptable to most concerned parties, but unfortunately the solutions for this problem have also often proven to be fraught with issues. These solutions have included extensive and invasive surgeries, opioids, repetitive injections, and other passing trends that have not stood the test of evidence-based examination.

The continued quest to relieve pain and suffering in the twenty-first century has brought a desire for physicians, engineers, and industry to work together to achieve a goal of less invasive and more efficacious options for patients who suffer from spine-related maladies. This illustrated atlas is a modern update of these newly developed, cutting-edge procedures. Each chapter has an objective to create a roadmap to give optimal instruction regarding techniques, complication mitigation, and patient selection for better outcomes. This allows the physician to consider the critical steps of each method and the pearls of each treatment option. This layout allows for advancement of the physician who is learning these therapies such as residents and fellows but also allows for patient care improvement in the experienced hands of a seasoned doctor. This book goes beyond perceived boundaries of specialties, providing critical information and guidance to invasive pain specialists, anesthesiologists, physiatrist, neurosurgeons, and orthopedic spine surgeons.

In this colorful atlas, we examine minimally invasive options for treatment of ailments caused by the disc, nerve, joint, ligament, and combined disease states involving multiple structures. For each procedure, we go by a step-by-step approach to help make the review of these methods easier for reference in the daily performance of these techniques.

We are very proud of this atlas and greatly acknowledge the work of the many excellent physicians, researchers, and colleagues who participated in this book. Not only does their scholarly work make this book an excellent resource that should be in all libraries of those treating spinal disease, but the work of these amazing physicians advances the field daily in the United States and throughout the international community. We also acknowledge the critical eye and timely editorial guidance given to this project by Lee Klein, who did an extraordinary job.

We are hopeful that this illustrated atlas meets our primary goal. That objective is to elevate patient care and improve outcomes. This goal of helping our patients is why we continue to strive continuously to improve care and to serve those who need our assistance to reduce suffering and improve quality of life.

New York, NY, USA — Sudhir Diwan
Charleston, WV, USA — Timothy R. Deer

Contents

Section Editors

Kenneth M. Aló, MD The Methodist Hospital Research Institute, Texas Medical Center Houston, TX, USA

Timothy Davis, MD Orthopedic Pain Specialists, Santa Monica, CA, USA

Steven M. Falowski, MD Department of Neurosurgery, St. Luke's University Health Network, Bethlehem, PA, USA

Corey W. Hunter, MD Ainsworth Institute of Pain Management, New York, NY, USA

Department of Physical Medicine and Rehabilitation, Mount Sinai Hospital, New York, NY, USA

Leonardo Kapural, MD, PhD Wake Forest School of Medicine, Carolinas Pain Institute, Winston-Salem, NC, USA

Jason E. Pope, MD Summit Pain Alliance, Santa Rosa, CA, USA

Contributors

Kenneth M. Aló, MD The Methodist Hospital Research Institute, Texas Medical Center, Houston, TX, USA

Kasra Amirdelfan, MD IPM Medical Group, Inc., Walnut Creek, CA, USA

Miguel D. Attias, MD Tampa Pain Relief Center, Palm Harbor, FL, USA

Nyla Azam Division of Pain Medicine, Weill Cornell Medical College, New York, NY, USA

Nomen Azeem, MD Department of Neurology, University of South Florida, Tampa, FL, USA

Javid Baksh, DO Premier Pain Solutions, Asheville, NC, USA

Brenda Beck, DO Department of Anesthesiology and Pain Management, University Hospitals Cleveland Medical Center, Cleveland, OH, USA

Lora L. Brown, MD TruWell, PLLC, St. Petersburg, FL, USA

Abram H. Burgher, MD The Pain Center, Scottsdale, Arizona, USA

Allen W. Burton, MD Divisional vice President and Medical Director, Neuromodulation, Abbott, Plano, TX, USA

Lucas W. Campos, MD, PhD Summit Pain Alliance, Santa Rosa, CA, USA

Jonathan D. Carlson, MD Arizona Pain/Pain Doctor, Glendale, AZ, USA

Christopher J. Centeno, MD The Centeno-Schultz Clinic, Broomfield, CO, USA

Ronil V. Chandra, MBBS, MMed, FRANZCR School of Clinical Sciences, Monash University, Melbourne, VIC, Australia

Grant H. Chen, MD, DABA Department of Anesthesiology and Critical Care, Memorial Sloan Kettering Cancer Center, New York, NY, USA

Kenneth Sunghoon Choi, MD Olympus Pain and Orthopedics, Dallas, TX, USA

Harold Cordner, MD Florida Pain Management Associates, Sebastian, FL, USA

William F. Cusack, DO Abbott Laboratories, Plano, TX, USA

Christopher J. Czura, PhD The Feinstein Institute for Medical Research, Northwell Health, Manhasset, NY, USA

Houman Danesh, MD Integrative Pain Management, Department of Anesthesiology, Perioperative and Pain Medicine, Mount Sinai Hospital, New York, NY, USA

Timothy Davis, MD Orthopedic Pain Specialists, Santa Monica, CA, USA

Timothy R. Deer, MD The Center for Pain Relief, Charleston, WV, USA

Michael J. DePalma, MD Virginia iSpine Physicians, PC, Richmond, VA, USA

Sudhir Diwan, MD, FIPP, DABIPP Lenox Hill Hospital, New York, NY, USA

Manhattan Spine and Pain Medicine, New York, NY, USA

Priyal Fadadu, BS Orthopedic Pain Specialists, Fremont, CA, USA

Steven M. Falowski, MD Department of Neurosurgery, St. Luke's University Health Network, Bethlehem, PA, USA

Michael A. Fishman, MD, MBA Center for Interventional Pain and Spine, Exton, PA, USA

Jason R. Fritz, MSBE Center for Bioelectronic Medicine, The Feinstein Institute for Medical Research, Manhasset, NY, USA

Arun Ganesh, MD Department of Anesthesiology, Duke University, Durham, NC, USA

Tony Goldschlager, MBBS, PhD, FRACS Department of Neurosurgery, Monash Health, Melbourne, VIC, Australia

Department of Surgery, Monash University, Melbourne, VIC, Australia

Maged Guirguis, MD Department of Anesthesiology and Critical Care Medicine, Ochsner Health System, New Orleans, LA, USA

University of Queensland Ochsner Medical School, Brisbane, QLD, Australia

Jennifer M. Hah, MD, MS Division of Pain Medicine, Department of Anesthesiology, Perioperative, and Pain Medicine, Stanford University, Palo Alto, CA, USA

Maged Hamza, MD Virginia Innovative Pain and Spine Center, Richmond, VA, USA

Lewis Hanna, PhD Cytonics Corporation, Jupiter, FL, USA

Nathan J. Harrison, MD Department of Anesthesia and Pain Management, Ochsner Health System, New Orleans, LA, USA

Salim M. Hayek, MD Department of Anesthesiology and Pain Management, University Hospitals Cleveland Medical Center, Cleveland, OH, USA

Lee P. Hingula, MD Division of Pain Management, Department of Anesthesiology and Critical Care Medicine, Memorial Sloan-Kettering Cancer Center, New York, NY, USA

Joshua A. Hirsch, MD NeuroEndovascular Program, Harvard Medical School, Massachusetts General Hospital, Boston, MA, USA

Corey W. Hunter, MD Ainsworth Institute of Pain Management, New York, NY, Australia

Department of Physical Medicine and Rehabilitation, Mount Sinai Hospital, New York, NY, USA

Jared M. Huston, MD, FACS Surgery and Science Education, Hofstra Northwell School of Medicine, Center for Bioelectronic Medicine, The Feinstein Institute for Medical Research, Manhasset, NY, USA

Matthew W. Hyzy, DO The Centeno-Schultz Clinic, Broomfield, CO, USA

Navdeep Singh Jassal, MD Florida Pain Medicine, Department of Neurology/Pain, University of South Florida, Wesley Chapel, FL, USA

Matthew P. Jaycox, MD Department of Anesthesiology, Rush University Medical Center, Chicago, IL, USA

Leonardo Kapural, MD, PhD Wake Forest School of Medicine, Carolinas Pain Institute, Winston-Salem, NC, USA

Daniel L. Kline, MD Valley Health Interventional Spine, Winchester, VA, USA

David Kloth, MD Connecticut Pain Care, Danbury, CT, USA

Jeffrey Kramer, MD University of Illinois, College of Medicine, Chicago, IL, USA

Eric T. Lee, MD, MA Musculoskeletal Care and Regenerative Medicine, Summit Pain Alliance, Santa Rosa, CA, USA

Michael S. Leong, MD Division of Pain Medicine, Department of Anesthesiology, Perioperative, and Pain Medicine, Stanford University, Palo Alto, CA, USA

Thabele M. Leslie-Mazwi, MD NeuroEndovascular Program, Harvard Medical School, Massachusetts General Hospital, Boston, MA, USA

Timothy R. Lubenow, MD Department of Anesthesiology, Rush University Medical Center, Chicago, IL, USA

Paul J. Lynch, MD Arizona Pain Specialists, Scottsdale, AZ, USA

Tory L. McJunkin, MD Arizona Pain Specialists, Scottsdale, AZ, USA

W. Porter McRoberts, MD Holy Cross Hospital, Anodyne Research, University of Miami, School of Medicine, Miami, USA

Mahesh Mohan, MD ORA Orthopedics, Moline, IL, USA

Azmi N. Nasser, DO Arizona Pain Treatment Centers, Scottsdale, AZ, USA

Kevin Pauza, MD Texas Spine and Joint Hospital, Tyler, TX, USA

Jason E. Pope, MD Summit Pain Alliance, Santa Rosa, CA, USA

Scott Pritzlaff, MD Division of Pain Medicine, Department of Anesthesiology, Perioperative, and Pain Medicine, Stanford University, Palo Alto, CA, USA

Louis J. Raso, MD Broward General Hospital, New York, USA

Dawood Sayed, MD Division of Pain Meidicne, University of Kansas Medical Center, Kansas City, KS, USA

Michael Cody Scarbrough, MD Department of Anesthesia and Pain Management, Ochsner Health System, New Orleans, LA, USA

Gaetano J. Scuderi, MD Department of Orthopedic Surgery, Jupiter Medical Center, Jupiter, FL, USA

Jasmine Silva, DO IPM Medical Group, Inc., Walnut Creek, CA, USA

Lee-Anne Slater, MBBS, FRANZCR Interventional Neuroradiology Service, Monash Imaging, Monash Health, Melbourne, VIC, Australia

Edward L. Swing, PhD Arizona Pain Specialists, Scottsdale, AZ, USA

Christopher J. Williams, MD The Centeno-Schultz Clinic, Broomfield, CO, USA

Andrea C. Wong, MD, MPH University at Buffalo Neurosurgery, Williamsville, NY, USA

Ajax Yang, MD, MPT Department of Rehabilitation Medicine, Icahn School of Medicine at Mount Sinai, New York, NY, USA

Michael Yang, MD Summit Pain Alliance, Santa Rosa, CA, USA

Adam C. Young, MD Department of Anesthesiology, Rush University Medical Center, Chicago, IL, USA

Greg Zakas, DO The C.O.R.E. Institute, Mesa, AZ, USA

Part I
Advanced Spinal Interventions

Steven M. Falowski and Kenneth M. Aló

The subspecialty of minimally invasive surgery (MIS) for the treatment of pain has been practiced in various forms for decades, but never has it undergone such simultaneous growth and transformation. The MIS neurosurgeon of old has evolved into today's MIS pain management interventionalist thanks to the advent of miniaturized optics, implants, electrodes, batteries, and endoscopic portals; high-resolution stereotaxy, perioperative mapping, and neurophysiologic monitoring systems; and directional, multichannel catheters with real-time intraoperative imaging. Transformed by these innovations, physicians are now focused on objective, compassionate, less traumatic, and advanced surgical care, as well as continuous, advanced training and education. Minimally invasive access, technology, and tools are changing rapidly with options that will soon fit in the hands of all pain specialists. It is therefore fitting that this new *Atlas*, in part dedicated to minimally invasive spinal education, arrives to help advance the field and future of minimally invasive surgery for the management of pain.

Chapter 1
Advanced Spinal Mapping: An Interventional Continuum for Axial, Radicular, and Dorsal Root Ganglion–Related Pain

Jonathan D. Carlson and Kenneth M. Aló

1.1 Indications

The anatomy of the spine can undergo numerous changes that result in pain. Various forms of chronic pain, including pain of the neck, back, or extremities, may indicate one or more spinal pathologies. Differing treatments may be used depending on the pain generator, including radiofrequency neurotomy, corticosteroid injection, decompression, and neurostimulation. Utilizing an appropriate treatment may be challenging, given frequently comorbid spinal pathologies and potentially overlapping symptoms. Spinal mapping enables the identification and treatment of the appropriate pain generator. Spinal mapping and subsequent treatments can be used for a number of varying indications:

- Facet arthropathy
- Posterior disc herniation or extrusion
- Anterior disc herniation or extrusion
- Central canal stenosis
- Lateral canal stenosis
- Neuroforaminal stenosis
- Chemical disruption of the disc
- Intradiscal pressure
- Annular disc tear
- Dorsal root ganglion (DRG) mapping to optimize DRG stimulation

J.D. Carlson (✉)
Arizona Pain/Pain Doctor, Glendale, AZ, USA
e-mail: jcarlsonmd@gmail.com

K.M. Aló
The Methodist Hospital Research Institute, Texas Medical Center, Houston, TX, USA
e-mail: aglioolio@gmail.com

S. Diwan, T.R. Deer (eds.), *Advanced Procedures for Pain Management*,
https://doi.org/10.1007/978-3-319-68841-1_1

1.2 Relevant Anatomy

Denis' three-column theory divides the anatomy of the spine into three parallel vertical columns [1]:

- Anterior column
- Middle column
- Posterior column

The anterior column includes the anterior longitudinal ligament (ALL) and the anterior half of the vertebral body and intervertebral disc. The middle column includes the posterior half of the vertebral body and intervertebral disc, as well as the posterior longitudinal ligament (PLL). The posterior column includes everything posterior to the PLL: the ligamentum flavum, pedicles, facet joints, and the neural arch and supraspinous ligaments.

1.3 Contraindications

Most spinal mapping techniques and associated interventional procedures tend to be minimally invasive, with low risk, but as with any spinal intervention, each patient must be carefully examined for any associated pathophysiological conditions or other contraindications to their use:

- Coagulopathy, platelet count of less than 100,000
- Implants (pacemaker, neural implants, etc.)
- Skin infection over placement site
- Allergic reaction to local anesthetics or any other medication provided during procedure
- Malignancy near placement site
- Hypovolemia
- Sepsis
- Spinal abnormalities or decreased spinal stability
- Pregnancy
- Renal insufficiency
- Chronic liver dysfunction
- Cerebrovascular disease
- Increased intracranial pressure
- Patient refusal

1.4 Preoperative Considerations

- The patient should receive an explanation of the procedure and all risks and sign an informed consent form.
- Patient must be able to remain in a prone position for the entire duration of the procedure.
- A complete preoperative checklist should be followed, including reports of medications such as anticoagulants.
- The needle placement site should be examined to ensure that no negative skin conditions are present.
- Intravenous access should be established for IV fluid and medication, in case the patient experiences a vasovagal reaction.

1.5 Fluoroscopic Views

Classic fluoroscopic views for selective nerve root block (SNRB) are utilized: anteroposterior (AP), oblique, and lateral views.

1.6 Positioning of the Patient

Patient positioning is a very important component of the procedural process. Incorrect patient positioning can lead to various problems and even bodily damage. A significant portion of epidurals, medial branch blocks, and radiofrequencies require patients to be on their abdomen in a prone position. When the patient is prone, it is best to provide support under the abdomen to reduce lumbar lordosis; this can be achieved by using a pillow. Furthermore, a pillow should be placed under the feet (upper foot) as a form of comfort. If the patient is placed laterally—such as during a cervical medial branch block and/or radiofrequency—then a pillow should be placed under the head to keep the cervical spine aligned and minimize lateral flexion.

1.7 Equipment

Standard radiofrequency ablation (RFA) equipment, probes, and needles are used for spinal nerve root mapping (Figs. 1.1 and 1.2).

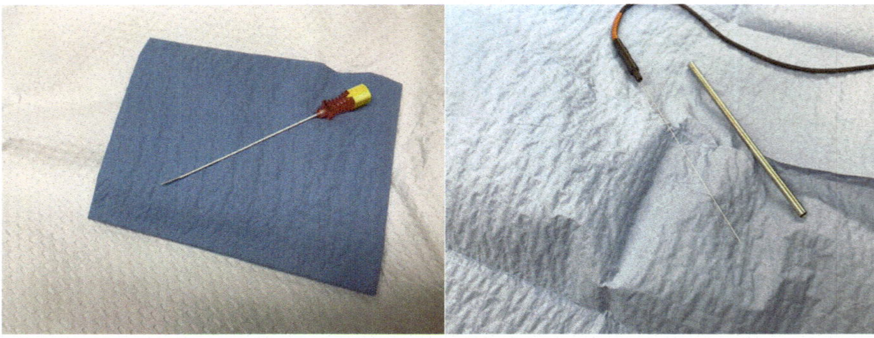

Fig. 1.1 *Left*, Standard radiofrequency ablation (RFA) needle with 10-mm active tip. *Right*, RFA probe

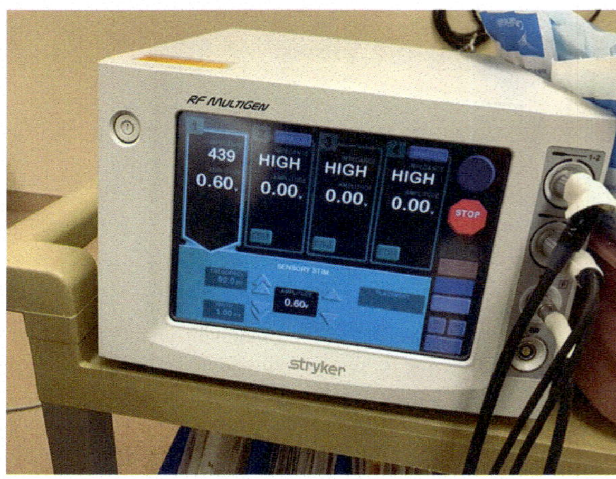

Fig. 1.2 Standard RFA machine with sensory program used for spinal nerve root mapping

1.8 Technique

Interventional treatments for chronic pain originating in the spine involve the localization of pain to the anterior or posterior column of one or more segments of the spine (Figs. 1.3 and 1.4). This mapping has traditionally involved either the selective injection of an anesthetic at the medial branch or spinal nerve roots (allowing a pain generator to be identified at a specific vertebral level) or provocative discography with pressure manometry to identify a pain generator at a specific intervertebral disc. There are some limitations with these traditional spinal mapping techniques. Pain relief provided by the anesthetics is usually delayed, meaning that the patient will not be able to provide immediate feedback on whether the targeted region is actually painful. Furthermore, several of these mapping techniques require structural imaging (MRI, CT, or xeroradiography) in order to identify potentially painful regions. These techniques suffer from additional disadvantages, including overlapping clinical presentations of facet-based and radicular pain, variance in patients'

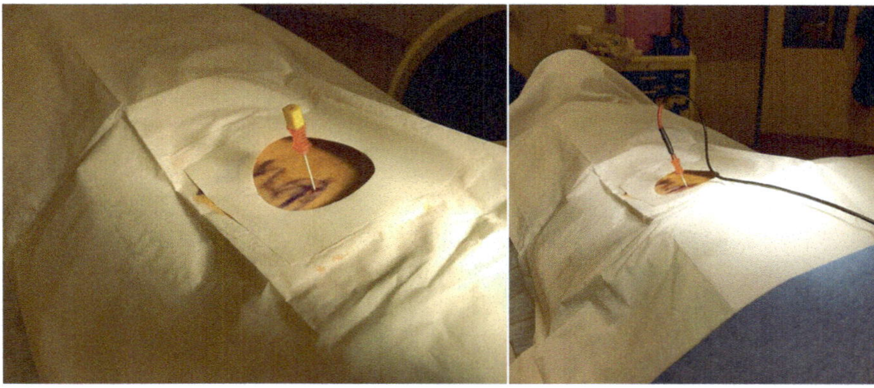

Fig. 1.3 Needle and probe placement for lumbar spinal nerve root mapping

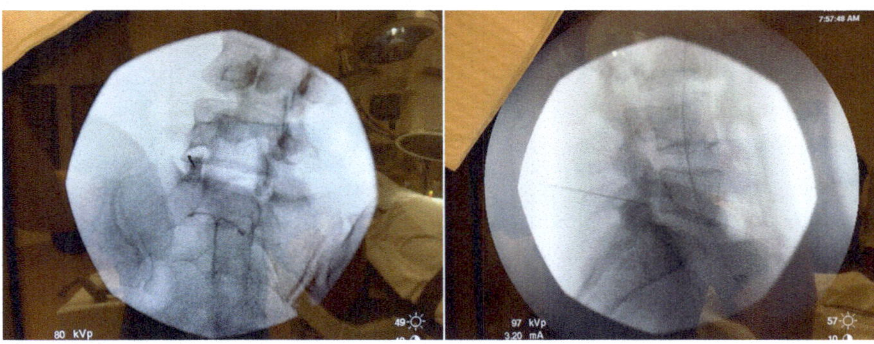

Fig. 1.4 Anteroposterior (AP) and lateral fluoroscopic views showing an example of needle placement for left L5 spinal nerve root mapping

pain reporting, and complications when attempting to identify the relationship between symptoms and structural imaging.

More recently, additional techniques have been introduced for the localization of pain generators. One such technique is radiofrequency needle stimulation [2]. Needle quantity varies by case, based on the number of regions being targeted. Radiofrequency stimulation can be used to generate paresthesia in multiple anatomical regions. Patients can provide immediate feedback on whether the affected region(s) are concordant with their pain. Additionally, this stimulation allows differentiation between radicular and segmental pain [3]. When concordant paresthesia is achieved through stimulation, anesthetic can be introduced to the corresponding nerves. A positive response to both radiofrequency needle stimulation and anesthetics should be followed by radiofrequency neurotomy [4, 5].

Despite its efficacy, radiofrequency stimulation has a few limitations. It requires multiple needle placements to examine the various levels, which generally requires multiple needle punctures, though it is possible to map multiple levels from a single incision by administering radiofrequency stimulation through an epidural catheter

[3]. The epidural catheter would allow for radiofrequency stimulation mapping of the dorsal ganglion and spinal root at numerous levels both bilaterally and ipsilaterally.

Another limitation of radiofrequency stimulation is that nerve branches at adjacent levels have overlapping areas of neural innervation. This can leave some ambiguity about the anatomical pain generator. Diagnostic epiduroscopy allows for the direct visualization of the epidural space. This technique allows for greater localization of pain generators. In the case of radiofrequency nerve stimulation, one can identify either dermatomal or sclerotomal pain patterns [6]. Diagnostic epiduroscopy can localize pain to either the anterior or posterior epidural space. New interventional techniques, such as new forms of decompression, new electrode designs for spinal cord stimulation, and new stimulation waveforms, can potentially take advantage of the more precise localization provided by advances in spinal pain mapping.

1.9 Middle Column/Anterior Column: Posterior Epidural Space

Fibrosis or the thickening and scarring of connective tissues has been treated in a multitude of ways. One popular treatment of choice for fibrosis within the posterior epidural space has been chemical adhesionolysis. Paired with fluoroscopy and enhanced with an endoscopic camera, epiduroscopic chemical adhesionolysis provides physicians with a better ability to penetrate through scarred tissue [7]. Though positive results have been found with the use of epiduroscopic chemical adhesionolysis, problems such as root compression and scarring can occur. Additionally, even though epiduroscopy provides visualization of change in inflammation within the epidural space, it has been limited by its poor optics and insufficient steering capability of the catheter(s) [8]. To ameliorate these epiduroscopy challenges, multiport endoscopes have been developed for the posterior epidural space, which allow increased instrumentation range and clearer and more precise visualization [9].

1.10 Anterior Epidural Space

Chronic pain can result from various pathologic changes of the anterior epidural space, such as acute neovascularization, annular disc tears, anterior disc herniations or extrusions, and chronic scar tethering. The anterior epidural space and disc-nerve interface can be directly visualized and accessed through an expanded in-line laminotomy and release of the filum terminale [10]. Alternatively, the anterior epidural space can be accessed through the sacral hiatus with a flexible endoscope [6]. The endoscope can be used to introduce balloons, stimulating catheters, laser waveguide fibers, and quantum molecular resonance fibers for both diagnosis and treatment. This approach has been used to successfully deliver decompression of the anterior epidural space [11].

1.11 Post-procedure Considerations

The patient should be contacted via telephone the day after the procedure to check for any potential complication that might have arisen. The patient should also be questioned about pain relief secondary to the local anesthetics. For interventional pain procedures, the patient should be reminded that relief may take several days (as for the anti-inflammatory effects of a steroid injection) or weeks (as for radiofrequency neurotomy). The patient should be monitored closely and should contact the pain clinic if he or she experiences any procedure-related complications or unexpected neurologic deficits:

- Urinary or bowel incontinence
- Bleeding
- Persistent nausea or vomiting
- Fever
- Severe site pain
- Paresthesia
- Weakness

1.12 Potential Complications

The procedures discussed in this chapter are primarily less invasive than other operations. They require percutaneous needle placement, but with the use of precise needle-placement techniques, complications associated with these procedures are rare. Site infections are a potential complication, but they can be easily circumvented by following sufficient aseptic guidelines. Other complications are also possible:

- Bruising of placement site
- Hematoma
- Paresthesia
- Nerve damage/injury
- Adverse injectate reaction
- Severe allergic reaction to local anesthetics
- Confusion
- Dural puncture headaches
- Chronic adhesive arachnoiditis

1.13 Clinical Pearls and Pitfalls

- Managing patient expectations and patient education are essential. Although nerve root mapping can help in elucidating which spinal nerve roots are affected, it is important to correlate the direct afferent and local anesthetic phase responses. The clinical diagnosis and decision-making on which nerve(s) may be affected is ultimately at the discretion of the provider.
- If intravenous sedation is to be used, it is important let the anesthesiologist know that the patient must be able to maintain meaningful communication throughout the entire procedure, for both safety and diagnostic purposes.
- It is very important to educate the patient that the important question is not how "intense" the sensory perception or paresthesia is when electrical stimulation is implemented, but rather whether it covers the area of the patient's pain (concordant paresthesia, etc.).
- Sensory stimulation of the intended spinal nerve root should ideally be done between 0.5 and 1.0 V, or the needle should be adjusted to optimize paresthesia perception.
- Once spinal nerve root mapping is complete, performing a concurrent selective nerve root block at the nerve root that may be the most affected should be considered, to further confirm the findings of the nerve root mapping.

References

1. Denis F. The three column spine and its significance in the classification of acute thoracolumbar spinal injuries. Spine. 1983;8:817–31.
2. Markman JD, Philip A. Interventional approaches to pain management. Anesthesiol Clin. 2007;25:883–98.
3. Alò K, Abramova M, Redko V, Williams J, McKee M, Noto D, et al. Technical update in spinal mapping, epidural disc and neural decompression, and neurostimulation: an interventional continuum for axial and radicular pain. Minim Invasive Surg Pain. 2013;1:54–62.
4. Dreyfuss P, Bogduk N. Lumbar medial branch neurotomy. In: Schmidt RF, Willis WD, editors. Encyclopedia of pain. New York: Springer; 2007. p. 1076–9.
5. Mikeladze G, Espinal R, Finnegan R, Routon J, Martin D. Pulsed radiofrequency application in treatment of chronic zygapophyseal join pain. Spine J. 2003;3:360–2.
6. Alò K, Abramova M, Cantu F, DeAndres J, Lierz P, Manchiaro P, et al. Technical update: axial and radicular pain. Recent advances in spinal pain mapping, epidural decompression and neurostimulation. Region Anesth Pain Med. 2011;36:45–9.
7. Manchikanti L, Boswell MV, Rivera JJ, Pampati VS, Damron KS, McManus CD, et al. A randomized, controlled trial of spinal endoscopic adhesiolysis in chronic refractory low back and lower extremity pain. BMC Anesthesiol. 2005;5:10.
8. Heavner J, Chokhavatia S, Kizelshteyn G. Percutaneous evaluation of the epidural and subarachnoid space with a flexible fiberscope. Reg Anesth. 1991;15(Suppl 1):85.
9. Raffaeli W, Caminiti A. L'endoscopia dello spazio epidurale – periduroscopia. Pathos. 2007;14(Suppl 1):61–5.
10. Richter E, Abramova M, Mussell J. Current trends in minimally invasive spinal surgery. J Neurosurg Rev. 2011;1(Suppl 1):1–13.

11. Richter EO, Abramova MV, Cantu F, DeAndres J, Lierz P, Manchiaro PL, et al. Anterior epiduroscopic neural decompression: eight-center experience in 154 patients. Eur J Pain Suppl. 2012;5:401–7.

Suggested Reading

Alò K, Abramova M, Richter E. Percutaneous peripheral nerve stimulation. Prog Neurol Surg. 2011;24:41–57.

Alò K, Abramova M, Redko V, Williams J, McKee M, Noto D, et al. Technical update in spinal mapping, epidural disc and neural decompression, and neurostimulation: an interventional continuum for axial and radicular pain. Minim Invasive Surg Pain. 2013;1:54–62.

Raffaeli W, Righetti D, Andruccioli J, Sarti D. Epiduroscopy and radiofrequency technique: the Raffaeli-Righetti technique. Pain Clin. 2007;19:1–7.

Saberski LR, Kitahata LM. Direct visualization of the lumbosacral epidural space through the sacral hiatus. Anesth Analg. 1995;80:839–40.

Chapter 2
MILD: Percutaneous Lumbar Decompression for Spinal Stenosis

Sudhir Diwan, Timothy R. Deer, Leonardo Kapural, and Jason E. Pope

2.1 Introduction

Lumbar spinal stenosis (LSS), or the narrowing of the spinal canal and neuroforamina, is secondary to degenerative changes in the spine, causing hypertrophy of the ligamentum flavum, degenerative disc disease, facet arthropathy, and osteophyte formation (Fig. 2.1). Central LSS leads to compression of the spinal cord, and foraminal stenosis causes compression of exiting nerve root causing radiculopathy. The hallmark symptom of LSS is neurogenic claudication (NC), which is pain aggravated by axial extension and relieved by forward flexion. Patients with LSS may also present with radiculopathy described as radiating pain in a dermatomal distribution. LSS generally affects men and women after age 50.

Lumbar spinal stenosis is defined as decrease in caliber of the spinal canal.

- Absolute spinal stenosis: 10 mm midsagittal lumbar canal diameter on CT
- Relative spinal stenosis: 13 mm midsagittal lumbar canal diameter on CT

S. Diwan (✉)
Lenox Hill Hospital, New York, NY, USA

Manhattan Spine and Pain Medicine, New York, NY, USA
e-mail: Sudhir.diwan63@gmail.com

T.R. Deer
The Center for Pain Relief, Charleston, WV, USA
e-mail: tdeermd@centerforpainrelief.com

L. Kapural (✉)
Wake Forest School of Medicine, Carolinas Pain Institute, Winston-Salem, NC, USA
e-mail: lkapural@ccrpain.com

J.E. Pope (✉)
Summit Pain Alliance, Santa Rosa, CA, USA
e-mail: popeje@me.com

S. Diwan, T.R. Deer (eds.), *Advanced Procedures for Pain Management*,
https://doi.org/10.1007/978-3-319-68841-1_2

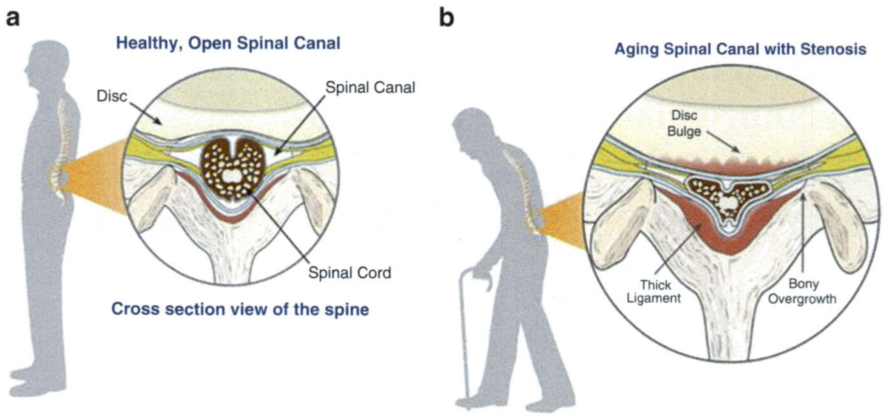

Fig. 2.1 (**a**, **b**) Comparing healthy open spinal canal with spinal canal stenosis with ligamentum flavum hypertrophy (*Courtesy of* Vertos Medical Inc.; Aliso Viejo, CA, USA)

The initial clinical presentation of LSS is insidious, and treated with conservative management including physical therapy, nonsteroidal anti-inflammatory and analgesic medications, and epidural steroid injections. The epidural steroid injections provide only short-term relief of radicular pain and are generally less effective in treating painful NC, which is not caused by central canal stenosis secondary to hypertrophied ligamentum flavum. Unfortunately, if the epidural steroid injections fail to provide adequate pain relief, the next step is surgical laminectomy decompression of the lumbar spinal canal with or without spinal fusion.

However, the quest for less invasive surgical techniques continues to shorten recovery times, decrease complication rates, and reduce tissue trauma, iatrogenic instability, and adjacent level disease secondary to extensive fusion. Percutaneous lumbar decompression of LSS is performed in an ambulatory set-up. The decompression of narrow spinal canal is achieved by removing small portions of lamina and ligamentum flavum (LF). The minimally invasive lumbar decompression (MILD) procedure is performed through a 6-gauge port under fluoroscopic guidance, with minimal tissue disruption. There is plenty of evidence in literature for the safety and clinical efficacy of this procedure, which virtually eliminates the possibility of serious complications including dural tear, blood loss requiring transfusion, and neurological complications.

2.2 Causes of Symptomatic LSS

- Ligamentum flavum hypertrophy (Fig. 2.2).
- Ligamentum flavum buckling
- Facet joint hypertrophy
- Vertebral body osteophytosis

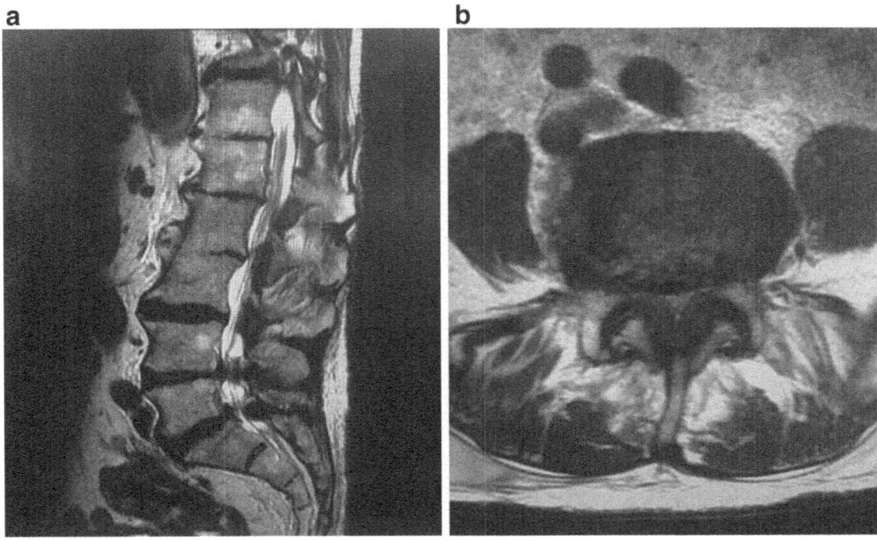

Fig. 2.2 (**a**, **b**) Severe spinal stenosis in sagittal (**a**) and axial (**b**) views

- Bulging and herniated discs
- Spondylolisthesis

2.3 Surgical Treatment of Central LSS

- Lumbar laminectomy
- Laminectomy with fusion
- Discectomy with laminectomy and fusion
- Interspinous space distraction

MILD procedure is a minimally invasive therapeutic option for LSS. It debulks the ligamentum flavum and portions of the lamina to restore space in the spinal canal. The restoration of space in the canal can be confirmed during the procedure utilizing the epidurogram (Fig. 2.2).

2.3.1 Epidurogram

The epidurogram is a key aspect of the MILD procedure. It is important for the safety during the procedure allowing decompression while ensuring that the rongeur or sculpter does not contact the dura, preventing potential patient injury. It should be performed at the same level and on the ipsilateral side of the level being treated. It is recommended to use the contralateral oblique fluoroscopic view to

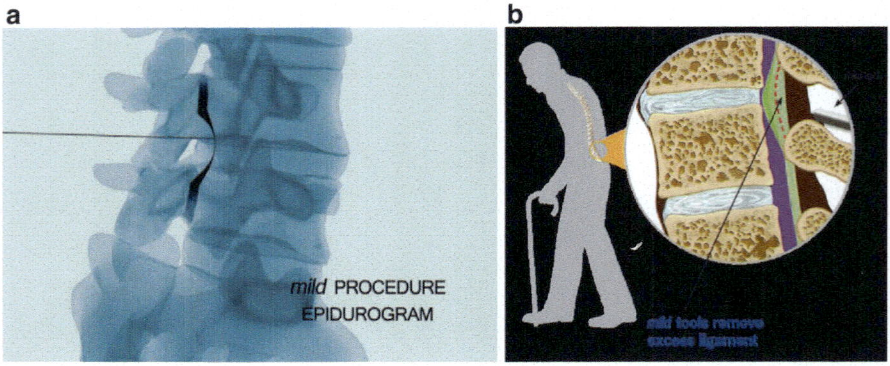

Fig. 2.3 Pre-procedure epidurogram (**a**) and hypertrophic ligament flavum (**b**) causing severe stenosis before MILD. (*Courtesy of* Vertos Medical Inc.)

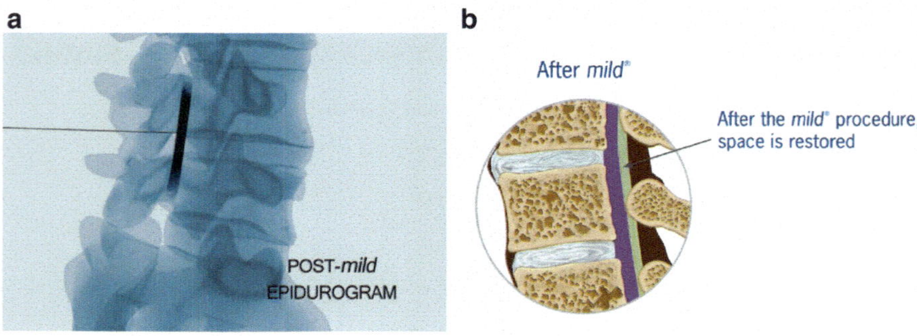

Fig. 2.4 (**a**) Epidurogram after MILD. (**b**) Space is restored, pressure reduced, and spinal canal mobility is restored after the procedure. (*Courtesy of* Vertos Medical Inc.)

visualize the epidurogram at the treatment site during decompression of the ligamentum flavum. The epidurogram provides an anterior safety margin that should be recognized at all times. The entire decompression procedure should be posterior to the epidurogram line to protect the spinal canal and neural structures.

In the contralateral view, the epidurogram presents as a clear line representing the posterior border with a "scalloped" appearance secondary to enlarged ligamentum flavum (Fig. 2.3). Reduction in the "scalloped" appearance, and thickening and straightening of the epidurogram line, indicate adequate decompression of the ligamentum flavum tissue (Fig. 2.4).

The MILD procedure only provides decompression.

- Removes only a small portion of the lamina to get access to the ligament
- 5.1 mm MILD portal minimizes tissue and muscle disruption
- Debulks the ligamentum flavum and decompresses the neural structures
- Leaves anterior fibers of the ligament flavum intact
- Supports structures like spinous process, facets, and the majority of the lamina is left intact

2.3.2 Fluoroscopic Guidance

Fluoroscopy is a necessary imaging tool to perform the MILD procedure. Align the inferior endplate of the level being treated in anteroposterior (AP), and open the interlaminar space for placement of the epidural needle for epidurogram. The epidural needle should be positioned in the ipsilateral side of the interlaminar space of the level being treated. The AP and contralateral oblique views are used for portal placement. The entire debulking procedure should be performed under the contralateral oblique view. AP view is used during resection to confirm medial-lateral instrument positioning. The contralateral oblique fluoroscopic view is obtained by rotating the C-arm to 40°–45° oblique on the contralateral side of the treatment side. The depth of instrument placement during the MILD procedure is observed in the contralateral oblique fluoroscopic view. All advancement of instruments, and the entire decompression procedure, should be performed utilizing this view.

2.4 Patient Selection for the MILD Procedure

2.4.1 Inclusion Criteria

Ideal candidates for the MILD procedure would be patients with symptomatic LSS and dorsal element hypertrophy. Nearly all selected patients experienced prior failure of conservative therapy that included physical therapy, medications, and/or epidural steroid injections. Typically, patients would experience back and/or leg pain with or without unilateral or bilateral numbness that occurs with axial loading especially when walking or prolonged standing. There should be radiologic evidence of LSS/ligamentum flavum thickness >2.5 mm and typically reduction of dural sac cross-sectional area to $\leq$100 mm^2.

2.4.2 Exclusion Criteria

There should not be anterior listhesis of >5.0 mm. The MILD procedure is avoided at prior decompression surgery level. During MIDAS studies history of recent spinal fractures with concurrent pain symptoms and disabling back or leg pain from causes other than LSS were considered exclusion criteria and should be considered relative contraindications for the procedure. Other exclusion criteria include a significant or symptomatic disc protrusion or osteophyte formation, as well as symptomatic facet hypertrophy at the targeted level.

In addition to MILD-specific exclusion criteria, general spinal surgery exclusion criteria also apply, like bleeding disorders, use of anticoagulants within 3–7 days of procedure, use of ASAs and/or NSAIDs within 7 days prior to treatment.

Lastly, inability of the patient to lie prone with anesthesia support and any pathologies affecting wound healing should be considered exclusion criteria for the MILD procedure as well.

2.5 MILD Procedure Equipments (Fig. 2.5)

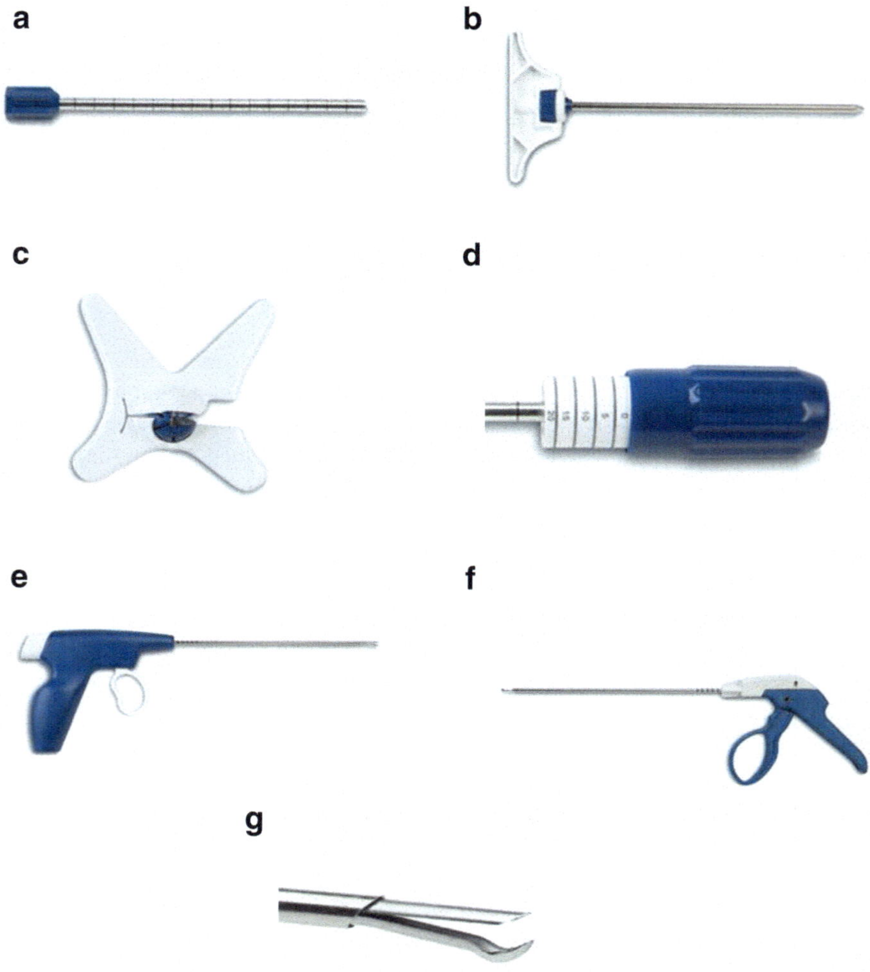

Fig. 2.5 (**a**) Portal. 5.1-mm portal minimizes tissue disruption. (**b**) Trocar and handle. (**c**) Portal stabilizer to minimizes medial and lateral movement. (**d**) Depth guide to ensure depth of cutting device. (**e**) Bone sculpter rongeur. (**f**) Tissue sculpter allows resection and retraction of ligamentous tissue. (**g**) Close-up of tissue sculpter. Top cutting surface cuts only at correct angle, and spoon-bill cuts only at correct angle. (*Courtesy of* Vertos Medical Inc.)

2.6 Technical Steps of the MILD Procedure

2.6.1 Patient Position

Patient is placed in a prone position with pillows under the abdomen to reduce lumbar lordosis (Fig. 2.6).

2.6.2 Fluoroscopy

Under fluoroscopic guidance, the midline with spinous process and bilateral medial pedicular lines are identified and marked at the intended level. The skin markings are useful guides for the trajectory and orientation of the instruments.

2.6.3 Epidurogram

The fluoroscope is positioned with the perfectly alligned inferior endplate of the level to be treated in order to open the superior aspect of the intervertebral space (Fig. 2.7). An epidural needle is positioned high to target intervertebral space close to midline and ipsilateral to the treatment side. Epidural space is accessed using loss of resistance technique and fluoroscopic guidance. Proper needle placement is assured by injecting and then confirming epidural spread of a small amount of non-ionized contrast in the contralateral oblique fluoroscopic view. Intravenous (IV) extension tubing should be used for contrast injection.

2.6.4 Determine the Trajectory

Identify the skin entry site, usually one and one half levels below, or at the level of the pedicle one level down the treatment site on the ipsilateral side, and usually about 15° off of the midline. By using a 5″ 22G spinal needle, first infiltrate skin with local anesthetic and advance the needle under fluoroscopic guidance while anesthetizing inferior lamina.

Use an AP fluoroscopic view to direct the needle to determine the medial to lateral trajectory needed at this level on this side. Once the trajectory of the needle is determined, the fluoroscopic view is changed to the contralateral oblique view to advance the lamina to visualize the portal depth. Do not advance the instrument unless utilizing direct visualization in the contralateral oblique view.

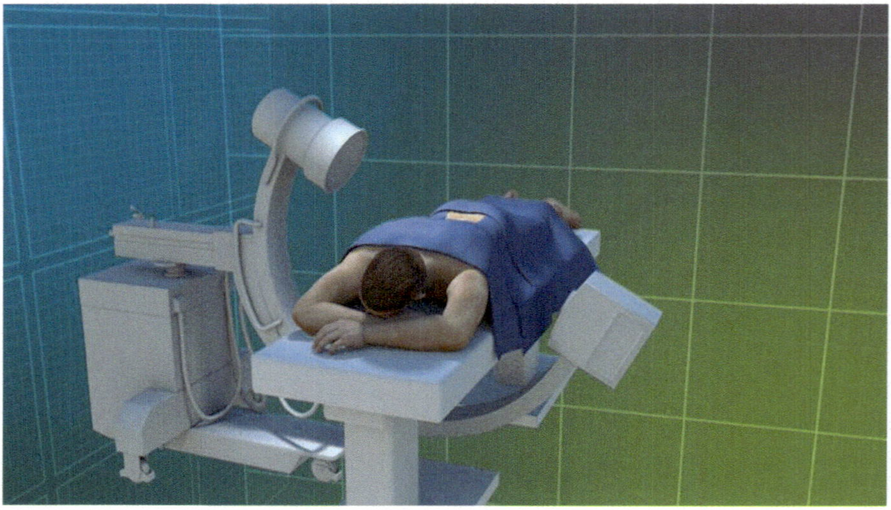

Fig. 2.6 Patient in prone position with contralateral fluoroscopic view. (*Courtesy of* Vertos Medical Inc.)

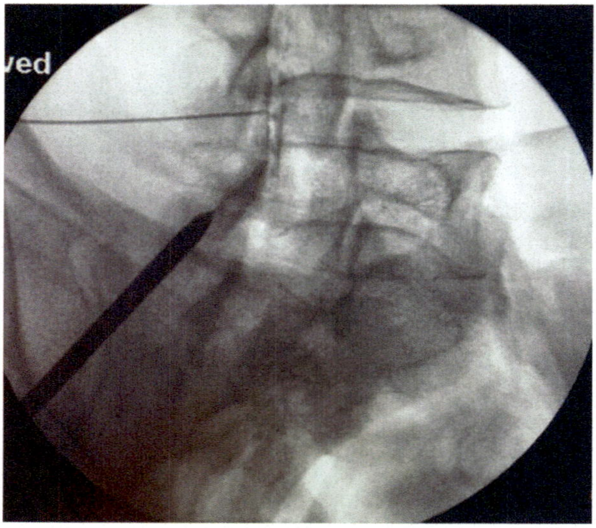

Fig. 2.7 This epidurogram line in contralateral fluoroscopic view. (*Courtesy of* Vertos Medical Inc.)

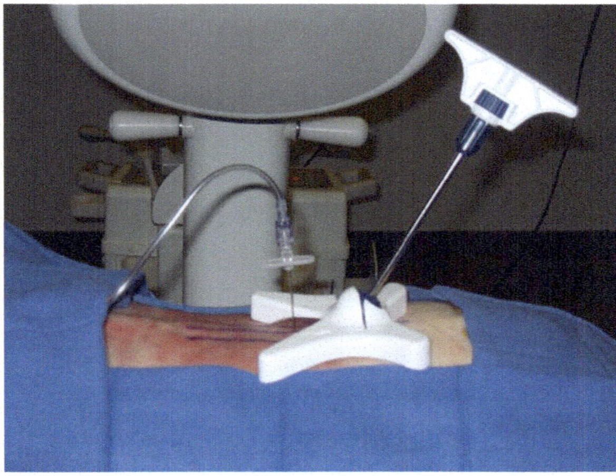

Fig. 2.8 Epidural needle connected to extension tubing, and trocar-portal unit with portal stabilizer. (*Courtesy of* Vertos Medical Inc.)

2.6.5 Insertion of Assembled Trocar-Portal Unit

Once the trejactory of the portal is decided, make a stab-incision with the #15 blade, insert the assembled trocar-portal unit, also known as the MILD tissue access device (Fig. 2.8). Advance the access device under contralateral oblique fluoroscopic view along the predetermined trajectory until the distal end touches the superior surface of the inferior lamina, within the posterior half of the lamina. Then release the locking screw on the handle and remove the trocar. Next, slide the portal stabilizer over to the portal and snap it into place to stabilize the cannula to facilitate tissue removal.

2.6.6 Depth Guide Insertion

The depth guide is then attached to the distal end of the portal to provide a stop to limit the depth of instruments inserted into the portal. The dial on the depth guide allows instruments to advance in 5-mm increments beyond the tip of the port and into the interlaminar space (Fig. 2.9).

2.6.7 Removal of Chips of Lamina

Next, insert the bone rongeur through the port to remove the chips of inferior lamina (Fig. 2.10). Withdraw the rongeur from the port and remove the chips after each pass. Start at the medial surface of the inferior lamina and work toward the lateral end. Then begin at the medial surface of the superior lamina and work toward the lateral end (Fig. 2.11).

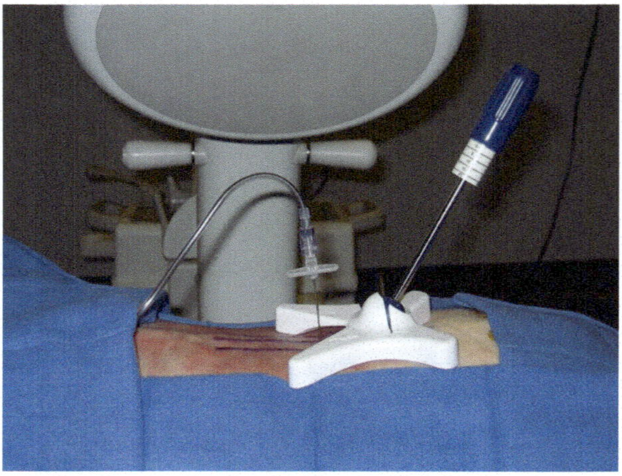

Fig. 2.9 Depth guide attached to distal end of the portal with the dial showing 5 mm increments. (*Courtesy of* Vertos Medical Inc.)

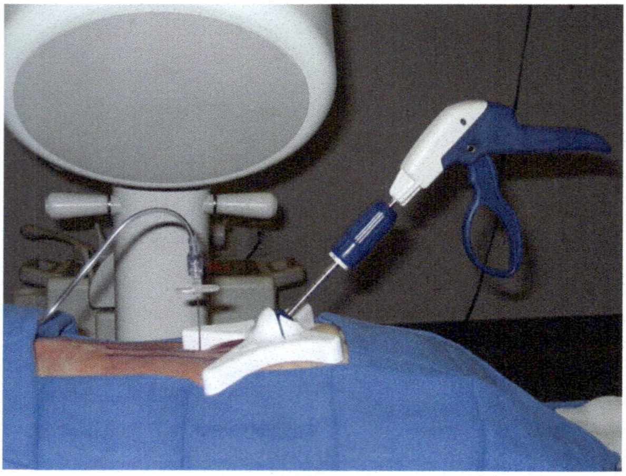

Fig. 2.10 Bone rongeur in place to remove bone chips. (*Courtesy of* Vertos Medical Inc.)

2.6.8 Debulking of Ligamentum Flavum

This is the critical step. Once an adequate amount of bone has been resected, the tissue sculptor is placed within the port to resect ligamentum flavum tissue. The sculptor is used for multiple bites and withdrawn from the port regularly to dislodge tissue to avoid overfilling. The debulking procedure is performed by scooping in upward motion from inferior to superior direction combined with activation of the trigger which provides the cutting of the ligamentous tissue. Reposition the tissue sculptor with each cut ensures additional tissue resection. The tissue resection

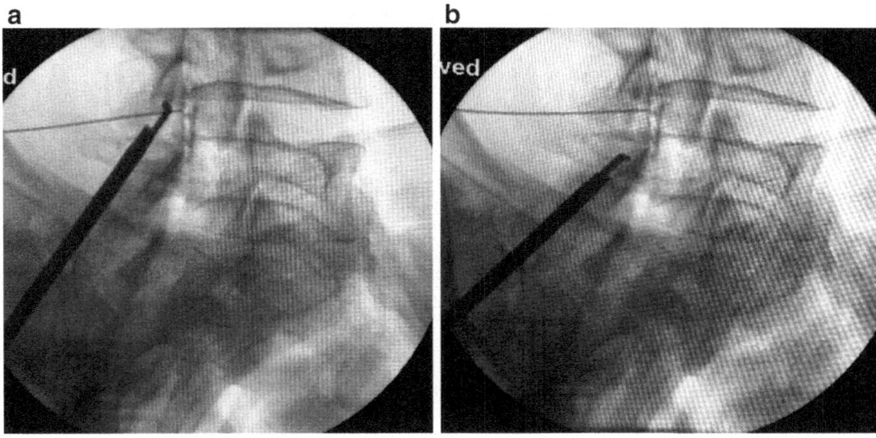

Fig. 2.11 Bone rongeur working on inferior (**a**) and superior lamina (**b**). (*Courtesy of* Vertos Medical Inc.)

should be carried out beginning at the medial aspect of the interlaminar space and working laterally. It is critical to use real-time fluoroscopic visualization of the epidurogram throughout the procedure. Extreme care is taken to remain posterior and avoid advancing the tissue sculptor beyond the epidurogram (Fig. 2.12).

2.6.9 Post-debulking Epidurogram

Repeat the epidurogram through the extension tubing to assess if the adequate ligamentum flavum tissue was resected by observing a thicker and straighter epidurogram indicating decompression (Fig. 2.13). This indicates completion of lumbar decompression procedure. The access portal is removed. Look for any potential bleeding through the stab incision, and close the wound by using a sterile adhesive strip and a sterile dressing.

2.7 Potential Complications

- Any procedure can result in three overarching complications: bleeding, infection, and nerve injury
- Dural tear is an uncommon complication and has clinically only been reported in few cases
- Neurologic injury with the mild procedure has not been reported to date
- Infection has not been reported
- Incision pain (or post-surgical pain) typically resolves within the first 48–72 h

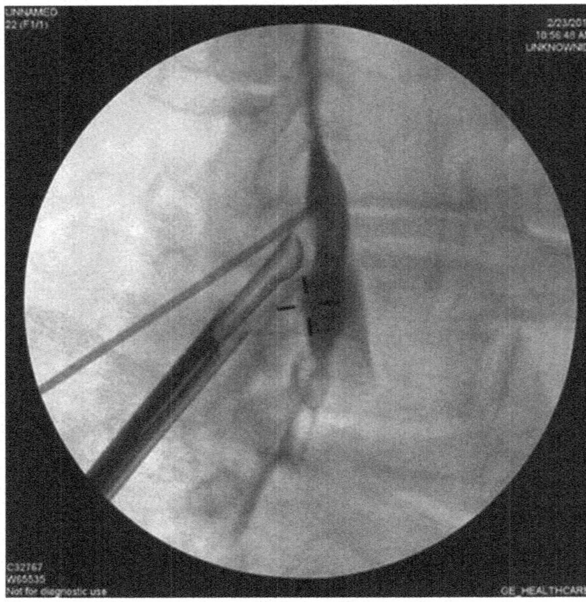

Fig. 2.12 Tissue sculptor debulking ligament flavum with thick epidurogram, indicating adequate decompression

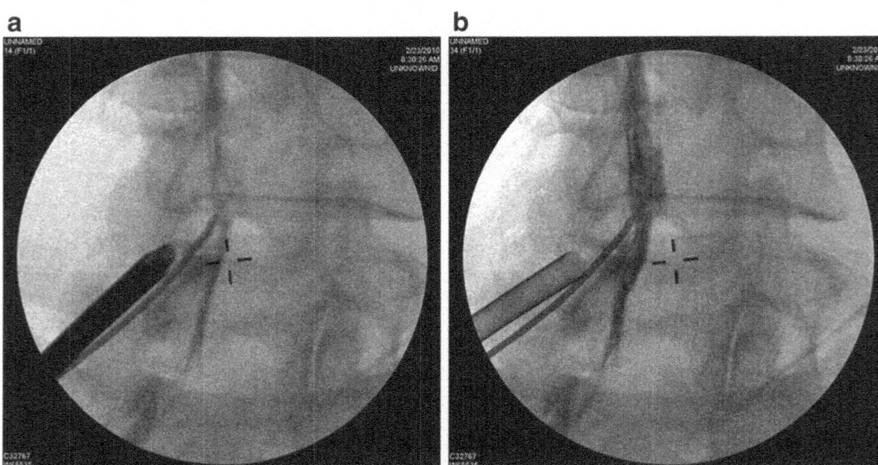

Fig. 2.13 The pre-procedure epidurogram (**a**) indicating stenosis and post-procedure epidurogram (**b**) indicating adequate decompression

2.8 Clinical Pearls

- Ipsilateral epidurogram with placement of the epidural needle at the level of decompression is desired
- Proper trajectory planning is critical to access the epidural space and can be mapped preoperatively with marking and employing a 22G 3.5-in. needle to topicalize the trocar tract
- When performing the ligamentum flavum tissue removal, lateral removal of the ligament is critical, staying medial to the facet line
- Post-operative epidurogram improvement is desired but does not correlate with clinical improvement as defined by standing and walking intolerance
- Patient selection is critical and neurogenic claudication in the presence of single- or two-level ligamentum flavum hypertrophy

Suggested Reading

Abbas J, Hamoud K, Masharawi YM, May H, Hay O, Medlej B, et al. Ligamentum flavum thickness in normal and stenotic lumbar spines. Spine. 2010;35(12):1225–30.
Basu S. Mild procedure: single-site prospective IRB study. Clin J Pain. 2012;28(3):254–8.
Chopko B, Caraway D. MiDAS I (mild Decompression Alternative to Open Surgery): a preliminary report of a prospective, multi-center clinical study. Pain Physician. 2010;13:369–78.
Chopko BW. A novel method for treatment of lumbar spinal stenosis in high-risk surgical candidates: pilot study experience with percutaneous remodeling of ligamentum flavum and lamina. J Neurosurg Spine. 2011;14:46–50.
Deer TR, Kapural L. New image-guided ultra-minimally invasive lumbar decompression method: the mild® procedure. Pain Physician. 2010;13:35–41.
Kreiner DS, MacVicar J, Duszynski B, Nampiaparampil DE. The mild® procedure: a systematic review of the current literature. Pain Med. 2014;15(2):196–205.
Lingreen R, Grider J. Retrospective review of patient self-reported improvement and post-procedure findings for mild® (minimally invasive lumbar decompression). Pain Physician. 2010;13:555–60.
Mekhail N, Vallejo R, Coleman MH, Benyamin RM. Long-term results of percutaneous lumbar decompression mild® for spinal stenosis. Pain Pract. 2012;12(3):184–93.
Schomer D, Solsberg D, Wong W, Chopko B. mild® lumbar decompression for the treatment of lumbar spinal stenosis. Neuroradiol J. 2011;24(4):620–6.
Weinstein JN, Tosteson TD, Lurie JD, Tosteson AN, Blood E, Hanscom B, et al. Surgical versus nonsurgical therapy for lumbar spinal stenosis. N Engl J Med. 2008;358:794–810.

Chapter 3
Superion: An Indirect Lumbar Decompression

Sudhir Diwan, Timothy R. Deer, Harold Cordner, Dawood Sayed, Jonathan D. Carlson, and Tory L. McJunkin

3.1 Introduction

Lumbar spinal stenosis (LSS) is a condition in which the spinal canal becomes narrowed from various causes such as degenerative facet arthropathy, disc degeneration, spondylolisthesis, and thickening of the ligamentum flavum [1]. These conditions can occur in combination or as a singular cause of the disease state. The most common manifestation of spinal stenosis is neurogenic claudication. Neurogenic claudication manifests itself as pain in the lower back and extremities, impaired walking, and other forms of disability in the elderly. Lumbar spinal stenosis is the most frequent indication for spinal surgery in those over 65 [2].

S. Diwan (✉)
Lenox Hill Hospital, New York, NY, USA

Manhattan Spine and Pain Medicine, New York, NY, USA
e-mail: Sudhir.diwan63@gmail.com

T.R. Deer
The Center for Pain Relief, Charleston, WV, USA
e-mail: tdeermd@centerforpainrelief.com; doctdeer@aol.com

H. Cordner
Florida Pain Management Associates, Sebastian, FL, USA
e-mail: DrC@floridapain.com

D. Sayed
Division of Pain Meidicne, University of Kansas Medical Center, Kansas City, KS, USA
e-mail: dsayed1@yahoo.com

J.D. Carlson
Arizona Pain /Pain Doctor, Glendale, AZ, USA
e-mail: jcarlsonMD@gmail.com

T.L. McJunkin
Arizona Pain Specialists, Scottsdale, AZ, USA
e-mail: Dr.McJunkin@ArizonaPain.com; torymcj@gmail.com

S. Diwan, T.R. Deer (eds.), *Advanced Procedures for Pain Management*,
https://doi.org/10.1007/978-3-319-68841-1_3

As increasing numbers of people in the aging population suffer from the debilitating symptoms of LSS, great interest has focused on minimally invasive treatments.

Conservative or nonsurgical management remains the front-line approach for patients suffering from mild-to-moderate symptoms of LSS. Conservative measures include physical therapy, medications, lumbar orthotics, and epidural steroid injections. Due to the mechanical compressive nature of LSS, conservative measures often fail to provide durable long-term relief, especially as symptoms progress.

Open lumbar laminectomy has long been accepted as the standard of care for patients with severe symptoms from LSS [3]. Cauda Equina syndrome remains the only absolute indication for decompression in LSS. All other open laminectomies are performed electively to improve the quality of life for these individuals who have disabling back and leg pain and significant limitations in walking tolerance [4]. The treatment algorithm for those with mild-to-moderate LSS has been less well defined. Patients with mild-to-moderate LSS may obtain partial relief from conservative measures but remain dissatisfied with their outcomes, or they may have failed an extended course of non-surgical management but are unable or unwilling to undergo traditional laminectomy and the considerable risks it entails. Open lumbar laminectomy has been shown to be associated with postoperative complication rates ranging from 12 to 29%, depending on comorbidity status. This is particularly important since LSS is predominantly a disease of the elderly, a demographic inherently associated with higher rates of comorbidities [5].

Indirect spinal decompression via interspinous spacer is a novel technique in the management of patients with mild-to-moderate LSS. While different options exist to accomplish this procedural goal, this chapter focuses on the spacer that, via studies monitored by the Food and Drug Administration, has the highest level of evidence-based support at this time.

The Superion® IDS is a minimally-invasive spinal implant that treats LSS symptoms by limiting extension at the symptomatic level that compresses the neural elements, and is designed for percutaneous surgical placement (Fig. 3.1). The device

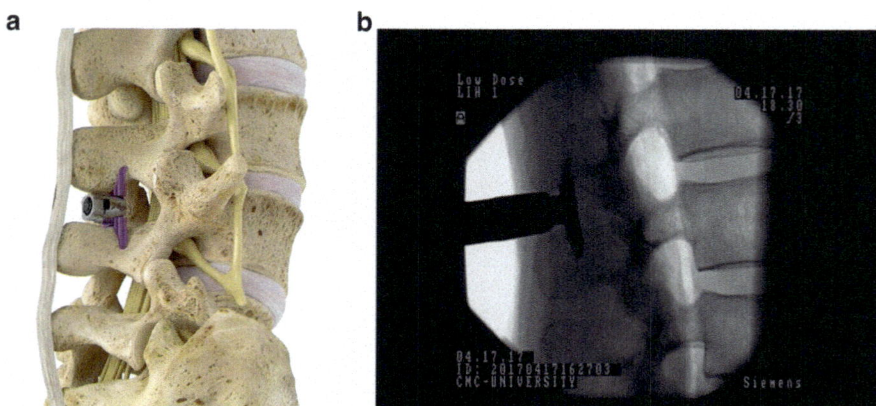

Fig. 3.1 (**a**, **b**) Superion implants

is intended to treat moderate spinal stenosis in the adult spine and can be implanted under general anesthesia, monitored anesthesia care, or local anesthesia with or without neuromonitoring.

3.2 Indications

Indirect Decompression System indications:

- Neurogenic intermittent claudication (NIC) secondary to lumbar spinal stenosis (LSS) presenting with leg and/or buttock pain that is relieved with flexion
- Moderately to severely impaired physical function
- Diagnosis of LSS defined as narrowing among the central, lateral, and/or foraminal spinal canal
- Radiographic confirmation of moderate LSS, as 25–50% reduction in canal area vs. adjacent level(s)
- Symptomatic with history of conservative management ≥6 months
- Male or female that is skeletally mature
- May be implanted at up to two adjacent levels from L1-L5

Indirect Decompression System contraindications:

- Unremitting buttock and/or leg pain in any spinal position that is not relieved with forward flexion
- Axial low back pain
- Spondylolisthesis or degenerative spondylolisthesis >grade 1.0
- Significant dynamic instability of the lumbar spine defined as ≥3 mm translation or ≥5° angulation on flexion/extension
- Significant scoliotic changes defined as lateral curvature >10° at level of intended treatment
- Sustained pathologic fracture of the vertebrae or multiple fracture of the vertebrae and/or hips
- Baastrup's disease (kissing spine syndrome): adjacent spinous processes in close approximation secondary to spine degeneration
- An allergy to titanium or titanium alloy
- Spinal anatomy or disease that would prevent implantation of the device or cause the device to be unstable in situ, such as:
  - Instability of the lumbar spine, e.g., isthmic spondylolisthesis or degenerative spondylolisthesis greater than grade 1 (on a scale of 1–4)
  - An ankylosed segment at the affected level(s)
  - Fracture of the spinous process, pars interarticularis, or laminae (unilateral or bilateral)
  - Scoliosis (Cobb angle >10°)

- Cauda equina syndrome defined as neural compression causing neurogenic bladder or bowel dysfunction
- Diagnosis of severe osteoporosis, defined as bone mineral density (from DEXA scan or equivalent method) in the spine or hip that is more than 2.5 S.D. below the mean of adult normal
- Active systemic infection, or infection localized to the site of implantation
- Prior fusion or decompression procedure at the index level
- Morbid obesity defined as a body mass index (BMI) of greater than 40

3.3 Relative Contraindications

- Severe spinal stenosis with neurologic deficit
- More than two levels of symptomatic lumbar spinal stenosis
- Prior lumbar surgery at affected levels
- Paget's disease or vertebral metastases

Spinous process fractures can occur with Superion® IDS implantation. Potential predictors for spinous process fractures include:

- Thin, or "gracile" spinous processes: if a spinous process is unusually thin, or measures less than 20 mm in superior-inferior dimension, the likelihood of a postoperative spinous process fracture may be increased.
- "Kissing" spinous processes: is the spinous processes are in very close approximation, or are in contact (i.e., "kissing"), increased difficulty may be experienced in placement of the Cannula. Where spinous processes do not "open up" in flexion, the likelihood of a spinous process fracture may be increased (Fig. 3.2).

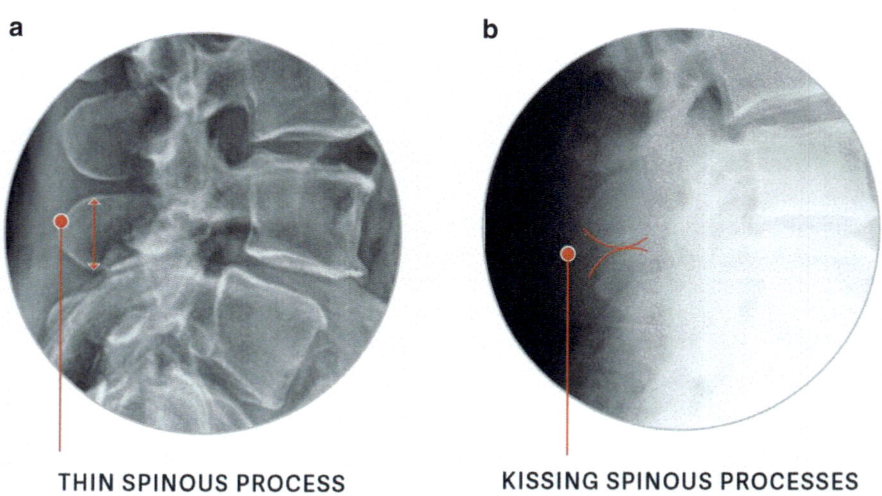

Fig. 3.2 (**a**) Thin spinous process. (**b**) "Kissing spine"

- If the Superion® Implant is placed in a "shallow" or more dorsal position, the likelihood of a postoperative spinous process fracture may increase by a factor >4. To reduce the potential for postoperative fracture, be certain to locate the implant body sufficiently anterior, and confirm implant position in lateral view of fluoroscopy.

3.4 Risks and Complications

Inherent risks and complications are those associated with any other surgical procedure, including:

- Anesthesia-related complications
- Blood loss, blood vessel damage, and hematoma
- Phlebitis or deep vein thrombosis, pulmonary embolism
- Blood transfusion related complications
- Cardiovascular and pulmonary complications
- Injury to muscle, soft tissue, or nerves
- Fever or infection, pneumonia
- Wound seroma, drainage, or delayed Healing
- Discomfort and rehabilitation associated with surgery
- Stroke or death

Risks associated with lumbar spine implants and associated instruments include:

- Sensitivity or allergy to the implant material
- Failure of the device and/or procedure to improve symptoms and/or function
- Pain and discomfort at the operative site secondary to presence of implants
- Implant malposition or incorrect orientation or cam lobes fracture
- Spinous process fracture
- Production of wear debris which may damage soft tissues including muscles or nerves
- Formation of hypertrophic scar tissue at implant site
- Migration or dislodgement of the implant from the original position, losing the effectiveness or causing damage to adjacent bone, soft tissues, or nerves
- Loosening, fatigue, deformation, breakage or disassembly of the implant, which may require another operation to remove the implant

Risks associated with lumbar spine surgery include:

- Damage to nerve roots to the spinal cord causing partial or complete sensory or motor loss
- Loss of bladder and/or bowel functions
- Dural leaks and tears in the tissue surrounding and protecting the spinal cord
- Instruments used during surgery may break or malfunction, which may cause damage to the operative site or adjacent structures
- New or worsened back or leg pain
- Surgery at the incorrect location or level

3.5 The Superion Implants

The implants are made of biocompatible strong titanium, with a high ratio of contact area to implant size, and contoured cam lobes correspond to spinous process anatomy (Fig. 3.3).

Equipment kit (Fig. 3.4): The Superion kit contains sharp and notched tip dilator 1, a main dilator 2, interspinous gauge, an inserter, a driver, a mallet, a radiolucent handle, a ring forceps and a self-retaining retractor.

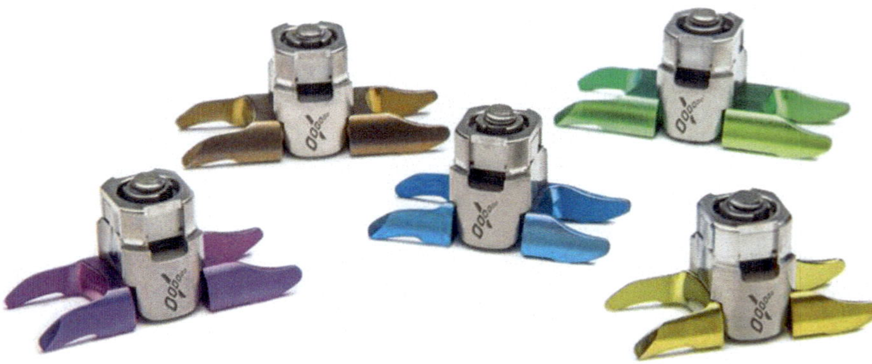

Fig. 3.3 Superion implants available in five color-coded sizes (8, 10, 12, 14, and 16 mm)

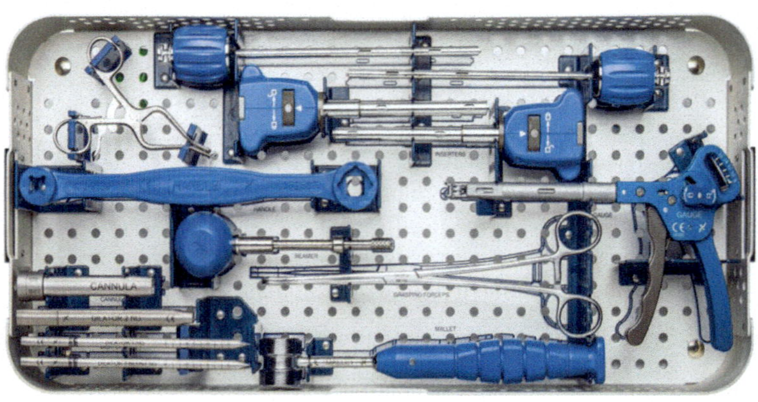

Fig. 3.4 The Superion instrument tray

3.6 Surgical Procedural Steps

3.6.1 Patient Positioning

Place the patient in prone position on a fluoroscopic table over a Wilson frame to ensure adequate flexion of lumbar spine, and to separate spinous processes to facilitate introduction of dilators. Follow the usual operating room discipline, wear appropriate surgical attire, and maintain strict sterile conditions to perform the procedure (Fig. 3.5).

3.6.2 Placement of Incision

Identify correct level and confirm midline and axial position in AP and lateral position. Make a 12–15 mm vertical incision at the operative level to expose superior spinous ligament (SSL). Confirm midline scalpel position under fluoroscopy before the incision (Fig. 3.6).

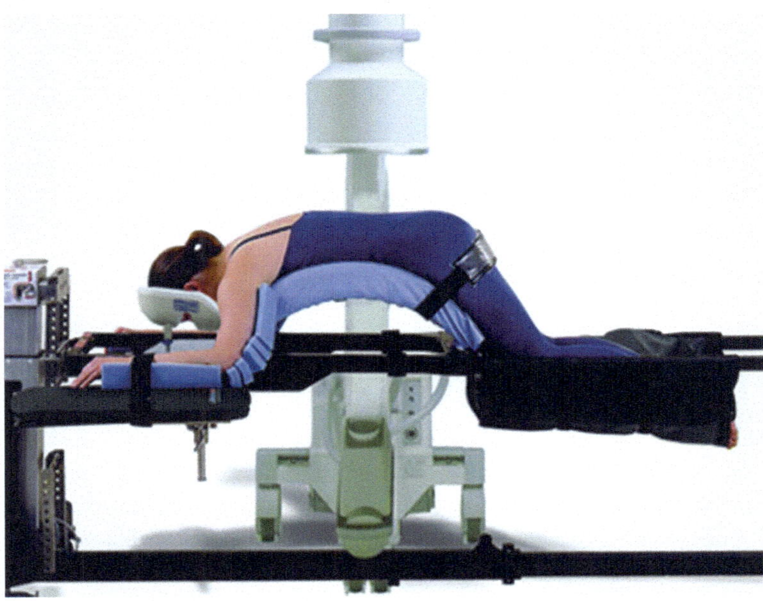

Fig. 3.5 Patient position on Wilson frame for spinal surgery

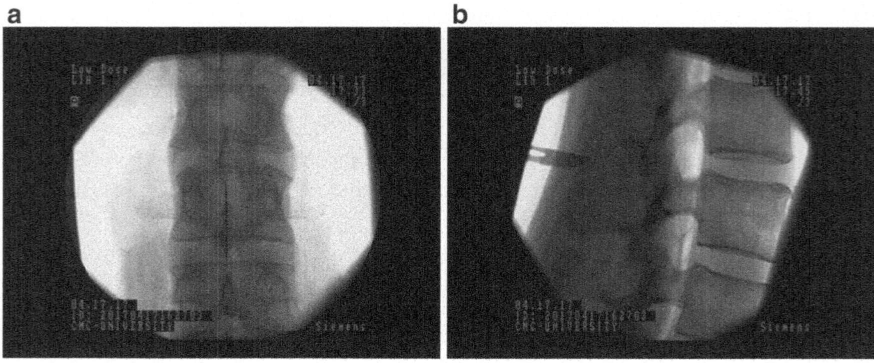

Fig. 3.6 (**a**, **b**) Confirm the position of scalpel before placing the incision

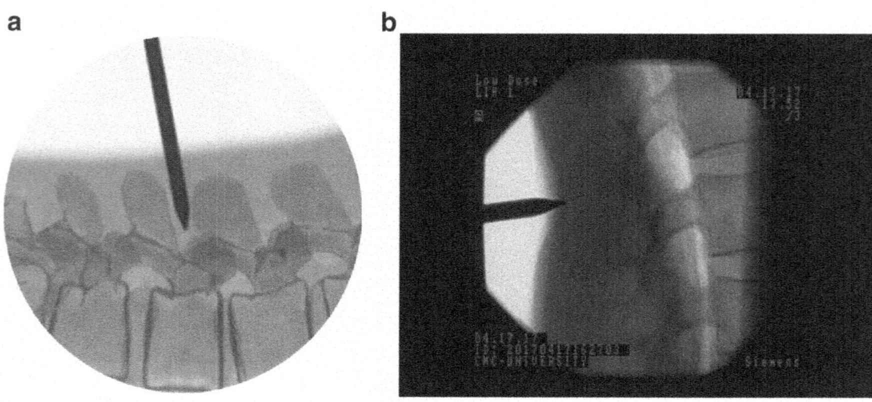

Fig. 3.7 (**a**, **b**) Insertion of dilator 1

3.6.3 Insertion of Sequential Dilators 1 and 2

Insert sharp tip dilator and advance it under lateral fluoroscopic guidance just ventral to SSL. Then using mallet, advance it up to posterior aspect of spino-laminar junction. Insert larger dilator 2 over dilator 1. Align dilator channels with superior and inferior spinous processes. Remove dilator 1, and advance dilator 2 by using radiolucent handle and mallet (Fig. 3.7).

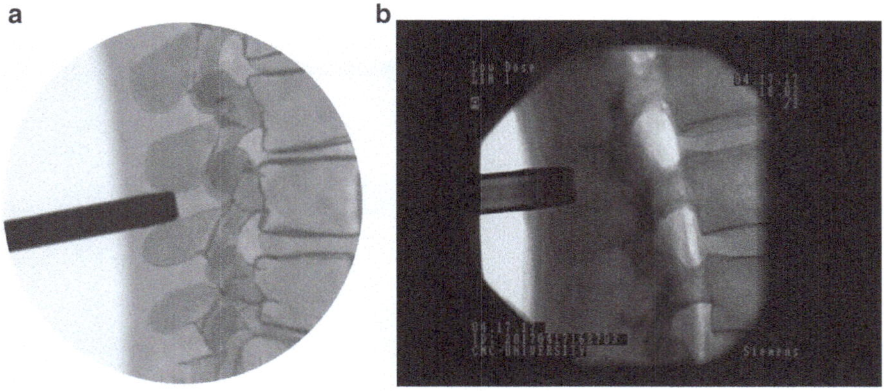

Fig. 3.8 (a, b) Insertion of cannula

3.6.4 Insertion of Cannula

Ensure the dilator 2 channels are aligned with superior and inferior spinous processes, insert the cannula over dilator 2, and advance it anterior to SSL under lateral fluoroscopy. Confirm the placement of cannula in midline in AP view and 2–5 mm anterior to SSL in lateral view (Fig. 3.8).

3.6.5 Placement of Interspinous Gauge

Insert the interspinous gauge through the cannula with handle directed laterally, and advance it until the shaft is flush with the proximal end of the cannula. Advance the gauge in lateral view to confirm the depth, with dorsal tip contacting spinolaminar junction of superior spinous process (Fig. 3.9).

3.6.6 Measuring Appropriate Size of the Implant

After optimal gauge positioning under live fluoroscopy, actuate the trigger until resistance is encountered at the distal tip, and lock the interspinous gauge. Note the measurement at the proximal end of the gauge handle corresponding to 8, 10, 12, 14, and 16 (Fig. 3.10).

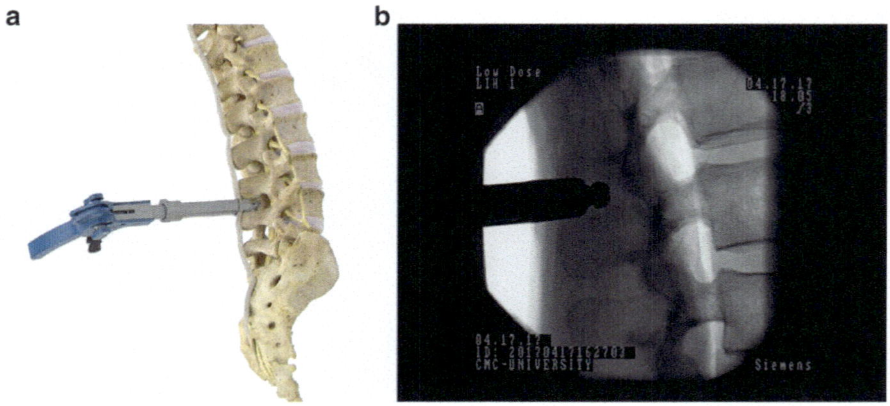

Fig. 3.9 (a, b) Placement of interspinous gauge

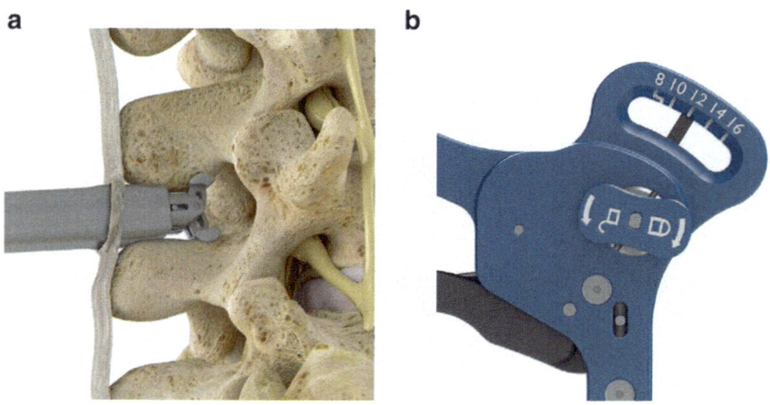

Fig. 3.10 (a, b) Measuring appropriate size of the implant

3.6.7 *Loading of Properly Sized Implant*

Ensure the inserter dial to unlocked position. Align the corresponding arrows on body of implant and the distal end of the inserter. Turn the inserter dial to finger-tight locked position. Place the driver inside the inserter and rotate until seats into the implant and is flush with proximal end of inserter (Fig. 3.11).

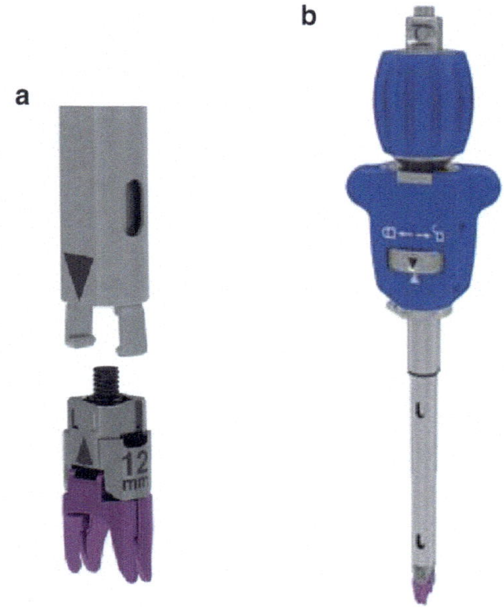

Fig. 3.11 (**a**, **b**) Loading of properly sized implant

3.6.8 Deployment of the Implant

Place the inserter and driver into the cannula, then align the arrow, pointing cephalad. Deploy the implant by turning the driver clockwise and assess the position under AP and lateral fluoroscopy. Do not force to deploy implant if you encounter resistance, but reposition and redeploy. Under AP fluoroscopy, the cam lobes should be capturing the superior and inferior spinous processes. Under lateral fluoroscopy, confirm the implant is not too far anterior to superior and inferior lamina. Reposition the redeploy if the implant is too far ventral or too far dorsal to spinolaminar junction. After confirming appropriate placement, continue rotating the driver until cam lobes are completely deployed (Fig. 3.12).

3.6.9 Confirmation of Final Position of Implant

It is crucial that the superior cam lobes rest ventrally against superior lamina confirmed under lateral view. If the implant is too far dorsally, will increase the likelihood of spinous process fracture by a factor of >4. In the final position, the superior and inferior spinous processes should be contained within the cam lobes in AP view, and should be positioned ventrally contacting the spinolaminar junction in lateral view (Figs. 3.13 and 3.14).

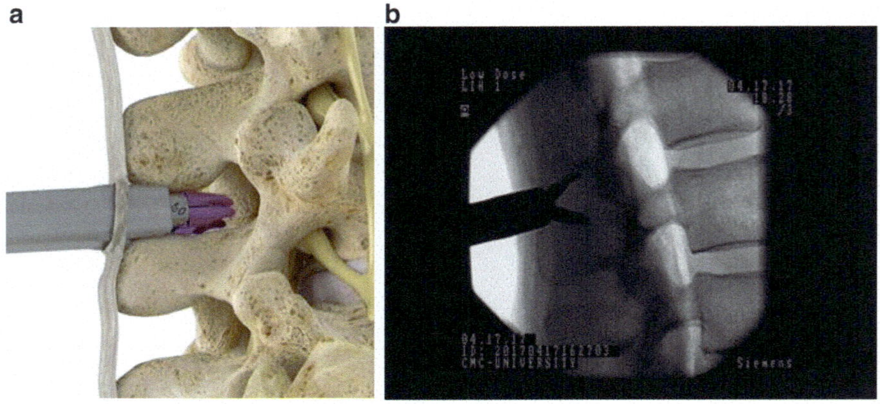

Fig. 3.12 (a, b) Deployment of the implant

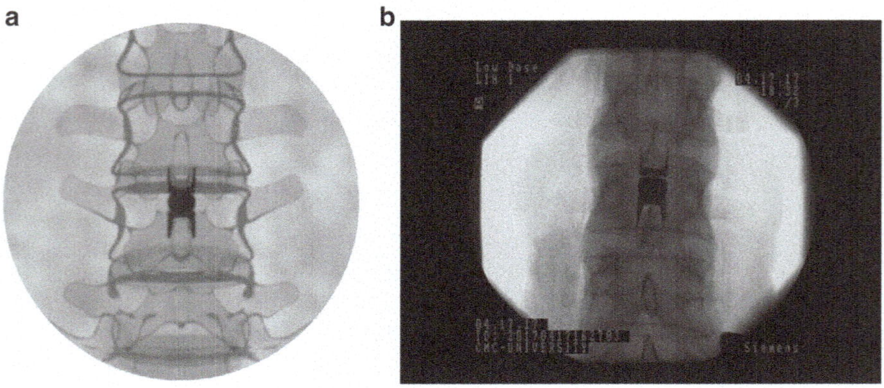

Fig. 3.13 (a, b) Final position of implant in AP view

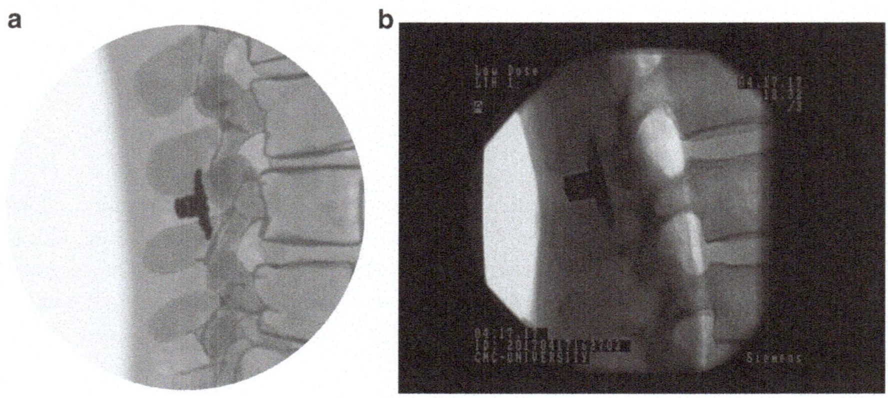

Fig. 3.14 (a, b) Final position of implant in lateral view

Removal of instruments and incision closure: Remove driver first, and then turn the inserter dial to unlock position and remove inserter. Remove the cannula and close the incision in usual fashion.

3.7 Clinical Pearls Superion

- Patient selection is critical for the success of this procedure. Neurogenic (arising from the nervous system) claudication (leg pain, heaviness, or weakness with walking) and relief with flexion are the most important clinical presentations.
- Up to two levels can be performed in the lumbar spine (excluding L5-S1).
- One must review the patient's imaging (MRI, CT, X-rays) to look for any contraindication to performing the procedure. Examples include Baastrup's disease (kissing spine syndrome), which may make the procedure technically impossible, and thin or gracile spinous processes that may make a spinous process fracture more likely.
- Patient positioning for the procedure with exaggerated lumbar flexion is important to maximize the interspinous space at the targeted level(s). Consider use of a Wilson frame or similar for positioning.
- A Body Mass Index (BMI) less than 35 is ideal. BMI greater than 35 can be done, but the most important factor is adequate visualization of the spinal structures in a lateral fluoroscopic view. If this view is negatively impacted by body habitus the procedure is relatively contraindicated.
- Only advance the cannulas in a lateral fluoroscopic view. To avoid injury to the dura, never advance the cannulas past the intralaminar junction.
- The initial angle of approach is critical between the superior and inferior targeted spinous process. Frequent AP and lateral x-rays are used to slowly guide the sequential dilating cannulas to the correct location with the correct trajectory. Care should be taken to avoid placing these cannulas obliquely off to the side of midline, as this makes the ultimate deployment of the Superion device difficult. It is important to ensure that your incision through the interspinous ligament is in midline and sufficiently deep and large enough to accommodate the dilator.
- Once the Superion device is fully deployed, ensure that it is in a deep anterior position adjacent to the lamina. If the device is more posterior, it increases the likelihood of a spinous process fracture.
- Best Practices for sterility and preventative precautions similar to those for a spinal cord stimulation implant should be used to prevent infection, as this an implant. For example, limit room traffic, double gloving, pre-op antibiotics, wound irrigation, full closure of the wound, and post-op antibiotics.

3.8 Evidence for Superion Therapy: Investigational Device Exemption (IDE) Pivotal Trial

A prospective, multicenter (29 sites), randomized controlled FDA-IDE pivotal trial of 391 patients compared Superion interspinous spacers (N = 190) to the control X-STOP spacer group (N = 201) [6]. Two years' results were published in *Spine* and the primary endpoints were met showing the Superion group was noninferior to the X-STOP spacer group. The predominant patient complaint of leg pain secondary to moderate LSS with intermittent neurogenic claudication was decreased in severity by 70% in both groups as indicated by mean visual analogue scores (VAS). The following was achieved in 2 years: Mean VAS scores demonstrated 77% pain relief for leg pain and 68% pain for back pain for both groups. Oswestry Disability Index (ODI) showed clinical results with a greater than 15%-point improvement in 65% of the patients [1]. Unfortunately, in 2015, the control comparator X-STOP became no longer commercially available in the United States. From the same clinical IDE study, Superion 4-year clinical data was published in *World Neurosurgery* [7]. The study indicated sustained relief of leg pain (78% VAS), back pain (66% VAS), and ODI 62% when compared to baseline [2]. At the time of this chapter completion, the Superion 5-year clinical data was recently accepted in the peer-reviewed journal *Clinical Interventions in the Aging* with similar sustained clinical results for leg and back VAS scores and ODI when compared to baseline.

In summary, the use of interspinous spacers is an option for minimizing the invasiveness of surgical treatment of Lumbar Spinal Stenosis. Proper patient selection, careful attention to procedural detail, and appropriate follow-up in the post-procedural period are each essential steps to an optimal outcome. This evidence-based treatment is an important part of the treatment algorithm, and the minimally invasive nature of the procedure is helpful in reducing risks to patients.

Acknowledgment *All images courtesy of Vertiflex Inc. (Carlsbad, CA, USA); www.vertiflexspine.com*

References

1. Katz JN, Harris MB. Clinical practice. Lumbar spinal stenosis. N Engl J Med. 2008;358:818–25.
2. Lee SI, Campion A, Huang A, Park E, Garst JH, Jahanforouz N, et al. Identifying predictors for postoperative clinical outcome in lumbar spinal stenosis patients using smart-shoe technology. J Neuroeng Rehabil. 2017;14(1):77.
3. Aalto TJ, Malmivaara A, Kovacs F, Herno A, Alen M, Salmi L, et al. Preoperative predictors for postoperative clinical outcome in lumbar spinal stenosis: systematic review. Spine (Phila Pa 1976). 2006;31(18):E648–63.
4. McNeill TW. Decompressive laminectomy. In: Andersson GB, McNeill TW, editors. Lumbar spinal stenosis. St. Louis: Mosby Year Book; 1991. p. 339.
5. Benz RJ, Ibrahim ZG, Afshar P, Garfin SR. Predicting complications in elderly patients undergoing lumbar decompression. Clin Orthop Relat Res. 2001;384:116–21.

6. Patel VV, Whang PG, Haley TR, Bradley D, Nunley PD, Davis RP, et al. Superion interspinous process spacer for intermittent neurogenic claudication secondary to moderate lumbar spinal stenosis. Spine (Phila Pa 1976). 2015;40(5):275–82.
7. Nunley PD, Patel VV, Orndorff DG, Lavelle WF, Block JE, Geisler FH. Superion interspinous spacer treatment of moderate spinal stenosis: 4-year results. World Neurosurg. 2017;104:279–83.

Chapter 4
Minimally Invasive Discectomy: Transforaminal Approach

Abram H. Burgher, Kenneth M. Aló, and Azmi N. Nasser

Disc prolapse resulting in back and leg pain is a common and often disabling condition. Treatment includes open microdiscectomy, which is a highly effective therapy in the short term for properly selected patients. Open microdiscectomy carries risk, however, requires a convalescent period, and demonstrates a diminishing effect over time relative to observation. For these reasons, there has been increasing interest in minimally invasive techniques such as endoscopic discectomy, which attempts to achieve results similar to those of open microdiscectomy while reducing risk and the recovery period. The most widely accepted endoscopic discectomy techniques utilize a transforaminal approach to access the target area. This chapter discusses two specific approaches to transforaminal endoscopic discectomy commonly referred to as "inside-out" and "outside-in".

4.1 Introduction

Back and neck pain affects more than two thirds of the population at some point, and it is the most common cause of disability in working-age people [1]. Pain from the spine has a number of discrete etiologies, including acute or subacute strain, lumbar facet syndrome, degenerative disc disease, and spinal stenosis, among

A.H. Burgher
The Pain Center, Scottsdale, Arizona
e-mail: ABurgher@ThePainCenter.com

K.M. Aló (✉)
The Methodist Hospital Research Institute, Texas Medical Center, Houston, TX, USA
e-mail: aglioolio@gmail.com

A.N. Nasser
Arizona Pain Treatment Centers, Scottsdale, AZ, USA
e-mail: drazminasser@yahoo.com

S. Diwan, T.R. Deer (eds.), *Advanced Procedures for Pain Management*,
https://doi.org/10.1007/978-3-319-68841-1_4

others. Back and leg pain due to disc prolapse has a prevalence of 1–3% in adults, making it a specific and common condition resulting in visits to healthcare providers and in many cases, surgery [2].

Though surgical care with microdiscectomy has been associated with more rapid symptom improvement than conservative measures, the effect diminishes with time; after 1 year, patients who have received surgery tend to fare no better than those who have not [3]. Surgery also requires a recovery period, resulting in additional disability, and it carries risks not associated with conservative care, including nerve injury, infection, dural tear with spinal headache, and intraspinal scar formation, among others [4]. Because surgical discectomy does appear to have clear early benefits, efforts have been made to devise minimally invasive discectomy approaches with lower complication rates and a quicker recovery period [5]. As techniques and technology have advanced over the past two decades, endoscopic techniques to decompress disc material have gained in popularity and are now employed with reasonable frequency. Many specific endoscopic techniques have evolved, with the most common approaches involving either an interlaminar or transforaminal approach. This chapter describes patient selection and technique for two different transforaminal techniques, commonly referred to as "inside-out" and "outside-in." The difference between these two approaches rests in the placement of the instruments and the primary locale of the procedure. When the instruments are placed inside the disc itself, and the discectomy primarily involves the debulking of the nucleus pulposis, it is an "inside-out" approach. By contrast, if the instruments remain primarily posterior to the disc, and the decompressive procedure occurs in the canal, neuroforamen, or extraforaminal zone, it is an "outside-in" approach.

4.2 Patient Positioning and Setup

These procedures can be performed with the patient in a prone or lateral position, depending on the preference of the proceduralist and the location of the target herniation. For paracentral protrusions or extrusions and unilateral symptoms, lateral decubitus positioning is often used, with the target side up. Lateral decubitus may help the traversing nerves to fall away from the target disc. An optional myelogram at the level above the target may be performed under fluoroscopic guidance to help visualize the thecal sac under fluoroscopy, reducing the risk of dural tear or nerve injury.

For patients who have protrusions or extrusions that cross the midline, a prone position is often preferred, particularly if symptoms are bilateral.

Conscious sedation or general anesthesia can be used. When general anesthesia is used, continuous neuromonitoring is recommended to reduce the risk of neural injury. If the patient is awake, he or she may be able to report neurologic or radicular symptoms much like neuromonitoring [6]. In addition, if the patient is awake and in lateral decubitus position, a straight leg raise test may be done to determine if sufficient decompression has been performed.

4.2.1 Anatomic Considerations

Before using this approach, the proceduralist must consider the patient habitus and instrument compatibility, as larger or obese patients may require longer instruments. The iliac crest must be cleared, and if it obstructs access to the L5-S1 disc, the patient may not be a candidate for transforaminal endoscopic discectomy at that level. Central and paracentral, nonmigrated disc herniations can otherwise generally be accessed through Kambin's triangle [7]. Central herniations require an approach more lateral from midline than paracentral or lateral disc herniations. For extrusions, a steeper approach, either cephalocaudad or caudocephalad, may be necessary [8].

Under fluoroscopy, the safe zone on the posterolateral surface of the annulus adjacent to the spinal canal, known as the *triangular working zone* or *Kambin's triangle*, may be identified [9].

4.3 Transforaminal "Inside-Out" Approach

This technique is illustrated in a patient with L4-5 right paracentral disc protrusion (Fig. 4.1). In this patient, needle placement is directed to the right dorsolateral quarter of the disc, with the distal needle tip anterior to the protrusion and in the vicinity of the nuclear-annular interface. An epiduroscope (Fig. 4.2) may be passed from caudal to rostral. The epiduroscope can be used to assist with mechanical disruption of scar tissue, identification of inflammatory foci, and identification of extruded components of disc, among other things. Use of the epiduroscope is beyond the scope of this chapter.

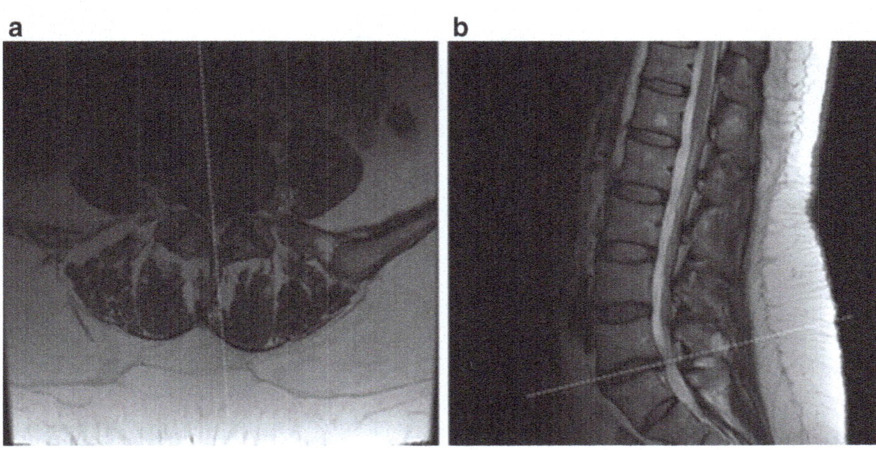

Fig. 4.1 Axial (**a**) and sagittal (**b**) T2-weighted MR images of L4-5 right paracentral protrusion

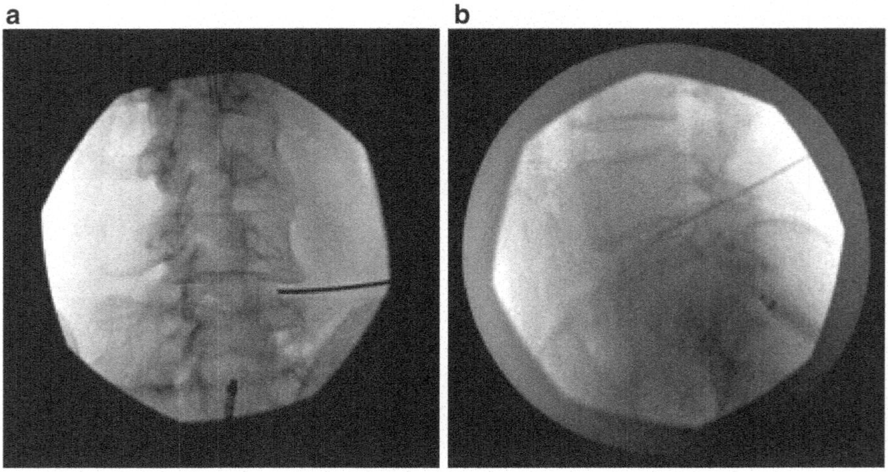

Fig. 4.2 In the same patient as in Fig. 4.1, oblique (**a**) and lateral (**b**) fluoroscopy views demonstrate needle placement directed to the right dorsolateral quarter of the disc. Also seen is an epiduroscope, passed from caudal to rostral

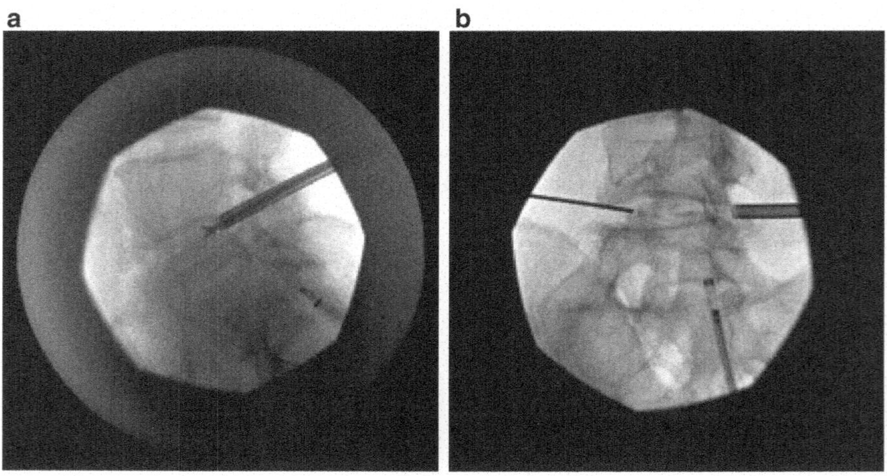

Fig. 4.3 (**a**) Seldinger technique is used to place serial dilators. The dilator shown has an internal diameter of 6 mm. (**b**) Also shown is needle placement on the contralateral side, as typically done for protrusions that come close to or cross the midline

Seldinger technique is used to place serial dilators (Fig. 4.3). Dilators of varying sizes can be used, depending on the size of the target protrusion. For most protrusions, the final dilator size is in the range of 4–8 mm. Forceps are used to create a cavity "beneath" the protrusion. For small protrusions, 0.5 g or less of tissue is removed, but large protrusions may require excision of 1.0 g of nuclear and internal

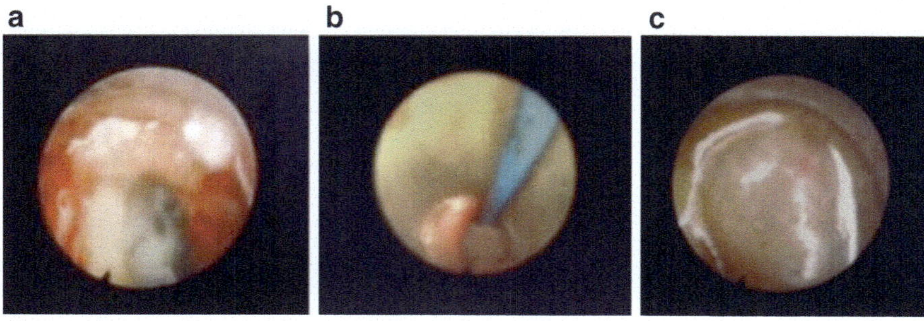

Fig. 4.4 Use of an endoscope to assist with identification of the cavity and the nuclear-annular interface. (**a**, **b**) Cautery (in this case a thulium laser) promotes collapse of the cavity created beneath the protrusion, thereby reducing the protrusion yet preserving most of the annulus. (**c**) The surface of the disc as the dilator is withdrawn

annular tissue. Needle placement on the contralateral side (*see* Fig. 4.3b) is typically done for protrusions that come close to or cross the midline.

An endoscope can be used to assist with identification of the cavity and the nuclear-annular interface (Fig. 4.4). The use of cautery promotes collapse of the cavity created beneath the protrusion, thereby reducing the protrusion yet preserving most of the annulus.

4.4 Transforaminal "Outside-In" Approach

The surgical site may be determined with anteroposterior (AP) and lateral fluoroscopy, using a long needle or Steinman pin on the skin over the target disc to draw index lines helping to direct the needle toward the target disc [10]. Another technique to determine the surgical site is using an in-line "tunnel" or "gun-barrel" fluoroscopic view, commonly used by interventional pain physicians for other transforaminal procedures. In this technique, the angle is reduced (from a lateral view) until the targeted superior articular process is in line with the posterior disc herniation located on presurgical MRI or CT imaging (Fig. 4.5).

A needle is docked on the superior articular facet (Fig. 4.6). The needle may then be directed and engaged onto the annulus, or into the disc for an optional discogram with indigo carmine to stain pathologic disc and help guide discectomy. Using basically a Seldinger technique, a flexible guidewire and sequential dilators are inserted.

Foraminotomy can be done with fluoroscopically guided sequential bone reamers, if needed (Fig. 4.7). Great care is needed to keep the instruments posterior in the foramen, along the facet, and to avoid exiting or transiting nerves. The foraminotomy should be limited to the medial pedicular line, or should be limited if neurologic signs are reported by the patient or by neuromonitoring. The medial pedicular line is closer to the thecal sac at upper lumbar levels, and slightly more lateral at lower levels, which may permit more reaming.

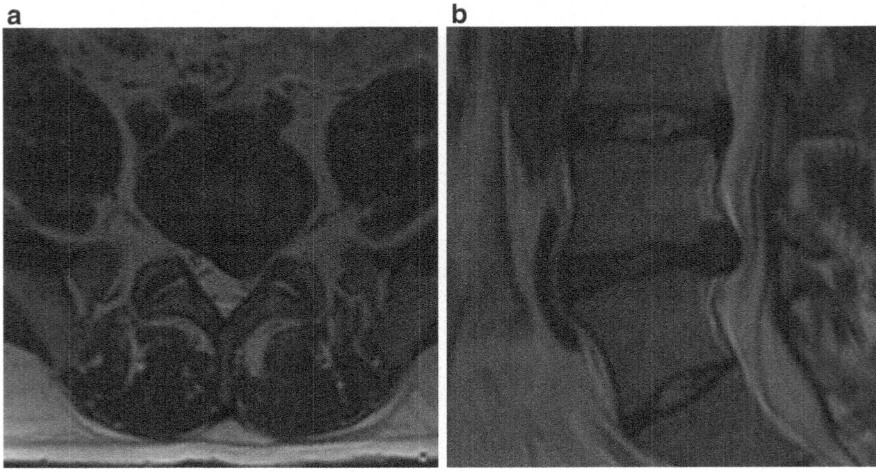

Fig. 4.5 Axial (**a**) and sagittal (**b**) T2-weighted MR images of L5-S1 left paracentral extrusion severely narrowing the lateral recess and displacing the S1 nerve root

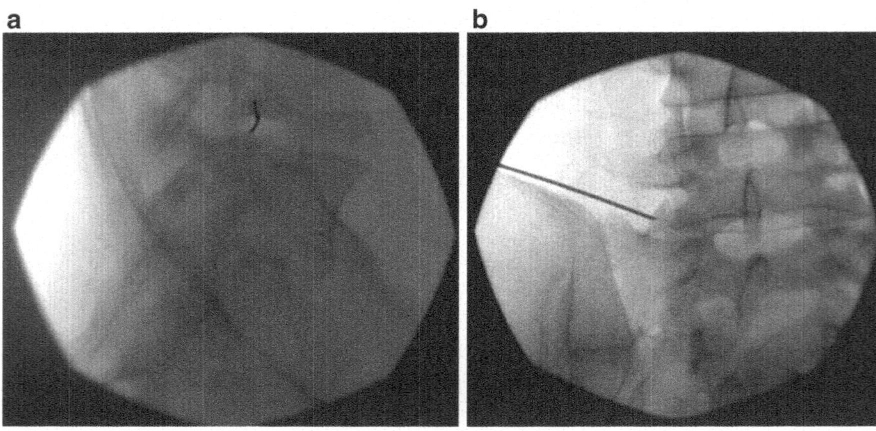

Fig. 4.6 (**a**) In the same patient, the needle is docked on the superior articular facet of S1. (Notice that the level of the iliac crest permits L5-S1 transforaminal access.) (**b**) The needle can then be directed and engaged onto the annulus

Over the largest dilator, insert a beveled working tube (Fig. 4.8) and confirm its placement posterior to the disc and over the site of disc herniation as previously identified. Instruments allow for further medial access into spinal canal. A steeper cephalo-caudad approach, with "joystick" manipulation of the working tube and articulating instrument (Fig. 4.9), may be used to help reach a migrated extrusion.

After initial tissue and disc removal the working tube is directed into the spinal canal (Fig. 4.10a). Further partial discectomy is performed and the traversing nerves are decompressed (Fig. 4.10b).

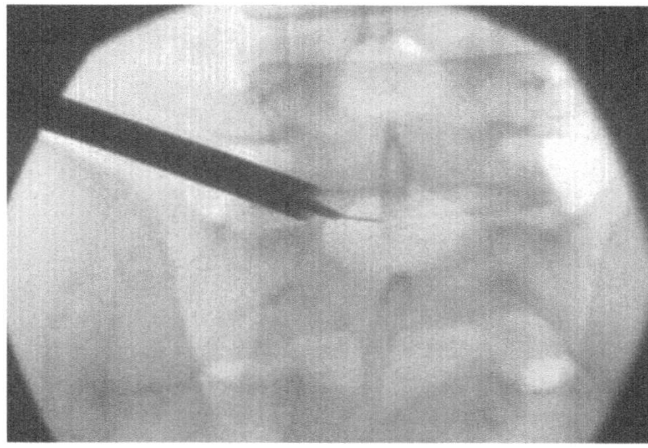

Fig. 4.7 Foraminotomy can be done with fluoroscopically guided sequential bone reamers, shown in the same patient as in Figs. 4.5 and 4.6

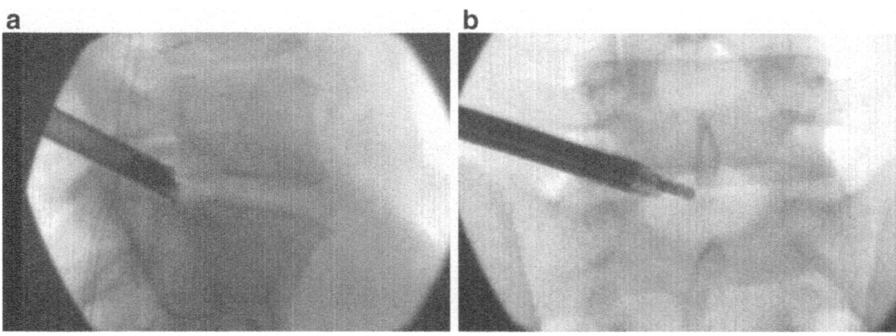

Fig. 4.8 (**a**, **b**) Over the largest dilator, insert a beveled working tube. The one pictured (in the same patient) has an outer diameter of 8 mm. Using lateral fluoroscopy, confirm placement posterior to the disc and over the site of disc herniation identified on presurgical MRI or CT with AP view

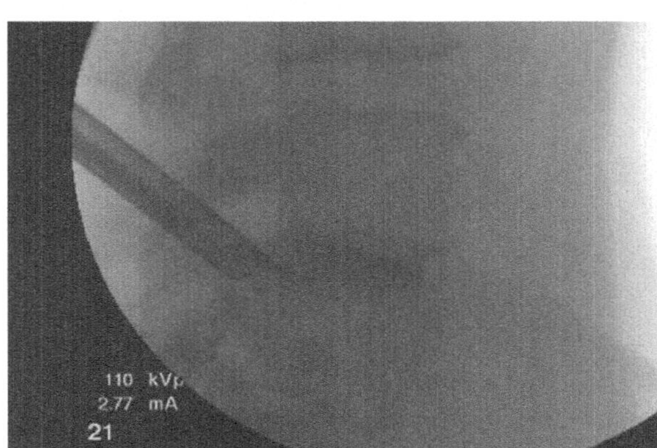

Fig. 4.9 Fluoroscopic image of a different patient, demonstrating a steeper cephalo-caudad approach to help reach migrated extrusion

a b

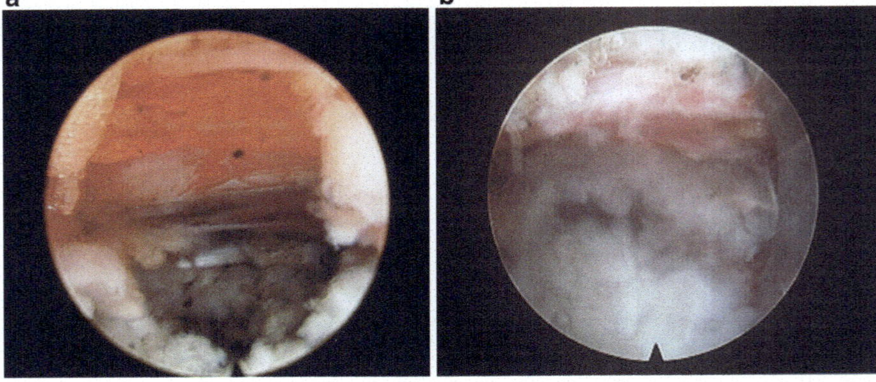

Fig. 4.10 Endoscopic view of the same patient as in Figs. 4.5, 4.6, 4.7 and 4.8. After initial tissue and disc removal, note the decompressed traversing nerves at the top (posterior) and partially resected (**a**) and resected (**b**) disc at the bottom (anterior)

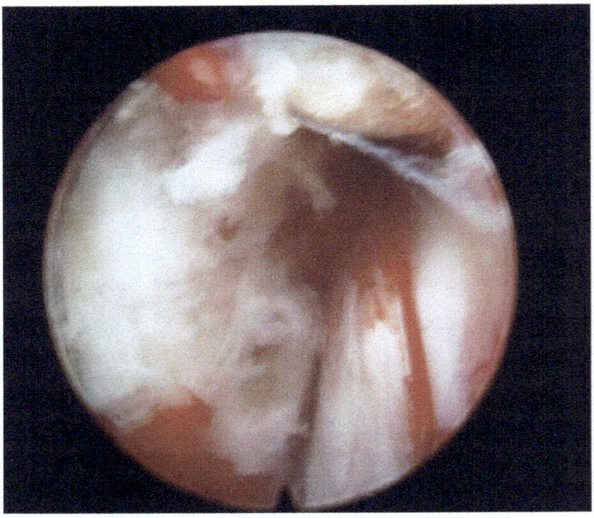

Fig. 4.11 Endoscopic view in a different case, inside the neuroforamen, with the disc *(left)* and exiting nerve root (*right*) visible

As shown in another case, the working tube can be positioned in the neuroforamen (Fig. 4.11), allowing disc and exiting nerve root to be visualized.

4.5 Conclusions

Minimally invasive endoscopic techniques for intraspinal decompression of protruded or herniated disc material have evolved significantly. The approach may vary depending on patient's anatomy and pathology, preference, and the experience of the surgeon. Given the clear short-term benefits of even traditional open surgical techniques for prolapsed disc with radiculopathy, additional study is needed to assist in determining which patients are appropriate for minimally invasive techniques.

References

1. Deyo RA, Weinstein JN. Low back pain. N Engl J Med. 2001;344:363–70.
2. Mazanec D, Okereke L. Interpreting the Spine Patient Outcomes Research Trial. Medical vs surgical treatment of lumbar disk herniation: implications for future trials. Cleve Clin J Med. 2007;74:577–83.
3. Peul WC, van Houwelingen HC, van den Hout WB, Brand R, Eekhof JA, Tans JT, et al. Surgery versus prolonged conservative treatment for sciatica. N Engl J Med. 2007;356:2245–56.
4. Weinstein JN, Lurie JD, Tosteson TD, Tosteson AN, Blood EA, Abdu WA, et al. Surgical versus nonoperative treatment for lumbar disc herniation: four-year results for the Spine Patient Outcomes Research Trial (SPORT). Spine (Phila Pa 1976). 2008;33:2789–800.
5. Dasenbrock HH, Juraschek SP, Schultz LR, Witham TF, Sciubba DM, Wolinsky JP, et al. The efficacy of minimally invasive discectomy compared with open discectomy: a meta-analysis of prospective randomized controlled trials. J Neurosurg Spine. 2012;16:452–62.
6. Jasper GP, Francisco GM, Telfeian A. Outpatient, awake, ultra-minimally invasive endoscopic treatment of lumbar disc herniations. R I Med J (2013). 2014;97:47–9.
7. Choi G. Percutaneous endoscopic lumbar discectomy (PELD). Hanyang Med Rev. 2008;28:4–17.
8. Jasper GP, Francisco GM, Telfeian AE. Endoscopic transforaminal discectomy for an extruded lumbar disc herniation. Pain Physician. 2013;16:E31–5.
9. Kambin P. Arthroscopic and endoscopic anatomy of the lumbar spine. In: Kambin P, editor. Arthroscopic and endoscopic spinal surgery: text and atlas. 2nd ed. Totowa: Humana Press; 2005. p. 29–48.
10. Kambin P. Herniated lumbar disc and lumbar radiculopathy. In: Kambin P, editor. Arthroscopic and endoscopic spinal surgery: text and atlas. 2nd ed. Totowa: Humana Press; 2005. p. 61–118.

Chapter 5
Minimally Invasive Percutaneous Endoscopic Discectomy: Transdiscal Approach

Ajax Yang and Sudhir Diwan

Since Kambin performed the first endoscopic discectomy in 1983 [1], various minimally invasive surgical techniques have been developed to mitigate the deleterious effects of disc herniation and nerve root compression. The current minimally invasive discectomy approaches are interlaminar, transforaminal, and transdiscal. Regardless of the approach, the goal is the resection of a herniated disc under direct endoscopic visualization. Compared with open discectomy, minimally invasive methods have been shown to eliminate cutting of muscles, reduce the rate of infection, shorten operating time, minimize blood loss, and decrease the incidence of cerebral spinal fluid leak and other major complications [2–5]. Although the routine use of endoscopic discectomy for the lumbar and cervical spine remains controversial [6–13], future high-quality research will help to delineate optimal treatment algorithms. This chapter presents the current concepts of the most commonly performed endoscopic spinal surgery [14–17]—the transdiscal approach. Relevant spinal anatomy, patient selection, clinical considerations, and the detailed surgical techniques are discussed.

A. Yang
Department of Rehabilitation Medicine, Icahn School of Medicine at Mount Sinai, New York, NY, USA
e-mail: ajax.yang@mountsinai.org; yang.ajax@gmail.com

S. Diwan (✉)
Lenox Hill Hospital, New York, NY, USA

Manhattan Spine and Pain Medicine, New York, NY, USA
e-mail: Sudhir.diwan63@gmail.com

S. Diwan, T.R. Deer (eds.), *Advanced Procedures for Pain Management*,
https://doi.org/10.1007/978-3-319-68841-1_5

5.1 Spinal Anatomy

Intervertebral discs consist of a slightly posteriorly positioned nucleus pulposus enclosed by the annulus fibrosus on the periphery. The nucleus pulposus contains crisscrossing collagenous and elastin fibers immersed in mucoid polysaccharides. The annulus fibrosus is made of fibrocartilaginous laminas that are subdivided into outermost, middle, and innermost layers. These layers are arranged in a concentric fashion. The annulus fibrosus firmly attaches to epiphyseal rings of the adjacent vertebral bodies. The discs attenuate the axial force in the vertebral column and allow flexion and extension motions. The discs account for 25% of the total spinal column height.

Even though the intervertebral discs are avascular, each disc is innervated by multiple nerves. Sinuvertebral nerves innervate the posterior lumbar disc and posterior longitudinal ligament (PLL). The posterolateral disc is supplied by the adjacent ventral primary rami and the grey rami communicantes. The lateral portion of the disc receives fibers from the rami communicantes [18]. Following acute disc injuries, pro-inflammatory interleukins and nerve growth factors are released; these have been linked to axial back pain and the degenerative process [19]. When the intradiscal material comes in contact with the dorsal root ganglion following an injury, radicular symptoms may be present without mechanical nerve root compression.

In addition to the strong anterior longitudinal ligament (ALL), the anterior and middle fibers of the annulus are most abundant anteriorly and laterally, which contribute to the anterior column stability. Posteriorly, the PLL is thin, and the annulus fibers are deficient. Therefore, the posterior region of a disc is most prone to mechanical deformation. A disc herniation is defined as a focal deformation of the disc (less than 25% of the circumference of the disc) extending beyond the normal intervertebral disc space. Herniated disc material may include nucleus pulposus, cartilage, fragmented apophyseal bone, or annulus fibrosus tissue [20]. The morphology of disc herniation usually presents as a narrow neck with a "mushroom" head of nucleus pulposus impinging the nerve roots. Herniated discs may be further grouped into contained and uncontained herniations. Containment is determined by the presence of disc materials held within an intact outermost annulus fibrosis and PLL. An uncontained herniation is defined by the absence of intact annulus fibrosis and/or PLL. A central disc herniation will cause compression of the traversing nerve root exiting the foramen at the level below, whereas a far lateral disc herniation is likely to affect the nerve root at the level of the herniated disc, with corresponding neural tension signs and dermatomal, myotomal, and reflex changes. Furcal nerves, primarily sensory, are found in roughly 15% of individuals at L4-5. These furcal nerves may traverse the L4 foramen far laterally and exit with the L5 nerve root, so that a far lateral disc herniation can cause L4-5 radicular symptoms.

Each foramen is made up of pedicles (cranial and caudal), the intervertebral body and disc (anterior), and the facet joint (posterior). The ligamentum flavum courses between the laminas and forms the posterior wall of the spinal canal. Spinal nerve root, radicular vasculatures, and meningeal nerves exit the foramen below the corresponding vertebral body in the lumbar spine. Kambin's triangle delineates an area

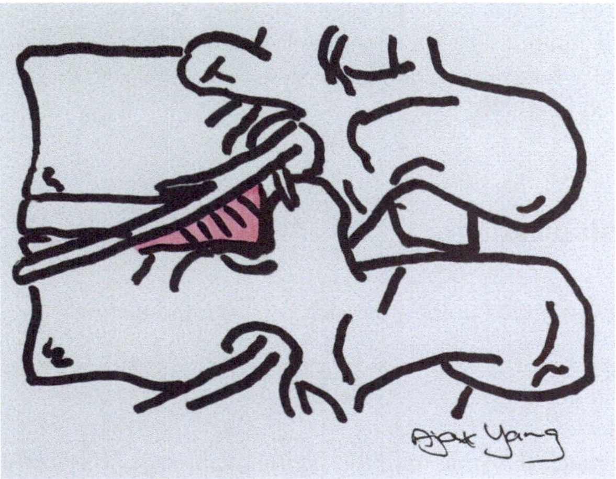

Fig. 5.1 Kambin's triangle (shaded in *pink*)

in this region formed by the exiting nerve root (hypotenuse), the superior end plate of the caudal vertebra (base), and the superior articular process (height) (Fig. 5.1). Kambin's triangle serves as an important landmark in interventional spine procedures, but it is important to be mindful that when the disc herniation is more apical, the Kambin's triangle is reduced, as the nerve becomes displaced more inferiorly. A calcified annulus fibrosus, osteophytes, facet joint hypertrophy, and vertebral body osteochondrosis can all make disc access difficult. A thorough knowledge of Kambin's triangle prevents unnecessary complications.

5.2 Patient Selection

Appropriate patient selection is imperative for favorable outcomes. Generally, the patient must demonstrate signs and symptoms consistent with mechanical impingement of a nerve root. The following are important considerations for planning endoscopic percutaneous discectomy procedure by the transdiscal approach:

- Contained herniated or bulging disc with radicular symptoms
- Positive neural tension signs (*eg*, positive straight leg raise test) accompanied by unrelenting monoradicular pain consistent with imaging findings (MRI, CT, discography)
- Radicular symptoms relieved by a diagnostic block of the suspected nerve root
- Unilateral radicular pain greater than low back pain
- Failure for at least 6 weeks of conservative management such as oral medications, physical therapy, and epidural steroid injections
- Confirmed electromyography studies
- Facet joint ruled out as a source of pain
- Greater than one half of disc height preserved

Evidence suggests that in the hands of an experienced surgeon, a large, uncontained herniated lumbar disc fragment (6–12 mm) and far lateral disc herniations can be sufficiently removed via an endoscopic discectomy procedure by a transforaminal approach [21].

5.3 Contraindications

The following conditions are considered contraindications for this type of procedure:

- Cauda equina syndrome
- Coagulopathy
- Herniation greater than one third the sagittal diameter of the spinal canal
- Calcified intervertebral disc herniation
- Concurrent spinal fracture, structural instability, tumor, pregnancy, or active infection
- Advanced degenerative joint disease, osteophytes, multilevel disc bulge, ligamentum flavum hypertrophy, or severe foraminal and spinal stenosis
- Psychiatric disorder, substance abuse, or lack of capacity to consent

5.4 Preoperative Planning and Patient Education

Thorough physical and neurological examination and diagnostic imaging are performed to establish the indication for the surgery. MRI is helpful to confirm the diagnosis. In equivocal situations, a diagnostic block is helpful to rule out other spinal conditions that mimic the symptoms of disc herniation. If other comorbidities are present, medical optimization should be achieved prior to surgery, such as the safe correction of anticoagulant status and evaluation for contrast allergy. Because the procedure is performed under local anesthesia with or without conscious sedation, the patient must be able to tolerate lying prone.

Patients must be educated on the benefits, risks, and alternatives to a percutaneous endoscopic discectomy (PED) procedure. Similar to open spinal surgeries, there are risks of infection, bleeding, nerve injury, paresthesia, disc collapse, dural tears, scar tissue formation, vertebral endplate damage, spinal instability, and damage to surrounding structures. Patients should understand that in the event of disc reherniation, future revision and open spinal surgery may be required. It is important to set realistic expectations, as long-term nerve compression with associated chronic swelling and perineural fibrosis may not have the same rapid improvement as acute disc herniation.

Postoperative plans and expectations should be discussed with the patient prior to the surgery. A comprehensive rehabilitation program will optimize functional mobility, core strengthening, and overall physical conditioning. The patient should be advised to adhere to a spinal mobility and strengthening routine to ensure long-term spine health.

5.5 The Transdiscal Approach

Because the PED procedure depends on proper positioning of the portal to ensure optimal access and sufficient visualization of the target disc and foramen, the success of the procedure is greatly influenced by the point of entry needle placement. During the transdiscal approach, the cannula normally is inserted similar to the discography approach. The entry point can be ipsilateral or contralateral, depending on the disc material to be removed, using an anteroposterior (AP) view with cranial-caudad adjustments to the fluoroscopic beam to square off the disc to be treated. The scope is then rotated to obtain an oblique view that clearly bisects the superior endplate with articular elements.

The skin entry point is marked just lateral to the superior articular process of the inferior vertebral body. Patients with body mass index greater than 40 present a unique challenge for the transdiscal approach. To reach the neural foramen at 45° in a morbidly obese patient, the needle length would have to be at least 21 cm (≥8 in.), which renders the transdiscal approach impractical. Similarly, in male patients with high iliac crests, approaching the L5-S1 foramen may pose a significant challenge, as the target foramen is embedded deeply in the pelvis, and the iliac crest obstructs the posterolateral trajectory to the disc space. The superior S1 endplate is at risk of injury if nonflexible instruments are used while adhering to the transdiscal approach. To create an optimal view at the L5-S1 level, the oblique fluoroscopic view requires the most amount of cranial tilt to place the superior articular process of S1 at the midpoint of the disc with clear visualization of the endplates. This oblique view will decrease the risk of injury by ensuring that the needle trajectory does not cross the nerve root.

5.6 Discography

Provocative discography is recommended to confirm the source of radicular symptoms. It is performed before or at the same time as the planned PED procedure. If planned at the time of the PED procedure, the water-soluble contrast is mixed with indigo carmine dye to provide visible radiopacity on the discography under fluoroscopy, and intraoperative light-blue chromatization of the disc tissue and annular tears. Depending on the disc pathology seen on the discogram, the transdiscal approach can be further subdivided into an inside-out technique [22] or outside-in technique [23]. The inside-out technique is appropriate for treating internal disc disruption, tears, and contained herniation in the foramen. The location of the disc herniation is of less concern with the inside-out technique, but this technique may remove too much normal disc tissue in minor disc herniation. For the outside-in technique, the opening of the access cannula is positioned in the foramen and does not enter the target disc space [23]. The outside-in technique is considered when treating foraminal disc herniation.

5.7 Uniportal Percutaneous Endoscopic Discectomy Technique

The patient is placed in the prone position on the operating room table, with pillows or a bolster placed beneath the lumbosacral area to reduce lumbar lordosis. Additionally, the knees are gently flexed, with pillows supporting the patient's ankles to improve positional comfort. The skin overlying the target area will be thoroughly cleaned and draped, with strict aseptic techniques. Intravenous administration of 1–2 g of cefazolin or 600 mg of clindamycin is recommended 30 min prior to the procedure.

The sterile draped C-arm is used to obtain an AP view of the spinous process centered between the pedicles of the target spinal segments. The fluoroscopic beam should be adjusted with an appropriate amount of cranial-caudal tilt until the target vertebral bodies and their end-plates are clearly in focus. Lines connecting the spinous processes and across the disc space are drawn. The C-arm is then repositioned to obtain a lateral view. Disc inclination angles are drawn and the cranial/caudal entry point is determined by the intersection of those lines. The skin and subcutaneous tissue are adequately anesthetized with 1% lidocaine infiltration. A 16-gauge, 6-inch-long spinal needle is then inserted into the skin, directed towards Kambin's triangle. The needle is usually angled 60° in the sagittal plane and advanced in the anteromedial direction towards the disc. In a larger patient, however, the needle entry point must be placed further laterally. Careful attention should focus on the needle trajectory, as the beveling of the needle may cause it to deviate away from the intended path as it pierces the soft tissues. Sufficient local anesthetic should be administered along the needle path down to Kambin's triangle to minimize intraoperative and postoperative pain. The safe annular entry point is confirmed on the AP and lateral view. On the AP view, the needle should be aligned with the posterior vertebral bodies at the inner pedicle line, with the tip nearly touching the posterior annulus (Fig. 5.2a). On the lateral view, the needle should be positioned on the posterior one third of the pedicle line (Fig. 5.2b). Under direct AP fluoroscopic visualization, the needle is carefully advanced until the tip is through the annular layer (Fig. 5.3). The final needle position is also confirmed on the lateral view. The lateral view confirms that an appropriate needle penetration depth is achieved, preventing over-penetration into the anterior nucleus or annulus. With the needle tip inside the disc, contrast (a combination of Omnipaque™ [iohexol] and indigo carmine dye) is introduced. This contrast mixture will aid in direct and fluoroscopic visualization of the diseased nucleus pulposus and annulus defects.

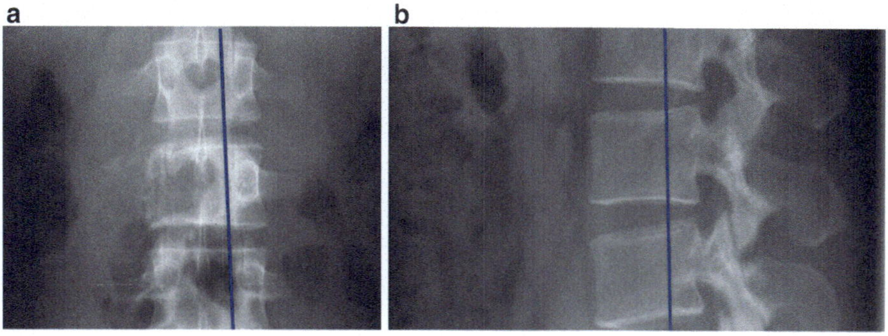

Fig. 5.2 (**a**) Anteroposterior (AP) fluoroscopic view with medial pedicle line drawn. (**b**) Posterior one third of the pedicle line on lateral view

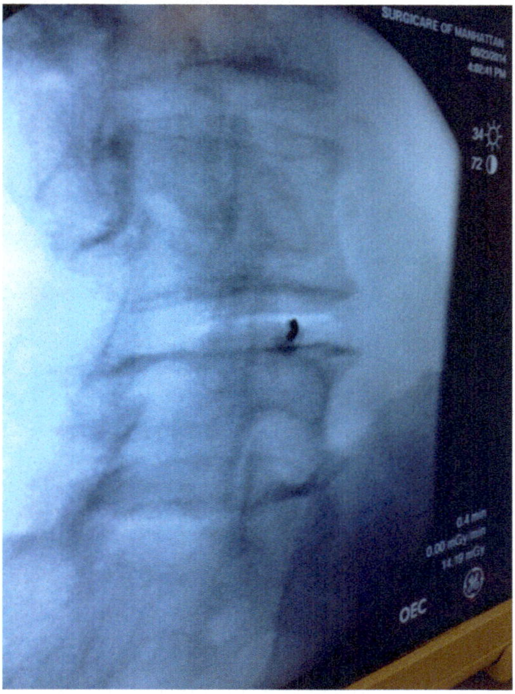

Fig. 5.3 AP fluoroscopic view of needle entry into the annular layer of the target disc

The next series of steps involve sequential inserting and retrieving of the needle, guide wire, blunt dilator, and beveled access cannula (Fig. 5.4). The guide wire is inserted through the spinal needle until it is 1–2 cm into the annulus. Once the guide wire is firmly held in place, the spinal needle is retrieved. The next step is to make a 2 cm skin incision with a #15 blade to allow the blunt dilator to be introduced over the

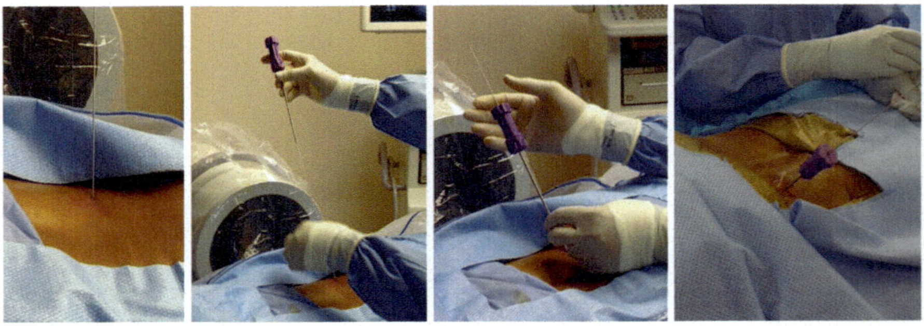

Fig. 5.4 Stepwise progression (*left* to *right*): Guide wire is in place; an access portal is inserted over the guide wire, toward the target disc space

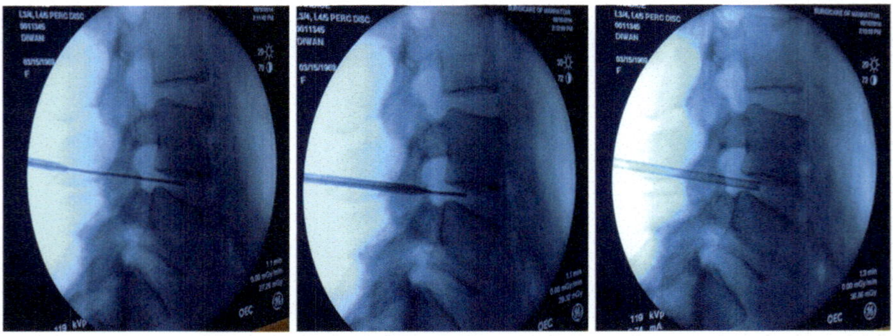

Fig. 5.5 Fluoroscopic views of accessory portal placement of the guide wire via the transdiscal approach (*left* to *right*). Note that the final portal tip is in line with the posterior one-third line

guide wire and securely engaged at the annular window. A mallet may be used to assist the annular fenestration process. After confirming that the dilator tip adequately embedded into the annulus on AP and lateral views, the access cannula is then slid over the dilator until the access cannula is deep in the annular window. At this point, the exiting nerve root is posterior to the access cannula. Care should be taken to secure the access cannula while the dilator is removed, because periannular bleeding will obscure endoscopic visualization. Finally, the trephine is inserted and then removed through the access cannula to perform an annulotomy. Under direct visualization, grasping forceps can be used to remove degenerated annular material in view.

Following sufficient annulotomy, the guide wire, dilator, and cannula are sequentially re-inserted and exchanged until the cannula is positioned in the center of the nucleus pulposus under fluoroscopic control (Fig. 5.5). Tissue debulking graspers are inserted through the access cannula to perform nucleotomy (Fig. 5.6). The annulotomy is expanded medially to the base of the herniation via cutting forceps to release the annular layer and allow extruded disc material to be removed adequately. A large amount of nucleus with blue dye is usually visible directly under the herniation.

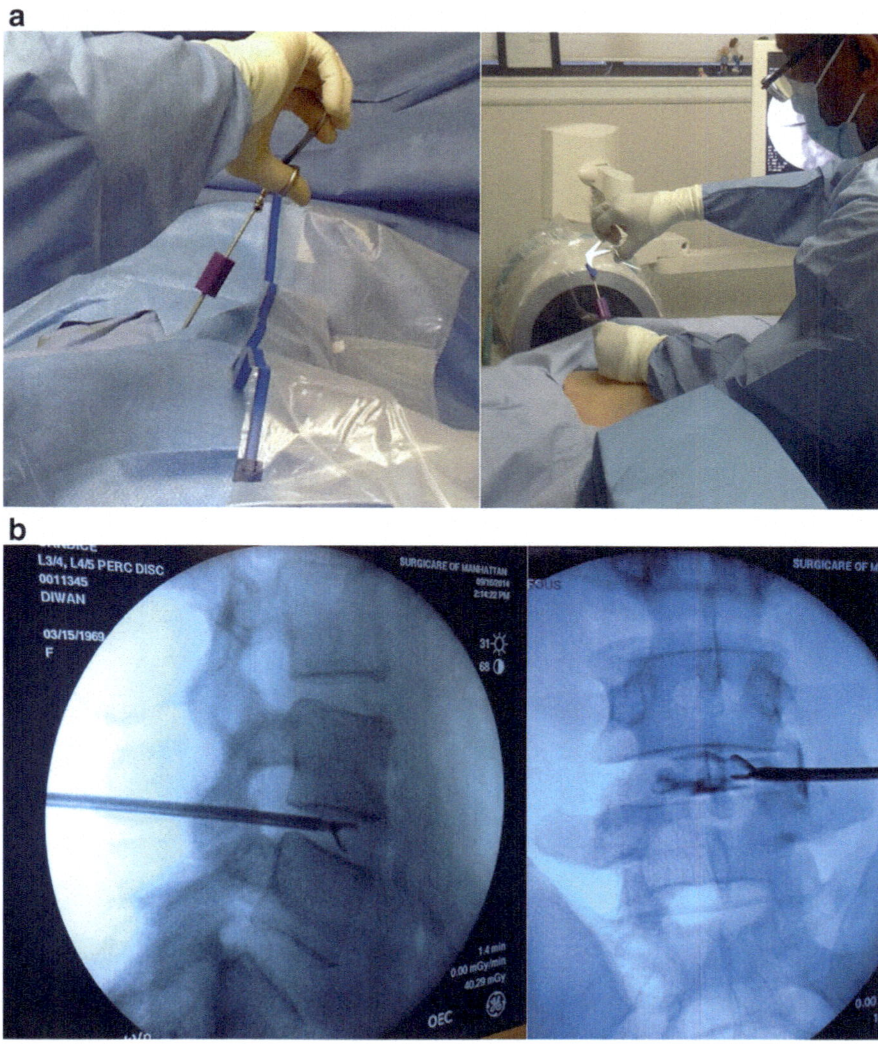

Fig. 5.6 (**a**) Nuclear debulking forceps are used to remove herniated disc material. (**b**) Fluoroscopic lateral view (*left*) and AP view (*right*) of the debulking forceps in the desired intradiscal space

5.8 Annulus Modulation

Once the herniated disc materials have been removed, the flexible steerable bipolar radiofrequency (RF) probe is used to shrink and thicken the herniation site (Fig. 5.7). The flexible RF probe is advanced towards the posterior or posterolateral aspect of the nucleus pulposus and positioned adjacent to the annular tears. AP and lateral fluoroscopic views should be obtained as needed for safety and efficacy. Small bleeding vessels are cauterized with the RF probe to achieve sufficient hemostasis. Optional endoscopic visualization is performed inside the newly created disc cavity.

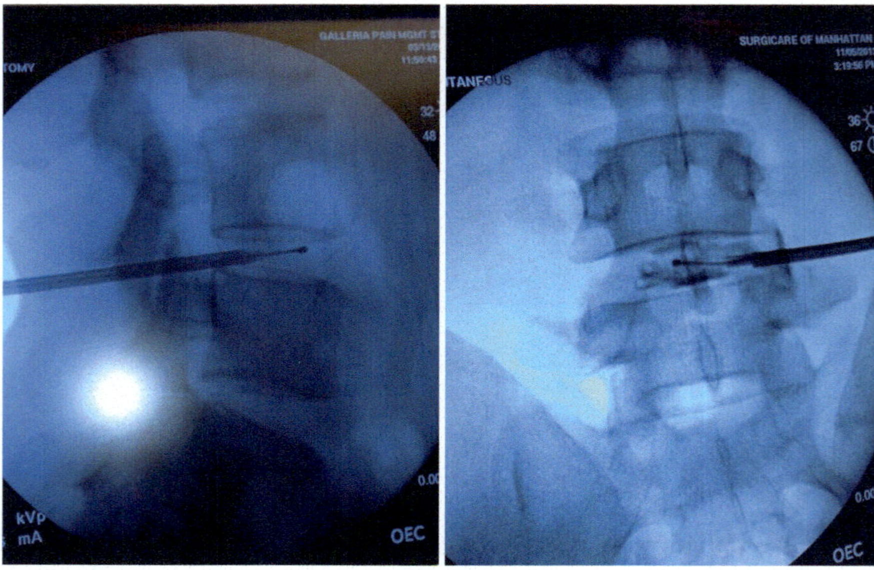

Fig. 5.7 Lateral (*left*) and AP (*right*) views of transdiscal radiofrequency (RF) probe

The access cannula and the endoscope can be retracted 2–3 mm to inspect the exiting nerve in the epidural space. The procedure site is irrigated before retrieving the endoscope and the blunt nerve retractor. An adhesive dressing is applied to close the skin stab wound.

5.9 Postoperative Care and Rehabilitation

Minimally invasive endoscopic discectomy is an outpatient procedure. The patient is discharged home on the same day with analgesics and anti-inflammatory medications. A follow-up visit is scheduled in 7–10 days. Signs of infection and bleeding should be closely monitored. The patient should be advised to minimize activities that increase intradiscal pressure. Postures such as sitting, slouching, and lifting should be avoided during the initial recovery period. If the patient shows improvement, a progressive rehabilitation protocol and neuromuscular re-education can be initiated under physical therapy supervision. A post-procedure back brace may be prescribed for a week or two to aid with instability and provide posterolateral support. The orthosis decreases axial loading and helps to improve functional status. The patient is encouraged to participate in aquatic exercises followed by progressive lumbar and core strengthening exercises, and to integrate good body mechanics and postural awareness into activities of daily living.

Even if the patient does not report significant improvement, the procedure should not be considered a failure until at least 6 weeks from the date of the procedure. If the patient shows signs and symptoms consistent with an inflamed nerve root, an image-guided selective nerve block may be considered.

5.10 Discussion

Current evidence supports the use of PED as a method for treating radicular pain caused by disc herniation [24–28]. Because this technology requires only local anesthesia with conscious sedation, it provides an opportunity for patients who are unable to tolerate general anesthesia to undergo open surgical discectomy. Thorough knowledge of Kambin's triangle and the surrounding neurovasculature is a cornerstone of the procedure. Appropriate patient selection, coupled with skilled access cannula placement and surgical techniques, drive the safety and effectiveness of this surgical procedure. Minimally invasive endoscopic discectomy offers the advantages at the cost of the surgeon's commitment to mastering the skills of negotiating instruments with a two-dimensional field of view. Future technical advancement through continued effort in research will improve our understanding and ability to treat disc herniation and other spinal disorders via minimally invasive endoscopic techniques.

References

1. Kambin P, Gellman H. Percutaneous lateral discectomy of the lumbar spine: a preliminary report. Clin Orthop Relat Res. 1983;174:127.
2. Ohya J, Oshima Y, Chikuda H, Oichi T, Matsui H, Fushimi K, et al. Does the microendoscopic technique reduce mortality and major complications in patients undergoing lumbar discectomy? A propensity score-matched analysis using a nationwide administrative database. Neurosurg Focus. 2016;40:E5.
3. Wong AP, Shih P, Smith TR, Slimack NP, Dahdaleh NS, Aoun SG, et al. Comparison of symptomatic cerebral spinal fluid leak between patients undergoing minimally invasive versus open lumbar foraminotomy, discectomy, or laminectomy. World Neurosurg. 2014;81:634–40.
4. Rahman M, Summers LE, Richter B, Mimran RI, Jacob RP. Comparison of techniques for decompressive lumbar laminectomy: the minimally invasive versus the "classic" open approach. Minim Invasive Neurosurg. 2008;51:100–5.
5. O'Toole JE, Eichholz KM, Fessler RG. Surgical site infection rates after minimally invasive spinal surgery. J Neurosurg Spine. 2009;11:471–6.
6. Evaniew N, Khan M, Drew B, Kwok D, Bhandari M, Ghert M. Minimally invasive versus open surgery for cervical and lumbar discectomy: a systematic review and meta-analysis. CMAJ Open. 2014;2:E295–305.
7. Lubelski D, Mihalovich KE, Skelly AC, Fehlings MG, Harrop JS, Mummaneni PV, et al. Is minimal access spine surgery more cost-effective than conventional spine surgery? Spine (Phila Pa 1976). 2014;39:S65–74.

8. Mu X, Wei J, Li P. What were the advantages of microendoscopic discectomy for lumbar disc herniation comparing with open discectomy: a meta-analysis? Int J Clin Exp Med. 2015;8:17498–506.
9. Gibson JN, Cowie JG, Iprenburg M. Transforaminal endoscopic spinal surgery: the future 'gold standard' for discectomy?—a review. Surgeon. 2012;10:290–6.
10. Ruan W, Feng F, Liu Z, Xie J, Cai L, Ping A. Comparison of percutaneous endoscopic lumbar discectomy versus open lumbar microdiscectomy for lumbar disc herniation: a meta-analysis. Int J Surg. 2016;31:86–92.
11. Anichini G, Landi A, Caporlingua F, Beer-Furlan A, Brogna C, Delfini R, Passacantilli E. Lumbar endoscopic microdiscectomy: where are we now? An updated literature review focused on clinical outcome, complications, and rate of recurrence. Biomed Res Int. 2015;2015:417801.
12. Ahn SS, Kim SH, Kim DW, Lee BH. Comparison of outcomes of percutaneous endoscopic lumbar discectomy and open lumbar microdiscectomy for young adults: a retrospective matched cohort study. World Neurosurg. 2016;86:250–8.
13. Dohrmann GJ, Mansour N. Long-term results of various operations for lumbar disc herniation: analysis of over 39,000 patients. Med Princ Pract. 2015;24:285–90.
14. Tsou PM, Alan Yeung C, Yeung AT. Posterolateral transforaminal selective endoscopic discectomy and thermal annuloplasty for chronic lumbar discogenic pain: a minimal access visualized intradiscal surgical procedure. Spine J. 2004;4:564–73.
15. Ruetten S, Komp M, Merk H, Godolias G. Use of newly developed instruments and endoscopes: full-endoscopic resection of lumbar disc herniations via the interlaminar and lateral transforaminal approach. J Neurosurg Spine. 2007;6:521–30.
16. Lühmann D, Burkhardt-Hammer T, Borowski C, Raspe H. Minimally invasive surgical procedures for the treatment of lumbar disc herniation. GMS Health Technol Assess. 2005;1:Doc07.
17. Yeung AT, Tsou PM. Posterolateral endoscopic excision for lumbar disc herniation: surgical technique, outcome, and complications in 307 consecutive cases. Spine (Phila Pa 1976). 2002;27:722–31.
18. Bogduk N, Tynan W, Wilson AS. The nerve supply to the human lumbar intervertebral discs. J Anat. 1981;132:39–56.
19. Alkhatib B, Rosenzweig DH, Krock E, Roughley PJ, Beckman L, Steffen T, et al. Acute mechanical injury of the human intervertebral disc: link to degeneration and pain. Eur Cell Mater. 2014;28:98–110; discussion 110–1.
20. Fardon DF, Williams AL, Dohring EJ, Murtagh FR, Gabriel Rothman SL, Sze GK. Lumbar disc nomenclature: version 2.0: recommendations of the combined task forces of the North American Spine Society, the American Society of Spine Radiology and the American Society of Neuroradiology. Spine J. 2014;14:2525–45.
21. Hussein M, Abdeldayem A, Mattar MM. Surgical technique and effectiveness of microendoscopic discectomy for large uncontained lumbar disc herniations: a prospective, randomized, controlled study with 8 years of follow-up. Eur Spine J. 2014;23:1992–9.
22. Gore S, Yeung A. The "inside out" transforaminal technique to treat lumbar spinal pain in an awake and aware patient under local anesthesia: results and a review of the literature. Int J Spine Surg. 2014;8. https://doi.org/10.14444/1028.
23. Lewandrowski KU. "Outside-in" technique, clinical results, and indications with transforaminal lumbar endoscopic surgery: a retrospective study on 220 patients on applied radiographic classification of foraminal spinal stenosis. Int J Spine Surg. 2014;8. https://doi.org/10.14444/1026.
24. Singh V, Piryani C, Liao K. Role of percutaneous disc decompression using coblation in managing chronic discogenic low back pain: a prospective, observational study. Pain Physician. 2004;7:419–25.

25. Alò KM, Wright RE, Sutcliffe J, Brandt SA. Percutaneous lumbar discectomy: clinical response in an initial cohort of fifty consecutive patients with chronic radicular pain. Pain Pract. 2004;4:19–29.
26. Manchikanti L, Singh V, Calodney AK, Helm S 2nd, Deer TR, Benyamin RM, et al. Percutaneous lumbar mechanical disc decompression utilizing Dekompressor®: an update of current evidence. Pain Physician. 2013;16:SE1–24.
27. Zhou Y. Diagnosis and minimally invasive treatment of lumbar discogenic pain. In: Smith HS, editor. Current therapy in pain. Philadelphia: Saunders Elsevier; 2009. p. 620–5.
28. Hellinger S. Treatment of contained lumbar disc herniations using radiofrequency assisted micro-tubular decompression and nucleotomy: four year prospective study results. Int J Spine Surg. 2014;8. https://doi.org/10.14444/1024.

Chapter 6
Minimally Invasive Facet Fusion

Louis J. Raso

Low back pain is one of the most common complaints given at a doctor's office, and it remains one of the more costly medical expenditures in modern society. Approximately 80% of all individuals will experience low back pain at some time, with costs in the million of dollars [1]. When conservative measures such as exercise, physical therapy, and injection therapy have failed, more aggressive treatments of these back complaints are needed.

Facet fusions were first used in 1949 as a means to treat mechanical low back pain. Since that time, many techniques for facet fusion have been developed [2]. Some companies have recently developed minimally invasive techniques involving use of an allograft to achieve stability and fusion. Such techniques are used to treat facet-mediated pain and instability due to Grade 1 spondylolisthesis, either as a stand-alone technique or in conjunction with a more invasive procedure. This chapter focuses on the minimally invasive stand-alone technique.

Facet fusion works by temporarily stopping spinal facet joints from moving until natural healing fuses the facet joints together by growing bone into bone dowels that are placed during the procedure [2]. It is used as an alternative to the use of metal screws to hold the joints together, preventing movement [3].

6.1 Basic Concerns

In facet disease, the cartilage in the joints is worn down as a result of wear and tear, aging, injury, or misuse. Another cause of facet disease is spondylolisthesis. Symptoms of facet joint problems are usually localized to the area of the facet joint [4]. When affected in the lumbar region, the patient experiences lower back pain

L.J. Raso (✉)
Broward General Hospital, New York, USA
e-mail: lraso@aol.com

S. Diwan, T.R. Deer (eds.), *Advanced Procedures for Pain Management*,
https://doi.org/10.1007/978-3-319-68841-1_6

radiating to the buttocks and upper thighs. Patients initially try physical therapy, NSAIDS, other medications, steroid injections, and radiofrequency ablation [5]. When these therapies fail, facet fusion becomes an option.

6.2 Indications for Facet Fusion

- Degenerative disc disease (back pain of discogenic origin confirmed by radiographic studies)
- Degenerative disease of the facet joints with pain and/or instability on plain flexion/extension radiographs with movement greater than 4 mm
- Trauma (fracture/dislocation)
- Spondylolisthesis
- Spondylolysis
- Pseudoarthrosis or failed previous fusion [2]

6.3 Contraindications

A number of conditions can be considered contraindications to minimally invasive facet fusion [2]:

- Patients with intolerance to materials used in the device
- Patients with active infection, pregnancy, or other medical conditions prohibiting performance of the procedure
- Congenital abnormalities
- Rapid joint disease, bone absorption, or osteopenia (Osteoporosis is a relative contraindication)
- Inadequate tissue coverage or bone stock or quality
- Re-operation

6.4 Minimally Invasive Techniques

Two current systems are discussed in this chapter, the TruFUSE® system (minSURG Corp.; Clearwater, FL) and the Zyfix™ system (X-spine Systems; Miamisburg, OH).

The TruFUSE® system, which uses precision-machined allograft dowels and matching surgical instrumentation, is a unique approach to posterior spinal fusion. Performed in a minimally invasive fashion, the tapered dowel design is impacted into the facet joint, providing immediate spinal stabilization by employing a classic wedge fixation, optimizing the potential for fusion (Fig. 6.1) [6].

The Zyfix™ system is a technique featuring a hollow, fenestrated titanium compression screw for autogenous bone graft introduction. The implant is packed with bone graft and creates a fusion mass across the facet joint, imparting long-term stability (Fig. 6.2).

Facet fusion is typically used early in the continuum of care as an intermediate, conservative measure to address or prevent minor instability [2], mechanical back pain, or degenerative joint disease. It can be used as a stand-alone procedure for facet-based pain or as a supplement to major fusion surgeries. One of the technique's primary attractions is that it is minimally destructive and does not preclude future surgical options for the patient, if warranted.

Minimally invasive facet fusion techniques have a number of benefits when compared with more invasive procedures:

- Less nerve and tissue damage.
- Less blood loss
- Low theoretical risk of adjacent segment disease
- Reduced hospitalization time
- Less postoperative pain
- Improved postoperative range of motion
- Less postoperative rehabilitation

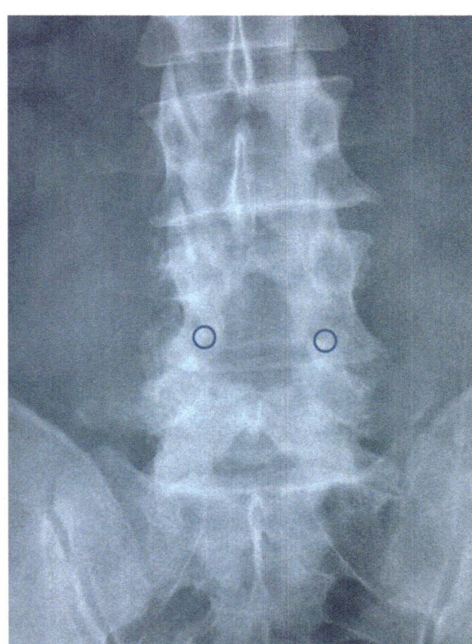

Fig. 6.1 AP view of bone dowels in place

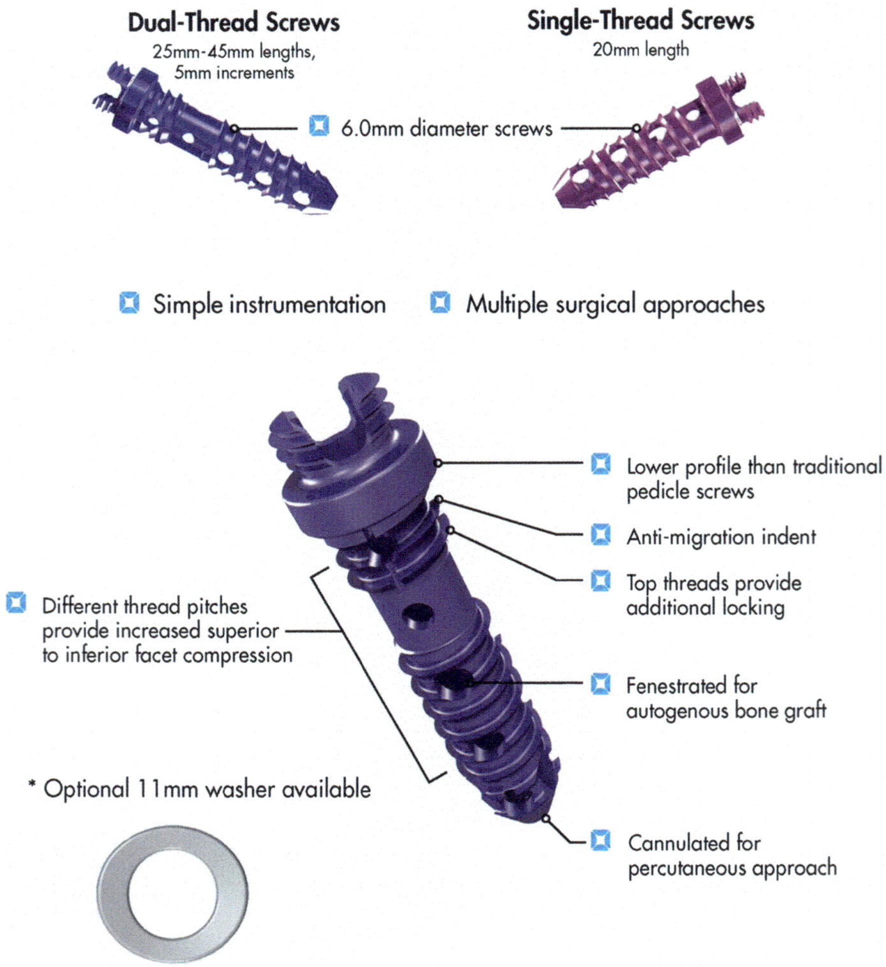

Fig. 6.2 Zyfix threaded compression screw

6.4.1 *TruFUSE® Technique*

The TruFUSE® technique involves using fluoroscopy to locate the midpoint of the affected facet joint and inserting a Steinmann pin. A cannulated spatula is placed over the Steinmann pin, which helps align the drill guide into the facet joint. A specialized reamer is then used to create a tapered void at the midpoint of the joint [6]. Finally, a bone dowel is impacted into the facet joint, thereby ensuring a tightly pressed fit (Figs. 6.3, 6.4, 6.5, 6.6 and 6.7).

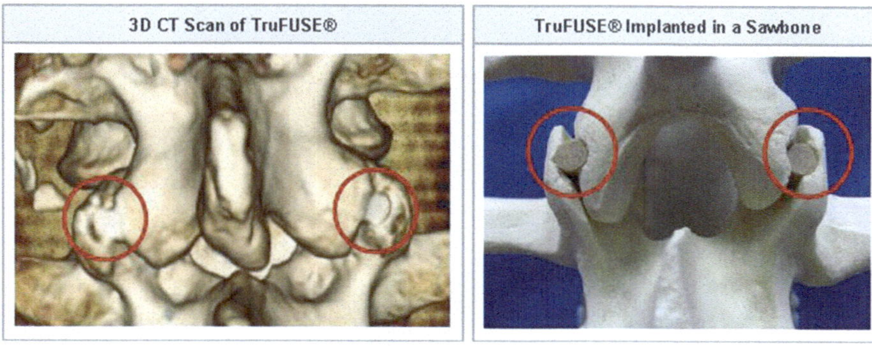

Fig. 6.3 CT scan postoperative and anatomical model view

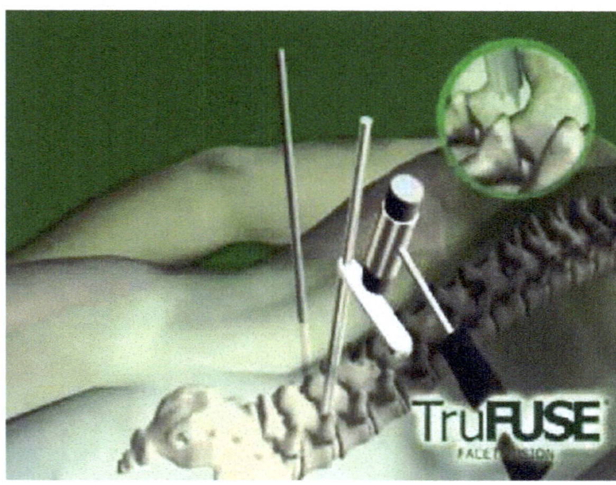

Fig. 6.4 Oblique approach to facet joints

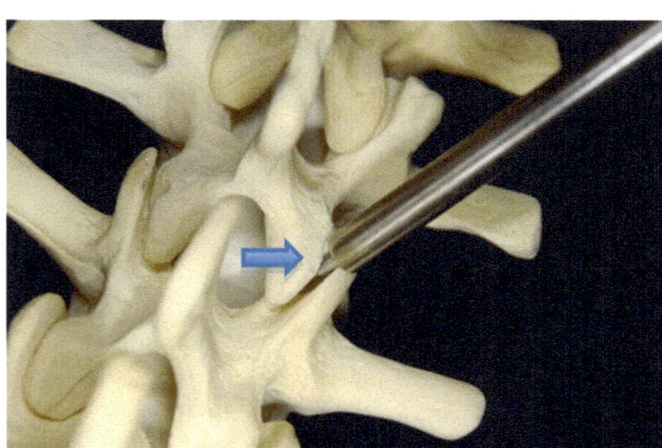

Fig. 6.5 Portal insertion and reaming of joint

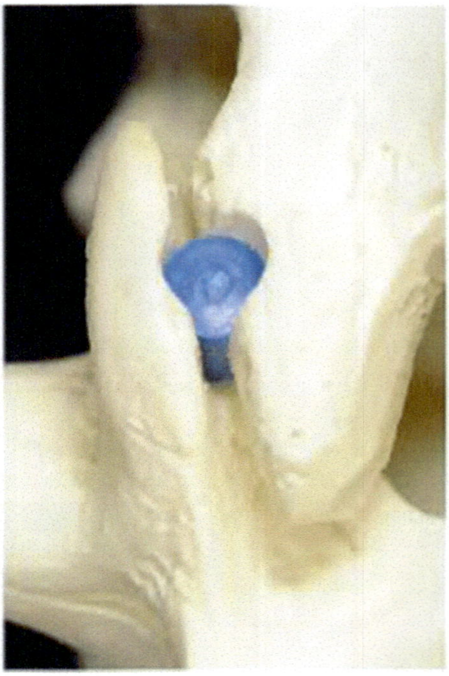

Fig. 6.6 Bone dowel in proper position

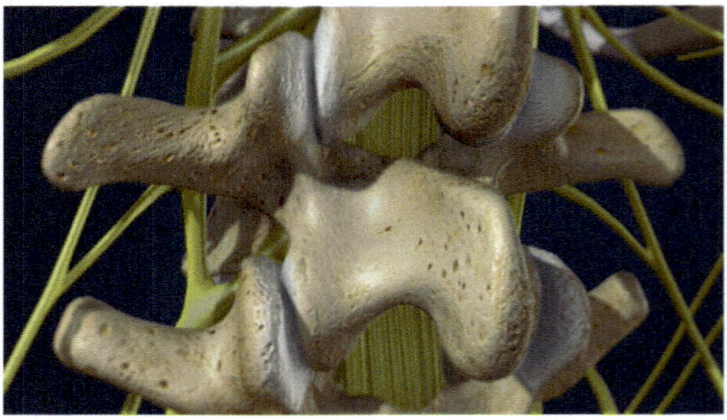

Fig. 6.7 Classic facet joint anatomy and orientation

The bone dowel performs several functions:

- Re-establishes natural joint orientation
- Separates the joint surfaces to reduce inflammation
- Stretches the anterior joint capsule and creates a press fit to enhance stability
- Optimizes the environment for fusion

The patient is placed prone on a standard operating table. Start with an anterior-posterior (AP) image of the corresponding facet joints in view. Rotate the beam in an oblique view to optimize and open up the facet joint at the desired level. Bilateral

Steinmann pins are advanced under fluoroscopic guidance into the midpoint of the desired facet joint. A stab wound is made adjacent to the pins. Beveled spatulas are advanced over the Steinmann pins and rotated. They are then tapped into place to open up the joint in the proper plane [6]. The drill guide is then inserted and the Steinmann pins and spatula are removed. It is also tapped into place to further widen the joint. The combination drill and compaction reamer is used to create a tunnel of subchondral bone; pulsed drilling is utilized to prevent heating. An impactor is attached to the bone dowel, which is placed and countersinked to a 2-mm depth. Most patients are discharged within 24 h. Bracing is recommended for 6 weeks postoperatively.

6.4.2 *Zyfix™ Technique*

The patient is again positioned prone on the operating table. Targeting of the facet joint anatomy is identical to the above technique. Instead of a Steinmann pin, a Jamshidi-type cannulated needle is advanced under fluoroscopic guidance. A K-wire is placed through the Jamshidi needle, and the needle is removed. Two dilators (inner and outer) are then threaded over the K-wire. The joint is then drilled over the K-wire and the long outer dilator, into the cortical bone margin. The screw is then loaded onto the screwdriver and placed within the drilled joint. Bone marrow aspirate is then placed within the screw and packed in place. All instruments are then removed and the surgical site is closed (Figs. 6.8, 6.9, 6.10, 6.11, 6.12 and 6.13) [7].

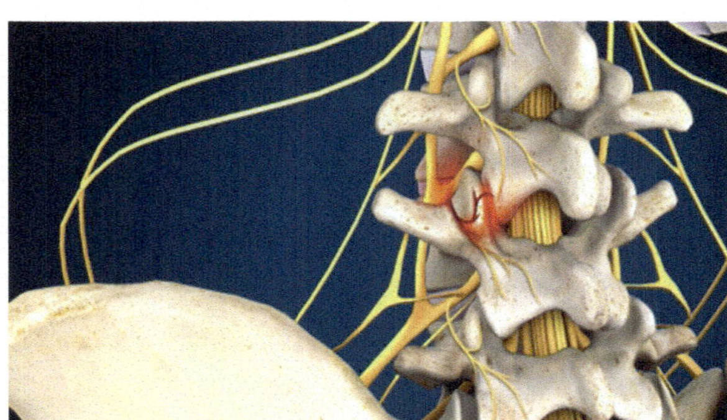

Fig. 6.8 Diseased facet joint and nerve supply

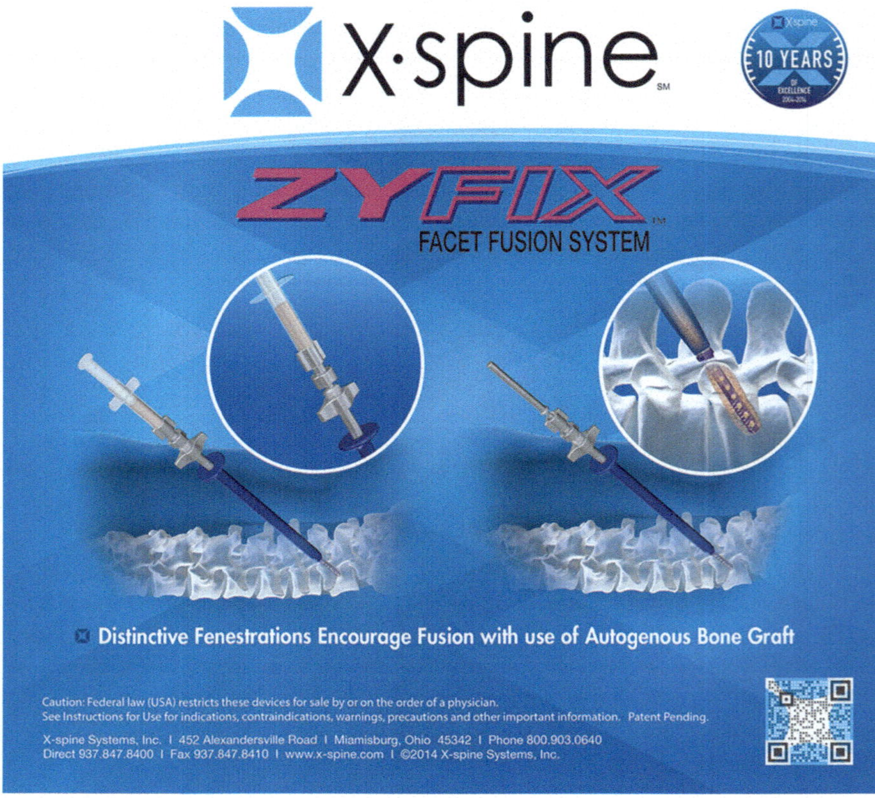

Fig. 6.9 Overview of Zyfix system

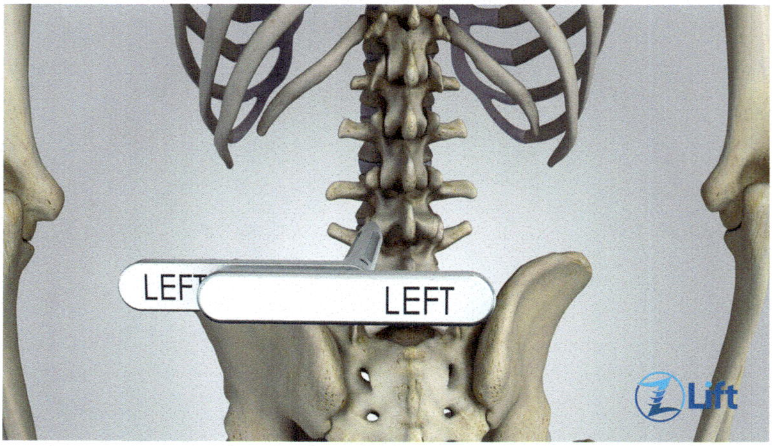

Fig. 6.10 Approach to left joint

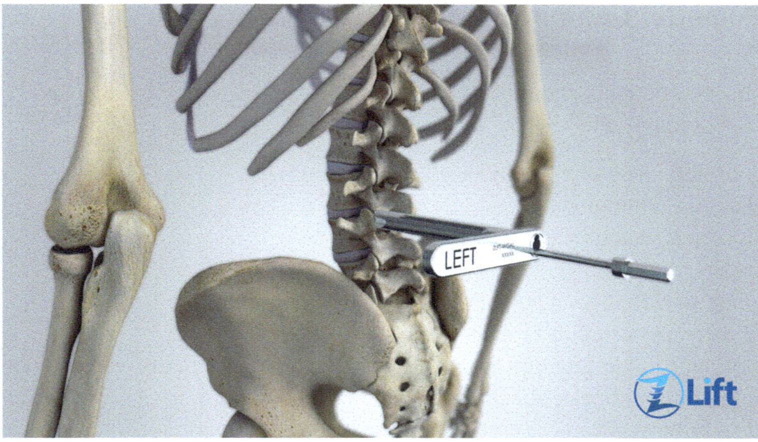

Fig. 6.11 Left facet with portal placement

Fig. 6.12 Normal facet anatomy

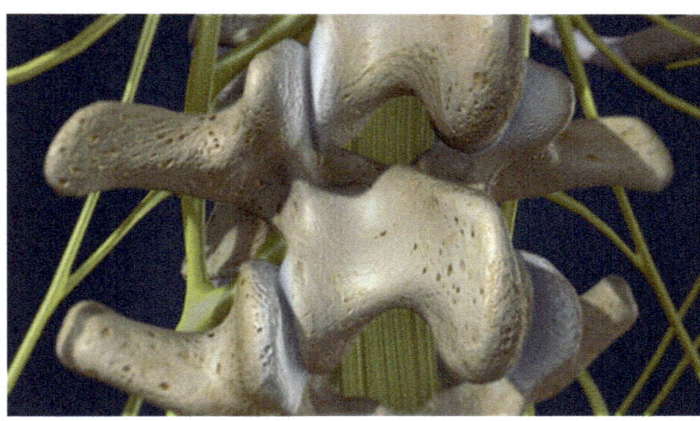

Fig. 6.13 Capsular orientation of facet joint

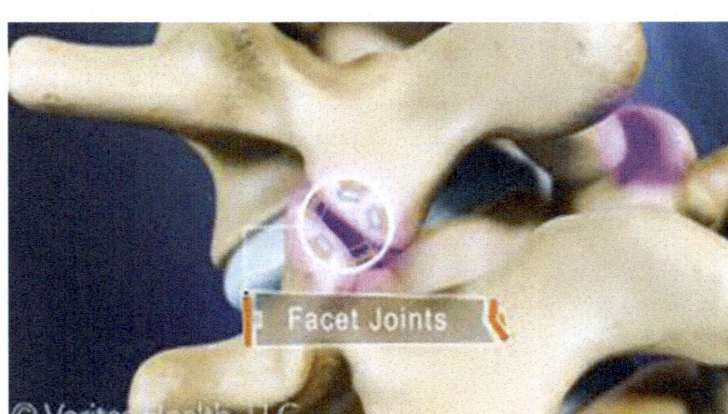

6.5 Potential Complications and Pitfalls

Physicians and patients should be aware of the potential complications and pitfalls of these techniques [2]:

- Early or late loosening of any or all components
- Breakage of components
- Foreign body reaction
- Infection
- Postoperative change in spinal curvature; loss of correction
- Dural tears, persistent CSF leakage, meningitis
- Loss of neurologic function including paralysis, radiculopathy, and/or continuation of pain; numbness, spasms, or sensory loss
- Cauda equina syndrome, paraplegia, reflex deficits, irritation, and/or muscle loss
- Fracture of any spinal bone
- Herniated nucleus pulposus or disc disruption (at, above, or below the level of surgery)
- Nonunion (pseudoarthrosis), delayed union, or malunion
- Loss or increase in spinal mobility
- Inability to perform activities of daily living
- Death

Acknowledgment *All images courtesy of minSURG Corporation (Clearwater, FL, USA); www.minsurg.com*

References

1. Kirkaldy-Willis WH, Wedge JH, Yong-Hing K, Reilly J. Pathology and pathogenesis of lumbar spondylosis and stenosis. Spine (Phila Pa 1976). 1978;3:319–28.
2. Maroon JC, Bost JW, LePere DB, Bost SM, Williams L, Amos AS. Clinical evaluation of TruFUSE® lumbar facet fusion system. Surg Sci. 2013;4:166–75.
3. Dreyer SJ, Dreyfuss PH. Low back pain and the zygapophysial (facet) joints. Arch Phys Med Rehabil. 1996;77:290–300.
4. Mooney V, Robertson J. The facet syndrome. Clin Orthop Relat Res. 1976;(115):149–56.
5. Fujiwara A, Tamai K, Yamato M, An HS, Yoshida H, Saotome K, Kurihashi A. The relationship between facet joint osteoarthritis and disc degeneration of the lumbar spine: an MRI study. Eur Spine J. 1999;8:396–401.
6. TruFUSE® Instructions for use. Clearwater: minSURG Corp.
7. Zyfix™ Facet fusion system information sheet and procedure instruction. Miamisburg: X-spine Systems.

Chapter 7
Vertebral Augmentation: Vertebroplasty and Kyphoplasty

Ronil V. Chandra, Lee-Anne Slater, Tony Goldschlager, Thabele M. Leslie-Mazwi, and Joshua A. Hirsch

Vertebroplasty and kyphoplasty are minimally invasive vertebral augmentation procedures that involve percutaneous image-guided injection of cement into the vertebral body. In general, most are performed for symptomatic vertebral fractures that fail conservative management. Augmentation is also common for symptomatic neoplastic fractures, osteolytic metastasis, symptomatic neoplasm, or vascular tumor. The definition of failure of conservative management is variable, but it generally is considered to have occurred when pain persists at a level that severely compromises the patient's mobility or activities of daily living despite a reasonable therapeutic trial of analgesic therapy, or if such therapy produces unacceptable side effects, such as excessive sedation or confusion from the level of analgesia required to maintain the pain at a tolerable level.

Randomized controlled trials have produced sufficient data to support the use of both vertebroplasty and kyphoplasty in carefully selected patients who fail conservative treatment and have severe pain and disability from osteoporotic or

R.V. Chandra (✉)
School of Clinical Sciences, Monash University, Melbourne, VIC, Australia
e-mail: ronil.chandra@monash.edu

L.-A. Slater
Interventional Neuroradiology Service, Monash Imaging, Monash Health, Melbourne, VIC, Australia
e-mail: LeeAnne.Slater@monashhealth.org

T. Goldschlager
Department of Neurosurgery, Monash Health, Melbourne, VIC, Australia

Department of Surgery, Monash University, Melbourne, VIC, Australia
e-mail: tony.goldschlager@monash.edu

T.M. Leslie-Mazwi • J.A. Hirsch
NeuroEndovascular Program, Harvard Medical School, Massachusetts General Hospital, Boston, MA, USA
e-mail: tleslie-mazwi@mgh.harvard.edu; jahirsch@mgh.harvard.edu

S. Diwan, T.R. Deer (eds.), *Advanced Procedures for Pain Management*,
https://doi.org/10.1007/978-3-319-68841-1_7

neoplasm-related vertebral fractures [1–4]. These trials have limitations, however, and further trials continue to assess the safety and effectiveness of vertebral augmentation. Until further data are available, continued careful patient selection combined with meticulous technique will help practitioners achieve high levels of safety and effectiveness as they integrate vertebral augmentation into their armamentarium of procedures for pain management.

7.1 The Procedures

Vertebroplasty involves the introduction of a percutaneous needle into the vertebral body and injection of cement directly into the vertebra (Fig. 7.1). Kyphoplasty involves an additional step in which a cavity is created within the vertebral body by inflating a balloon tamp. After deflation and withdrawal of the balloon tamp, cement is injected into the cavity created (Fig. 7.2). Operator preference generally dictates the choice of vertebroplasty or kyphoplasty. Recent data suggest that there is no difference in pain and disability outcomes or symptomatic complications between vertebroplasty and kyphoplasty for osteoporotic fractures [5, 6].

7.2 Indications

Vertebroplasty or kyphoplasty may be indicated for the treatment of symptomatic osteoporotic vertebral body fractures that are refractory to conservative management, or for the treatment of symptomatic vertebral bodies weakened or fractured owing to neoplasia, also refractory to conservative management.

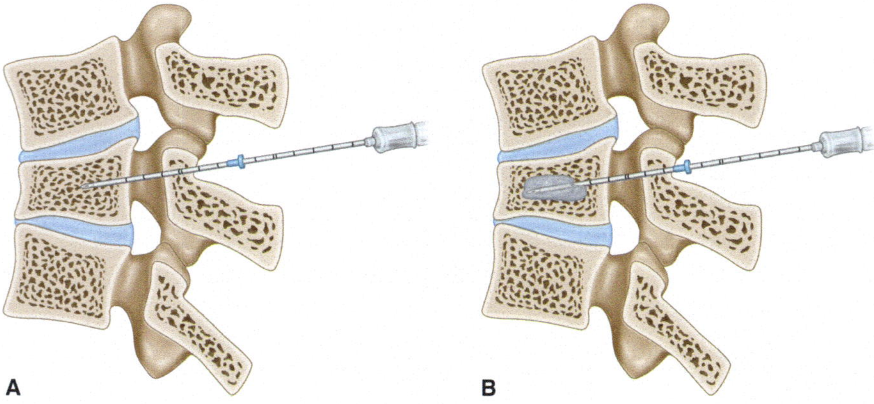

Fig. 7.1 Vertebroplasty involves introduction of a percutaneous needle into the vertebral body (**a**) and injection of cement directly into the vertebra (**b**)

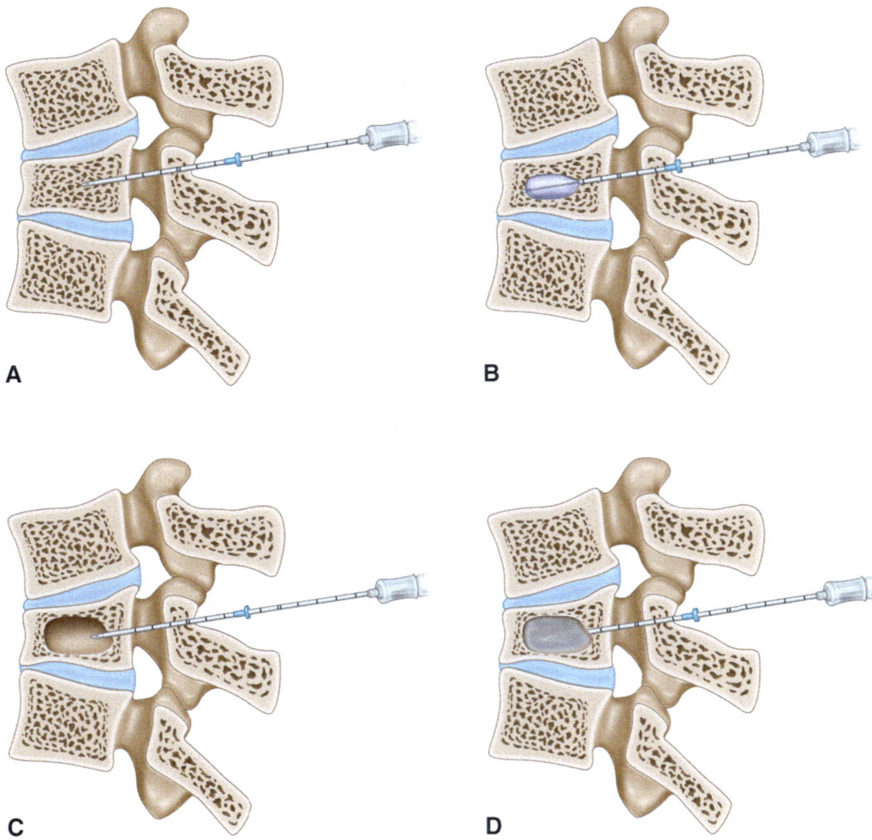

Fig. 7.2 Kyphoplasty. After introduction of a percutaneous needle into the vertebral body (**a**), a balloon tamp is inflated within the vertebral body (**b**). Deflation and withdrawal of the balloon tamp leaves a cavity (**c**), into which cement can be injected (**d**)

7.3 Contraindications

These procedures have several absolute contraindications:

- Known allergy to bone cement
- Irreversible bleeding disorder
- Inability to safely tolerate sedation or general anesthesia, from a cardiorespiratory perspective
- Active infection, especially spinal infection
- Compressive myelopathy resulting from fracture retropulsion

Other conditions are relative contraindications. Patients with these conditions present a greater risk of complications, and the procedures are best performed by experienced operators:

- Cervical or high thoracic (T1–T4) vertebral augmentation
- Vertebra plana or near plana
- Marked tumor destruction of vertebral body walls
- Poor visualization of osseous structures on fluoroscopy because of marked osteopenia or tumor destruction
- Complete disruption of the posterior vertebral body cortex
- Retropulsion of the posterior vertebral body cortex and associated canal stenosis
- Extension of tumor through the posterior vertebral body and into the epidural space

7.4 Preprocedural Workup

The goal of the preprocedural workup is to select patients who are likely to benefit from treatment and to screen for contraindications. The decision to treat should be based on factors in the history and physical examination, as well as appropriate investigations.

7.4.1 History and Physical Examination

- The classic symptom is sudden-onset deep midline pain. Note that fractures in osteoporotic or pathological bone may occur with little or no trauma.
- The pain is typically "mechanical"—that is, exacerbated by motion and axial loading (worse with weight-bearing and at least partially relieved by recumbency). There may be some lateral radiation, but this should not be the dominant feature of the pain.
- Standardized pain and disability scores should be documented, as well as the current analgesic regimen. These will be re-assessed after the procedure to determine whether there has been a satisfactory treatment response.
- Failure of conventional management and/or intolerance to current analgesia should be documented. A reasonable trial of conservative management is 4–6 weeks, as fracture pain usually resolves within this time [7]. It is reasonable to consider earlier treatment for patients requiring parenteral narcotics or analgesic infusions, or patients requiring hospitalization due to severe pain [7, 8].
- The physical examination should typically reveal midline tenderness over the fractured vertebra, but often patients may have subjective off-midline tenderness and still gain significant benefit [9]. Nonetheless, if there clear disconcordance between examination findings and imaging, vertebral augmentation should not be performed (Fig. 7.3).
- Baseline lower-limb neurologic function should be documented in all patients.

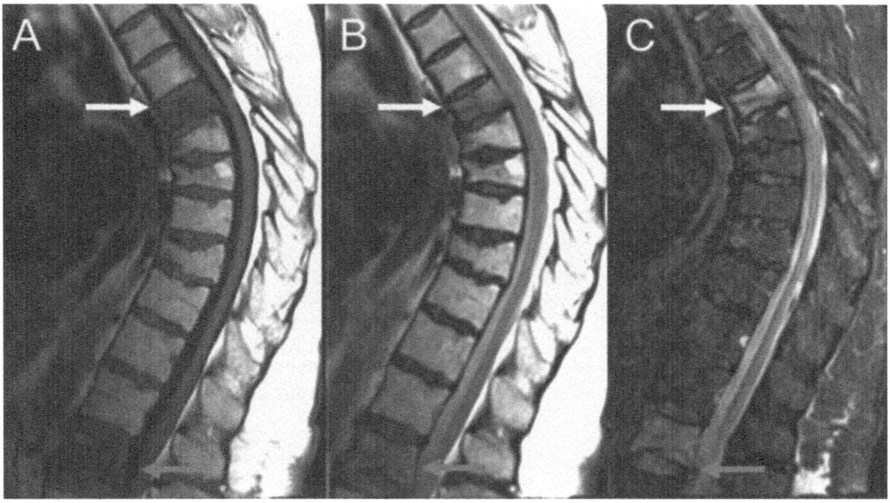

Fig. 7.3 Importance of physical correlation with imaging. T1-weighted MRI (**a**) shows low signal in the acute T5 (*white arrow*) and L1 (*dotted arrow*) vertebral body fractures. T2-weighted MRI (**b**) and short-tau inversion recovery (STIR) MRI (**c**) show corresponding marrow edema, indicating acute fractures. However, the patient did not have pain in the upper thoracic spine and was not tender over the T5 fracture. She did have pain in the upper lumbar spine and was tender over the L1 fracture. It is reasonable to exclude the T5 fracture from treatment since the clinical features do not correlate with imaging

7.4.2 Investigations

- Basic preprocedural laboratory investigations should screen for coagulopathy, systemic infection, and significant metabolic abnormality. Operator preference and patient characteristics generally dictate whether additional tests such as urinalysis, electrocardiogram (ECG), or chest radiography are performed before the procedure.
- Imaging of the spine should be performed in all patients. The goal of imaging is to identify the fracture level, assess the acuity of the fracture, identify potential technical challenges, and aid in procedural planning.
- Though radiographs are the most common initial imaging performed, they are limited in identifying the acuity of the index fracture and for undisplaced fractures. MRI is the investigation of choice and should be obtained if there are no contraindications. Short tau inversion recovery (STIR) or fat-saturated T2-weighted sequences are ideal in identifying pathological bone marrow edema, which is present in recent vertebral fractures (Fig. 7.3). Moreover, if there is no recent fracture, MRI may identify alternative pain generators, such as spinal canal compromise and/or compression of the spinal cord or nerve roots.
- If there is a contraindication to MRI, or in patients who may not be able to tolerate the examination due to severe pain, nuclear scintigraphic bone scan with single-photon emission computed tomography (SPECT) is the test of choice. SPECT allows good anatomical localization of the fracture location and can predict a positive clinical response to vertebral augmentation.

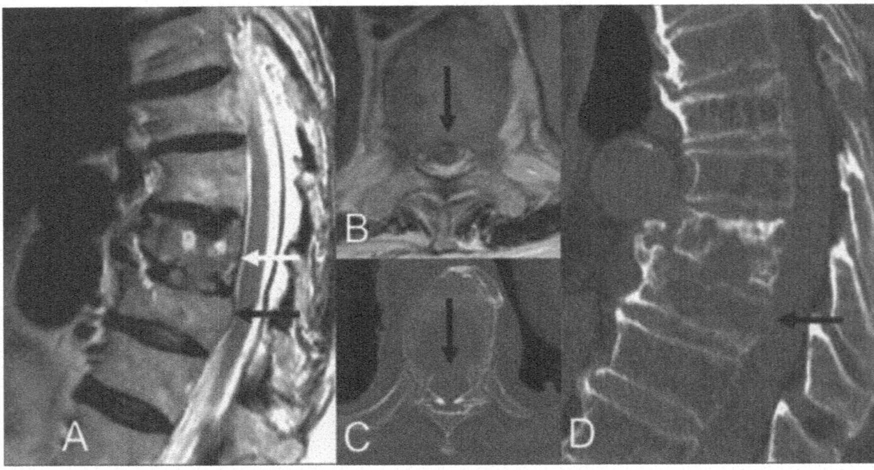

Fig. 7.4 Assessment of the posterior vertebral body cortex. T2-weighted MRI (**a**) shows altered signal in the T9 (*white arrow*) and T10 (*black arrow*) vertebral bodies from tumor replacement. Axial T2 MRI (**b**) demonstrates mild epidural extension, but the posterior vertebral body wall integrity is difficult to assess (*arrow*). Axial CT (**c**) and sagittal CT (**d**) better show the loss of integrity of part of the vertebral body cortex, which should be taken into account when considering vertebral augmentation

- CT scans are often complementary to MRI and can be particularly useful for preprocedural planning in certain contexts, such as evaluation of the integrity of the posterior vertebral body cortex (Fig. 7.4). This evaluation is more important for cancer-related vertebral fractures; it will also help define the extent of tumor sclerosis, which increases the technical difficulty of the procedure.

7.5 Technique

7.5.1 Procedure Preparation

- Confirm the patient identity and consent as per local hospital practices and processes. Preprocedural imaging available in the procedure room facilitates rapid correlation to ensure that the correct vertebral levels are treated.
- Imaging guidance is required. Operator preference dictates the use of fluoroscopic or CT guidance. Advantages of fluoroscopic guidance include real-time needle positioning and adjustment, and cement injection under direct fluoroscopic vision. Advantages of CT guidance include the greater surrounding anatomical bone and soft tissue detail, which facilitates accurate needle trajectory planning. Most operators use fluoroscopic guidance for thoracic and lumbar vertebroplasty.

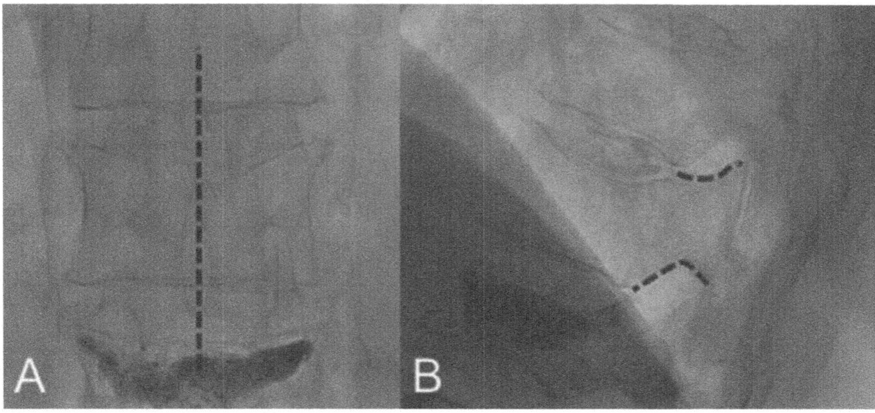

Fig. 7.5 Preparation for needle access. (**a**) Anteroposterior (AP) view. Rotate the image intensifier to a true AP position with the spinous process (*dotted line*) in the middle of the vertebral body. (**b**) Lateral view. Align the pedicles (*dotted lines*) to a true lateral position. Note that because of patient scoliosis the ribs may not be aligned, but the pedicle must be aligned for accurate trajectory planning

- Analgesia is required. In most cases, vertebroplasty can be performed under local anesthesia and moderate conscious sedation, or monitored anesthesia care. General anesthesia may be required for patients with significant narcotic analgesic requirements, or those who are unable to tolerate prone or oblique prone positioning.
- Continuous ECG, pulse oximetry, and blood pressure monitoring should be performed.
- Use standard guidelines for operator and assistant scrub, sterile gowns, masks, and gloves to minimize risk of infection. Prepare the skin in sterile fashion and drape appropriately Administer intravenous antibiotic prophylaxis using either cefazolin (1–2 g) or clindamycin (600 mg, if there is a penicillin allergy).
- Rotate the image intensifier (II) to a true AP position, and if using biplane fluoroscopy, align the pedicles to a true lateral position (Fig. 7.5).

7.5.2 Needle Placement

- Bring the pedicles to the mid-section of the vertebral body by adjusting the cranio-caudad angulation. Decide on either an AP view for planning the needle trajectory, or an end-on ("down the barrel") view. The "down the barrel" view requires ipsilateral oblique II rotation to place the needle trajectory and x-ray trajectory parallel so the needle appears as a dot end-on. Alternatively, an oblique view, between the AP and "down the barrel" views, is often satisfactory.
- Decide on a transpedicular or parapedicular needle trajectory (Fig. 7.6). A transpedicular trajectory passes through the entire length of the pedicle into the verte-

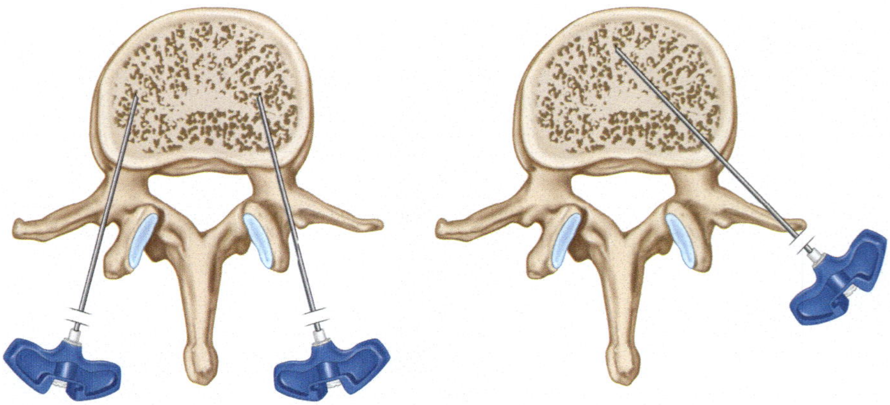

Fig. 7.6 Transpedicular and parapedicular needle trajectories. (**a**) A transpedicular trajectory passes through the entire length of the pedicle into the vertebral body. This intraosseous path protects adjacent neural and vascular structures, but it can limit the ability to achieve midline needle tip position. (**b**) The parapedicular trajectory penetrates the lateral wall of the pedicle along its path or at the junction of the pedicle and vertebral body, so it is easier to achieve midline needle tip position with a single needle

bral body. This intraosseous path protects adjacent neural and vascular structures, but can limit the ability to achieve midline needle tip position. The parapedicular trajectory penetrates the lateral wall of the pedicle, and thus it is often easier to achieve midline needle tip position with a single needle.

- Place a 22-gauge spinal needle onto the target entry position and anesthetize the periosteum (Fig. 7.7).
- Place the vertebroplasty needle along the same trajectory, and ensure that the planned needle trajectory remains superior to the inferior cortex and lateral to the medial cortex of the pedicle to prevent needle entry into the neural foramen or spinal canal. This is particularly important until secure access into the vertebral body is achieved (Fig. 7.8). Ultimately, either a unipedicular or bipedicular approach is utilized to achieve the final needle tip position in the anterior third of the vertebral body (Fig. 7.9).

7.5.3 Vertebroplasty

- When the operator is almost ready for cement injection, the cement should be prepared. Overall working time with the cement varies from 10 to 20 min, depending on temperature and the specific formulation being used. The ideal consistency for injection is typically close to the consistency of toothpaste.
- Prior to injection, remove the inner stylet of the needle and inject a small volume of saline into the vertebral body. This ensures that there will be no pressurized injection of air or air embolus, and also that there will not be any rapid or uncon-

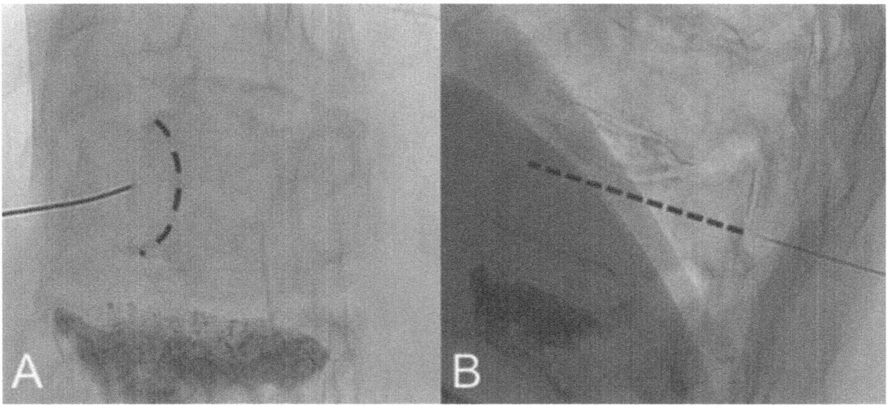

Fig. 7.7 Anesthetizing the periosteum with a 22-gauge spinal needle. (**a**) Oblique view. Note that the cranio-caudad angulation of the II has been adjusted to bring the pedicles within the vertebral body and rotates obliquely to clearly identify the medial border of the pedicle for unipedicular access. Aim to enter the pedicle at the 3 o'clock position for the left pedicle, or the 9 o'clock position for the right pedicle. (**b**) Lateral view. The trajectory of the 22-gauge spinal needle (*dotted line*) helps plan the trajectory for the vertebroplasty needle

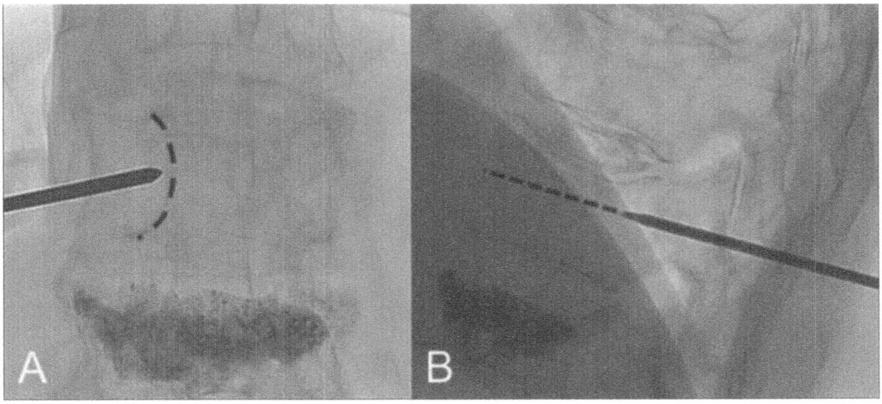

Fig. 7.8 Ensuring a safe needle trajectory. (**a**) Oblique view. The needle trajectory must remain superior to the inferior cortex and lateral to the medial cortex (*dotted line*) of the pedicle until secure access into the vertebral body is achieved. (**b**) Lateral view. The tip of the vertebroplasty needle is now at the junction of the pedicle and the vertebral body. The trajectory should be extrapolated (*dotted line*) to estimate the final needle position

trolled pressure buildup during initial cement injection, due to fragments of bone or marrow at the needle tip.

- Operators may use manual bone filler devices or cement injector systems to deliver the cement. The preferred delivery system is connected to the cannula and the cement is slowly injected under fluoroscopic guidance. Slowly inject the cement, monitoring the deposition with continuous fluoroscopic imaging. Ideally, the cement should remain within the vertebra and fill the fracture line (Fig. 7.10).

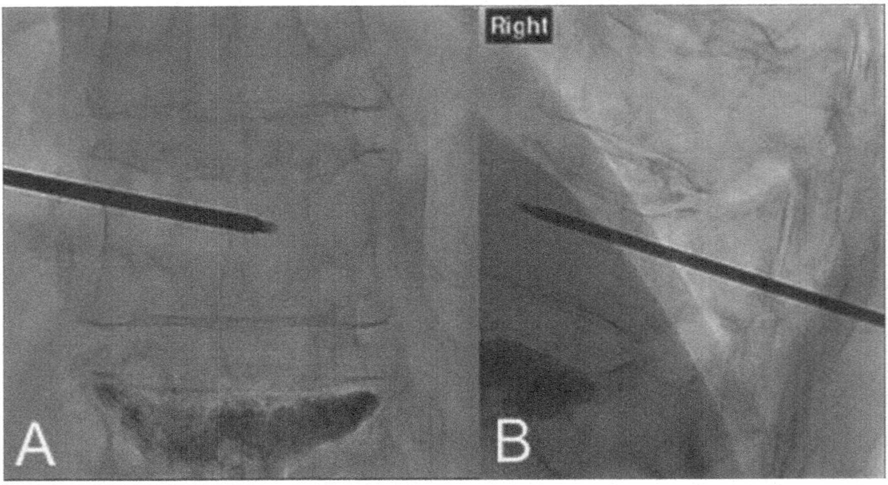

Fig. 7.9 Final needle tip position, with a unipedicular approach. (**a**) AP view. The needle tip lies at or just beyond the midline of the vertebral body. (**b**) Lateral view. The needle tip lies in the anterior third of the vertebral body. The previously planned needle trajectory has been achieved

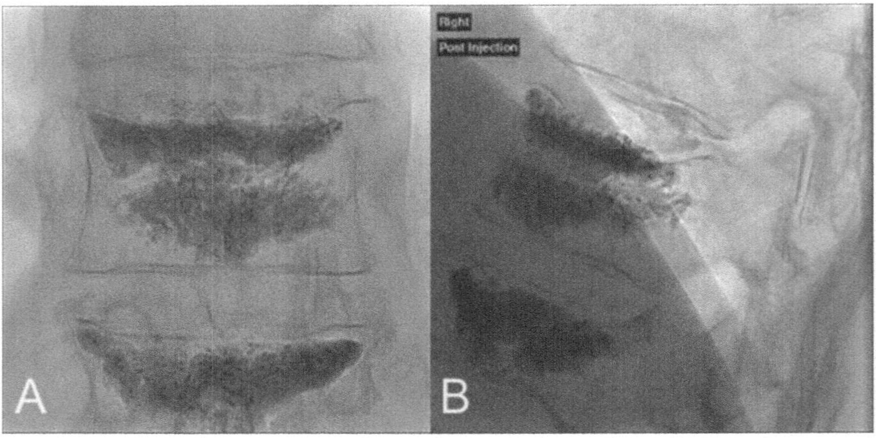

Fig. 7.10 Final cement fill via a unipedicular approach. (**a**) AP view. The cement has filled across the midline into both right and left compartments of the vertebral body from the midline tip position. (**b**) Lateral view. The fracture cleft paralleling the superior endplate has been filled, as well as the bony trabeculae in the inferior half of the vertebral body

- There is debate on the exact endpoints and volume of cement injection. Nevertheless, cement extravasation beyond the marrow space should be avoided. Volumes as low as 0.5 mL have achieved satisfactory pain relief in published series [10].
- Alternative techniques:
  - Unipedicular needle access can reduce procedure time and avoid the risks of placing a second needle for bipedicular needle access.

- Curved vertebroplasty needles can allow needle redirection into fracture lines or tumor compartments without relying on cement migration from a single cement delivery point.
- Thicker and more viscous cement preparations may reduce the risk of cement extravasation beyond the marrow space, and may be useful for cancer-related fractures in which there may be destruction of the vertebral body walls.

7.5.4 *Kyphoplasty*

- Kyphoplasty involves the additional step of cavity creation within the vertebral body, into which cement is injected.
- The needle is pulled back to the posterior part of the vertebral body to create room for the insertion of a balloon tamp. Monitor advancement of the balloon tamp along the needle tract, and position the balloon in the anterior part of the vertebral body (Fig. 7.11a).
- Slowly inflate the balloon tamp with iodinated contrast under continuous fluoroscopic monitoring (Fig. 7.11b). Continue to inflate until the target inflation volume is reached, the attached manometer indicates significant pressure or the patient experiences some discomfort.
- The balloon tamp is then deflated, the needle is primed with saline, and cement is injected into the cavity. The low pressure in the cavity allows for injection of more viscous cement than is used for vertebroplasty. The cement generally fills the cavity, either matching or slightly exceeding the inflated balloon tamp volume (Fig. 7.12).

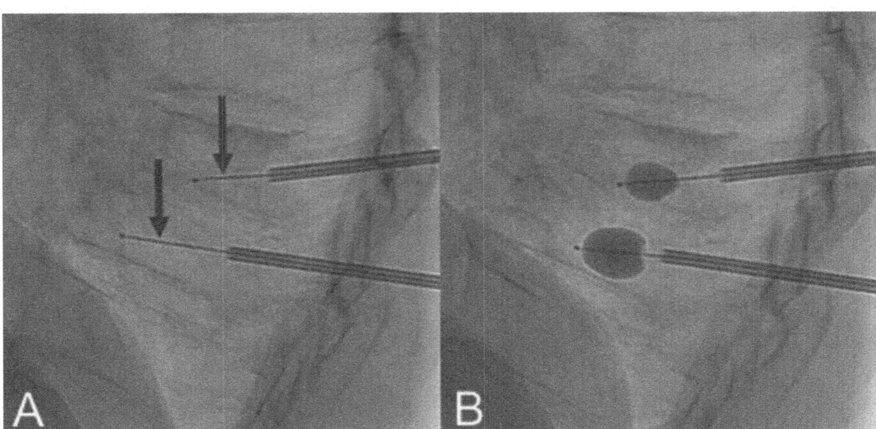

Fig. 7.11 Kyphoplasty, lateral views. (**a**) The vertebroplasty needles have been pulled back to the posterior part of the vertebral body to create room for the insertion of the uninflated balloon tamps (*arrows*), which have been inserted into the anterior part of the vertebral bodies. (**b**) The balloon tamps are inflated to create a cavity within the vertebral body. Gentle and slow inflation is suggested for cancer-related fractures, to avoid tumor displacement

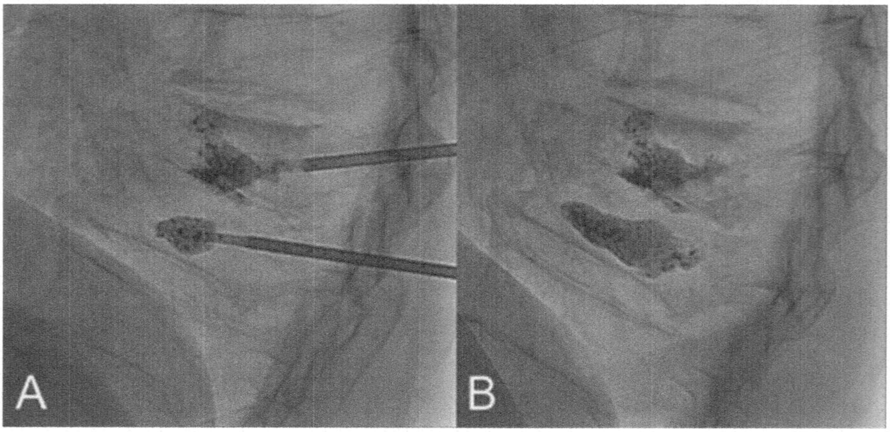

Fig. 7.12 Kyphoplasty: lateral views of cement injection. (**a**) The cement generally fills the cavity, initially matching and then exceeding the inflated balloon tamp volume. (**b**) Final cement deposition. Note that care is taken to prevent any cement leak posteriorly into the spinal canal

- The combination of the cavity and more viscous cement reduces the risk of cement extravasation beyond the marrow space.

7.6 Complications

Potential complications should be explained to the patient:

- Symptomatic cement leakage into the neural foramen, spinal canal, or adjacent vascular structures
- Nerve or spinal cord damage
- Vessel injury leading to bleeding
- Failure to improve pain or worsened pain
- Paraspinal hematoma
- New fracture of the rib, pedicle, or vertebral body
- Pneumothorax
- Pulmonary embolus
- Hypotension or depressed myocardial function due to cement injection
- Anaphylaxis from the cement

The overall permanent major complication rate should be less than 1% for osteoporotic fractures and less than 5% for cancer-related fractures [11].

7.7 Tips to Minimize Risk of Complications

- Ensure appropriate and careful patient selection.
- Use meticulous technique.
- Biplane fluoroscopy is invaluable in monitoring cement injection and reduces overall procedural time.
- Provide adequate analgesia and sedation to reduce patient motion.
- Take spot radiographs or increase the radiation dose temporarily to aid in identification of bony landmarks when there is marked osteopenia or tumor destruction.
- Turn down ambient light and use your assistant to help identify any cement extravasation during injection.
- Avoid cement injection into the posterior third of the vertebral body, where there are higher risks of venous extravasation, particularly into the basivertebral and epidural veins.
- If there is extra-osseous extravasation, cease cement injection temporarily, allow the cement to harden, and then inject again slowly to see if the cement now fills a different fracture compartment.
- Have a low threshold to cease the cement injection.

7.8 Post-procedure Management

Patients should have a short period of bed rest and observation (often 2–3 h), which can be tailored to the clinical circumstance and operator preference. Vital signs and lower extremity neurological function should be assessed at regular intervals and compared with pre-procedural findings. After an appropriate duration of observation, supervised ambulation is permitted; a support brace is typically not required. Most patients can be discharged the same day. If there is any clinical deterioration, appropriate imaging and management should be rapidly instituted.

Post-procedure follow-up should be performed, with reassessment of previously recorded pain and disability scores and analgesic use. There should be continual monitoring of procedural clinical effectiveness and safety, ideally within a quality improvement program.

7.9 Conclusion

There are sufficient data to support the use of vertebroplasty and kyphoplasty in carefully selected patients with osteoporotic or cancer-related vertebral fractures who have severe pain and disability that is refractory to conservative management. However, published trials have limitations, and further trials are ongoing. Nonetheless, continued careful patient selection, combined with meticulous technique, will help practitioners achieve successful outcomes for their patients.

References

1. Barr JD, Jensen ME, Hirsch JA, McGraw JK, Barr RM, Brook AL, et al. Position statement on percutaneous vertebral augmentation: a consensus statement developed by the Society of Interventional Radiology (SIR), American Association of Neurological Surgeons (AANS) and the Congress of Neurological Surgeons (CNS), American College of Radiology (ACR), American Society of Neuroradiology (ASNR), American Society of Spine Radiology (ASSR), Canadian Interventional Radiology Association (CIRA), and the Society of NeuroInterventional Surgery (SNIS). J Vasc Interv Radiol. 2014;25:171–81.
2. Chandra RV, Meyers PM, Hirsch JA, Abruzzo T, Eskey CJ, Hussain MS, et al. Vertebral augmentation: report of the Standards and Guidelines Committee of the Society of NeuroInterventional Surgery. J Neurointerv Surg. 2014;6:7–15.
3. Chandra RV, Yoo AJ, Hirsch JA. Vertebral augmentation: update on safety, efficacy, cost effectiveness and increased survival? Pain Physician. 2013;16:309–20.
4. Berenson J, Pflugmacher R, Jarzem P, Zonder J, Schechtman K, Tillman JB, et al. Balloon kyphoplasty versus non-surgical fracture management for treatment of painful vertebral body compression fractures in patients with cancer: a multicentre, randomised controlled trial. Lancet Oncol. 2011;12:225–35.
5. Evans AJ, Kip KE, Brinjikji W, Layton KF, Jensen ML, Gaughen JR, Kallmes DF. Randomized controlled trial of vertebroplasty versus kyphoplasty in the treatment of vertebral compression fractures. J Neurointerv Surg. 2016;8:756–63.
6. Gu CN, Brinjikji W, Evans AJ, Murad MH, Kallmes DF. Outcomes of vertebroplasty compared with kyphoplasty: a systematic review and meta-analysis. J Neurointerv Surg. 2016;8:636–42.
7. Kallmes DF, Jensen ME. Percutaneous vertebroplasty. Radiology. 2003;229:27–36.
8. Stallmeyer MJB, Zoarski GH, Obuchowski AM. Optimizing patient selection in percutaneous vertebroplasty. J Vasc Interv Radiol. 2003;14:683–96.
9. Rad AE, Kallmes DF. Pain relief following vertebroplasty in patients with and without localizing tenderness on palpation. AJNR Am J Neuroradiol. 2008;29:1622–6.
10. Kaufmann TJ, Trout AT, Kallmes DF. The effects of cement volume on clinical outcomes of percutaneous vertebroplasty. AJNR Am J Neuroradiol. 2006;27:1933–7.
11. McGraw JK, Cardella J, Barr JD, Mathis JM, Sanchez O, Schwartzberg MS, et al. Society of Interventional Radiology quality improvement guidelines for percutaneous vertebroplasty. J Vasc Interv Radiol. 2003;14(9 Pt 2):S311–5.

Part II
Advanced Neuromodulation

Jason E. Pope and Leonardo Kapural

Neuromodulation, both chemical and electrical, affords the ability to treat difficult pain presentations from multiple etiologies. Growing evidence generation, novel targets, novel pulse trains, with a focus on patient safety and durable efficacy, have allowed for earlier placement in the treatment algorithm. In this new *Atlas*, we hope to help guide clinicians by offering strategies to refine surgical technique and peri-operative planning, optimize the pairing of device selection, disease indication, and patient selection, while working toward maximizing patient outcomes. Our field is on the front line of community health and we hope you enjoy this information as much as we did creating it.

Chapter 8
Neuromodulation: Mechanisms of Action

Nomen Azeem and Miguel D. Attias

Neuromodulation may refer to spinal cord stimulation (SCS), peripheral nerve stimulation (PNS), or peripheral nerve field stimulation for the treatment of chronic pain. All neurostimulation treatments share common mechanisms of action that affect the nervous system in order to suppress pain, but each modality seems to have its own unique and particular mechanisms. Multiple clinical and animal studies to date have revealed that neurostimulation therapy involves a complex interaction with multiple structures in the nervous system, with the effect not just attributed to the gate control theory, as initially believed. Improved understanding has led to the development of high-frequency, burst waveform, and dorsal root ganglion (DRG) stimulation.

8.1 Introduction

Neuromodulation or neurostimulation has been employed since the ancient Egyptians reportedly used an electrogenic fish to treat ailments 4500 years ago [1]. Later, the ancient Greeks and Romans recorded the medical use of the torpedo fish to treat gout, arthritis, and other disease states [2]. Over time, neurostimulation has been used as treatment for ailments that range from psychiatric disorders to pain symptoms. In 1967, Dr. C. Norman Shealy implanted the first unipolar spinal cord stimulator in the intrathecal space adjacent to the dorsal columns; this provided

N. Azeem (✉)
Department of Neurology, University of South Florida, Tampa, FL, USA
e-mail: azeemnx@gmail.com

M.D. Attias
Tampa Pain Relief Center, Palm Harbor, FL, USA
e-mail: doctorattias@gmail.com

S. Diwan, T.R. Deer (eds.), *Advanced Procedures for Pain Management*,
https://doi.org/10.1007/978-3-319-68841-1_8

adequate cancer and neuropathic pain relief [3]. Today, electric neuromodulation or neurostimulation refers to spinal cord stimulation (SCS), peripheral nerve stimulation (PNS), and peripheral nerve field stimulation, among other modalities.

In 1965, a neurophysiologist, Ron Melzack, and a psychologist, Patrick Wall, published a landmark paper describing the gate control theory of pain. It suggested that pain is a complex neurologic and perceptual phenomenon, and that pain perception is in part a function of the balance between the impulses transmitted to the spinal cord through both the larger, myelinated nerve fibers and the smaller pain fibers, both of which synapse on the dorsal horn of the spinal cord [4]. It is postulated that a "gate" in the dorsal horn of the spinal cord is responsible for relaying transmission of neural activity signaling pain in the central nervous system. The gate opens to transmit a pain signal when there is more small-fiber activity than large-fiber activity, and it closes to inhibit transmission of the pain signal when the opposite occurs. Over the past 40 years, this theory has been the mainstay of the proposed mechanisms of action for neuromodulation. Based on this mechanism of action, it is understood that paresthesias secondary to large-fiber activity must be induced over the painful areas in order to provide effective pain blockade. In recent years, however, owing to clinical and basic science observations, it is thought that that the neuromodulation of pain is much more complex than originally believed. For example, neurostimulation is most effective for neuropathic or sympathetically mediated ischemic pain, but not so effective for nociceptive pain. Also, neurostimulation alleviates chronic pain but does not effectively suppress acute pain. Thus, a sole mechanism of analgesia from neuromodulation based on the gate control theory does not fully account for these clinical observations. Research groups utilizing computational models have challenged this theory and introduced novel paradigms with the aid of neural circuitry simulation [5].

8.2 Spinal Cord Stimulation

Since its inception, there have efforts to explain the physiologic basis for the pain-suppressive effects of SCS. Research using animal models has suggested that the effects of SCS are the consequence of a complex set of interactions at several levels of the nervous system, including the dorsal horn of the spinal cord and supraspinal components. According to a literature review by Oakley and Prager [6], a significant component of the SCS effect is eliminated in animal models with dorsal column lesions, which suggests that at least a portion of the SCS effect is mediated through the dorsal columns. In other animal models, the effects of the SCS are further reduced if the spinal cord is transected above the level of electrode placement, suggesting that both supraspinal and segmental mechanisms are in use. A study of SCS effects on brain stem activity in animals shows the activation of the anterior pretectal nucleus [7], which involves the descending pain inhibitory pathways. It is thought that the activation of this structure is responsible for the relief of pain that outlasts the period of stimulation in humans [4].

In the 1970s and 1980s, some research groups were very actively exploring the mode of action of SCS, but the design of these studies was not specific to neuropathic pain [8]. In 1994, the effect of SCS was first studied in animal models specific to neuropathic pain [9], and over the years, the Karolinska group has enriched the literature with multiple publications studying the neurobiology of SCS in neuropathic pain [10]. An extensive electrophysiological study performed by Guan et al. (with Dr. Srinivasa Raja as a senior researcher) demonstrated that bipolar electrical stimulation at the dorsal column or lumbar dorsal roots attenuated dorsal horn neuronal hyperexcitability in nerve-injured rats and inhibited short-term neuronal sensitization [11].

The evidence found in these and other studies demonstrates that SCS attenuates the response to nerve injury in which wide-dynamic-range (WDR) neurons, known to play a role in central sensitization, become hyperexcitable in the dorsal horn [4]. Although the validity of translating experimental results to the clinical setting is unclear, it may be suggested that by altering the characteristics of WDR cells, SCS may provide relief not only from allodynia but also from spontaneous neuropathic pain [12].

Although there is not much data from human research, it has been found that administering naloxone, an opioid receptor antagonist, to patients along with SCS does not diminish the effect of SCS-induced analgesia. This finding illustrates that SCS does not provide pain relief via opioid receptors. Neurochemically, experimental evidence in animal models with SCS revealed increased levels at the dorsal horn of gamma-aminobutyric acid (GABA), which may inhibit the spinothalamic pain tract, and adenosine, which may inhibit neuropathic pain (Fig. 8.1). There were also increases in serotonin and norepinephrine, which have long been thought to play a role in supraspinal descending pain modulation. Furthermore, it was found that there is a decrease in the levels of both glutamate and aspartate, which are excitatory neuromediators in the dorsal horn [6].

The analgesic effect of SCS on sympathetic-mediated ischemic pain is thought to occur through inhibition of efferent sympathetic activity, resulting in a decrease in peripheral vasoconstriction and relief of pain by restoring a balance of oxygen demand and supply. Also, activation of the antidromic mechanisms below the motor threshold may result in the release of peripheral calcitonin gene-related peptide (CGRP) and nitric oxide (NO) with subsequent peripheral vasodilation [13].

8.3 High-Frequency Stimulation

Although there seems to be lack of consensus about what the term *high-frequency stimulation* (HFS) actually means, in clinical practice today this term is most frequently used to refer to the 10 kHz frequency rate, versus the traditional frequencies below 1200 Hz. There is currently only one commercial system capable of delivering such a pulse rate, which has had CE Marking since 2010 and was approved by the FDA in May 2015. The Senza™ system (Nevro Corp., Menlo Park, CA, USA)

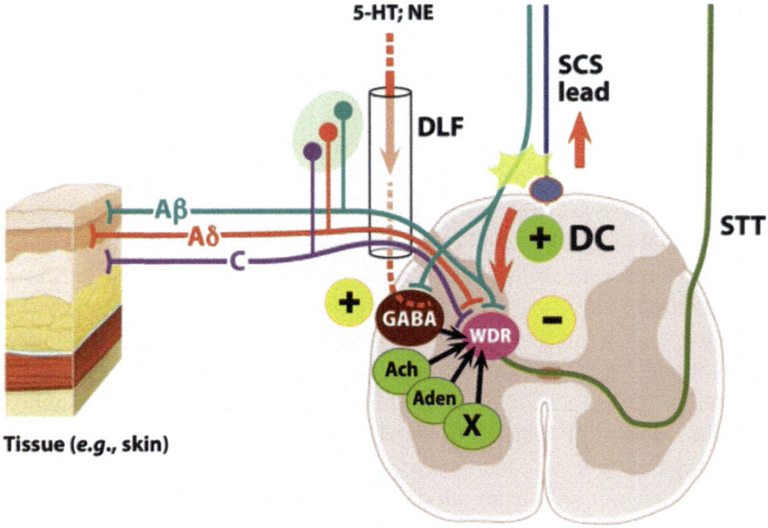

Fig. 8.1 Schematic representation of spinal transmitters possibly involved in the spinal cord stimulation (SCS) effect in neuropathic pain based on current knowledge derived predominantly from experiments performed on animal (rat) models of mononeuropathy. Antidromic activation of dorsal columns (DC) is, *via* collaterals, destined to the dorsal horns, establishing contact with a multitude of neurons, among them wide-dynamic-range (WDR) neurons and GABAergic interneurons. A stimulation-induced release of gamma-aminobutyric acid (GABA), binding preferentially to $GABA^B$ receptors, may result in a decreased release of glutamate. Additional effects involve increased release of acetylcholine (Ach) binding to muscarinic M4 receptors and adenosine (Aden) binding to A1 receptors. An important mechanism is activation of descending controls *via* serotonergic and noradrenergic pathways contained in the dorsolateral funiculus (DLF) originating in supraspinal, brainstem centers. (Many of the mechanisms of action are still unknown [X].) *NE* norepinephrine, *STT* spinothalamic tract. (*Reproduced with permission from* Linderoth B, Meyerson BA. Spinal cord stimulation: exploration of the physiological basis of a widely used therapy. Anesthesiology. 2010;113:1265–7)

allows this frequency of stimulation to be delivered to the spinal cord without inducing paresthesia [14], and its effectiveness was presented in two robust clinical trials [15, 16]. Although there is strong evidence of clinical efficacy, there have been few publications attempting to elucidate the basic mechanisms of action involved in kilohertz-frequency stimulation.

A few hypotheses about the mechanism of pain modulation induced by HFS have been suggested [17]:

- Temporal summation, in which multiple pulses build on each other to achieve neuronal activation
- Depolarization blockade, in which propagating action potentials are blocked by the HFS
- Desynchronization, in which the HFS results in pseudo-spontaneous neuronal activity

Clinical experience and computational studies [18] suggest that the first two hypotheses are less likely.

An animal study that used a rat L5 nerve ligation model [19] demonstrated for the first time that SCS frequencies in the kilohertz range alleviate neuropathic mechanical hypersensitivity in a time course and magnitude that differs from conventional (50-Hz) SCS. Compared with conventional stimulation, HFS had an earlier onset of effect and required a lower intensity to block peripheral Aβ fibers; however, it failed to significantly inhibit windup in spinal WDR neurons. The authors suggested, based on their experience and previous publications, that kilohertz-level stimulation may cause activation of afferent fibers, dorsal horn and dorsal column neurons, and neurons in supraspinal pain modulatory structures in a not-precisely-predictable (stochastic), asynchronous manner hypothetically exerting different pain-inhibitory effects from those produced when nerves fire synchronously at lower rates of stimulation. Another, more recently published report [20] studied rat models of different types of pain, comparing the effects of HFS at 500, 1000, or 10,000 Hz *versus* conventional SCS; it reported similar reductions in hypersensitivity due to nerve lesion with conventional SCS at 50 Hz. Furthermore, microrecordings of afferent activity in the gracile nucleus showed that conventional SCS produced massive activation in the nucleus, but they showed no activation during the high-frequency SCS. As no activity was conveyed rostrally in subparesthetic, high-frequency SCS, the authors hypothesized that its mechanisms of action are primarily segmental.

Although it seems that more questions than answers are being generated regarding the mode of action of HFS, it is clear that the seeds have been planted in the quest for further clues that should reconcile the basic science data with the positive clinical results obtained with this mode of stimulation.

8.4 Burst Waveform Stimulation

Traditionally, SCS is delivered via tonic stimulation, a consistent stream of single pulses at a pre-set amplitude, frequency, and pulse width. With the goal of improving both patient satisfaction and clinical outcomes, these basic elements of electrical stimulation can be modified to result in new electrical stimulation patterns or waveforms.

A burst waveform consists of multiple packets of high-frequency impulses that are delivered periodically, followed by a single repolarization period. It has been found that burst is a naturally occurring signaling modality in human physiology [21–24]. Thalamic cells can fire in tonic or burst patterns, but ascending action potentials are more likely to be routed to the cortex when the thalamus is firing in burst pattern [25–27].

The burst SCS waveform introduced by Dr. De Ridder et al. in 2010 [28] consists of a series of five pulses, each with a duration of 1000 ms and a pulse frequency of 500 Hz, followed by a single repolarization pulse and delivered in trains repeated at

40 Hz. De Ridder demonstrated, via source-localized EEG, that burst stimulation produces significantly more alpha activity in the dorsal anterior cingulate than tonic stimulation [29]. This observation correlates well with the finding that burst stimulation reduces attention to pain, as this is mediated by the same structure [30].

In 2013, de Vos, De Ridder, et al. [31] assessed the effectiveness of burst stimulation in three groups of patients with chronic pain who were users of conventional-frequency tonic SCS. They showed that burst stimulation significantly reduced pain for almost all patients in the study. Furthermore, when compared with conventional SCS, burst stimulation led to a significant additional pain reduction. Most patients also preferred the presence of little or no paresthesia with burst stimulation, although some preferred tonic stimulation apparently because the paresthesia assured them that the SCS device was actually working.

The hypothesis of an exploratory study using EEG as a measurement technique suggested a mode of action of burst stimulation in humans [32]. The conclusion was that both burst and tonic SCS modulate the ascending lateral pathway and descending pain inhibitory pathway, but burst stimulation exerts further modulatory effects upon the medial pain pathway, possibly by a direct effect on the spinothalamic pathways. In this manner, it normalizes an imbalance between ascending pain input via the medial system and descending pain inhibitory activity. This mechanism could explain the superior results reported by burst SCS in comparison with tonic stimulation [28, 29, 31, 33–35].

A systematic review of the literature was published in 2016 [36], considering the available evidence for burst SCS in treating chronic, intractable pain. In this report, only five papers met inclusion criteria, so the statistical conclusion was naturally limited, given the small sample size. At the time of the writing of this manuscript, the period since CE approval had been short and FDA approval and large-scale clinical implementation of burst stimulation was still pending. The positive results of a prospective, randomized multicenter study designed to support approval of burst stimulation in the United States were presented during a plenary session at the 19th annual meeting of the North American Neuromodulation Society (NANS) in Las Vegas, Nevada. The SUNBURST (Success Using Neuromodulation with BURST) study is sponsored by St. Jude Medical. Further research is needed to elucidate the mechanisms and further support the clinical efficacy of this promising novel waveform.

8.5 Dorsal Root Ganglion Stimulation

The dorsal root ganglion (DRG) is a collection of pseudo-unipolar cell bodies of neurons surrounded by glial cells and axons that form the primary afferent sensory nerve. The DRG cell bodies are a component of the primary sensory neurons that are involved in pain transmission and modulation. There are about 15,000 neurons per DRG at the segmental levels where a major plexus innervates the limbs [37]. Previous reports have implicated the DRG in the development and maintenance of chronic pain [38, 39]. In animal models, several pathophysiologic changes were identified in the DRG, including altered electrophysiological membrane properties [40], changes in the expression of integral membrane proteins [41], and altered gene expression [42]. These changes may explain how the DRG can significantly contribute to chronic pain states [38].

The T-junction is the branch of the DRG neuron that connects the cell body to the axon; it plays an important role in the modulation of pain signals that are sent to the CNS. According to a study done by Gemes and associates [43], a significant reduction in action potential was found when ganglia excised from rats had stimulation applied to the DRG. Because of its somatotopic arrangement, stimulation of the DRG can provide more precise localization of stimulation based on dermatomal mapping. In addition, the limited amount of cerebrospinal fluid surrounding the DRG allows the placement of a percutaneous lead closer to neural targets, which limits energy dissipation.

Electrical stimulation of the DRG counteracts the abnormal changes that occur within the DRG as a result of peripheral afferent fiber injury. By stabilizing and decreasing hyperexcitability of DRG neurons, stimulation decreases neuropathic pain. Many hypotheses have been formulated to explain the mechanisms of action [44]:

- Modification of abnormal growth factor release in the DRG
- Reversal of microglial activation within the DRG, causing inhibition of the cytokine cascade and therefore decreased inflammation and pain
- Downstream effects of vasodilation and stabilization of sensitized peripheral nociceptors
- Upstream effects that deactivate sensitized WDR neurons within the spinal cord and turn off brain centers activated by peripheral neuropathic activity
- Rectification of abnormal electrical activity patterns within the DRG
- Downregulation of abnormal ion channels and restitution of normal ion flux
- Filtering of electrical impulses traveling from the peripheral nociceptor on the way to the spinal cord

Although DRG stimulation has been utilized for years in Australia and Europe, with multiple studies validating its efficacy, research in DRG stimulation began in the U.S. within the past few years. According to the work done by Dr. Levy and Deer in the ACCURATE study, a prospective, randomized multicenter, controlled clinical trial, 12-month outcome data demonstrated sustained pain relief superior to that of conventional SCS, with improved therapeutic targeting. This evidence of superiority was utilized in order to obtain FDA approval for DRG stimulation in April 2016 [45].

The promising results of DRG stimulation witnessed thus far are encouraging. Further positive long-term data will solidify the role of DRG stimulation in certain patients with chronic pain. Although the current approved indications for DRG stimulation (complex regional pain syndrome [CRPS] types 1 and 2) are limiting, further clinical trials will assist in expanding the approved indications for DRG stimulation.

8.6 Peripheral Nerve Stimulation

It is thought that there are overlapping mechanisms of action for both SCS and PNS. Chung et al. [46] showed that applying a 5-min conditioning stimulus to a peripheral nerve produces a profound inhibition in primate spinothalamic tract cells in response to both noxious electrical and thermal stimuli. However, direct stimulation of the peripheral nerve has been theorized to act by creating a change in nerve transmission or a balance of Aδ and C fiber response compared with other nociceptors [46]. Ignelzi and Nyquist [47] recorded single-fiber activity in the cat superficial radial nerve and found that, after repetitive high-frequency electrical stimulation of the nerve, there were transient excitability changes in both large- and small-diameter afferent fibers that consisted of slowing in single-fiber conduction velocity and an increase in electrical threshold. They concluded that clinical electroanalgesia is mediated by a direct change in peripheral nerve excitability [47]. Campbell and Taub confirmed that human subjects experience sensory loss in the distribution of a peripheral nerve stimulated transcutaneously. The onset of analgesia was associated with the loss of the Aδ component in the compound action potential recording, suggesting a peripheral axonal blockade [48].

8.7 Peripheral Nerve Field Stimulation

Peripheral nerve field stimulation theoretically may operate by one or more of the following mechanisms [49]:

- Impact on local blood flow
- Blocking of cell membrane depolarization
- Change in neurotransmitter levels
- Change in the levels of localized and systemic endogenous endorphins
- Change in the message at the spinal cord level

8.8 Outlook for the Future

Our understanding of the mechanisms of action underlying neuromodulation is still in its infancy; it is far from being fully explained. A better understanding of the complex interaction of physiologic effects on the nervous system by SCS and PNS is still needed to further improve and expand current applications. A number of proposed mechanisms have led the way to allow patients to benefit from neuromodulation therapy over the past several decades, and research in recent years has led to the development of new technologies such as high-frequency, burst waveform, and DRG stimulation to improve pain blockade in patients. Although we have made progress, more large-scale studies are needed in order to truly understand the effects of neuromodulation and further improve long-term outcomes.

References

1. Kane K, Taub A. A history of local electrical analgesia. Pain. 1975;1:25–138.
2. Miles J. Electrical stimulation for the relief of pain. Ann R Coll Surg Engl. 1984;66:108–12.
3. Shealy CN, Taslitz N, Mortimer JT, Becker DP. Electrical inhibition of pain: experimental evaluation. Anesth Analg. 1967;46:299–305.
4. Melzack R, Wall PD. Pain mechanisms: a new theory. Science. 1965;150:971–9.
5. Arle JE, Carlson KW, Mei L, Iftimia N, Shils JL. Mechanism of dorsal column stimulation to treat neuropathic but not nociceptive pain: analysis with a computational model. Neuromodulation. 2014;17:642–55; discussion 655.
6. Oakley J, Prager J. Spinal cord stimulation—mechanism of action. Spine. 2002;27:2574–83.
7. Roberts MHT, Rees H. Physiological basis of spinal cord stimulation. Pain Rev. 1994;1:184–98.
8. Handwerker HO, Iggo A, Zimmermann M. Segmental and supraspinal actions on dorsal horn neurons responding to noxious and non-noxious skin stimuli. Pain. 1975;1:147–65.
9. Meyerson BA, Herregodts P, Linderoth B, Ren B. An experimental animal model of spinal cord stimulation for pain. Stereotact Funct Neurosurg. 1994;62:256–62.
10. Linderoth B, Meyerson BA. Dorsal column stimulation: modulation of somatosensory and autonomic function. Semin Neurosci. 1995;7:263–77.
11. Guan Y, Wacnik PW, Yang F, Carteret AF, Chung C-Y, Meyer RA, Raja SN. Spinal cord stimulation-induced analgesia: electrical stimulation of dorsal column and dorsal roots attenuates dorsal horn neuronal excitability in neuropathic rats. Anesthesiology. 2010;113:1392–405.
12. Linderoth B, Foreman RD. Mechanisms of spinal cord stimulation in painful syndromes: role of animal models. Pain Med. 2006;7:S14–26.
13. Stojanovic MP, Abdi S. Spinal cord stimulation. Pain Physician. 2002;5:156–66.
14. Van Buyten JP, Al-Kaisy A, Smet I, Palmisani S, Smith T. High-frequency spinal cord stimulation for the treatment of chronic back pain patients: results of a prospective multicenter European clinical study. Neuromodulation. 2013;16:59–65; discussion 65–6.
15. Kapural L, Yu C, Doust MW, Gliner BE, Vallejo R, Sitzman BT, et al. Novel 10-kHz high-frequency therapy (HF10 therapy) is superior to traditional low-frequency spinal cord stimulation for the treatment of chronic back and leg pain: the SENZA-RCT randomized controlled trial. Anesthesiology. 2015;123:851–60.
16. Kapural L, Yu C, Doust MW, Gliner BE, Vallejo R, Sitzman BT, et al. Comparison of 10-kHz high-frequency and traditional low-frequency spinal cord stimulation for the treatment of chronic back and leg pain: 24-month results from a multicenter, randomized, controlled pivotal trial. Neurosurgery. 2016;79(5):667–77.
17. Miller JP, Eldabe S, Buchser E, Johanek LM, Guan Y, Linderoth B. Parameters of spinal cord stimulation and their role in electrical charge delivery: a review. Neuromodulation. 2016;19:373–84.
18. Lempka SF, McIntyre CC, Kilgore KL, Machado AG. Computational analysis of kilohertz frequency spinal cord stimulation for chronic pain management. Anesthesiology. 2015;122:1362–76.
19. Shechter R, Yang F, Xu Q, Cheong YK, He SQ, Sdrulla A, et al. Conventional and kilohertz-frequency spinal cord stimulation produces intensity- and frequency-dependent inhibition of mechanical hypersensitivity in a rat model of neuropathic pain. Anesthesiology. 2013;119:422–32.

20. Song Z, Viisanen H, Meyerson BA, Pertovaara A, Linderoth B. Efficacy of kilohertz-frequency and conventional spinal cord stimulation in rat models of different pain conditions. Neuromodulation. 2014;17:226–34; discussion 234–5.
21. Amir R, Michaelis M, Devor M. Burst discharge in primary sensory neurons: triggered by subthreshold oscillations, maintained by depolarizing after potentials. J Neurosci. 2002;22:1187–98.
22. Emmers R. Thalamic mechanisms that process a temporal pulse code for pain. Brain Res. 1976;103:425–41.
23. Radhakrishnan V, Tsoukatos J, Davis KD, Tasker RR, Lozano AM, Dostrovsky JO. A comparison of the burst activity of lateral thalamic neurons in chronic pain and non-pain patients. Pain. 1999;80:567–75.
24. Lenz FA, Garonzik IM, Zirh TA, Dougherty PM. Neuronal activity in the region of the thalamic principal sensory nucleus (ventralis caudalis) in patients with pain following amputations. Neuroscience. 1998;86:1065–81.
25. Jahnsen H, Llinás R. Voltage-dependent burst-to-tonic switching of thalamic cell activity: an in vitro study. Arch Ital Biol. 1984;122:73–82.
26. Swadlow HA, Gusev AG. The impact of 'bursting' thalamic impulses at a neocortical synapse. Nat Neurosci. 2001;4:402–8.
27. Sherman SM. A wake-up call from the thalamus. Nat Neurosci. 2001;4:344–6.
28. De Ridder D, Vanneste S, Plazier M, van der Loo E, Menovsky T. Burst spinal cord stimulation: toward paresthesia-free pain suppression. Neurosurgery. 2010;66:986–90.
29. De Ridder D, Plazier M, Kamerling N, Menovsky T, Vanneste S. Burst spinal cord stimulation for limb and back pain. World Neurosurg. 2013;80:642–9.
30. Kulkarni B, Bentley DE, Elliott R, Youell P, Watson A, Derbyshire SW, et al. Attention to pain localization and unpleasantness discriminates the functions of the medial and lateral pain systems. Eur J Neurosci. 2005;21:3133–42.
31. de Vos CC, Bom MJ, Vanneste S, Lenders MW, De Ridder D. Burst spinal cord stimulation evaluated in patients with failed back surgery syndrome and painful diabetic neuropathy. Neuromodulation. 2014;17:152–9.
32. De Ridder D, Vanneste S. Burst and tonic spinal cord stimulation: different and common brain mechanisms. Neuromodulation. 2016;19:47–59.
33. Schu S, Slotty PJ, Bara G, von Knop M, Edgar D, Vesper J. A prospective, randomized, double-blind, placebo-controlled study to examine the effectiveness of burst spinal cord stimulation patterns for the treatment of failed back surgery syndrome. Neuromodulation. 2014;17:443–50.
34. De Ridder D, Vanneste S, Plazier M, Vancamp T. Mimicking the brain: evaluation of St Jude Medical's Prodigy Chronic Pain System with Burst Technology. Expert Rev Med Devices. 2015;12:143–50.
35. De Ridder D, Lenders MW, De Vos CC, Dijkstra-Scholten C, Wolters R, Vancamp T, et al. A 2-center comparative study on tonic versus burst spinal cord stimulation: amount of responders and amount of pain suppression. Clin J Pain. 2015;31:433–7.
36. Hou S, Kemp K, Grabois M. A systematic evaluation of burst spinal cord stimulation for chronic back and limb pain. Neuromodulation. 2016;19:398–405.
37. Hogan Q. Labat lecture: the primary sensory neuron: where it is, what it does and why it matters. Reg Anesth Pain Med. 2010;35:306–11.
38. Sapunar D, Kostic S, Banozic A, Puljak L. Dorsal root ganglion—a potential new therapeutic target for neuropathic pain. J Pain Res. 2012;5:31–8.
39. Van Zundert J, Patijn J, Kessels A, Lame I, van Suijlekom H, van Kleef M. Pulsed radiofrequency adjacent to the cervical dorsal root ganglion in chronic cervical radicular pain: a double blind sham controlled randomized clinical trial. Pain. 2007;127:173–82.
40. McCallum JB, Kwok WM, Sapunar D, Fuchs A, Hogan QH. Painful peripheral nerve injury decreases calcium current in axotomized sensory neurons. Anesthesiology. 2006;105:160–8.

41. Rush AM, Dib-Hajj SD, Liu S, Cummins TR, Black JA, Waxman SG. A single sodium channel mutation produces hyper- or hypoexcitability in different types of neurons. Proc Natl Acad Sci U S A. 2006;103:8245–50.
42. Fields RD. New culprits in chronic pain. Sci Am. 2009;301:50–7.
43. Gemes G, Koopmeiners A, Rigaud M, Lirk P, Sapunar D, Bangaru ML, et al. Failure of action potential propagation in sensory neurons: mechanisms and loss of afferent filtering in C-type units after painful injury. J Physiol. 2013;591:1111–31.
44. Krames ES. The dorsal root ganglion in chronic pain and as a target for neuromodulation: a review. Neuromodulation. 2015;18:24–32.
45. St. Jude Medical. A safety and effectiveness trial of spinal cord stimulation of the dorsal root ganglion for chronic lower limb pain (ACCURATE). https://clinicaltrials.gov/ct2/show/NCT01923285
46. Chung JM, Fang ZR, Hori Y, Lee KH, Willis WD. Prolonged inhibitor of primate spinothalamic tract cells by peripheral nerve stimulation. Pain. 1984;19:259–75.
47. Ignelzi RJ, Nyquist JK. Excitability changes in peripheral nerve fibers after repetitive electrical stimulation. Implications in pain modulation. J Neurosurg. 1979;51:824–33.
48. Campbell JN, Taub A. Local analgesia from percutaneous electrical stimulation. A peripheral mechanism. Arch Neurol. 1973;28:347–50.
49. Abejon D, Deer T, Verrills P. Subcutaneous stimulation: how to assess optimal implantation depth. Neuromodulation. 2011;14:343–8.

Chapter 9
Anatomy of Neuromodulatory Targets: Central Nervous System and the Periphery

Scott Pritzlaff, Jennifer M. Hah, Michael A. Fishman, and Michael S. Leong

Current neuromodulatory targets have advanced from the dorsal columns of the spinal cord to multiple areas of the body. This chapter describes traditional anatomic landmarks and why spinal cord stimulation leads are placed in regions that are different from dermatologic mapping. In addition, stimulation by body region and various pain conditions is introduced, explaining how neuromodulation differs in treatment from head to foot.

9.1 Central Nervous System (CNS)

A precise understanding of the three-dimensional architecture of the spine provides an important basis for neuromodulation techniques. Although the use of fluoroscopy imaging can delineate important bony structures for spinal cord stimulator (SCS) lead placement, optimal placement requires accurate inference of soft tissue structures.

S. Pritzlaff • J.M. Hah • M.S. Leong
Division of Pain Medicine, Department of Anesthesiology, Perioperative, and Pain Medicine, Stanford University, Palo Alto, CA, USA
e-mail: spritzla@stanford.edu; jhah@stanford.edu; msleong@stanford.edu

M.A. Fishman (✉)
Center for Interventional Pain and Spine, Exton, PA, USA
e-mail: MFishman@Centerisp.com

S. Diwan, T.R. Deer (eds.), *Advanced Procedures for Pain Management*,
https://doi.org/10.1007/978-3-319-68841-1_9

9.1.1 Spine Anatomy

The spinal cord extends from the brainstem proximally to the conus medullaris, comprised of the fibrous filum terminale and the neural cauda equina [1]. In adults, the spinal cord terminates at the caudal end of the L1 vertebral level [1]. The pia mater (innermost layer), arachnoid mater, and dura mater (outermost layer) surround the spinal cord (Fig. 9.1). The subarachnoid or intrathecal space contains cerebrospinal fluid (CSF) and is located between the pia and arachnoid mater. The choroid plexuses of the cerebral ventricles produce approximately 500 mL of CSF each day, of which 30–80 mL is located below the T11–T12 level in the subarachnoid space [1]. The subdural space, between the dura and arachnoid mater, contains minimal amounts of serous fluid [2].

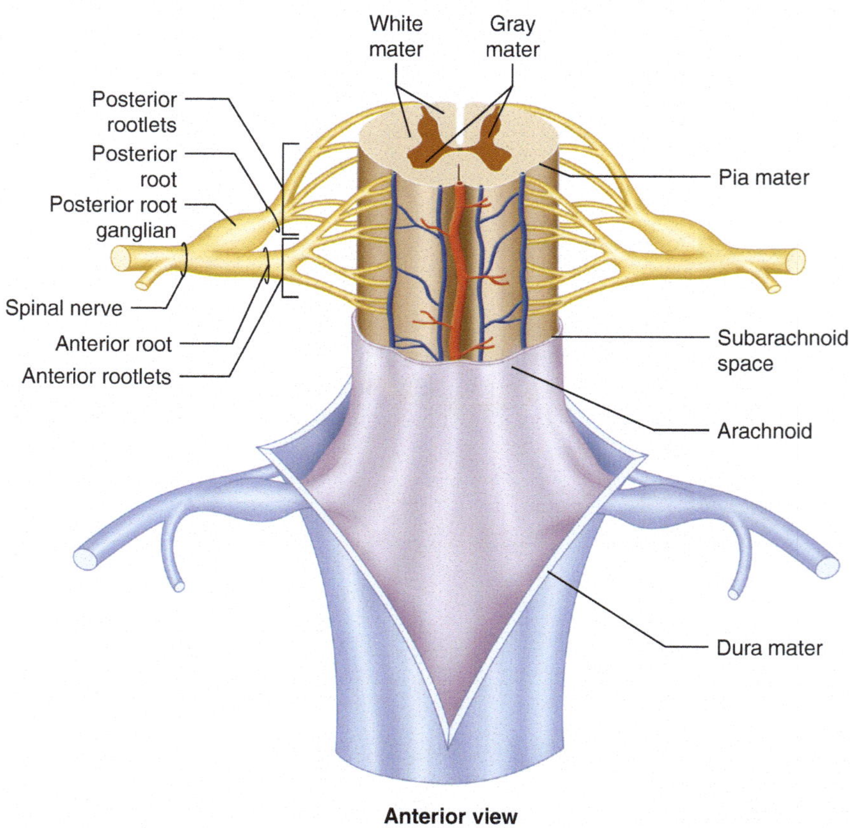

Fig. 9.1 Spinal cord meninges

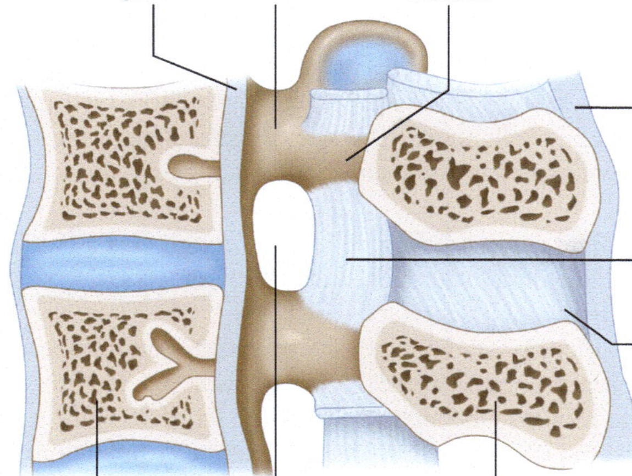

Fig. 9.2 Borders of the epidural space

The epidural space is superficial to the dura mater and extends from the foramen magnum to the sacral hiatus. The borders of the epidural space include the posterior longitudinal ligaments anteriorly, the pedicles and intervertebral foramina laterally, and the ligamentum flavum posteriorly (Fig. 9.2) [1]. In contrast to the subarachnoid space, the epidural space contains nerve roots and fat, areolar tissue, lymphatics, and blood vessels [3]. Epidural veins are situated anterolaterally within the epidural space, whereas epidural arteries are situated more laterally [2]. Though often thought of as a contiguous space, the epidural space contains meningo-vertebral ligaments that septate the epidural space into compartments of nonuniform size and shape [4]. These meningo-vertebral ligaments attach to the posterior dural sac and the ligamentum flavum or laminae, are localized to the posterior median or paramedian space, and run in a craniocaudal direction from the dural sac to the ligamentum flavum [5]. The distance between the ligamentum flavum and the dura mater is greatest (about 5–6 mm) at the L2 level. The distance decreases to 3–4 mm in the thoracic spine, and further decreases to 1.5–2 mm at C7 [2]. This variable distance between the ligamentum flavum and dura mater has important implications for SCS lead placement. Leads placed in the thoracic spine tend to exhibit higher impedance, stemming from less contact with the dura. Thus, systems placed in the thoracic spine may have a shorter battery life than those placed in the cervical spine [2]. Furthermore, the ligamentum flavum develops as a paired structure identifiable at 12 weeks gestational age, which ultimately fuses together at the midline [6]. At higher thoracic and cervical levels, midline gaps are often present from incomplete fusion of the left and right aspects of the ligament [6]. In addition, the gaps are most often located in the inferior aspect of the intervertebral space. Consequently, above the T4 level in the thoracic spine, palpation of the ligamentum flavum through a loss-of-resistance technique may not be a reliable method for epidural needle placement. Posterior to the ligamentum flavum lay the lamina and spinous processes of the vertebral bodies or the interspinous ligament. Immediately superficial to these structures is the supraspinous ligament, which spans the vertebral spines [1]. Thus, a needle must traverse skin, subcutaneous tissue, the supraspinous ligament, interspinous ligament, and ligamentum flavum to reach the epidural space.

Most of the electrical current during SCS runs through the CSF, with negligible conductivity through the dura mater, bone, and other contents of the epidural space [7]. White matter also exhibits conductivity during SCS. Thus, the width of the subarachnoid, CSF-filled space, determines current distribution. Because the width of subarachnoid space is greatest at the T3 to T6 level, SCS lead placement in the upper thoracic spine results in the highest perception thresholds (the minimum voltage at which paresthesias are perceived from electrical stimulation). In contrast, lead placement in the cervical spine results in the lowest perception thresholds.

Perception thresholds also vary with patient position changes and with dynamic activity by altering the thickness of the dorsal CSF layer. This effectively brings neural targets closer to or further away from the electrode, causing a dynamic change in the perception threshold. In other words, patients experience overstimulation if the neural target shifts closer to the electrode, and understimulation if it shifts away. The AdaptiveStim™ technology (Medtronic; Minneapolis, MN) uses a gyroscope to detect changes in body position and automatically adjust stimulation amplitude.

9.1.2 Dorsal Column Anatomy

The dorsal column comprises nerves engaged in sensory, motor, and proprioceptive functions, and is the target of spinal cord stimulation. These ascending tracts in the dorsal column pass without decussation to the gracile and cuneate nuclei of the medulla oblongata [8]. The large myelinated fibers of the dorsal column represent the central processes of primary afferent neurons. In general, stimulation of the dorsal column large myelinated fibers is more efficacious than dorsal root stimulation, which results in segmental motor stimulation before appropriate paresthesias can be achieved [7]. Understanding the somatotopic representation of the dorsal column can optimize SCS lead placement. Lateral fibers represent more rostral dermatomes, while medial fibers represent more caudal structures [2]. This organization results from sequential entry of dorsal root fibers from a caudal to rostral direction. Therefore, at any specific level, the dorsal column contains nerves from all dermatomes distal to that level (Fig. 9.3) [8]. Thus, specific vertebral levels can be targeted to achieve desired stimulation (C5–6 for upper extremity, T10–11 for lower extremity, T6–9 for low back, and C1–4 for neck) [7]. Although any given

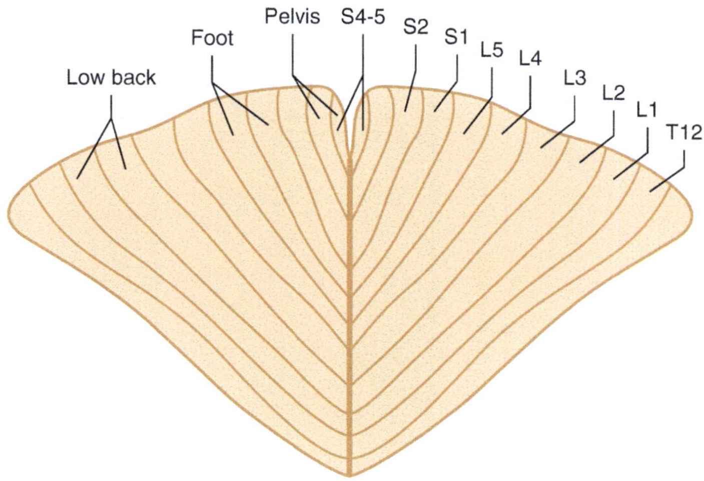

Fig. 9.3 Dorsal column somatotopic organization. Somatotopic representation of dermatomes at the level of the T11 dorsal columns [8]

spinal nerve has a vertebral entry point, the actual nerve root fibers enter the cord several segments more cranially [9]. To obtain a specific dermatomal level of stimulation, the dorsal column must be stimulated several segments above the vertebral level. Clinical neurostimulation typically recruits large myelinated fibers to a depth of 0.7 mm [9]. In addition, only about 1% of dorsal column fibers are large enough to be activated by SCS [9, 10].

9.1.3 Mechanisms of Neuromodulation

The concept of neuromodulation originated in response to Wall and Melzack's gate control theory of pain (Fig. 9.4) [11]. The concept that an imbalance between large fibers carrying innocuous input versus small fibers carrying peripheral nociceptive input laid the groundwork for the development of neuromodulation as an effective therapy for neuropathic, visceral, and nociceptive pain. Wall and Melzack's gate control theory of pain reduction described the idea of diminishing pain through selective activation of large-diameter fibers [11]. Pain signals are transmitted from nociceptors via A-delta and C-fibers, which are medium-diameter, lightly myelinated and small-diameter, nonmyelinated axons. The gate theory describes competitive input of large A-beta and smaller A-delta and C-fibers through a gate, with only one signal able to pass at a time. Thus, increasing the activity of large nerve fibers could close the gate to input from smaller pain fibers. Melzack and Wall described closing the gate to pain transmission through electrical stimulation of A-beta fibers [11].

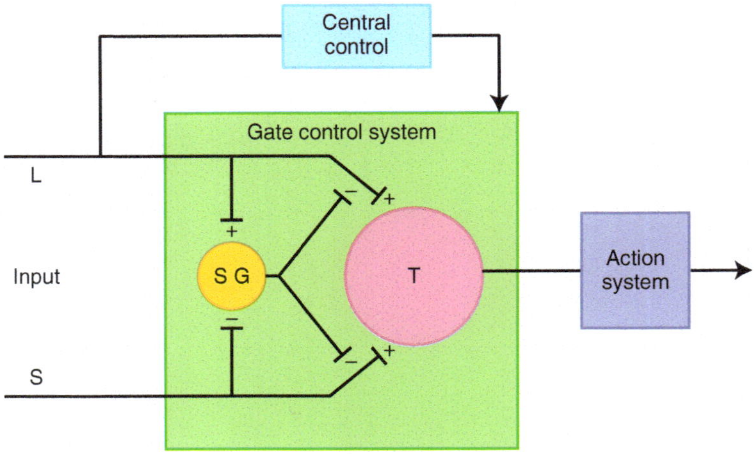

Fig. 9.4 The gate control theory of pain [11]. Large-diameter (L) and small-diameter (S) fibers project to the substantia gelatinosa (SG) and first central transmission (T) cells. The inhibitory effect exerted by SG on the afferent fiber terminals is increased by activity in L fibers and decreased by activity in S fibers. A line from the large-fiber system to the central control mechanisms represents the central control trigger. These mechanisms subsequently project back to the gate control system and the T cells project to the entry cells of the action system. + = excitation; − = inhibition

Specifically, Wall and Melzack proposed that the substantia gelatinosa functions as a modulator of afferent input, afferent patterns in the dorsal columns act as a CNS trigger for modulating properties of the gate control system, and central transmission cells in the dorsal horn activate neural mechanisms leading to response and perception [11].

Since the description of the gate control theory of pain, research has shown that additional mechanisms not described by this phenomenon are also involved in neuromodulation. This can be clinically demonstrated through continued analgesia even several hours after an SCS pulse generator is turned off [2].

Though neuromodulation has typically centered on electrical field coverage of pain regions, Foreman and Linderoth [12] have demonstrated that spinal cord stimulation affects wide dynamic range (WDR) neurons and must influence neurotransmitter levels at the spinal cord (Fig. 9.5). This graphic postulates mechanisms of action at the dorsal columns that could activate primary Aβ afferents and excite interneurons. This activation of interneurons would inhibit wide dynamic range (WDR) cells. This inhibition of WDR cells could account for the improvement of patients with neuropathic pain, peripheral vascular diseases, visceral (abdominal and pelvic) pain, and even nonanginal cardiac pain.

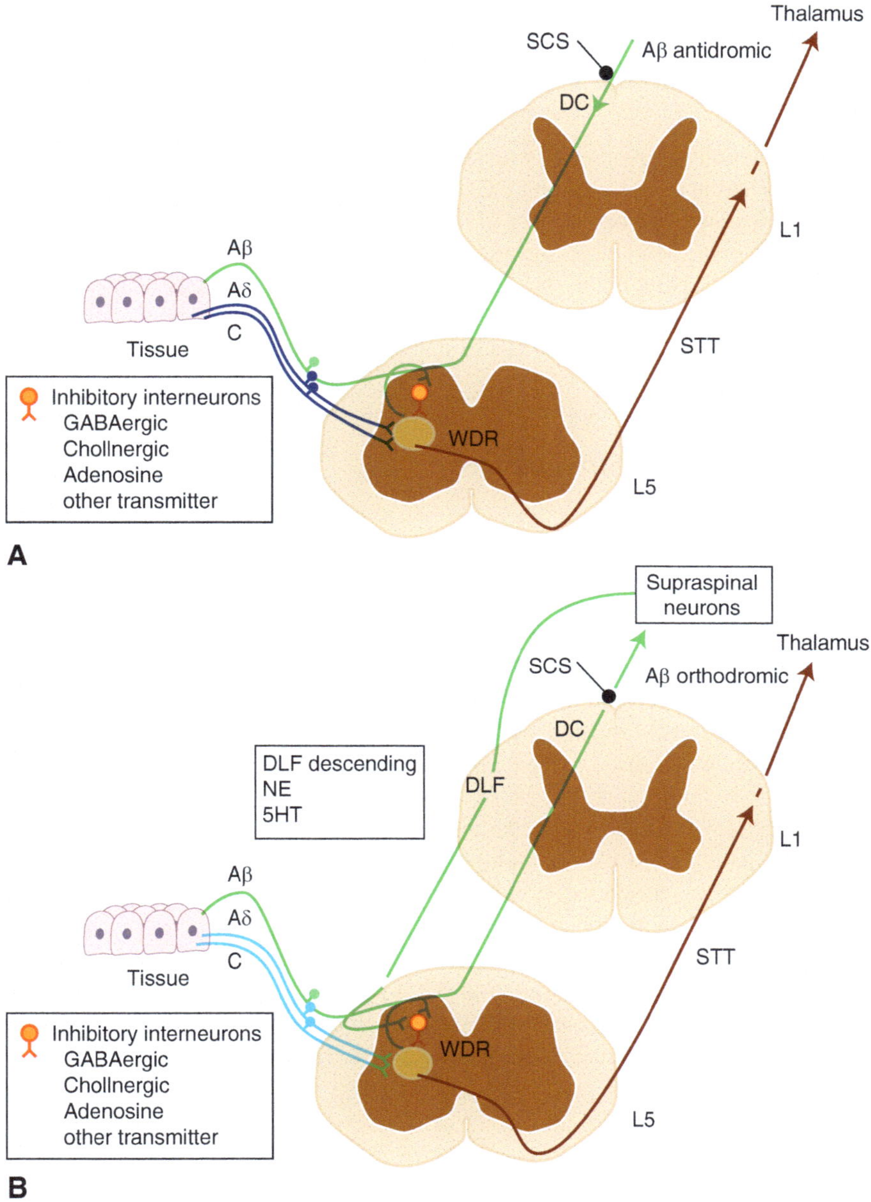

Fig. 9.5 Mechanisms of spinal cord stimulation (SCS) in neuropathic pain. SCS (*black ball at spinal segment L1*) activates dorsal columns antidromically (**a**) and orthodromically (**b**). (**a**) Antidromically transmitted action potentials activate collaterals of the primary Aβ afferents that excite interneurons (*red*). Activation of the interneurons inhibits wide dynamic range (WDR) cells. Numerous transmitters and modulators are involved in the modulation exerted by interneurons, as highlighted in the inset. The Aδ and C fibers from somatic structures (tissue) releasing glutamate and aspartate and that would excite WDR cells are inhibited, as mirrored in a decreased release of excitatory amino acids paralleled by an increase in GABA release. (**b**) Orthodromic activation of the primary afferent fibers with SCS evokes supraspinal relays (supraspinal neurons mainly in the brain stem) that transit information in descending pathways that release transmitters (DLF, dorsolateral funiculus; inset) to modulate WDR cells via segmental interneurons. Specific supraspinal relays are not shown because information about their organization is still evolving

9.2 Neuromodulatory Targets

Neuromodulation has evolved significantly in the 50 years since its initial treatment of back pain at the dorsal column by C. Norman Shealy in 1967. Spinal cord stimulation is now employed in a variety of conditions including neuropathic, ischemic, and visceral pain. Moreover, specific conditions such as postherpetic neuralgia, complex regional pain syndrome sacral and bladder pain, various headache syndromes, and even peripheral neuralgias are being increasingly treated with electrical stimulation. Specific targets and disease states are outlined in Table 9.1.

9.2.1 Spinal Cord Stimulation

Spinal cord stimulation (SCS) is the most common use of current implantable electrical stimulation systems for chronic pain management. The physiological and neuropharmacological mechanisms of action of SCS are complex and not well defined [13]. Nevertheless, SCS has been shown to be effective in treating back pain and CRPS. Newer experimental and clinical data show that SCS applied to different segments of the dorsal column elicits fundamentally different results on various target organs or parts of the body (Fig. 9.6).

Neuropathic pain caused by nerve dysfunction damage or altered nerve function is the main indication for SCS. Peripheral nerve injury, complex regional pain syndrome (CRPS) type I and II, peripheral neuropathy (idiopathic or diabetic), central neuropathic pain from stroke, or multiple sclerosis, spinal cord injury, and ischemia (cardiac as well as peripheral vascular disease) are good examples of conditions treated successfully with SCS [14].

The treatment of pain by applying electrical currents to the spinal cord, initially called dorsal column stimulation (DCS) but currently spinal cord stimulation (SCS), is delivered by electrodes over the dorsal columns of the spinal cord so as to modulate pain generation or processing. The goal of conventional SCS

Table 9.1 Targets of spinal cord stimulation

• Headache/cephalalgias
• Spinal disorders
• Angina
• Postherpetic neuralgia
• Abdominal pain
• Peripheral neuralgia/neuropathy
• Complex regional pain syndrome
• Bladder and pelvic pain

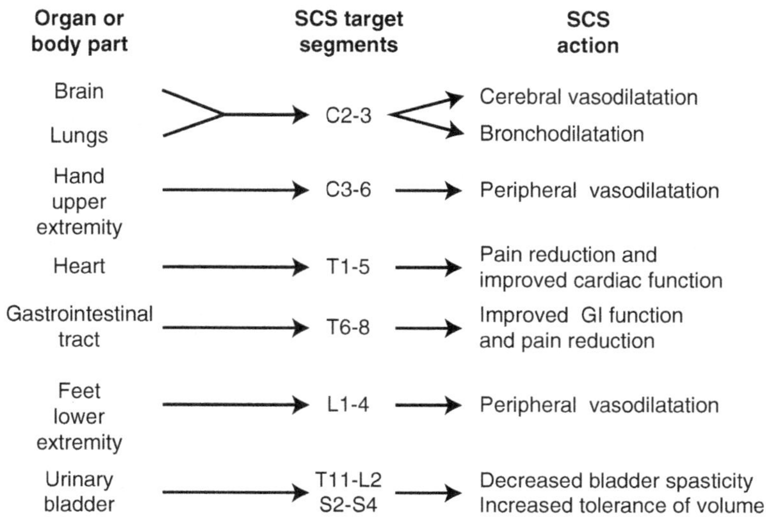

Fig. 9.6 Anatomic targets for spinal cord stimulation (SCS). This schematic diagram highlights different segments (not vertebral levels) of the spinal cord where SCS induces functional changes in target organs or body parts. Note that for the urinary bladder, T11–L2 segments modulate sympathetic control and S2–S4 segments modulate parasympathetic control [12]

(<1 kHz) is to replace the experience of pain with pleasant paresthesias targeted to the altered location [14]. Newer high-frequency (>10 kHz) stimulation devices, such as the Senza system, have become available in the United States since early 2015 [15]. The benefit to the high stimuli stimulation may include eliminating paresthesias, increasing tolerability but still providing excellent targeted pain control for patients.

Just outside of the spinal cord, dorsal root ganglion stimulation is proving to be a new region that may advance neuromodulation. A review by Krames [16] demonstrates why DRG stimulation may be an excellent target for decreasing hyperexcitability and chronic pain. Current existing devices developed by Spinal Modulation Inc. demonstrated efficacy in a multicenter, prospective trial in patients with painful regions of limb and/or trunk pain [17]. Moreover, DRG stimulation seems to prevent paresthesias due to positional changes while maintaining efficacy [18].

With emerging technology, SCS lead selection has become increasingly complex, as numerous SCS has evolved from monopolar or bipolar configurations. Complicated electrode arrays delivered either by percutaneously placed cylindrical platforms or surgically placed paddle platforms [13]. Common configurations for low back pain include two and three lead percutaneous cylindrical leads as well as paddle leads [14].

9.2.2 *Pain in the Chest: Neuromodulation for Refractory Angina*

Due to advances in modern medicine, the mortality from cardiovascular disease continues to decline. Revascularization procedures and medication have revolutionized treatment and increased survival. As a result of this, morbidity from cardiovascular disease has continued to rise.

Refractory angina (RA) has been defined as a chronic condition characterized by the presence of angina caused by coronary insufficiency in the presence of coronary artery disease which cannot be controlled by a combination of medical therapy, angioplasty and coronary bypass surgery. The presence of reversible myocardial ischemia should be clinically established to be the cause of the symptoms. Chronic is defined as a duration of more than 3 months [19]. Refractory angina pain can be a debilitating condition. Myocardial ischemia due to obstructive coronary disease activates both mechanical and chemical cardiac receptors. These receptors trigger the nerves which are conveying signals to the brain, where angina is ultimately 'felt'. In patients with refractory angina the high-threshold receptors in the myocardium have become low-threshold receptors. The subsequent sensitization of these receptors in the myocardium results in an altered angina threshold [19].

A variety of neuromodulatory techniques have been employed for angina. Transcutaneous electrical nerve stimulation (TENS) has been shown to be an effective method for treatment of angina, although there are technical limitations to this modality. The gel pads used to fix the electrodes to the skin can be cumbersome and have been known to cause dermatitis when used for a long period of time [20]. Patient compliance with TENS can also be a limiting consideration for this therapy.

Subcutaneous electrical nerve stimulation is an alternative to TENS and SCS. SENS electrodes are placed subcutaneously, at the side of the sternum in the area where the patient usually feels angina, and are connected to a pulse generator, which is implanted in the abdominal wall. This technique is easier and less invasive compared with SCS, thus reducing the risk of complications [21].

SCS is a proven effective therapy for RA with multiple trials supporting its use and proving its cost effectiveness [22]. It has been suggested that SCS produces its effects in refractory angina via an interaction of the following mechanisms: (1) pain reduction; (2) a reduction of sympathetic tone; (3) reduced myocardial oxygen demand; and (4) improved coronary microcirculatory blood flow, resulting in a lessening of myocardial ischemia [23].

SCS in RA patients is thought to be due to modification of the $\alpha 1$-adrenergic pathways leading to a sympatholytic and vasodilatory effect, which improves the microcirculation in the affected ischemic tissue [23]. Nitric oxide and calcitonin-gene-related peptide are also released, leading to vasodilation and improved microcirculation [24]. Other neurotransmitters such as acetylcholine, adenosine, and substance P are still subjects of ongoing investigations. Clinically reduced ulceration and oxygen demand have been observed in ischemic disease patients treated with SCS, which improves their pain and perfusion status significantly [25].

9.2.3 *Pain in the Head: Neuromodulation for Headache Disorders*

Primary headache disorders encompass a multitude of conditions that can be a source of significant disability for patients. Primary headache disorders frequently treated with neuromodulation include chronic migraine (CM), chronic tension-type headache, as well as the trigeminal autonomic cephalgias (TACs). TACs are a complex group of headache disorders that include cluster headache, paroxysmal hemicrania and short-lasting unilateral neuralgiform headache attacks with conjunctival injection and tearing/cranial autonomic features (SUNCT/SUNA). Other peripheral conditions that may contribute to chronic headache include occipital neuralgia (ON) and supraorbital neuralgia. These conditions may exacerbate underlying primary headache conditions such as CM or TACs, but they can also be the primary source of pain as well. Neuromodulation for headache disorders is best divided into two categories: central and peripheral modalities.

9.2.3.1 Central Stimulation

Deep brain stimulation (DBS) has been in practice since the 1950s and has been used for variety of neurologic conditions including epilepsy as well as chronic pain states. Deep brain stimulation consists of the placement of electrodes through the skull and cortex to the sub-cortical structures within the brain. The purpose is to stimulate these structures and modulate their function [26]. The electrode is placed ipsilateral to the attack, except for bilateral placement for conditions affecting both sides. The most common reported side effect of DBS is ophthalmoplegia and vertigo with higher stimulation amplitudes [27]. Recent data suggests that DBS has a systems effect rather than a localized deactivation effect in the posterior hypothalamic region, and may provide further insights into the disorder itself. The literature supports the use of DBS mainly in patients with TACS, primarily those affected by cluster headaches. There are some case reports of patients also receving DBS for SUNCT and paroxysmal hemicranias, but the results have shown mixed results [28].

9.2.3.2 Peripheral Stimulation

Considerable focus has also been devoted to peripheral nerve stimulation for headache syndromes. Currently, PNS is thought to modulate central pain processing by exploiting the anatomic and functional relationship of the peripheral sensory nerves of the head and neck to affect brainstem and higher cortical pain centers [29]. The current concept of the trigeminocervical complex describes the communications between the trigeminal nerve supplying sensation to the anterior head and face and the upper cervical nerves supplying sensation to the posterior head [28]. Percutaneous

Table 9.2 Percutaneous targets for peripheral nerve stimulation (PNS)

Lead placement	Benefit
Leads placed subcutaneously at the terminal branches of afferent nerves supplying the trigeminocervical complex	Chronic migraine and chronic tension-type headache
Occipital nerve stimulation (ONS): Applying an electrode impulse over the greater, lesser, or third occipital nerves (branches of C2–C3 cervical nerve roots)	Chronic migraine, hemicrania continua, chronic cluster headache, SUNCT, and paroxysmal hemicrania
Auriculotemporal nerve stimulation: Leads placed along bilateral auriculotemporal nerves	Chronic migraine (case reports only)
Sphenopalatine ganglion (SPG) stimulation: Efferents from the SPG innervate the dura and meninges, and initiate peripheral pain mechanisms of migraine, including neurogenic inflammation and vasodilatation. The parasympathetic outflow from the superior salivatory nucleus to the SPG from there, after synapsing, to target organs of the eye and sinuses is felt to be the pathway for most of the autonomic features of cluster headache	Chronic migraine and cluster headache
Supraorbital nerve stimulation (has been combined with ONS)	Chronic cluster headache and migraine headache (case reports only)

SUNCT Short-lasting unilateral neuralgiform headache attacks with conjunctival injection and tearing

stimulation of peripheral targets has been proven to be effective for headache syndromes are numerous (Table 9.2).

Noninvasive stimulation techniques for headache are also viable long term treatment options. The Cefaly™ device (CEFALY Technology; Belgium) is available by prescription in the USA and Europe and is the first device to use transcutaneous stimulation for targeted treatment of migraine (Fig. 9.7). The device consists of an electrode with skin adhesive placed on the forehead covering the sites of the supraorbital and supratrochlear nerves, both of which are branches of the ophthalmic nerve or the first branch of the trigeminal nerve. Biphasic rectangular impulses with an electrical mean of zero, impulse width of 250 μs, frequency of 60 Hz, and maximum intensity of 16 mA are generated with device activation. The relatively high frequency and low intensity is aimed to avoid crossing the pain threshold while still being able to activate Aβ afferents and leading to paresthesia in the distribution of the nerve and preventing the activation of Aδ and C fibers important in nociception and reducing hyperalgesia [29].

Vagal nerve stimulation (VNS) has also been a target for headache treatment. Current evidence for the use of VNS for pain indications is most robust, though still relatively limited, for the indication of chronic headaches and migraines [30]. Several noninvasive VNS (nVNS) devices are currently on the market. The NEMOS device (Cerbomed; Erlangen, Germany) provides transcutaneous VNS via the auricular branch of the vagus nerve. Its primary use has been for cluster headaches, episodic migraines, and chronic migraines. Reportable adverse events across several

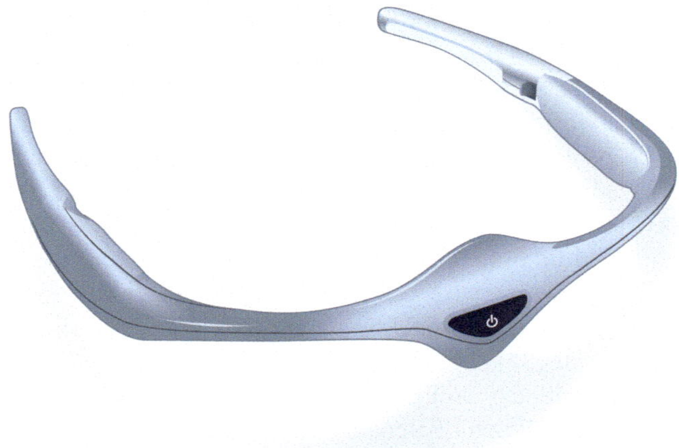

Fig. 9.7 The Cefaly™ device consists of an electrode with skin adhesive placed on the forehead covering the sites of the supraorbital and supratrochlear nerves

published studies include local discomfort, skin irritation, transient muscle stiffness, and pain that resolved with NSAID treatment.

9.2.4 Pain in the Limbs: Complex Regional Pain Syndrome, Peripheral Neuropathy, and Peripheral Vascular Disease

Complex regional pain syndrome (CRPS) a neuropathic pain condition characterized by vasomotor, sudomotor, sensory, and trophic signs and symptoms. CRPS is subdivided into CRPS type 1 and type 2. The signs, symptoms, and presentation of both types are very similar. CRPS-I, classically called reflex sympathetic dystrophy, is defined by the absence of injury to a major nerve. CRPS-II, known previously as causalgia, occurs following damage to a major nerve. Patients affected by CRPS can have a significant level of disability and mental distress. Traditionally, initial treatment of CRPS has focused on multidisciplinary care including treatment with medications like opioids, anticonvulsants, and tricyclic antidepressants. Physical and occupational therapy as well as intensive psychological therapy including cognitive behavioral therapy are also pillars of CRPS treatment. An interdisciplinary treatment protocol, developed under the aegis of IASP, recommends simultaneous psychological, rehabilitative, and interventional pain management with therapeutic options determined by the patient's clinical progress. The Neuromodulation Appropriateness Consensus Committee (NACC) recommends SCS for the treatment of CRPS-I and CRPS-II with pain of at least 3 months' duration or severe, rapidly progressing disease that is not responding to more conservative measures such as physical and occupational therapy [31].

The current conceptual model for SCS supports segmental inhibition as a tenet for analgesia. Data obtained from animal studies indicate that second-order neurons and interneurons can be affected by SCS, and that spinal and supraspinal inhibitory loops may account for the major effects of SCS in neuropathic pain [32–34]. Implanting a SCS is often considered both an expensive and an invasive treatment, and satisfactory lead placement is necessary for successful treatment. The technical goal of SCS is to achieve stimulation-induced paresthesias in the anatomical distribution of the affected limb. Despite the apparent upfront cost, if the treatment is appropriate and is shown to have good outcomes, overall costs, morbidity, and chronic decreased functionality would be significantly reduced with fewer ineffective treatments and tests [35]. Krames et al. [36] have introduced the SAFE principles as a way to appropriately ordinate therapies for the treatment of chronic pain. SAFE is an acronym standing for **S**afety, **A**ppropriateness, time to **F**iscal neutrality, and **E**fficacy (Fig. 9.8) [37]. These principles help to guide pain practitioners in their decision to consider SCS for CRPS patients.

Peripheral neuropathy can also be successfully treated with neuromodulation. The prevalence of diabetes and related complications continues to rise in the United States and throughout the world. Diabetic neuropathy is common problem in longstanding diabetics. Painful diabetic neuropathy (PDN) can interfere with mobility, quality of life, and overall well being. There is good data to show that when conservative measures failure including medications fail, SCS is a reasonable alternative therapy. In several recent studies, SCS resulted in clinical and statistical improvements in pain and quality of life of patients with painful diabetic neuropathy [38, 39].

Spinal cord stimulator is approved for the treatment of critical limb ischemia in Europe, but not currently in the United States. Currently, conservative management of chronic critical limb ischemia consists of analgesics, vasodilators, and anticoagu-

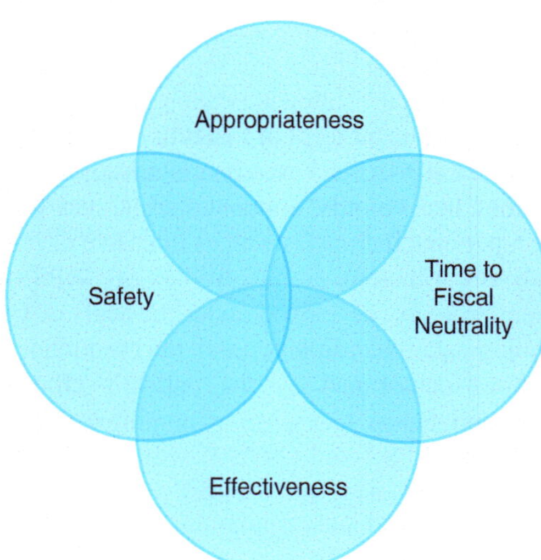

Fig. 9.8 *SAFE* analysis analyzes **S**afety, **A**ppropriateness, time to **F**iscal neutrality, and **E**fficacy [36]

lants. In those who are not surgical candidates, SCS is an alternative that may improve limb salvage. As with the therapeutic effects of SCS in CAD, it is hypothesized that SCS leads to improvement in critical limb ischemia due to vasodilation and subsequent improvement of blood flow. SCS may be a treatment option for those patients who are nonsurgical candidates and have critical limb ischemia [40]. According to the NACC, ischemia due to structural lesions (peripheral arterial occlusive disease or due to vasospasm like in Raynaud's disease) are well treated by SCS; however, venous engorgement has not been shown to respond. The NACC feels that the evidence supporting sympathectomy is very poor and recommends SCS be utilized prior to the irreversible approach of sympathectomy [31].

References

1. Miller RD. Miller's anesthesia. 8th ed. Philadelphia: Elsevier/Saunders; 2015.
2. Kreis P, Fishman S. Spinal cord stimulation: percutaneous implantation techniques. New York: Oxford University Press; 2009.
3. Boon JM, Prinsloo E, Raath RP. A paramedian approach for epidural block: an anatomic and radiologic description. Reg Anesth Pain Med. 2003;28:221–7.
4. Jiang H, Shi B, Xu S. An anatomical study of lumbar epidural catheterization. BMC Anesthesiol. 2015;15:94.
5. Shi B, Zheng X, Min S, Zhou Z, Ding Z, Jin A. The morphology and clinical significance of the dorsal meningovertebra ligaments in the cervical epidural space. Spine J. 2014;14:2733–9.
6. Yoon SP, Kim HJ, Choi YS. Anatomic variations of cervical and high thoracic ligamentum flavum. Korean J Pain. 2014;27:321–5.
7. Ramasubbu C, Flagg A 2nd, Williams K. Principles of electrical stimulation and dorsal column mapping as it relates to spinal cord stimulation: an overview. Curr Pain Headache Rep. 2013;17:315.
8. Feirabend HKP, Choufoer H, Ploeger S, Holsheimer J, Van Gool JD. Morphometry of human superficial dorsal and dorsolateral column fibres: significance to spinal cord stimulation. Brain. 2002;125:1137–49.
9. Foletti A, Durrer A, Buchser E. Neurostimulation technology for the treatment of chronic pain: a focus on spinal cord stimulation. Expert Rev Med Devices. 2007;4:201–14.
10. Yampolsky C, Hem S, Bendersky D. Dorsal column stimulator applications. Surg Neurol Int. 2012;3:S275–89.
11. Melzack R, Wall PD. Pain mechanisms: a new theory. Science. 1965;150:971–9.
12. Foreman RD, Linderoth B. Neural mechanisms of spinal cord stimulation. Int Rev Neurobiol. 2012;107:87–119.
13. Kapural L. Spinal cord stimulation for intractable chronic pain. Curr Pain Headache Rep. 2014;18:406.
14. Deer T, Pope J, Hayek S, Narouze S, Patil P, Foreman R, et al. Neurostimulation for the treatment of axial back pain: a review of mechanisms, techniques, outcomes, and future advances. Neuromodulation. 2014;17:52–68.
15. U.S. Food and Drug Administration. FDA approves spinal cord stimulation system that treats pain without tingling sensation. 8 May 2015. http://www.fda.gov/NewsEvents/Newsroom/PressAnnouncements/ucm446354.htm
16. Krames ES. The dorsal root ganglion in chronic pain and as a target for neuromodulation: a review. Neuromodulation. 2015;18:24–32.
17. Liem L, Russo M, Huygen FJ, Van Buyten JP, Smet I, Verrills P, et al. A multicenter, prospective trial to assess the safety and performance of the spinal modulation dorsal root ganglion

neurostimulator system in the treatment of chronic pain. Neuromodulation. 2013;16:471–82; discussion 482.
18. Kramer J, Liem L, Russo M, Smet I, Van Buyten JP, Huygen F. Lack of body positional effects on paresthesias when stimulating the dorsal root ganglion (DRG) in the treatment of chronic pain. Neuromodulation. 2015;18:50–57; discussion 57.
19. Mannheimer C, Camici P, Chester MR, Collins A, DeJongste M, Eliasson T, et al. The problem of chronic refractory angina; report from the ESC Joint Study Group on the Treatment of Refractory Angina. Eur Heart J. 2002;23:355–70.
20. Strobos MA, Coenraads PJ, De Jongste MJ, Ubels FL. Dermatitis caused by radio-frequency electromagnetic radiation. Contact Dermatitis. 2001;44:309.
21. De Decker K, Beese U, Staal MJ, Dejongste MJ. Electrical neuromodulation for patients with cardiac diseases. Neth Heart J. 2013;21:91–4.
22. Eldabe S, Thomson S, Duarte R, Brookes M, deBelder M, Raphael J, et al. The effectiveness and cost-effectiveness of spinal cord stimulation for refractory angina (RASCAL Study): a pilot randomized controlled trial. Neuromodulation. 2016;19:60–70.
23. Wu M, Linderoth B, Foreman RD. Putative mechanisms behind effects of spinal cord stimulation on vascular diseases: a review of experimental studies. Auton Neurosci. 2008;138:9–23.
24. Bernardini N, Neuhuber W, Reeh PW, Sauer SK. Morphological evidence for functional capsaicin receptor expression and calcitonin gene-related peptide exocytosis in isolated peripheral nerve axons of the mouse. Neuroscience. 2004;126:585–90.
25. Kinfe TM, Pintea B, Vatter H. Is spinal cord stimulation useful and safe for the treatment of chronic pain of ischemic origin? A review. Clin J Pain. 2016;32:7–13.
26. Jenkins B, Tepper SJ. Neurostimulation for primary headache disorders: part 2, review of central neurostimulators for primary headache, overall therapeutic efficacy, safety, cost, patient selection, and future research in headache neuromodulation. Headache. 2011;51:1408–18.
27. Goadsby PJ. Neurostimulation in primary headache syndromes. Expert Rev Neurother. 2007;7:1785–9.
28. Hong J, Ball PA, Fanciullo GJ. Neurostimulation for neck pain and headache. Headache. 2014;54:430–44.
29. Zhu S, Marmura MJ. Non-invasive neuromodulation for headache disorders. Curr Neurol Neurosci Rep. 2016;16:11.
30. Chakravarthy K, Chaudhry H, Williams K, Christo PJ. Review of the uses of vagal nerve stimulation in chronic pain management. Curr Pain Headache Rep. 2015;19:54.
31. Deer TR, Mekhail N, Provenzano D, Pope J, Krames E, Leong M, et al. The appropriate use of neurostimulation of the spinal cord and peripheral nervous system for the treatment of chronic pain and ischemic diseases: the Neuromodulation Appropriateness Consensus Committee. Neuromodulation. 2014;17:515–50; discussion 550.
32. El-Khoury C, Hawwa N, Baliki M, Atweh SF, Jabbur SJ, Saadé NE. Attenuation of neuropathic pain by segmental and supraspinal activation of the dorsal column system in awake rats. Neuroscience. 2002;112:541–53.
33. Williams KA, Korto K, Cohen SP. Spinal cord stimulation: "neural switch" in complex regional pain syndrome type I. Pain Med. 2009;10:762–6.
34. Dubuisson D. Effect of dorsal-column stimulation on gelatinosa and marginal neurons of cat spinal cord. J Neurosurg. 1989;70:257–65.
35. Goff BJ, Naber JW, McCallin JP, Lopez EM, Guthmiller KB, Lautenschlager KA, et al. Immediate return to ambulation and improved functional capacity for rehabilitation in complex regional pain syndrome following early implantation of a spinal cord stimulation system. Case Rep Anesthesiol. 2014;2014:784021.
36. Krames E, Poree L, Deer T, Levy R. Implementing the SAFE principles for the development of pain medicine therapeutic algorithms that include neuromodulation techniques. Neuromodulation. 2009;12:104–13.

37. Poree L, Krames E, Pope J, Deer TR, Levy R, Schultz L. Spinal cord stimulation as treatment for complex regional pain syndrome should be considered earlier than last resort therapy. Neuromodulation. 2013;16:125–41.
38. Duarte RV, Andronis L, Lenders MW, de Vos CC. Quality of life increases in patients with painful diabetic neuropathy following treatment with spinal cord stimulation. Qual Life Res. 2016;25:1771–7.
39. Slangen R, Schaper NC, Faber CG, Joosten EA, Dirksen CD, van Dongen RT, et al. Spinal cord stimulation and pain relief in painful diabetic peripheral neuropathy: a prospective two-center randomized controlled trial. Diabetes Care. 2014;37:3016–24.
40. Lee S, Abd-Elsayed A. Some non-FDA approved uses for neuromodulation: a review of the evidence. Pain Pract. 2016;16:935–47.

Chapter 10
Neuromodulation: Optimizing Surgical Outcomes and Risk Reduction

Nomen Azeem

Neuromodulation involves the minimally invasive permanent implantation of a neurostimulator to provide relief of chronic pain. To optimize surgical outcome, the implanting physician should be adequately trained, select appropriate patients, understand potential complications, and provide patient education, and medical wellness should be assured, to reduce risks for the surgery. Steps to reduce the potential for bleeding, infection, or paralysis should be taken by the implanting physician preoperatively, intraoperatively, and postoperatively.

Neuromodulation or neurostimulation, which includes both spinal cord stimulation and peripheral nerve stimulation, is a safe and reversible treatment option for patients with chronic pain due to disease processes of the central nervous system, the peripheral nervous system, or both. Conservative treatment options may have failed in these patients, who continue to have neuropathic or sympathetically mediated pain. Spinal cord and peripheral neurostimulation techniques for the relief of pain and improvement in organ function have been practiced since 1967 [1]. Most complications from neurostimulation implantation surgery are minor, are correctable, and do not increase morbidity and mortality rates. Extensive published reviews suggest that approximately 30–40% of patients treated with a spinal cord stimulator (SCS) will have a complication requiring a revision [2–6].

N. Azeem (✉)
Department of Neurology, University of South Florida,
Tampa, FL, USA
e-mail: azeemnx@gmail.com

S. Diwan, T.R. Deer (eds.), *Advanced Procedures for Pain Management*,
https://doi.org/10.1007/978-3-319-68841-1_10

10.1 Physician Training

In order to minimize technique-related complications, the physician must demonstrate competence for the appropriate surgical implantation of the neurostimulator device. The Neuromodulation Appropriateness Consensus Committee (NACC) of the International Neuromodulation Society (INS) recommends that improvement of outcomes for implanted neurostimulation devices must include setting higher standards for the training and quality of potential implanters [7]. Implanters should have undergone training in a recognized, high-volume center with proper credentialing. During formal training, the implanter should ideally perform a minimum of ten cases as the primary implanter and under supervision. Appropriate training should include patient selection and contraindications to intended procedures, the anatomy of the intended implant area, complication identification and management, and collaboration with colleagues. The implanter should be comfortable with troubleshooting during the implantation procedure and with the methods and techniques used to achieve proper stimulation, while maintaining patient and implanter safety. The implanter should be able to recognize and treat hardware-related and biological complications and should be able to recognize the benefits and pitfalls of various commercial leads and lead types and their specific indications [8].

10.2 Patient Selection

To optimize surgical outcome, steps for risk reduction should begin with the selection of patients for neurostimulation treatment. Appropriate patient selection is a complex process that begins with a detailed patient interview combined with a thorough physical examination conducted during an office visit in order to identify complaints, relevant history, and deficits. The physician should also inquire about coexisting medical conditions during the office visit and should obtain any pertinent diagnostic testing (spinal imaging, EMG/NCS, bloodwork). If the patient has multiple medical comorbidities, it is advisable to have the primary care specialist or subspecialist (*e.g.* cardiologist, hematologist, or infectious disease specialist) maximize the medical care of the patient prior to surgery.

Multiple indicators can help to determine the likely effectiveness of neuromodulation with SCS for appropriate patients. The indicators include the experience of the implanter, the etiology of the patient's pain, treatment closer to onset of pain, the existence of comorbidities that might cause failure or lead to complications, and a well-performed psychologic evaluation to rule out patients with psychologically caused pain, underlying psychoemotional distress, or schizophrenia [8]. Specifically, individuals with significantly depressed mood and those with low energy levels are at higher risk of failing their SCS trial [9]. In addition, a recent systematic review of 25 studies found that somatization, anxiety, and poor coping were important predictors of poor outcome [10]. In the setting of psychiatric or psychological disorders, the patient must be evaluated, stabilized, and obtain psychological clearance prior to surgery.

10.3 Patient Education

Once the patient has been selected for neurostimulation treatment, patient education is vital to optimize outcomes. During this time, expectations about results from neurostimulation treatment such as pain relief and improved quality of life, as well as the risk of complications, cosmetic concerns, and follow-up care should be discussed at length with the patient, family, and caregivers. Written instructions that include preoperative patient responsibilities can reinforce verbal instructions. Additional instructions should include the date, time, and location for the procedure and reminders to require the patient to stop specific medications before the trial and implant. The patient should also be advised to call to cancel the procedure if he or she becomes ill or chooses not to undergo the procedure, to bathe with appropriate prep material before surgery, and to arrange for transportation to and from the surgical suite. Discharge instructions for postoperative care can be distributed on the day of the trial or implant. The patient or caregivers should know how to contact the physician or clinic if questions arise or complications occur [8].

After deciding to move forward with treatment, the patient must undergo a 4- to 7-day trial period with placement of temporary percutaneous leads in order to determine the potential benefits of neurostimulation. The trial is done under conscious sedation with monitoring for patient comfort. Although the trial lead placement has lower risk than permanent placement, the patient should understand that the risk of the trial revolves around the lead, needle, and anesthesia [11].

The patient should also understand the different methods of permanent placement of a neurostimulation system. For example, there are two options for permanent SCS placement: percutaneous lead placement or surgical paddle lead placement. A percutaneous electrode offers relatively easy access to multiple spinal levels and thus facilitates paresthesia mapping. A surgical paddle electrode might be required for screening, however, if a percutaneous catheter electrode cannot access the epidural space satisfactorily, such as in a patient who has undergone a previous laminectomy or posterior fusion at the level of insertion. There is no inherent difference in the fracture rates for these two types of electrodes [7]. Percutaneous leads are cylindrical wire leads that have multiple contacts that can be manipulated to act as an anode or cathode. Percutaneous electrodes are considered easier to insert and cause less surgical trauma than the paddle type, which are inserted via incision, deep dissection, laminotomy, and removal of posterior spinal structures. If the patient is to have surgical lead placement, it should be advised that this is a more extensive surgical technique, which often requires general anesthesia and its possible added risks.

10.4 Understanding Complications

To improve surgical outcome and reduce risks, knowledge and understanding of potential complications is vital. Although a minimally invasive procedure, neurostimulator implantation complications have been a historical concern. In 2004, Cameron reviewed SCS complications over 20 years (1981–2003) in 51 papers that totaled 2972 patients. The most common complications were lead migration (13.2%), lead breakage (9.1%), infection (3.4%), hardware malfunction (2.9%), unwanted stimulation (2.4%), and battery failure (1.6%) [3]. Generally, complications of neurostimulator implant surgery can be categorized into hardware-related complications or biological complications.

10.4.1 Hardware Complications

Hardware complications include lead-related complications and battery failure. Lead migration and fracture are the most common SCS complications, which can result in a loss of paresthesia and pain relief. Lead migration may result from poor technique in anchoring or anchor failure. If reprogramming cannot recapture the paresthesia/pain overlap, then reoperation to replace the lead over the spinal target or level that produces a paresthesia/pain overlap may be needed [8]. Unexpected battery failure of a fully implantable pulse generator (IPG) occurred in 32 (1.7%) of the 900 cases reviewed by Cameron through 2004, although 22 of the 32 failures occurred after more than the expected 3-year battery duration [3]. Surgical revision with battery replacement is necessary for battery failure.

10.4.2 Biological Complications

Biological complications may include infection, neuraxial hematoma, dural puncture, neurologic injury, skin erosion, seroma, and pain over the implant. Infection rates associated with SCS systems vary and have been reported in the range of 3.4–4.6% from two large systematic reviews [3, 12]. Kumar et al. [13], in a multicenter randomized controlled trial comparing SCS with conventional medical management of neuropathic pain, reported an 8% rate of infection or wound breakdown. Biological complications are most prevalent within the first 3 months after implantation.

10.4.2.1 Surgical Site Infection (SSI)

The three major types of infection related to SCS implantation include superficial infections, deep infections, and epidural abscesses. Superficial SSIs involve the skin and subcutaneous tissue surrounding an incision and are defined as infections occurring within 30 days after the operation [14]. A deep incisional infection related to surgery involves the deep soft tissue, including muscle and fascia. When an implant is involved, the timeframe for a deep infection is up to 1 year after surgery [14]. Turner et al. [12] reported that a majority of infections associated with SCS systems are superficial infections (4.5% superficial SSIs and 0.1% deep SSIs). Follett et al. [15] reported that most infections (54%) occur at the generator site and that infection rates are lower at the SCS electrode implant site (17%) and with the lumbar incision (8%). The most common organisms to cause postoperative infections are *Staphylococcus aureus* (20%), coagulase-negative staphylococci (14%), *Enterococcus* (12%), *Escherichia coli* (8%), and *Pseudomonas aeruginosa* (8%) [16]. Prophylactic antibiotic therapy should be utilized and has been shown to reduce the risk of SSIs in both animal and clinical studies [17–19]. Furthermore, antibiotic prophylaxis has been shown to be an effective intervention for preventing postoperative wound infection, independent of surgery type, resulting in an approximately 50% reduction in the incidence of wound infections [20]. Patients should be administered intravenous antibiotics such as a single dose of cephalosporin (clindamycin if allergic to cephalosporin) or vancomycin (for methicillin-resistant *S. aureus*) 30–120 min prior to surgery, to prevent infection. The current preoperative dosing of cefazolin, based on weight, is 1 g for individuals weighing less than 80 kg, 2 g for individuals 81–160 kg, and 3 g for individuals >160 kg. For individuals with a beta-lactam allergy, clindamycin (600–900 mg based on weight) or vancomycin (1 g) may be used [8]. No advantages have been documented for antibiotic use following SCS implantation [21]. In addition, in other surgical specialties, prolonged antibiotic use in the postoperative period has not been shown to improve outcomes and in some studies resulted in poor outcomes [22, 23].

In the setting of a neurostimulator implant, the greatest concern regarding SSIs is the potential for progression to an epidural abscess. An epidural abscess may present with acute neurologic deficit (weakness, sensory changes, radicular pain, saddle anesthesia, incontinence) plus fever, leukocytosis, and severe pain. Immediate neurosurgical evacuation of the epidural abscess and explantation of the device, followed by antibiotic therapy, is recommended.

10.4.2.2 Hematoma Formation

Although rare, epidural hematoma formation following the placement of SCS leads (whether percutaneous or surgical) is a neurosurgical emergency. In a series of 509 paddle electrodes, Barolat [24] reported one case of epidural hematoma resulting in paraplegia. In a 20-year review of the literature, Cameron [3] estimated the risk of epidural hematoma development at 0.3% and paralysis at 0.03%. Levy and colleagues [25] reported on a sample of 44,587 cases, among whom 0.25% had major neurologic deficit. Of these 111 patients, 61 (0.14%) had limited motor deficit, six had autonomic changes (0.013%), 46 had sensory deficits (0.10%), and 21 had CSF leakage due to dural puncture. The same series reported 16 epidural hematomas with limited motor deficit, 15 hematomas without motor deficit (0.034%), and 52 hematomas with major motor deficits (0.12%) [25]. More recent case reports describe hematomas with implantation of either paddle or percutaneous leads as a result of lead migration and not due to anticoagulant/antiplatelet medications [25–30].

The highest risk for bleeding is during placement and removal of the device and within the first 24 h after the procedure. The patient should be advised to call the physician immediately for any acute neurologic change. An epidural hematoma may result from puncture of a blood vessel when placing neurostimulator leads in the epidural space and is a potential neurosurgical emergency. In most cases, bleeding of these epidural vessels does not lead to a space-occupying lesion, but intrinsic clotting disorders, liver disease, or medications that affect clotting may increase the risk. Thus the current recommendations for standard of care call for the discontinuation of any anticoagulant or antiplatelet therapy, and it is crucial that such patients consult with the prescribing provider to determine their suitability for anticoagulation cessation and the need for bridging before placement of a temporary or permanent SCS system [8]. The fact that there are no published guidelines regarding anticoagulated patients and SCS has prompted many implanters to adopt and accept guidelines for the anticoagulated patient undergoing regional anesthesia [8]. In accordance with the NACC recommendations, anticoagulation or antiplatelet therapy should be held for the duration of any neurostimulator trial period and restarted 24 h after lead removal or 24 h after permanent implantation of the neurostimulator [8].

The onset of symptoms of an epidural hematoma can be immediate and drastic, presenting as acute neurologic deficit (weakness, sensory changes, radicular pain, saddle anesthesia, incontinence). An immediate CT scan of the spine should be ordered to confirm the diagnosis, followed by a neurosurgical decompression.

The best treatment of incision-site hematoma is prevention by vigilant hemostasis during dissection and careful wound handling before closing. If the patient presents with purple discoloration over the incision site that is painful and solid to palpation, monitor for expanding hematoma and/or infection. Most hematomas resolve without intervention but may have to be evacuated if they persist or worsen.

10.4.2.3 Dural Puncture or Neurologic Injury

Dural puncture occasionally occurs during epidural needle placement for lead positioning. The result can be symptoms of post–dural puncture headache (PDPH) as well as CSF leakage into the wound. The incidence of dural puncture has been estimated at 0–0.3% [8]. The incidence of CSF leak following traditional paddle lead placement was reported to be 0.05% [3, 25]. Risk factors for dural puncture include previous surgery at the location of needle entry into the epidural space, a calcified ligamentum flavum, spinal stenosis at the site of needle entry into the epidural space, and an uncooperative patient [8].

Patients who develop PDPH may suffer from a positional headache, diplopia, tinnitus, neck pain, and/or photophobia. These symptoms are typically self-resolving and may also respond to caffeine. If the symptoms persist, then an autologous epidural blood patch may be utilized therapeutically. Care must be taken when performing the blood patch to match the volume of autologous blood injected to the level of puncture, with smaller volumes required for more cephalad punctures in the thoracic and cervical spine [31].

Neurologic injury is a serious potential complication of SCS implantation and can occur from direct trauma to nerves and spinal cord during placement of a needle, percutaneous lead, or paddle leads. Meyer et al. [32] reported a case of quadriplegia following inadvertent intramedullary percutaneous lead placement in a patient under general anesthesia. In a MAUDE (FDA Manufacturer and User Facility Device Experience) database review, Levy et al. [25] recently investigated neurologic injury following traditional paddle lead placement. In a 3-year period, 44,587 paddles were implanted in as many patients. Neurologic complications occurred in 260 patients, for a rate of 0.58%. Motor dysfunction without epidural hematoma occurred at a rate of 0.13% for paddle leads introduced by laminotomy [33].

10.4.2.4 Skin Erosion

Skin erosions are typically a consequence of superficial lead placement and are more often a consequence of peripheral nerve stimulation (PNS) or peripheral nerve field stimulation (PNFS), usually centering on the distal end of the lead [4]. Skin erosion of leads or hardware is an uncommon complication of SCS; overall, Cameron reported a 0.2% incidence of skin erosion [3]. In contrast, Verrills et al. [34] reported an incidence of 7% for hardware erosion in 100 cases using PNFS [34]. IPG battery erosion or dehiscence can be reduced by appropriate placement away from mobile or osteal locations and by careful layered closure, with avoidance of suture lines over the implanted device.

Management of skin erosion complications differs for SCS and PNS/PNFS systems, concerns being stratified by the development of the surgical emergent epidural abscess, a serious infection of septic joints, or easily treatable superficial cellulitis [8]. The NACC recommends removal of the SCS device if a deep infection occurs that involves the device pocket, regardless of whether there are systemic infection symptoms, and salvage attempts are discouraged [8].

10.4.2.5 Seroma Formation

A seroma is a collection of serosanguinous fluid at an incision site, which may result from excessive intraoperative tissue trauma and excessive use of electrocautery or excessive blunt dissection. Seromas may delay wound healing and may present as a red, swollen wound without a fever (or with minimal fever). Diagnosis can be confirmed by aspiration with culture and sensitivity. The treatment for a seroma includes a pressure bandage, aspiration, or incision and drainage. The risk of pathogen introduction is critical and should govern the algorithmic risk-benefit assessment for invasive treatment.

If a seroma persists in spite of treatment, reoperation may be advisable to reduce the amount of dead space by paying attention to appropriate closure techniques [8].

10.4.2.6 Pain over the Implant Site

Patients implanted with neuromodulation devices often report pain related to the site of device components, such as pain around the IPG site or pain over the lead-anchor site or lead-extension junctions. In SCS studies, the incidence of component pain is generally low. North et al. [5], Kumar et al. [13] reported no cases of device-related discomfort. Cameron [3] reported 24 cases of device-related discomfort from a total of 2753 (0.9%). IPG site pain may resolve with time and can be treated with topical medications such as lidocaine or capsaicin for symptomatic pain relief. If pain persists over the IPG site or the lead anchor site, then a revision surgery may be necessary.

All components of the patient's health should be optimized prior to moving forward with the implantation, as risk reduction is an easier method of achieving a good outcome than having to manage complications [10].

10.5 Perioperative and Postoperative Care

At the time of the permanent placement surgery, the patient should be assessed for any skin lesions or infections at or near sites of needle entry or incisions. Once in the operating room, the patient should be carefully prepped (using chlorhexidine, betadine, alcohol) over an area greater than 6 cm from the proposed surgical site, and then draped [35]. Povidone-iodine and chlorhexidine-based solutions are two agents commonly utilized for skin preparation [36]. These products are often combined with isopropyl alcohol, which is an effective bactericidal agent that disorganizes cell membrane lipids and denatures cellular proteins. Isopropyl alcohol has been shown to increase the antimicrobial activity of both products. In clinical studies, chlorhexidine-based products were superior to povidone-iodine–based products [37, 38]. Darouiche et al. [37] examined the SSI rates of patients who underwent surgery in six hospitals and were assigned to skin preparation with either chlorhexidine and alcohol or povidone-iodine. The overall rate of SSIs was significantly lower in the chlorhexidine-alcohol group (9.5%) than in the povidone-iodine group (16.1%).

Intraoperatively, careful attention should be given to lead anchoring, to reduce the risk for lead migration. Wound closure is also a very important component in postoperative infection prevention. The incidence of wound infection is generally quoted at 4.5%, but outliers do exist in some practices [39]. The surgical wound should be sutured in multiple layers to appropriately approximate the wound and to minimize any dead space. Skin can be closed with surgical staples or subcuticular suture. Once incisions are closed, a nonocclusive dressing should be applied over the wound and left in place. Surgical incisions should be protected with an occlusive sterile dressing for 24–48 h (CDC Recommendation Category IB) [40–42]. In the recovery area, the patient should be monitored for any neurological changes. Once determined to be medically stable, the patient may be discharged home or to an inpatient postsurgical unit in the hospital, based on the type of neurostimulation device implanted. The patient should be advised to apply ice packs to the area of incisions if experiencing local pain and swelling.

Following the implant of the neurostimulator system, the patient should be advised to call the implanting physician's office for further evaluation if there is a fever of 100 °F or higher, chills, nausea, vomiting, or lethargy. The patient must be evaluated for surgical site redness, warmth, swelling, or drainage from the surgical incision consistent with wound infection. If infection is suspected, baseline laboratory studies should be ordered, including complete blood count (CBC), erythrocyte sedimentation rate (ESR), and C-reactive protein (CRP). Also, if the wound is draining, a specimen should be obtained and sent for culture and sensitivity. If infection is confirmed but is extraneural, oral or intravenous antibiotics can be started. Some cases may require an incision and drainage or even removal of the neurostimulator device to limit the spread of infection (especially epidural spread with SCS). Once the device has been removed and the wound irrigated thoroughly, the wound may be closed with a JP drain or left open to close by secondary intention. A wound care consult and surgery consult should be considered.

Other postoperative complications include wound dehiscence. Wound dehiscence can occur between 5 and 8 days postoperatively and is more common in patients who are diabetic, uremic, immunosuppressed, or smokers [43]. Iatrogenic causes include poor wound closure technique or improper suture selection. If there are no signs of infection, the patient can be taken to the operating room for irrigation and reclosure, but if there is a sign of infection, the system must be explanted [44].

The patient should be instructed to avoid vigorous activity (including not lifting anything heavier than a gallon of milk) and excessive bending or twisting for 6–8 weeks to allow for epidural scar formation to prevent lead migration. The patient should be scheduled to return to the office in 7–14 days for a wound check and/or removal of staples or sutures.

10.6 Conclusions

Neurostimulation is an exceptional option for chronic pain relief in appropriately selected patients. Neuromodulation, when applied responsibly in properly chosen patients by an adequately trained implanter, should have a low complication rate. Institutional educational requirements and interventional society and consensus guidelines, when followed, should protect patients against the misuse of the technology [45]. As with any surgical procedures, there are inherent risks and potential complications that should be discussed with the patient prior to proceeding with implantation of a neurostimulation device. By being vigilant and taking the appropriate precautions preoperatively, intraoperatively, and postoperatively, however, the implanting physician can optimize surgical outcome.

References

1. Shealy CN, Mortimer JT, Reswick J. Electrical inhibition of pain by stimulation of the dorsal column: preliminary clinical reports. Anesth Analg. 1967;46:89–91.
2. Eldrige JS, Weingarten TN, Rho RH. Management of cerebral spinal fluid leak complicating spinal cord stimulator implantation. Pain Pract. 2006;6:285–8.
3. Cameron T. Safety and efficacy of spinal cord stimulation for the treatment of chronic pain: a 20-year literature review. J Neurosurg. 2004;100:254–67.
4. Kumar K, Buchser E, Linderoth B, Meglio M, Van Buyten JP. Avoiding complications from spinal cord stimulation: practical management recommendations from an international panel of experts. Neuromodulation. 2007;10:24–33.
5. North RB, Kidd DH, Farrokhi F, Piantadosi SA. Spinal cord stimulation versus repeated lumbosacral spine surgery for chronic pain: a randomized, controlled trial. Neurosurgery. 2005;56:98–107.
6. Rosenow JM, Stanton-Hicks M, Rezai AR, Henderson JM. Failure modes of spinal cord stimulation hardware. J Neurosurg Spine. 2006;5:183–90.
7. Deer TR, Mekhail N, Provenzano D, Pope J, Krames E, Leong M, et al. The appropriate use of neurostimulation of the spinal cord and peripheral nervous system for the treatment of chronic pain and ischemic diseases: the Neuromodulation Appropriateness Consensus Committee. Neuromodulation. 2014;17:515–50; discussion 550.
8. Deer TR, Mekhail N, Provenzano D, Pope J, Krames E, Thomson S, et al. The appropriate use of neurostimulation: avoidance and treatment of complications of neurostimulation therapies for the treatment of chronic pain. Neuromodulation. 2014;17:571–98.
9. Olson KA, Bedder MD, Anderson VC, Burchiel KJ, Villanueva MR. Psychological variables associated with outcome of spinal cord stimulation trials. Neuromodulation. 1998;1:6–13.
10. Celestin J, Edwards RR, Jamison RN. Pretreatment psychosocial variables as predictors of outcomes following lumbar surgery and spinal cord stimulation: a systematic review and literature synthesis. Pain Med. 2009;10:639–53.
11. Deer T, Stewart D. Complications of spinal cord stimulation: identification, treatment, and prevention. Pain Med. 2008;9:S93–101.
12. Turner JA, Loeser JD, Deyo RA, Sanders SB. Spinal cord stimulation for patients with failed back surgery syndrome or complex regional pain syndrome: a systematic review of effectiveness and complications. Pain. 2004;108:137–47.

13. Kumar K, Taylor RS, Jacques L, Eldabe S, Meglio M, Molet J, et al. Spinal cord stimulation versus conventional medical management for neuropathic pain: a multicentre randomised controlled trial in patients with failed back surgery syndrome. Pain. 2007;132:179–88.
14. Mangram AJ, Horan TC, Pearson ML, Silver LC, Jarvis WR. Guideline for prevention of surgical site infection, 1999. Hospital Infection Control Practices Advisory Committee. Infect Control Hosp Epidemiol. 1999;20:250–78.
15. Follett KA, Boortz-Marx RL, Drake JM, DuPen S, Schneider SJ, Turner MS, Coffey RJ. Prevention and management of intrathecal drug delivery and spinal cord stimulation system infections. Anesthesiology. 2004;100:1582–94.
16. Bjerk N, Hobson DW, Seal LA. Preoperative skin preparation: a systems approach. Infect Control Today. 2001;1–5.
17. Beer GM, Wallner H. Prevention of seroma after abdominoplasty. Aesthet Surg J. 2010;30:414–7.
18. Kumar K, Wilson JR, Taylor RS, Gupta S. Complications of spinal cord stimulation, suggestions to improve outcome, and financial impact. J Neurosurg Spine. 2006;5:191–203.
19. Fletcher N, Sofianos D, Berkes MB, Obremskey WT. Prevention of perioperative infection. J Bone Joint Surg Am. 2007;89:1605–18.
20. Bowater RJ, Stirling SA, Lilford RJ. Is antibiotic prophylaxis in surgery a generally effective intervention? Testing a generic hypothesis over a set of meta-analyses. Ann Surg. 2009;249:551–6.
21. McDonald M, Grabsch E, Marshall C, Forbes A. Single- versus multiple-dose antimicrobial prophylaxis for major surgery: a systematic review. Aust N Z J Surg. 1998;68:388–96.
22. Ohtori S, Inoue G, Koshi T, Yamashita M, Yamauchi K, Suzuki M, et al. Long-term intravenous administration of antibiotics for lumbar spinal surgery prolongs the duration of hospital stay and time to normalize body temperature after surgery. Spine. 2008;33:2935–7.
23. Nelson CL, Green TG, Porter RA, Warren RD. One day versus seven days of preventive antibiotic therapy in orthopedic surgery. Clin Orthop Relat Res. 1983;176:258–63.
24. Barolat G. Experience with 509 plate electrodes implanted epidurally from C1 to L1. Stereotact Funct Neurosurg. 1993;61:60–79.
25. Levy R, Henderson J, Slavin K, Simpson BA, Barolat G, Shipley J, North R. Incidence and avoidance of neurologic complications with paddle type spinal cord stimulation leads. Neuromodulation. 2011;14:412–22.
26. Santiago FM, Santiago J, Prieto M, García-Sánchez MJ, Sánchez-Carríon JM, Martínez-Tellería A, Garzón A. Dorsal epidural hematoma after implantation of a dorsal nerve stimulator. Rev Esp Anestesiol Reanim. 2005;52:440–1.
27. Smith CC, Lin JL, Shokat M, Dosanjh SS, Casthely D. A report of paraparesis following spinal cord stimulator trial, implantation and revision. Pain Physician. 2010;13:357–63.
28. Zan E, Kurt KN, Yousem DM, Christo PJ. Spinal cord stimulators: typical positioning and postsurgical complications. Am J Roentgenol. 2011;196:437–45.
29. Takawira N, Han RJ, Nguyen TQ, Gaines JD, Han TH. Spinal cord stimulator and epidural haematoma. Br J Anaesth. 2012;109:649–50.
30. Giberson CE, Barbosa J, Brooks ES, McGlothlen GL, Grigsby EJ, Kohut JJ, et al. Epidural hematomas following removal of percutaneous spinal cord stimulator trial leads: two case reports. Reg Anesth Pain Med. 2014;39:73–7.
31. Rai A, Carpenter J, Miele V. Epidural blood patch at C2: diagnosis and treatment of spontaneous intracranial hypotension. Am J Neuroradiol. 2005;26:2663–6.
32. Meyer SC, Swartz K, Johnson JO. Quadraparesis and spinal cord stimulation: case report. Spine. 2007;32:E565–8.
33. North RB, Recinos VR, Attenello FJ, Shipley J, Long DM. Prevention of percutaneous spinal cord stimulation electrode migration: a 15-year experience. Neuromodulation. 2014;17:670–6; discussion 676–7.
34. Verrills P, Vivian D, Mitchell B, Barnard A. Peripheral nerve field stimulation for chronic pain: 100 cases and review of the literature. Pain Med. 2011;12:1395–405.

35. Seal LA, Paul-Cheadle D. A systems approach to preoperative surgical patient skin preparation. Am J Infect Control. 2004;32:57–62.
36. Lio PA, Kaye ET. Topical antibacterial agents. Med Clin North Am. 2011;95:703–21.
37. Darouiche RO, Wall MJ Jr, Itani KM, Otterson MF, Webb AL, Carrick MM, et al. Chlorhexidine-alcohol versus povidone-iodine for surgical-site antisepsis. N Engl J Med. 2010;362:18–26.
38. Ostrander RV, Botte MJ, Brage ME. Efficacy of surgical preparation solutions in foot and ankle surgery. J Bone Joint Surg Am. 2005;87:980–5.
39. Torrens JK, Stanley PJ, Fagaunathan PL, Bush DJ. Risk of infection with electrical stimulation. Lancet. 1997;349(9053):729.
40. Chrintz H, Vibits H, Cordtz TO, Harreby JS, Waaddegaard P, Larsen SO. Need for surgical wound dressing. Br J Surg. 1989;76:204–5.
41. Hutchinson JJ, McGuckin M. Occlusive dressings: a microbiologic and clinical review. Am J Infect Control. 1990;18:257–68.
42. Hutchinson JJ, Lawrence JC. Wound infection under occlusive dressings. J Hosp Infect. 1991;17:83–94.
43. Kreis P, Fishman S. Spinal cord stimulation: percutaneous implantation techniques. New York: Oxford University Press; 2009. p. 135–8.
44. Mullholland MW, Doherty GM. Complications in surgery. Philadelphia: Lippincott Williams & Wilkins; 2006.
45. Krames ES, Monis S, Poree L, Deer T, Levy R. Using the SAFE principles when evaluating electrical stimulation therapies for the pain of failed back surgery syndrome. Neuromodulation. 2011;14:299–311.

Chapter 11
Extracranial Peripheral Nerve and Peripheral Nerve Field Stimulation for Headache: Trialing

Michael Yang

As with spinal cord stimulation (SCS), trialing is needed to test for efficacy prior to permanent implantation of peripheral nerve stimulation and peripheral nerve field stimulation. Though there are some similarities between SCS and peripheral nerve and peripheral nerve field stimulation, there are also unique differences in pre-trial preparation, patient selection, and particularly the techniques involved. This chapter discusses the various steps in successful peripheral nerve stimulation and peripheral nerve field stimulation trials.

11.1 Introduction

Peripheral nerve stimulation (PNS) is the direct electrical stimulation of specific nerves outside of the central nervous system; peripheral nerve field stimulation (PNfS) is the stimulation of an area where specific nerve(s) cannot be identified, using superficial, subcutaneous lead placement. The procedures and technique for both are very similar except for the primary targets: PNS procedures will target the specific nerve, whereas PNfs will target the approximate area of pain the patient experiences.

PNS can be performed through either an open surgical or a percutaneous technique, well described by Stanton-Hicks and Salamon [1]. The percutaneous technique is more common because of the ease of subcutaneous placement and the reduced risk to the patient. PNS and PNfs directly inhibit primary nociceptive afferents; thus, one can infer that central sensitization can be diminished or avoided by peripheral nociceptive suppression. Though multitudes of peripheral nerves can be affected, this chapter focuses mainly on the uses of PNS and PNfs for controlling

M. Yang (✉)
Summit Pain Alliance, Santa Rosa, CA, USA
e-mail: Michael.i.yang@gmail.com

S. Diwan, T.R. Deer (eds.), *Advanced Procedures for Pain Management*,
https://doi.org/10.1007/978-3-319-68841-1_11

headaches (migraine, trigeminal neuralgia, occipital neuralgia, supraorbital neuralgia, cervicogenic headache, and hemicrania continua) [2].

11.2 Pre-trial Preparation

As with SCS, patient selection in PNS and PNfs is vital to the success of the trial and permanent implant.

- As with all procedures, informed consent must be obtained. The patient should be informed the risks and benefits, dangers, and possible side effects of the procedure. Many percutaneous neuromodulatory stimulation devices are not approved for PNS or PNfS by the FDA, so thorough discussion with the patient regarding this "off-label" use is essential.
- A strong history of psychological pathology does confound the efficacy of stimulation therapy. Most insurance companies require psychological pre-screening prior to spinal cord stimulator trial. Comorbid psychiatric illness reduces interventional treatment success rates [3], but one should also appreciate the fact that approximately 20–45% of chronic pain patients have accompanying psychopathology [4].
- A thorough physical exam is necessary to document the pain patterns and determine whether the pain follows a specific peripheral nerve distribution or affects a generalized field where no specific nerve can be identified.
- Contraindications include local infection near the injection site, coagulopathy, cognitive inability to manage the stimulator, comorbidities or conditions that prevent fluoroscopic or ultrasound needle guidance, and inability to obtain consent [5].
- PNS and PNfs trial lead placement is superficial in nature, so the bleeding risk is attenuated compared with procedures inside the spinal canal. The American Society of Regional Anesthesia guidelines for preoperative anticoagulation are therefore less appropriate for guidance in these cases; nevertheless, sound clinical judgement should be applied despite a decreased risk of bleeding and/or permanent neurological damage.

11.3 Trial Lead Implantation

11.3.1 Supraorbital and/or Infraorbital Nerve Stimulation Trial

Slavin and Wess [6] described the most commonly employed technique for terminal branch trigeminal nerve stimulation. The patient is prepared in usual sterile fashion. Local anesthesia is used to infiltrate the skin after fluoroscopic confirmation of the

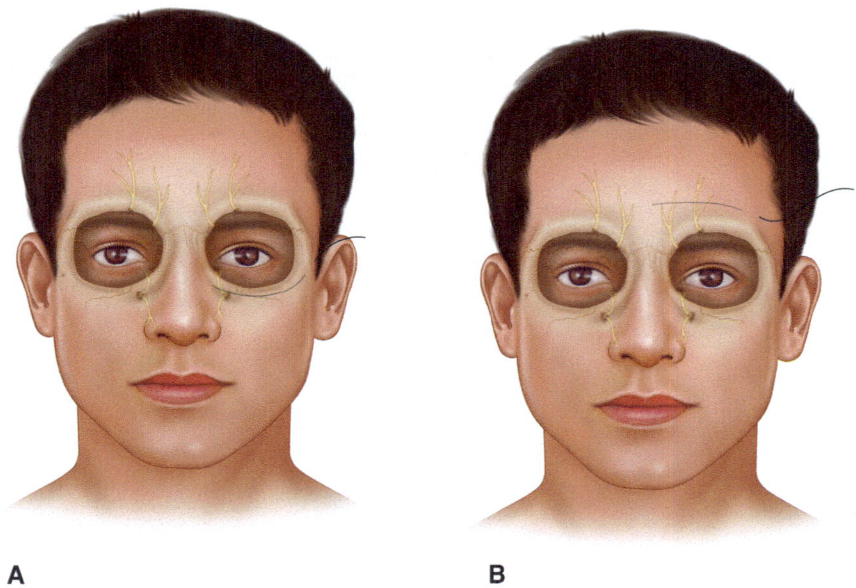

Fig. 11.1 Technique for infraorbital (**a**) and supraorbital (**b**) lead placement

site (3–4 cm lateral and 1–2 cm superior to the lateral corner of the eye). A small incision is then made, and a standard 14G Touhy needle is directed toward the midline approximately 1 cm above the supraorbital ridge until it is approximately 1 cm from the midline (Fig. 11.1). The needle should be bent to allow for the contour of the patient's face.

For the infraorbital nerve, the target site is the infraorbital foramen on fluoroscopy, which is approximately 1 cm below the orbit and just lateral to the ipsilateral nose. The entry point is lateral and inferior to the eye over the zygomatic arch (Fig. 11.1) [6]. It is important to keep the needle in the subcutaneous layer, avoiding too superficial placement (to prevent lead tip erosion) or too deep of placement (to avoid motor recruitment).

The stylet is removed, the percutaneous electrode is placed, and the needle is withdrawn to allow for intraoperative stimulation testing. Judicious use of local anesthetic only at the puncture site will allow for intraoperative testing.

Once the desired therapeutic paresthesia overlying the patient's pain is achieved, the needle is withdrawn and removed while performing serial fluoroscopic guidance to ensure that there is no inadvertent lead migration (Fig. 11.2). The externalized lead is then secured with the supplied plastic anchor of the surgeons choosing and nonabsorbable sutures. A sterile dressing is applied and the patient is taken to the recovery area.

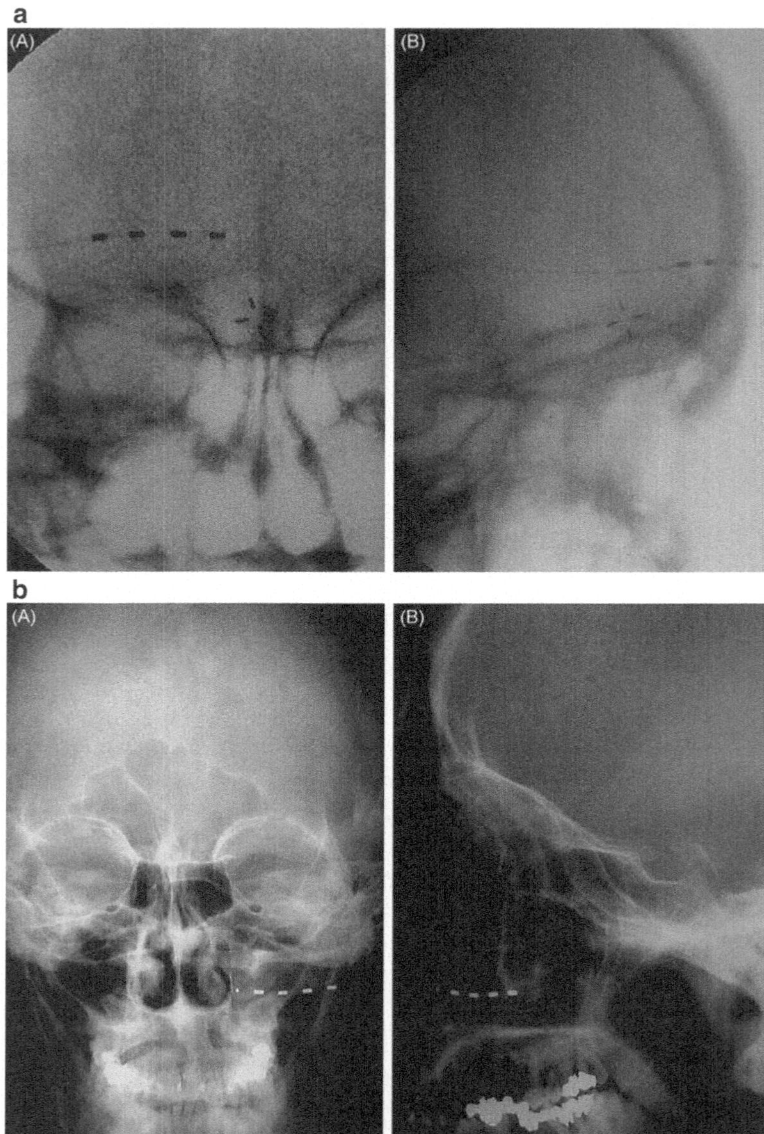

Fig. 11.2 Fluoroscopic images of supraorbital (**a**) and infraorbital (**b**) lead placement (Reprinted from Slavin and Wess [6]; with permission)

11.3.2 Greater Occipital Nerve Stimulation Trial

The greater occipital nerve is the medial branch of dorsal primary rami of C2; it has become a popular target for the treatment of cervicogenic headaches [7, 8]. Anatomic landmarks include the mastoid process and the occipital protuberance. It is generally found 1.5 cm lateral from the external occipital protuberance and 3.5 cm inferior. The nerve is always medial to the occipital artery (Fig. 11.3).

Many different techniques have been described to stimulate the greater occipital nerve. The main differences are percutaneous cylindrical versus paddle lead (Fig. 11.4), medial-to-lateral versus lateral-to-medial, or C1-2 versus nuchal ridge [8, 9].

Proponents of the paddle lead argue that the paddle lead, due to its unidirectional current, may cause less circumferential stimulation and thus less skin burning sensation. There may be an argument for less lead migration with the paddle lead as well, owing to its larger surface area. Depending on the needle trajectory and anatomical placement of the leads, muscle spasm may be avoided by placing the electrodes more superficially, but this may increase the chance of erosion and skin paresthesia [7–9].

The trial is performed with the patient in the prone position. The surgical site is prepared and draped in sterile fashion, leaving the entry site exposed. Image guidance is a prerequisite; fluoroscopy and/or ultrasound guidance is commonly used. After the target location is chosen, the incision site is identified and marked. Judicious local anesthetic should be used at the incision site while avoiding the greater occipital nerve. This chapter focuses on the medial, nuchal approach.

An incision is made in the mid-line just caudal to the occipital protuberance. The needle is bent to accommodate the contour of the head. Under fluoroscopic and/or ultrasound guidance, the needle is placed along the nuchal ridge ipsilateral to the target greater occipital nerve. Once an appropriate lead position is achieved, the needle is withdrawn slightly to allow for intraoperative stimulation testing. Once therapeutic stimulation is achieved, the needle is removed and the lead is secured using nonabsorbable suture. A sterile dressing is applied, and further programming and assessment is performed in the recovery room.

11.4 Post-implant Techniques and Complications

All the trial lead placements can be intraoperatively tested for the efficacy of the stimulation if judicious use of local anesthesia is applied only at the incision site. If there is accidental injection of the local anesthetic to the field or to the target peripheral nerve, then trial stimulation must be carried out postoperatively.

Postoperative prophylactic antibiotics are not usually necessary during the trial, a period typically lasting 4–7 days. Removal of the leads usually is the first course of action if infection is suspected. If signs of infection continue after lead removal,

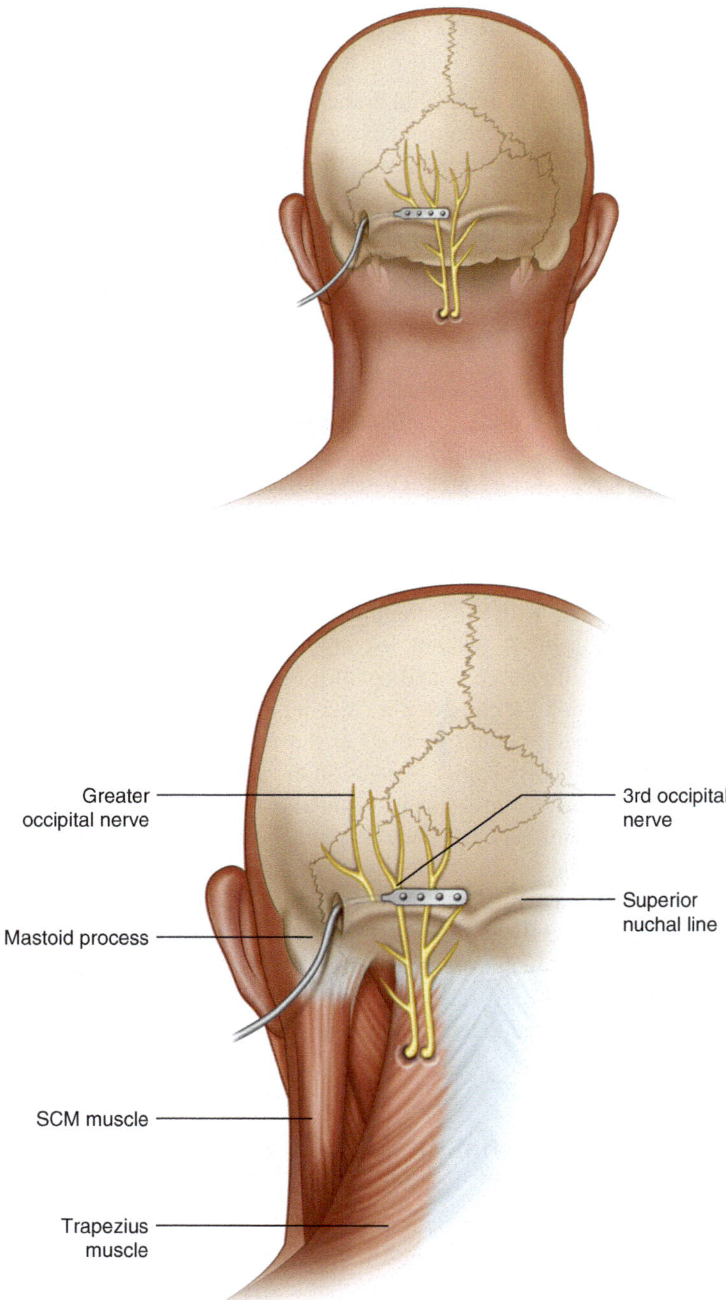

Fig. 11.3 Greater occipital nerve diagram. *SCM* sternocleidomastoid

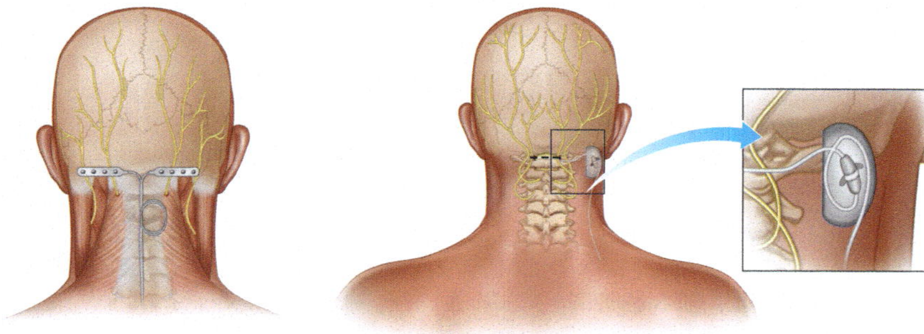

Fig. 11.4 Percutaneous and paddle occipital nerve stimulation lead placements

then a course of appropriate antibiotics is warranted. Some physicians may decide to have longer PNS and PNfs trial periods, as the procedural morbidity or mortality is very low because of the superficial nature of the lead placement. If the patient experiences more than 50% pain relief during the trial, it is deemed successful, and permanent device placement can be carried out 3–4 weeks later.

Potential complications include infection, lead migration, overstimulation, hardware malfunction, myofascial spasm or pain, and patient dislike of stimulation/paresthesia.

11.5 Clinical Pearls

- Thorough knowledge of peripheral nerve anatomy and use of fluoroscopic and/or ultrasound guidance is essential to the success of the trial lead implant.
- As with spinal cord stimulation, the most common complication is lead migration.
- Because PNS and PNfs are off-label uses of a device that was approved for spinal cord stimulation, judicious adaptation of the equipment is necessary to maximize efficacy. Bending the needle to fit the contour of the implant region is vital to placement of the leads in the subcutaneous layer.
- Placement that is too superficial may lead to skin burning sensation and/or lead tip erosion; placement too deep may lead to motor recruitment.
- Most insurance companies require psychological prescreening, as there are significant comorbidities associated with severe psychological pathology that will likely confound the success of the trial.
- Careful use of local anesthesia only at the needle's insertion site is paramount to enable intraoperative PNS and PNfS testing.
- PNS and PNfS procedures have low morbidity and mortality, owing to the superficial nature of the lead placement.

References

1. Stanton-Hicks M, Salamon J. Stimulation of the central and peripheral nervous system for the control of pain. J Clin Neurophysiol. 1997;14:46–62.
2. Bittar RG, Teddy PJ. Peripheral neuromodulation for pain. J Clin Neurosci. 2009;16:1259–61.
3. Fishbain DA, Goldberg M, Meagher BR, Steele R, Rosomoff H. Male and female chronic pain patients categorized by DSM-III psychiatric diagnostic criteria. Pain. 1986;26:181–97.
4. Gallagher R. Primary care and pain medicine: a community solution to the public health problem of chronic pain. Med Clin North Am. 1999;83:555–83.
5. Torrens K, Stanely PJ, Ragunathan PL, Bush DJ. Risk of infection with electrical spinal cord stimulation. Lancet. 1997;349:729.
6. Slavin KV, Wess C. Trigeminal branch stimulation for intractable neuropathic pain: technical note. Neuromodulation. 2005;8:7–13.
7. Oh MY, Ortega J, Bellotte JB, Whiting DM, Aló K. Peripheral nerve stimulation for the treatment of occipital neuralgia and transformed migraine using a c1-2-3 subcutaneous paddle style electrode: a technical report. Neuromodulation. 2004;7:103–12.
8. Hayek SM, Jasper JF, Deer TR, Narouze SN. Occipital neurostimulation-induced muscle spasms: implications for lead placement. Pain Physician. 2009;12:867–76.
9. Jasper JF, Hayek SM. Implanted occipital nerve stimulators. Pain Physician. 2008;11:187–200.

Chapter 12
Extracranial Peripheral Nerve Field and Peripheral Nerve Stimulation for Headache: Permanent Implant

Michael Yang and Lucas W. Campos

As with traditional spinal cord stimulation, after completing a successful trial with greater than 50% pain relief, the patient is eligible to proceed with placement of a permanent implant for peripheral nerve stimulation or peripheral nerve field stimulation. This chapter discusses the techniques used in the permanent implantation, as well as post-implantation protocols and follow-up.

12.1 Introduction

Disorders of the peripheral nervous system often present a unique challenge. Severe neuropathic pain can be extremely resistant to typical pain treatments. Painful peripheral nerve disorders often have pain in a particular nerve distribution. Thus, an optimal treatment modality should deliver targeted relief to the precise distribution of the pain. To be considered for peripheral nerve stimulation (PNS) or peripheral nerve field stimulation (PNfS), patients should have chronic, severe, disabling neuropathic pain refractory to other treatments, including medications, nerve blocks, and physical therapy [1]. Local anesthetic block may confirm which nerve is affected, but is not predictive of PNS success [2].

The ability to focus therapeutic stimulation into the distribution of a specific peripheral nerve without providing unwanted stimulation into other areas represents the primary advantage of PNS/PNfS [3]. Examples of indications for PNS/PNfS include postherpetic neuralgia, postsurgical neuropathic pain, and occipital, inguinal, and genitofemoral neuralgia [4]. PNS/PNfs is also used to treat migraine (both chronic and transformed), hemicrania continua, cluster headaches, and other chronic daily headaches [5].

M. Yang • L.W. Campos (✉)
Summit Pain Alliance, Santa Rosa, CA, USA
e-mail: Michael.i.yang@gmail.com; lwcamposmdphd@gmail.com

S. Diwan, T.R. Deer (eds.), *Advanced Procedures for Pain Management*,
https://doi.org/10.1007/978-3-319-68841-1_12

The success of the therapy hinges on appropriate candidate selection and optimal placement of the leads for most effective stimulation. Although PNS/PNfS has a lower risk of complications than spinal cord stimulation (SCS), infection, lead erosion, and mechanical issues must be considered. Patients with suboptimal outcomes may have unrealistic expectations for the device. The benefits and techniques for the implantation of the percutaneous, cylindrical leads have been described in the previous chapter. This chapter focuses on proper lead placement and implantation of the battery for the permanent implantation of PNS/PNfs systems, and minimizing of adverse events.

12.2 Pre-implant Preparation and Considerations

- A thorough physical examination is necessary to identify specific peripheral nerve involvement or to determine whether the pain is generalized to a specific field involving multiple nerve endings.
- As with all procedures, informed consent must be obtained. The patient should know the risks, benefits, and alternatives for the procedure. Although these were clearly delineated before the trial, they should be repeated before the implantation procedure.
- Diagnostic imaging and preoperative lab work should be reviewed to ensure the absence of any anatomic, hematologic, or metabolic pathology that would preclude implantation. BMI, diabetes control, MRI compatibility and the need for future MRIs should also be considered [6].
- A pretrial psychological screening should have been performed before the trial. This screening is meant to detect cognitive impairment or dementia, substance abuse, untreated anxiety or depression, or unrealistic expectations related to the stimulator [7].
- The use of preoperative antibiotics is well established and should be completed prior to incision [8, 9]. The choice of preoperative antibiotic administration should be based on local pathogens and sensitivity.
- Patients previously identified as carriers of methicillin-resistant *Staphylococcus aureus* (MRSA) are known to be at an increased risk for infection. A preoperative nasal swab should be incorporated into the selection process for these patients to confirm that MRSA is not present at the time of surgery [9, 10].

12.3 Placement of the Permanent Implant

- After prepping and draping the patient in usual sterile fashion, a skin wheal is raised. Careful attention is made to minimize the amount of local anesthetic, to avoid spread to the region of final lead placement, which would inhibit the patient's perception of paresthesia during intraoperative trial stimulation.

- Using a scalpel with a #11 blade, a puncture incision of approximately 5 mm is made to minimize tissue disruption. An appropriately curved Tuohy needle is advanced through the incision. A loss of resistance signifies entrance into the subcutaneous space.
- The interventionalist then grips the needle hub and applies slight posterior pressure. This creates a "tenting" of the tissue as the distal portion of the needle is raised below the skin surface. The free hand is used to palpate the skin surface and assess advancement of the needle as denoted by the tenting of the skin.
- When properly performed, minimal resistance is noted as the tip of the needle is advanced subcutaneously. If there is substantial resistance to advancement of the needle and if skin dimpling is produced, then the lead is too superficial, and the needle must be redirected into a deeper plane. If the needle tip cannot be palpated, it is too deep in the subcutaneous tissues and must be redirected superficially.
- The stylet is then removed from the introducer needle and the lead is advanced through the needle lumen.
- The needle is then withdrawn over the lead prior to performing intraoperative stimulation.
- After performing intraoperative stimulation, the leads are secured to the skin, either using an anchoring device or by suturing directly to the lead.
- As with the trial lead implantation, successful pain coverage is achieved by the positioning of the lead so that it is adjacent to (or at least very near) the target nerve.
- In PNfs, the lead is placed at the central, focal point of the pain region. The techniques and procedures used in the implantation of the lead(s) were explained in detail in the previous chapter.
- Once the leads are in place, they are tunneled subcutaneously to the battery site, where a subcutaneous pocket is created to house the implantable pulse generator (Figs. 12.1, 12.2, 12.3 and 12.4).

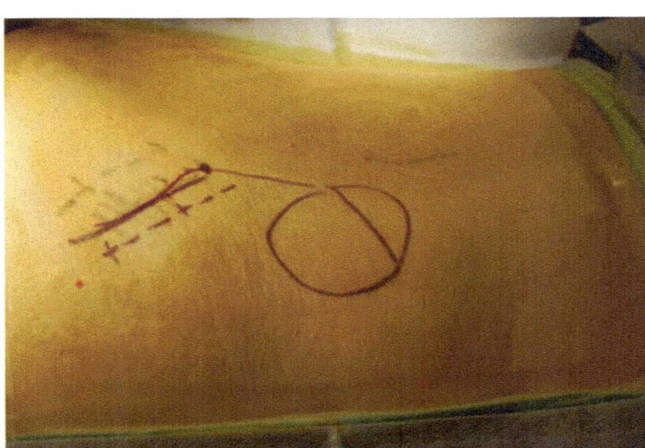

Fig. 12.1 When creating a pocket for the implantable pulse generator (IPG), the physician should carefully plan its location based on factors such as the lead target, the patient's body habitus, and patient function (*Reprinted from* Deer TR, Stewart CD. Pocketing techniques for spinal cord stimulation and peripheral nerve stimulation. In: Deer and Pope, eds. [14]; p 72; *with permission*)

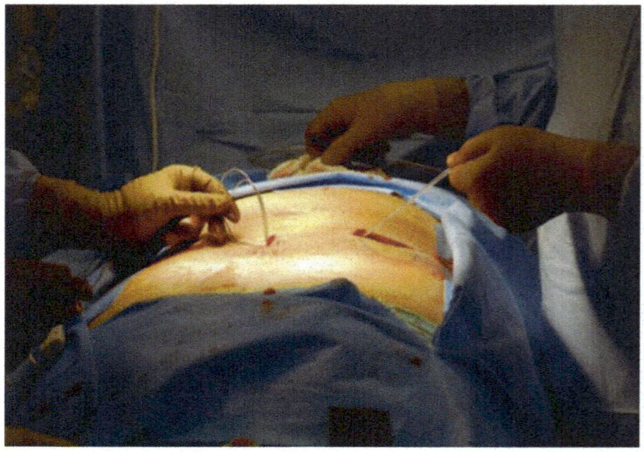

Fig. 12.2 After the pocket is created, the leads are tunneled into the pocket. Lead length should be long enough to create a strain relief loop, which reduces lead migration (*Reprinted from* Deer TR, Stewart CD. Pocketing techniques for spinal cord stimulation and peripheral nerve stimulation. In: Deer and Pope, eds. [14]; p 74; *with permission*)

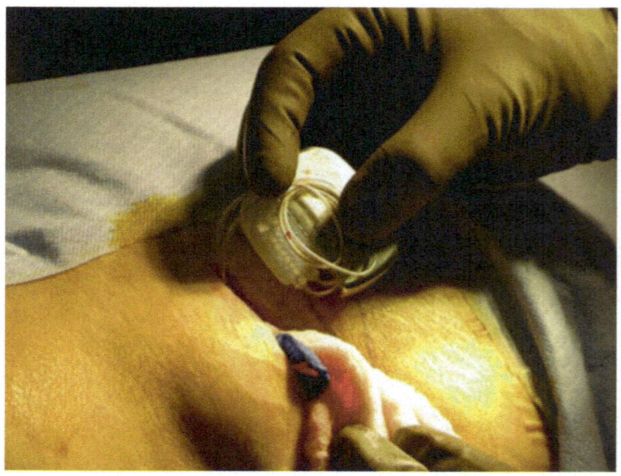

Fig. 12.3 Excess lead length should be secured using a strain relief loop at the surgical site of lead placement and at the pocket site, placing the wire below the generator (*Reprinted from* Deer TR, Stewart CD. Pocketing techniques for spinal cord stimulation and peripheral nerve stimulation. In: Deer and Pope, eds. [14]; p 72; *with permission*)

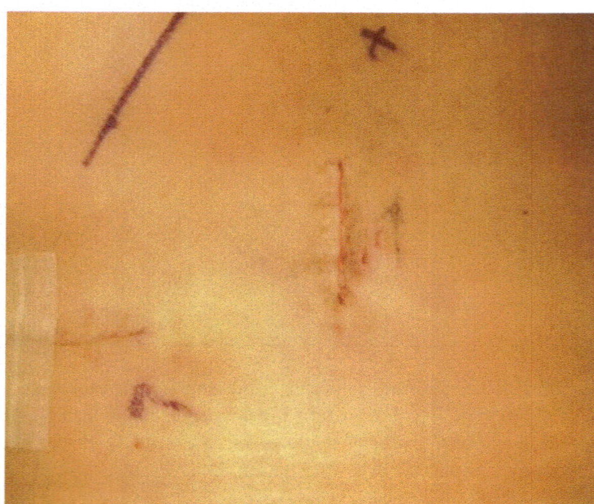

Fig. 12.4 Example of a well-healing IPG pocket site (*Reprinted from* Deer TR, Stewart CD. Pocketing techniques for spinal cord stimulation and peripheral nerve stimulation. In: Deer and Pope, eds. [14]; p 75; *with permission*)

12.4 Clinical Pearls

- Tunneling leads across joints and highly mobile regions of the body (*e.g.* neck, axilla, lower back) may increase the incidence of lead migration. If forced to cross a joint line, the range of motion in the joint and the overall length of the system (array to IPG) must be considered. Sufficient strain relief loop size must be made to allow for incomplete loop closure. Extreme joint extension or flexion should not tighten the loop to such a degree that a kink appears, or the lead will likely fracture.
- Pain relief requires attention to two fundamental details: lead depth and lead positioning into the region of maximal pain. Superficial lead placement results in painful dysesthesia (burning and stinging sensation) at low sensory thresholds. Deep placement may cause insertion into muscle tissue or inability to recruit terminal sensory afferents at low energies.
- If too much local anesthetic is placed at the stab wound, the needle may pull the local anesthetic deeper and anesthetize the target neural fibers. Occasionally blood or swelling around the lead array also will insulate it and diminish paresthesia. The interventionalist must simply wait and retest the array after the swelling or anesthetic effect abates and good paresthesia is felt without lead repositioning.

12.5 Post-implant Considerations

- Programming for PNS/PNfS systems is based on the target neural tissue and different impedance characteristics of the subcutaneous layer.
- Both conventional and advanced PNS/PNfS programming techniques can demand higher energy requirements for paresthesia and pain relief, depending on the area of coverage.
- Patients often report the area between multiple electrodes as one solid area of paresthesia, rather than distinctly different, smaller areas of paresthesia. Paresthesia does not appear to be diluted as the distance between electrodes increases, but increased power is required.
- Whether postoperative infections are reduced with the continued use of antibiotic prophylaxis remains controversial [11, 12]. Other postoperative measures to reduce infection risk may include utilization of dressings impregnated with silver [13].

References

1. Campbell JN, Long DM. Peripheral nerve stimulation in the treatment of intractable pain. J Neurosurg. 1976;45:692–9.
2. Soin A, Fang Z-P, Velasco J. Peripheral neuromodulation to treat postamputation pain. Prog Neurol Surg. 2015;29:158–67.

3. Petersen EA, Slavin KV. Peripheral nerve/field stimulation for chronic pain. Neurosurg Clin N Am. 2014;25:789–97.
4. Papuć E, Rejdak K. The role of neurostimulation in the treatment of neuropathic pain. Ann Agric Environ Med. 2013;1:14–7.
5. Reed KL, Black SB, Banta CJ II, Will KR. Combined occipital and supraorbital neurostimulation for the treatment of chronic migraine headaches: initial experience. Cephalalgia. 2010;30:260–71.
6. Manchikanti L. Evidence-based medicine, systematic reviews, and guidelines in interventional pain management, part I: introduction and general considerations. Pain Physician. 2008;11:161–86.
7. Campbell CM, Jamison RN, Edwards RR. Psychological screening/phenotyping as predictors for spinal cord stimulation. Curr Pain Headache Rep. 2013;17:307.
8. Epstein NE. Preoperative, intraoperative, and postoperative measures to further reduce spinal infections. Surg Neurol Int. 2011;2:17.
9. Follett KA, Boortz-Marx RL, Drake JM, DuPen S, Schneider SJ, Turner MS, Coffey RJ. Prevention and management of intrathecal drug delivery and spinal cord stimulation system infections. Anesthesiology. 2004;100:1582–94.
10. Rathmell JP, Lake T, Ramundo MB. Infectious risks of chronic pain treatments: injection therapy, surgical implants, and intradiscal techniques. Reg Anesth Pain Med. 2006;31:346–52.
11. Kakimaru H, Kono M, Matsusaki M, Iwata A, Uchio Y. Postoperative antimicrobial prophylaxis following spinal decompression surgery: is it necessary? J Orthop Sci. 2010;15:305–9.
12. Kanafani ZA, Dakdouki GK, El-Dbouni O, Bawwab T, Kanj SS. Surgical site infections following spinal surgery at a tertiary care center in Lebanon: incidence, microbiology, and risk factors. Scand J Infect Dis. 2006;38:589–92.
13. Epstein NE. Do silver-impregnated dressings limit infections after lumbar laminectomy with instrumented fusion? Surg Neurol. 2007;68:483–5; discussion 485.
14. Deer TR, Pope JE. Atlas of implantable therapies for pain management. 2nd ed. New York: Springer Science + Business Media; 2016.

Chapter 13
Intracranial Neuromodulation: Deep Brain Stimulation for Pain

Steven M. Falowski

Deep brain stimulation (DBS) is a form of intracranial stimulation in which electrical current can be delivered to deep nuclei. It is performed by the insertion of implanted electrodes via a burrhole to the subcortical targets, utilizing navigation. It is a reversible and adjustable procedure that falls under the category of neuromodulation; because it is less invasive than other neurosurgical procedures, it carries a low risk profile.

DBS has become a standard procedure performed by neurosurgeons for multiple indications. The most common indications include movement disorders such as Parkinson's disease, essential tremor, and dystonia. This indication gained Food and Drug Administration (FDA) approval in the United States in 1997, but even earlier, it had gained traction as a treatment option for chronic pain, and it has been utilized in this regard since the 1970s. It gained initial FDA approval following a multicenter trial for the treatment of chronic pain conditions, but this approval was retracted [1]. Further trials would be necessary to determine its efficacy and safety in this regard. Although considered investigational in the United States, it is a viable treatment option carrying significant response rates in those with peripheral neuropathic pain, nociceptive pain, failed back surgery syndrome (FBSS), phantom limb pain, and cephalalgias.

13.1 Indications

DBS carries favorable results for the treatment of chronic pain, with multiple chronic pain conditions reported in the literature that respond to the therapy. It carries favorable results for various indications and can be used when conservative

---

S.M. Falowski (✉)
Department of Neurosurgery, St. Luke's University Health Network, Bethlehem, PA, USA
e-mail: sfalowski@gmail.com

S. Diwan, T.R. Deer (eds.), *Advanced Procedures for Pain Management*,
https://doi.org/10.1007/978-3-319-68841-1_13

methods, medications, and extracranial procedures have not been successful. Indications have included FBSS, phantom limb pain, facial neuropathic pain, and peripheral neuropathic pain. The response rate is higher for those with nociceptive pain than for those with neuropathic pain. Cephalalgias have promising results, with cluster headaches carrying the best success rates. Its use has also been reported after amputation, brachial plexus injury, stroke, spine injury, and multiple sclerosis [2].

A meta-analysis of DBS for pain relief demonstrated long-term success in those with intractable low back pain (FBSS), as well as patients with phantom limb pain and neuropathies. Interestingly, DBS was more effective for nociceptive than for deafferentation pain [3]. An additional literature review found a range of success from 47 to 60% with up to 80 months' follow-up in the use of DBS for chronic pain [4]. Overall efficacy was also reported for refractory nociceptive pain (61%) and phantom limb pain (71%) [5].

A single study found that those patients with phantom limb pain or pain after brachial plexus injury and anesthesia dolorosa obtained the highest relief [6], with post-stroke pain responding in 70% of patients. Various reports in the literature have shown that DBS can be used in the treatment of other painful conditions, including post-herpetic trigeminal nerve pain [7]. It has also been found to be an effective treatment for cluster headaches, with an overall efficacy rate for primary headache disorders reported as 65% [8, 9].

DBS should be assessed and included in a treatment paradigm that involves other interventions such as spinal cord stimulation, peripheral nerve stimulation, and intrathecal therapy. In this vein, combination therapies have gained some traction in the treatment of FBSS, with the spinal cord stimulator (SCS) being able to treat the neuropathic leg pain, whereas the nociceptive back pain is relieved by DBS [10]. Supraorbital stimulation has been used in conjunction with DBS for the treatment of cluster headaches [11].

13.2 Targets

Multiple targets for DBS have been described in the literature. These have included the ventrocaudalis thalamic nucleus, globus pallidus, subthalamic nuclei, ventral striatum, periventricular grey (PVG), and periaqueductal grey (PAG) matter. The use of these targets is variable, especially in the face of complex pain patterns. Pain syndromes can be ill-defined and may include different combinations of pain. For example, FBSS patients may have both nociceptive low back pain and neuropathic leg pain.

Many authors favor the use of PAG/PVG stimulation in the treatment of nociceptive pain, whereas ventroposterolateral (VPL) and ventroposteromedial (VPM) stimulation is favored for those with neuropathic pain [4]. These targets carry long-term success for intractable low back pain, with a meta-analysis demonstrating the highest success with PVG/PAG stimulation [3].

Post-amputation phantom limb pain and post-stroke pain have been treated with DBS of the PVG, with the highest degree of pain alleviation [6]. Post-herpetic neuralgia of the trigeminal nerve is treated with stimulation of the PVG/PAG and/or the VPM nucleus of the thalamus [7]. Cluster headaches may carry the most significant success with DBS that commonly targets the ipsilateral posterior inferior hypothalamus [8, 9].

13.3 Surgical Technique and Complications

DBS is performed using stereotactic navigation for placement of the electrodes. Either a frame can be placed or other methods can be used that employ fiducial markers and platforms for the head. Stereotactic imaging can include CT scan imaging or MRI. Surgery is generally performed utilizing intravenous sedation with local anesthesia for the incisions.

Electrodes are commonly placed into subcortical targets using microelectrode recording, which gives the ability to "map out" the desired target nucleus. Additional test stimulation can be performed to confirm proper placement without unwanted side effects from adjacent structures [12]. As with other neuromodulation procedures, a trial period is needed to determine efficacy. Patients will therefore have these electrodes externalized for that period; if the treatment is successful, the patient returns within a week to have internalization of the electrodes and placement of generators. Figure 13.1 shows completed DBS placement.

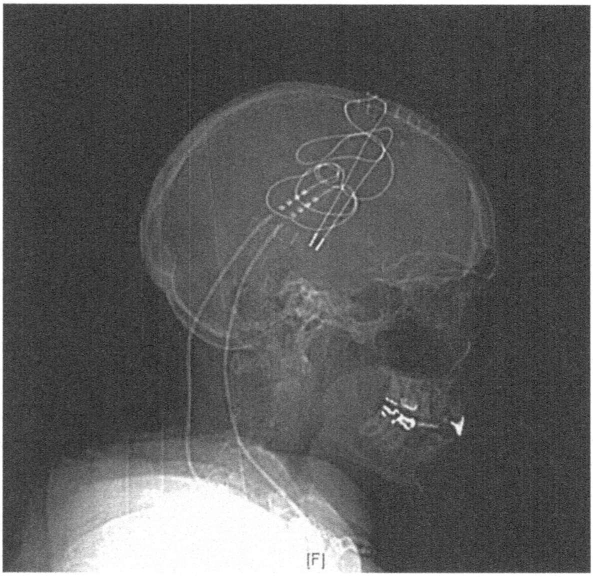

Fig. 13.1 Radiograph with bilateral DBS leads

Advancements in technology, as well as increased experience with DBS through its treatments for movement disorders, have led to a low risk profile for this therapy. Morbidity remains low and mortality is significantly rare. The most serious complications of DBS include an intracranial hemorrhage, with reports demonstrating an incidence of 1.9–4.1% of cases, as well as a permanent neurologic deficit, with reports ranging from 2.0 to 3.4% [4, 13, 14]. Infections carry an incidence of 3.3–13.3%, but more recent literature has demonstrated infection rates of 1.9% with the use of techniques to isolate the implants from skin incisions [13].

13.4 Conclusions

DBS for chronic pain is an essential part of the treatment paradigm that involves other interventions such as spinal cord stimulation, peripheral nerve stimulation, and intrathecal therapy. Although used since the 1970s and initially approved by the FDA, DBS had fallen out of favor and became investigational in the United States. More recently, interest has increased, given the success of DBS with movement disorders and as well as its low risk profile.

When viewed against other modalities in this difficult patient population, there are few that carry success rates similar to those of DBS, especially for FBSS, phantom limb pain, facial neuropathic pain, and nociceptive pain. Cephalalgias may carry the most promising results.

References

1. Hamani C, Schwalb JM, Rezai AR, Dostrovsky JO, Davis KD, Lozano AM. Deep brain stimulation for chronic neuropathic pain: long-term outcome and the incidence of insertional effect. Pain. 2006;125:188–96.
2. Levy RM, Deer T, Henderson J. Intracranial neurostimulation for pain control: a review. Pain Physician. 2010;13:157–65.
3. Bittar RG, Kar- Purkayastha I, Owen SL, Bear RE, Green A, Wang S, Aziz TZ. Deep brain stimulation for pain relief: a meta-analysis. J Clin Neurosci. 2005;12:515–9.
4. Levy RM, Lamb S, Adams JE. Treatment of chronic pain by deep brain stimulation: long term follow-up and review of the literature. Neurosurgery. 1987;21:885–93.
5. Parmar VK, Gee L, Smith H, Pilitsis JG. Supraspinal stimulation for treatment of refractory pain. Clin Neurol Neurosurg. 2014;123:155–63.
6. Owen SL, Green AL, Nandi DD, Bittar RG, Wang S, Aziz TZ. Deep brain stimulation for neuropathic pain. Acta Neurochir Suppl. 2007;97(Pt 2):111–6.
7. Green AL, Nandi D, Armstrong G, Carter H, Aziz T. Post-herpetic trigeminal neuralgia treated with deep brain stimulation. J Clin Neurosci. 2003;10:512–4.
8. Leone M, May A, Franzini A, Broggi G, Dodick D, Rapoport A, et al. Deep brain stimulation for intractable chronic cluster headache: proposals for patient selection. Cephalalgia. 2004;24:934–7.
9. Leone M, Franzini A, Broggi G, Bussone G. Hypothalamic deep brain stimulation for intractable chronic cluster headache: a 3-year follow-up. Neurol Sci. 2003;24:S143–5.

10. Chodakiewitz Y, Bicalho G, Chodakiewitz J. Multi-target neurostimulation for adequate long term relief of neuropathic and nociceptive chronic pain components. Surg Neurol Int. 2013;4:170–5.
11. Jenkins B, Tepper SJ. Neurostimulation for primary headache disorders: part 2, review of central neurostimulators for primary headache, overall therapeutic efficacy, safety, cost, patient selection, and future research in headache neuromodulation. Headache. 2011;51:1408–18.
12. Kumar K, Toth C, Nath RK. Deep brain stimulation for intractable pain: a 15-year experience. Neurosurgery. 1997;40:736–46.
13. Falowski S, Ooi YC, Smith A, Verhargen Metman L, Bakay RA. An evaluation of hardware and surgical complications with deep brain stimulation based on diagnosis and lead location. Stereotact Funct Neurosurg. 2012;90:173–80.
14. Deer TR, Mekhail N, Petersen E, Krames E, Staats P, Pope J, et al. The appropriate use of neurostimulation: stimulation of the intracranial and extracranial space and head for chronic pain. Neuromodulation Appropriateness Consensus Committee. Neuromodulation. 2014;17:551–70; discussion 570.

Chapter 14
Spinal Cord Stimulation, Cervical: Trialing

Matthew P. Jaycox, Adam C. Young, and Timothy R. Lubenow

14.1 Introduction

Much like with the lumbar and thoracic spine, spinal cord stimulation (SCS) of the cervical spine may be used to treat a variety of neuropathic pain conditions of the neck and upper extremities [1–5]. However, anatomical considerations unique to the cervical spine may present challenges to the interventional pain physician. This chapter discusses the relevant anatomy, describes the technique for cervical epidural lead placement and trialing, and suggests ways to minimize risks of complications.

14.2 Indications

Based on the anatomical location of pain, SCS of the cervical spine has a number of indications:

- Failed spine surgery syndrome of the cervical spine
- Neuropathic pain of the upper extremities, neck, and face
- Complex regional pain syndrome of the upper extremities
- Ischemic pain of the upper extremities

M.P. Jaycox • A.C. Young • T.R. Lubenow (✉)
Department of Anesthesiology, Rush University Medical Center, Chicago, IL, USA
e-mail: Matthew_Jaycox@rush.edu; mjaycox@earthlink.net; Adam_Young@rush.edu; dr.adam.young@gmail.com; timlubenowmd@gmail.com

S. Diwan, T.R. Deer (eds.), *Advanced Procedures for Pain Management*,
https://doi.org/10.1007/978-3-319-68841-1_14

14.3 Relevant Anatomy

The cervical spine is composed of seven cervical vertebrae, and there are eight cervical nerves. In contrast to the lumbar and lower thoracic region, the cervical epidural space is significantly narrower, which has implications for the placement of stimulator leads, particularly if two leads are desired. The cervical epidural space extends from the dura of the foramen magnum to the lower border of C7, at which point the thoracic epidural space begins at C7 and extends to the upper margin of L1. Sensation to the angle of the mandible arises from C1–C2. The occiput region receives sensation from the occipital nerves, which arise from the dorsal roots of C2 and C3. The regions of the neck receive sensory innervation along their respective dermatomes. The shoulder and arm receive innervation from the cervical roots, which give rise to the brachial plexus, roots C5–T1 [6].

Several relevant aspects of anatomy should be kept in mind when performing a cervical SCS trial:

- Cervical epidural space: At C7, the AP width from the ligamentum flavum to the dura mater is only 1.5–2 mm. With flexion, this may increase to 4 mm.
- The anatomic and physiologic midlines may differ by as much as 2 mm at all spinal cord levels.
- Because of the cervical lordosis and the shallow path necessary for the needle placement trajectory, the epidural space is typically cannulated below the level of T1-2, usually between T2-3 and T4-5.
- Epidural anatomy often makes advancement of electrode leads above C2 difficult.
- Exiting nerve roots from the cervical neuroforamina are larger in diameter in the lower four cervical roots when compared to the upper four roots.

14.4 Concerns and Contraindications

As with SCS in the lumbar and thoracic regions, a cervical SCS trial is utilized when more conservative options have failed. However, the nature and extent of conservative care is in debate, as data show that SCS can be more effective and safer than the alternatives of long-term opiate use, polypharmacy, and surgical reoperation. When there is neurological compromise, there are few good alternatives to spine surgery reoperation, but when the primary goal is pain relief, the outcomes of surgical re-operation in the cervical region are (as with lumbar surgery) fair at best. Therefore SCS of the cervical spine should be considered earlier in the treatment paradigm for cervical failed spine surgery syndrome when pain is the primary operative indication.

That being said, it should be noted that in the vast majority of cases, only patients who have undergone cervical spine surgery with an anterior approach (*e.g.* anterior cervical discectomy and fusion [ACDF]), would be able to undergo a cervical SCS trial. Patients with a history of posterior cervical spine surgery will have postsurgical anatomic changes that are likely to make percutaneous epidural lead placement impossible.

Several basic requirements are important in the selection of patients for a cervical SCS trial:

- Patients have demonstrable pathology and an objective rationale for their pain complaint.
- Patients have psychiatric or psychological clearance before the procedure [7].
- Conservative therapies have failed.
- Patients do not have serious drug habituation or abuse problems.
- The pain pattern is primarily radiating to the upper extremity.
- Surgical intervention is not indicated.

A cervical SCS trial can have several contraindications:

- Infection, systemic or localized
- Coagulopathy
- Severely distorted or complicated anatomy, including severe spinal stenosis (relative)
- Active psychosis

14.5 Preoperative Considerations

Preoperative steps and considerations are important:

- Informed consent and proper explanation of all potential complications
- Physical examination of the area for infection, skin ulceration or necrosis, and extent of disease
- Review of pertinent imaging of both the area to be entered and the area in which the leads will eventually be positioned
- Patient's ability to lie prone for the intended length of the procedure
- Intravenous access for IV fluid and medications for mild sedation

Fluoroscopic views should start with an anterior-posterior (AP) view centered over the T1-2 interspace. The patient's chest and spinous processes should be perfectly vertical. A very slight cephalad tilt can sometimes aid in "opening up" the intervertebral foramen. It is also critical to be able to visualize in a perfect, true lateral view, which allows one to accurately approximate the posterior epidural space and minimize risk of needle trauma to the cord.

14.5.1 Equipment

- 14-gauge modified Tuohy epidural needles in both straight and curved-tip (Coudé) configurations (provided by device manufacturer)
- 1 or 2 electrode arrays, 8–16 contacts each
- Standard implant accessories, including guidewires, anchors, electrode stylets, and stimulating box(es) with connection cables
- Loss-of-resistance syringe
- 10 mL syringe for local anesthetic
- 25G 1.5-in. needle for skin infiltration
- 2-0 silk suture on a needle for suturing lead anchors
- Needle driver
- Butterfly closures (Steri-Strips)
- Antiseptic disc such as Biopatch® (Ethicon)
- Occlusive dressing such as Tegaderm™ (3M)

14.5.2 Medications

- 1% lidocaine
- Iodinated contrast (*e.g.* Isovue-M® 300) (nonionic water-soluble contrast)
- IV antibiotic that covers Gram-positive cocci (*e.g.* Cefazolin)

14.6 Technique

14.6.1 Positioning

The chest should be elevated off the table with either a single vertical roll positioned on the sternum, or side-by-side rolls positioned in the mid-clavicular line. Care must be taken to ensure that the patient's breasts are not lying upon the rolls, in order to avoid pressure injury. A pillow may be placed under the hips to elevate the abdomen so the patient can breathe comfortably. The face should lie in a semirigid foam cradle in the neutral position, or with slight flexion in order to widen the cervical epidural space. As with all prone positioning, the eyes, nose, and mouth must be free. The arms can either be tucked at the sides or placed above the shoulders upon padded armrests that allow them to lie below the level of the C-spine. Whichever is chosen, it is critical that the arms do not obscure the lateral view of the spine. This positioning may require some refinement and adjustment to the individual patient.

14.6.2 Procedure

Antisepsis of the skin should commence following positioning. An abrasive scrub with an iodine-based solution or alcohol is ideal to clear gross contaminants such as dirt and sloughed skin. Then an alcohol-based prepping solution (*e.g.* chlorhexidine gluconate/isopropyl alcohol) is applied and allowed to dry completely [8]. If not allowed to dry, the solution is considered a potential fire hazard.

As with all trial SCS lead placement, the patient should be alert and communicative in order to ensure correct lead positioning [9, 10]. Although it is sometimes necessary to provide a modicum of sedation to assist with epidural cannulation and lead advancement, in our practice we avoid the use of propofol during cervical SCS trialing. It is preferable to make the patient comfortable with local anesthetic infiltration at the needle entry site. It is unwise to rely on excessive sedation to accomplish the job of local skin anesthesia. Alkalinization of the lidocaine can render it less noxious to the patient during infiltration.

After centering the fluoroscope over the T1-T2 interspace, the optimal site of entry should be determined. This will usually be between T2-T3 and T4-T5. Techniques that employ cannulating the lower thoracic epidural space with the goal of the threading the leads "all the way" to the cervical spine are often impractical and risk excessive lead migration, or even fracture.

Preoperative antibiotics should now be administered. After determining the most appropriate level for epidural needle entry (which is usually the level with the widest and most patent interspace), the skin should be marked and infiltrated with local anesthetic. A paramedian approach is most often employed, so the skin should be localized 1–2 cm off midline and two to three levels caudad to the intended epidural entry level. This requires a shallow approach of the needle, approximately 15°–30° off the skin. A shallow approach is necessary to ensure placement of the needle within the dorsal epidural space, and to assist with advancement of the stimulator lead. If it becomes necessary to take a more acute path with the needle, a curved-tip (Coudé) needle can be used, as the curved tip will still allow the electrode lead to advance within the posterior epidural space.

Using a shallow approach, one aims the needle at the target level, directed toward the painful side—that is, leftward needle for left-sided pain. If two leads are intended, then a bilateral paramedian approach is used with needle cannulation. It is our practice to contact the inferior lamina just caudad to the interspace, as this gives one a reliable indicator of anatomic depth. The needle may then be cautiously "walked off" in a cephalad fashion, and loss-of-resistance technique may be employed to identify the epidural space.

The fluoroscope is then positioned in the lateral fashion and the styleted needle is visualized. The needle is then advanced carefully to the region of the ligamentum flavum. An AP view should now be obtained to ensure that the needle has not advanced past midline. The stylet is now removed, a syringe is attached to the needle, and "loss-of-resistance" technique is used to access the epidural space.

Table 14.1 Targets for cervical spinal cord stimulation[a]

Level	Target
C1–C2	Face
C2–C3	Upper neck
C3–C4	Shoulder to hand
C4–C5	Forearm to hand, radial nerve
C5–C6	Forearm to hand, median nerve
C6–C7	Forearm to hand, ulnar nerve
C7–T1	Anterior shoulder, upper chest

[a]Variability exists, and repositioning based on patient response is often necessary

The syringe may be filled with either 3–4 mL of preservative-free saline, or 2–3 cm^3 of air. The needle is advanced in small increments, while testing the plunger resistance frequently, waiting for the loss of bounce. Loss of resistance is less subtle in the upper thoracic and cervical region than in the lumbar spine. As a result, it is necessary to frequently confirm the position of the needle tip in lateral view. When loss of resistance is encountered, the physician may then confirm placement of the needle within the epidural space by passing the epidural guidewire. It should pass easily within the posterior epidural space. Do not force the guidewire, as this can create channeling. If the guidewire does not pass freely, then it usually means that the very distal tip of the Tuohy needle has breached the ligamentum flavum, but not enough of the needle aperture lies within the epidural space. If this occurs, the needle should be advanced slightly or repositioned to allow easy passage of the guidewire, and ultimately of the electrode lead.

Using live or pulsed-live fluoroscopy, the lead should be advanced with great care, targeted at the appropriate level for the patient's individual pain pattern (Table 14.1). The lead should be positioned just off midline. If the patient has bilateral pain, a second lead is often placed to the opposite side. Although bilateral stimulation may be achieved with a single midline-placed electrode, placement of two electrode leads bilaterally allows for a greater variety and variability of stimulation patterns. When placing two leads for single-sided pain, one lead is placed off midline toward the painful side, and the second is placed in the midline.

Most eight-contact electrode arrays provide a broad enough area of coverage that sufficient stimulation can be achieved to all painful areas in the cervical spine. If a greater anatomic area of coverage is required, the leads may be apposed closely, and staggered. Some electrode arrays contain 16 points of contact and may provide larger areas of coverage utilizing a single lead. This has implications for patients with large areas of pain, bilaterally.

Once the lead(s) are placed at the appropriate site and level, they are connected to the temporary external power source via one or more connection boxes. Intraoperative testing then occurs. The patient should be completely awake and conversant at this point, and no further sedation should be given. If the patient does not experience adequate paresthesias and stimulation into their painful areas, the leads should be repositioned either cephalad, caudad, or laterally as appropriate, and retested.

Once the patient and the physician have determined that the degree of the coverage is satisfactory, the position of the leads is once again verified in AP and lateral views (Figs. 14.1 and 14.2). The needles are then cautiously removed so as not to disturb the final placement of the electrode leads. Manufacturer-supplied lead anchors are then utilized to secure the leads to the dorsum of the skin of the back. Anchors come in many styles, with newer generations of anchors poten-

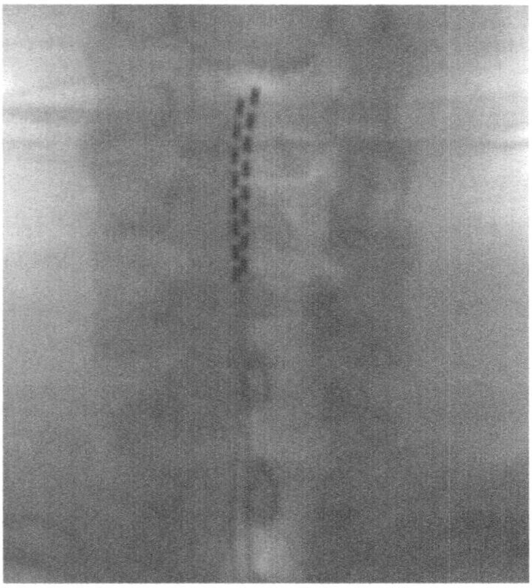

Fig. 14.1 Threading electrode through introducer needle

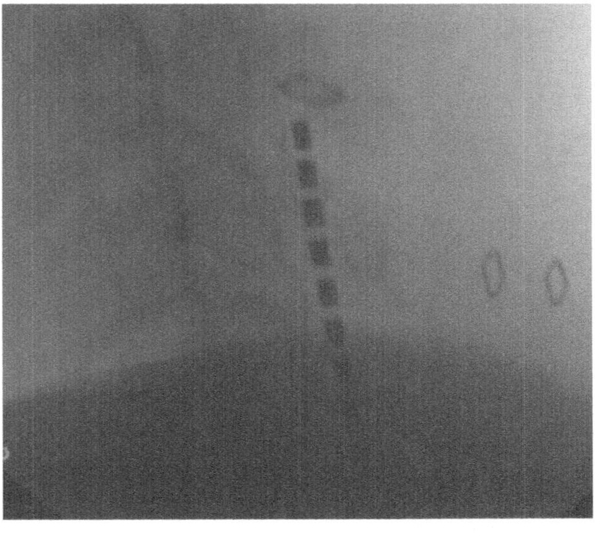

Fig. 14.2 Loss of resistance technique with glass syringe

tially offering lower rates of lead migration. With the anchors apposed to the skin, they are sutured in place. Two anchoring sutures per lead are sufficient. An antiseptic disc (*e.g.* Biopatch®) may be placed on the skin at the lead entry site to mitigate against infection. Steri-Strips can be used to further secure the leads in place. In our practice, we always secure our leads using both anchors and Steri-Strips. A tension-relief loop should be laid down to prevent lead movement. The leads and connection box(es) are now secured under an occlusive dressing such as Tegaderm™. The boxes should be padded against the skin of the patient with sterile gauze.

14.6.3 Post-procedure

With the patient supine and seated upright, the leads are again tested. It is not uncommon for stimulation patterns to change slightly as a result of the shift in position from prone to upright, and some reprogramming may be needed. Complete loss of coverage, however, warrants investigation into whether the leads have migrated substantially. Modern SCS trialing units come with a patient-held programmer that can accommodate multiple stimulation programs. A patient can ideally be provided with two or more programs to trial, and the individual programs may be suited to specific conditions and activity levels. Patients are then sent home to test the system for the next 4–7 days. They are instructed to go about their normal activities of daily living in order to determine if the SCS is effective under "real world" conditions. We find it helpful to have patients return to the office mid-trial for programming adjustments, if needed. Once the patient has clearly determined whether the trial SCS is (or is not) helping sufficiently and providing adequate analgesia, the sutures are cut, and then the anchors and leads are removed. Leads should be removed with a steady, constant force applied to the externalized ends. If appropriate, a date for permanent implantation is then set.

14.7 Post-procedure Follow-Up

The patient should be followed up by telephone 2–3 days after the conclusion of the procedure and queried about any of the following symptoms:

- Infection/temperature greater than 101 °F
- Bleeding
- Drainage from the entry sites
- Severe back pain or new-onset extremity weakness
- Photophobia or stiff neck

14.8 Clinical Pearls and Tips

- Placement of two leads allows for a greater degree of stimulation patterns (Figs. 14.3 and 14.4).
- Placing the leads in a slightly more lateral position can allow for direct nerve stimulation at the entry zone. This may be helpful in cases where specific nerve root involvement occurs as a result of the disease process.
- A curved-tip needle (Coudé) can allow for a more acute approach to the epidural space, while still allowing the lead to be passed within the dorsal epidural space.
- Having an assistant place his or her hands on either side of the Tuohy needle during epidural cannulation and applying downward pressure to compress the subcutaneous tissues of the thoracic paraspinal regions can allow for greater discrimination during loss-of-resistance technique.
- A small amount (2–3 mL) of iodinated contrast may be injected to confirm entry into the epidural space. Large volumes should not be injected so as to avoid spread to the cervical levels, which could interfere with stimulation testing.

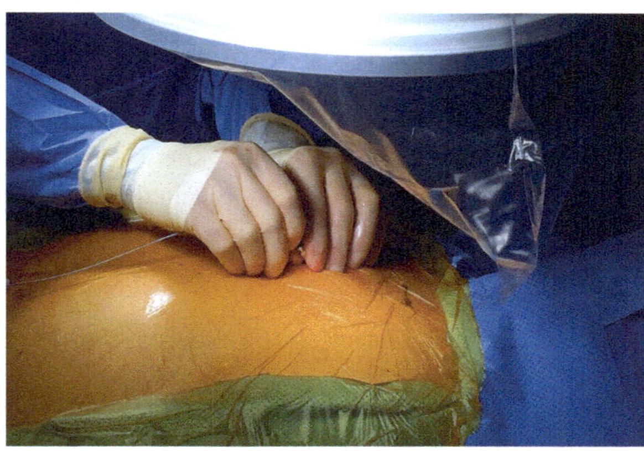

Fig. 14.3 Anterior-posterior view radiograph of cervical spine demonstrating location of stimulator leads

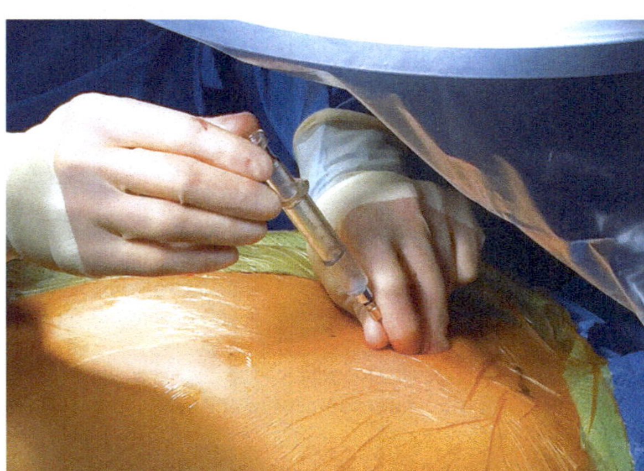

Fig. 14.4 Lateral view radiograph of cervical spine demonstrating dorsal location of stimulator leads

- Avoid opiate analgesics or ketamine intraoperatively, to avoid confounding during the initial phase of the trial.
- Consider placing the noninvasive blood pressure (NIBP) cuff on the leg or ankle, so as not to confuse the patient during limb stimulation testing.
- It is reasonable to extend the trial period by 1 or 2 days if the patient is unsure whether 50% relief of symptoms has been achieved. This assumes that no signs of infection are present.
- Leads should be removed with the patient's neck flexed and the upper back slightly bent over. Having the patient hug a pillow can assist.

14.9 Potential Complications and Pitfalls

Cervical SCS trials are prone to all the same risks as cervical epidural cannulation:

- Infection: Perioperative antibiotics should be used, and strict adherence paid to antisepsis during the procedure.
- Bleeding/hematoma: Guidelines of the American Society of Regional Anesthesia and Pain Medicine (ASRA) should be followed in the anticoagulated patient [11, 12].
- Subarachnoid puncture (wet tap): If the patient experiences a severe post–dural puncture headache (PDPH), the intensity may preclude his or her ability to provide an accurate assessment of the SCS trial's effectiveness. In this scenario, it may be best to terminate the trial prematurely, treat the PDPH, and trial again at a later date. We believe that performing an epidural blood patch with trial leads in place is not recommended, owing to the risk of infection.
- Nerve root irritation (neuritis)
- If the patient experiences any dysesthesias during lead advancement, stop, wait for it to resolve, and/or reposition the lead.
- If the patient experiences uncomfortable stimulation at very low amplitude levels, one or both leads are likely in the intrathecal space.
- If the patient experiences motor stimulation, either the amplitude settings are too high or the leads are too lateral and anterior and should be repositioned [13].
- Lead fracture or lead migration

References

1. North RB, Kidd D, Shipley J, Taylor RS. Spinal cord stimulation versus reoperation for failed back surgery syndrome: a cost effectiveness and cost utility analysis based on a randomized, controlled trial. Neurosurgery. 2007;61:361–8.
2. Taylor RS, Ryan J, O'Donnell R, Eldabe S, Kumar K, North RB. The cost-effectiveness of spinal cord stimulation in the treatment of failed back surgery syndrome. Clin J Pain. 2010;26:463–9.

3. Kemler MA, Raphael JH, Bentley A, Taylor RS. The cost-effectiveness of spinal cord stimulation for complex regional pain syndrome. Value Health. 2010;13:735–42.
4. Deer TR, Skaribas IM, Haider N, Salmon J, Kim C, Nelson C, et al. Effectiveness of cervical spinal cord stimulation for the management of chronic pain. Neuromodulation. 2014;17:265–71; discussion 271.
5. Kramer J, Vallejo R, Benyamin R. Neuromodulation of the cervical spinal cord in the treatment of chronic intractable neck and upper extremity pain: a case series review of the literature. Pain Physician. 2007;10:305–11.
6. Richardson J, Groen GJ. Applied epidural anatomy. Contin Educ Anaesth Crit Care Pain. 2005;5:98–100.
7. Beltrutti D, Lamberto A, Barolat G, Bruehl SP, Doleys D, Krames E, et al. The psychological assessment of candidates for spinal cord stimulation for chronic pain management. Pain Pract. 2004;4:204–21.
8. Darouiche RO, Wall MJ Jr, Itani KM, Otterson MF, Webb AL, Carrick MM, et al. Chlorhexidine-alcohol versus povidone-iodine for surgical-site antisepsis. N Engl J Med. 2010;362:18–26.
9. Abram SE, Francis MC. Hazards of sedation for interventional pain procedures. Anesthesia Patient Safety Foundation Newsletter. 2012;2:29–44.
10. Rathmell JP, Michna E, Fitzgibbon DR, Stephens LS, Posner KL, Domino KB. Injury and liability associated with cervical procedures for chronic pain. Anesthesiology. 2011;114:918–26.
11. Narouze S, Benzon HT, Provenzano DA, Buvanendran A, De Andres J, Deer TR, et al. Interventional spine and pain procedures in patients on antiplatelet and anticoagulant medications: guidelines from the American Society of Regional Anesthesia and Pain Medicine, the European Society of Regional Anaesthesia and Pain Therapy, the American Academy of Pain Medicine, the International Neuromodulation Society, the North American Neuromodulation Society, and the World Institute of Pain. Reg Anesth Pain Med. 2015;40:182–212.
12. Deer TR, Mekhail N, Provenzano D. The appropriate use of neurostimulation: avoidance and treatment of complications of neurostimulation therapies for the treatment of chronic pain. Neuromodulation Appropriateness Consensus Committee. Neuromodulation. 2014;17:571–97.
13. Barolat G, Massaro F, He J, Zeme S, Ketcik B. Mapping of sensory responses to epidural stimulation of the intraspinal neural structures in man. J Neurosurg. 1993;78:233–9.

Chapter 15
Spinal Cord Stimulation: Thoracic and Lumbar—Trial

Maged Guirguis, Michael Cody Scarbrough, and Nathan J. Harrison

15.1 Introduction

Neuromodulation is defined by the International Neuromodulation Society as the "therapeutic interaction with the central, peripheral, or autonomic nervous system for therapeutic effect by means of targeted electrical stimulation or pharmacological delivery from implanted devices," all with the aim of cost-effective, clinically relative treatment of refractory neuropathic pain [1–6]. Spinal cord stimulation (SCS) is the most established member of this family and has been in practice for nearly 50 years [7]. Beginning with the gate control theory proposed by Melzack and Wall in 1965 [8], the development and use of spinal cord stimulation has grown exponentially. The theory suggested that the stimulation of large non-nociceptive myelinated fibers of the peripheral nerves (A-β fibers) inhibited the activity of small nociceptive projections (A-δ and C) in the dorsal horn of the spinal cord. While the original gate theory seems to partially explain the effect of electrical stimulation on the dorsal column, complete understanding of the mechanism of action has not yet been elucidated. Proposed theories are mostly based upon the mechanism of pain which is targeted, such as stimulation-induced suppression of central excitability and release of neurotransmitters such as serotonin, gamma-amino butyric acid and substance P in neuropathic pain or inhibition of sympathetic vasoconstriction in ischemic

M. Guirguis (✉)
Department of Anesthesiology and Critical Care Medicine, Ochsner Health System, New Orleans, LA, USA

University of Queensland Ochsner Medical School, Brisbane, QLD, Australia
e-mail: drmagedaziz@yahoo.com

M.C. Scarbrough • N.J. Harrison
Department of Anesthesia and Pain Management, Ochsner Health System, New Orleans, LA, USA
e-mail: mscrbrgh@me.com; nathanha504@gmail.com

S. Diwan, T.R. Deer (eds.), *Advanced Procedures for Pain Management*,
https://doi.org/10.1007/978-3-319-68841-1_15

associated pain [9]. With the most recent advancements including high-frequency stimulation, burst stimulation, and precise dorsal root ganglion stimulation, spinal cord stimulation is a rapidly growing modality for pain management. Trial implantation of leads allows for patient response to be evaluated prior to permanent implantation. Additional advantages of percutaneous trials include: cost-effectiveness [10] when performed outside of the operating room in office-based procedures rooms [11], and determination of energy requirements for the individual patient, which assists in making the choice of battery type. Few treatment modalities in medicine offer the ability to trial the efficacy of intervention in a reversible and minimally invasive fashion prior to permanent implantation.

15.2 Patient Selection

One of the most important decision points in proceeding with spinal cord stimulation is appropriate patient selection, which is imperative for patient satisfaction and safety as well as key to building a successful neuromodulation practice. Several authors have put forth criteria to help practitioners decide which patients will qualify for, benefit from, and succeed from a dorsal column stimulation trial and ultimately proceed with permanent implantation. This is to be used only as a guide for determination, as not all patients will succeed the trial. Consensus has been established upon the following parameters [12, 13]:

- Patient agrees to proceed with trial after thorough explanation of risk/benefits and expectation.
- Conservative treatment of an underlying chronic painful pathology has failed.
- Surgical intervention is not, or is no longer, indicated.
- Psychological clearance has been obtained.
- Imaging modalities (preferably MRI) have been obtained and no anatomic abnormalities are identifiable.
- Lack of absolute contraindications including sepsis, coagulopathy, previous intervention or trauma obliterating the epidural space, local infection, presence of a demand pacemaker, or implanted defibrillator.

15.2.1 Selected Indications

Use of dorsal column stimulation in patients with failed back surgery syndrome (FBSS) has been shown to be particularly helpful. Notably, it is more cost-effective in the long term [14, 15], is more effective in relieving pain than medical management or repeat laminectomy, and decreases opioid consumption in comparison to repeat surgery [1, 5].

Literature also suggests that patients with complex regional pain syndrome (CRPS) have shown to benefit from spinal cord stimulation. Despite most studies being case series models, the overwhelming majority showed improvement in pain scores years post-implantation [2, 16–20].

In addition to treating the more common diagnoses, previously mentioned, neuromodulation has gained FDA approval for other painful disorders, albeit with reduced incidence of significant response. These include postherpetic neuralgia, post-thoracotomy pain, phantom limb pain, and spinal cord injuries.

Literature supports the use of stimulation for peripheral vasculopathies and chronic anginal pain [21–23]; these, however, have not yet gained FDA approval. Focal neuralgias, such as occipital nerve stimulation for prophylactic treatment of chronic migraines, are also being investigated as maladies receptive to treatment by neuromodulation [24, 25].

15.2.2 Trial Preparation

A successful trial of neuromodulation devices is not an infallible indicator of a successful outcome. Very careful screening of potential candidates is necessary.

Screening for the SCS trial requires a series of steps:

- Examine the MRI for any anatomical anomalies and determine whether spinal canal volume is adequate for the placement of trial leads into the epidural space.
- Examine the MRI for signs of instability of the spine, such as excessive anterolisthesis due to par interarticularis defects. A referral for a surgical consult should be done if any instability exists. Once any instability is treated, the patient may undergo an SCS trial.
- Perform a thorough physical exam to document the painful areas.
- Any signs of addiction, major depression, and other major psychological disorders should be treated and the patient re-evaluated for the SCS trial.
- Obtain informed consent with discussion of the benefits, alternatives, and risks, including infection at surgical sites, bleeding that may cause an epidural hematoma requiring emergent decompressive surgery, and damage to surrounding nerves.
- Follow guidelines regarding stopping and restarting any anticoagulation medication (i.e., ASRA guidelines). Consultation with the patient's cardiologist or neurologist may be necessary before stopping anticoagulation medication.
- Consider checking for evidence of active dermal, dental, or urological infectious etiologies and treat or consult accordingly (including urinalysis).

15.3 Techniques

The following steps describe the technique for placing a percutaneous SCS lead in the thoracic and lumbar spine [26]:

- Airway equipment and resuscitation drugs must be maintained and readily available.

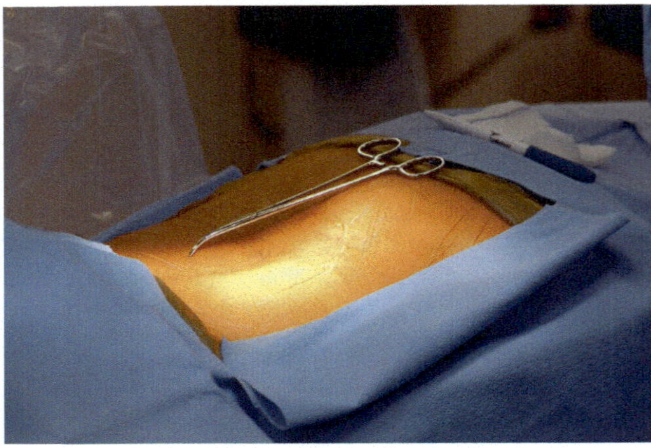

Fig. 15.1 After ensuring proper correction of lumbar lordosis and performing sterile preparation, fluoroscopic images are taken to plan initial skin entry site

- The physician may choose to provide a preoperative weight-based dose of intravenous antibiotics.
- Oral or IV analgesic and anxiolytic medications can be given preoperatively, but it is possible to perform a trial with local anesthetic only. Minimal sedation should be used during the procedure, as the patient must be alert and communicative during intraoperative stimulation to ensure proper lead placement.
- The patient is placed in a prone position with the arms abducted and flexed at the elbow to ensure that they are outside the fluoroscopic field. A pillow is placed beneath the abdomen to reduce lumbar lordosis, facilitating needle entry into the epidural space. The field is then prepared in sterile fashion (Fig. 15.1).
- Following intradermal and subcutaneous injection of local anesthetic, make a small stab incision with a #11 blade over the insertion site, which is typically one level caudad to the target interlaminar space (Fig. 15.2).
- A 14G Tuohy needle is inserted through the stab incision site at a 30°–45° angle to the skin. The needle is aimed toward the midline for optimal entry into the epidural space (Fig. 15.2).
- The needle should contact the lamina just below the target interlaminar entry site. The needle stylet can then be removed and a loss of resistance (LOR) syringe attached.
- The Tuohy should then be angled more steeply and walked down the bone to enter the epidural space. Once LOR occurs, the syringe is detached and a trial electrode lead is slowly advanced through the needle into the epidural space.
- Anteroposterior (AP) and lateral fluoroscopic guidance is used to verify that the lead is progressing cephalad in the dorsal epidural midline.
- If dual leads are going to be used during the trial, the second lead is usually placed on the opposite side or the same side as the entry point for the previous needle. At times when a parallel approach is not possible, an ipsilateral approach

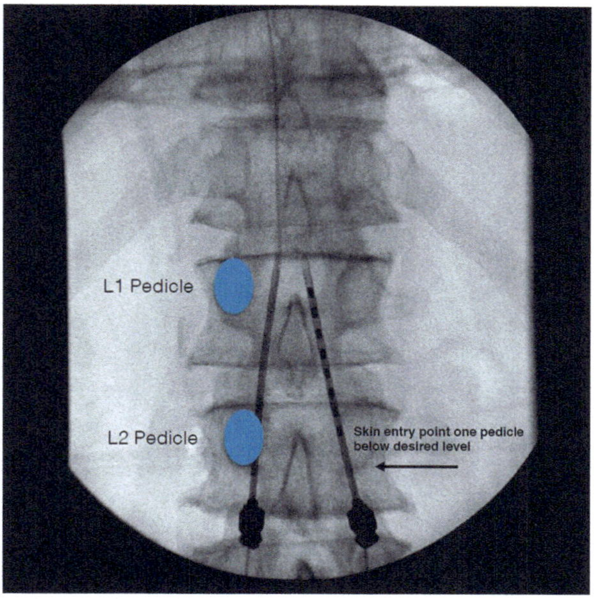

Fig. 15.2 Skin entry site is usually on the inferior border of the pedicle one level below the desired target. Needles are aimed to the arrive at the midline. Shown here is the parallel needle approach

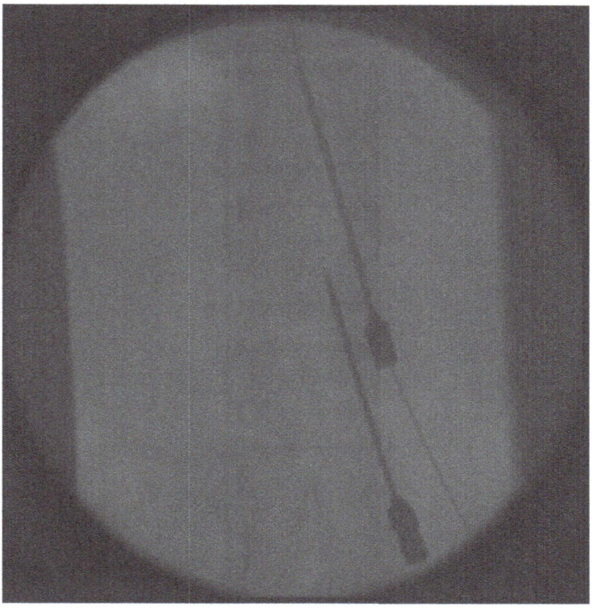

Fig. 15.3 Example of ipsilateral approach where Touhy needles are both placed on the same side but at two different levels

can be taken, with the second needle entering on the same side at the level above or below the first lead placement (Figs. 15.2 and 15.3).

- Most patients with lower back and leg pain find adequate coverage with a lead placed midline between T8 and T10. Placing two leads, each slightly off the physiologic midline to the right and left between T8 and T10, provides both back

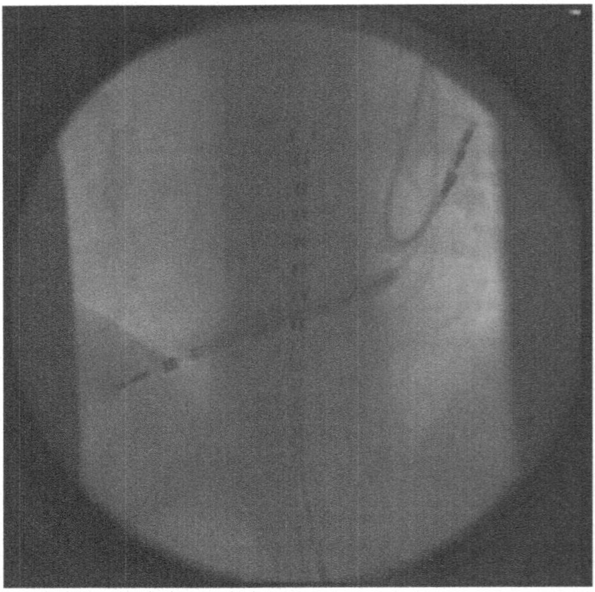

Fig. 15.4 Final position of dorsal column leads in midline covering T8 and T9 vertebral bodies. Horizontal wires seen here represent pacemaker wires

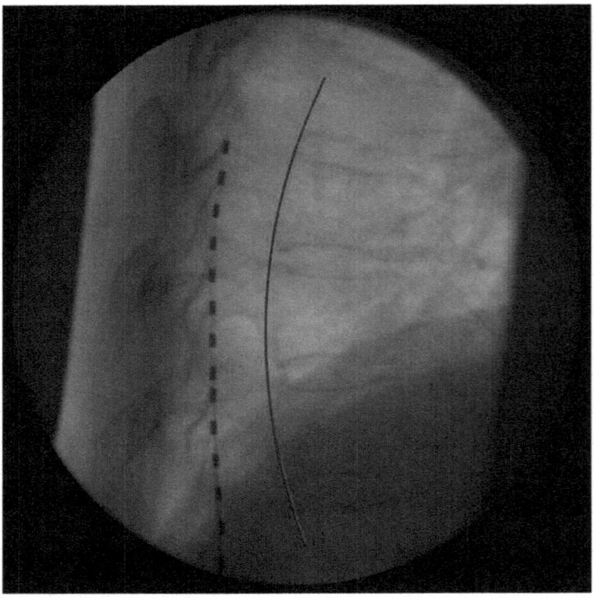

Fig. 15.5 A lateral fluoroscopic view is taken to ensure that leads lie in the posterior epidural space. The *red line* denotes anterior epidural space

and lower extremity stimulation, and allows for steering the stimulation pattern horizontally (Fig. 15.4) [27]. Leads should be no more than 2–4 mm off the midline. During the procedure and at the end, AP and lateral fluoroscopic images should be saved to document the level and the correct placement of the leads in the epidural space (Fig. 15.5).

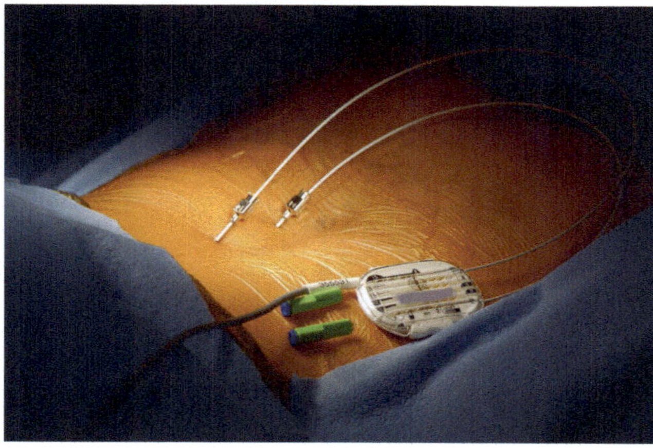

Fig. 15.6 Dorsal column leads are connected to temporary pulse generator for intraoperative testing

- Once the electrodes are in place, the manufacturer's representative calibrates the SCS to achieve a strong yet comfortable paresthesia over the painful area(s) (Fig. 15.6). The lead stylets are then carefully removed and a fluoroscopic record of the final electrode placement is obtained.
- The Tuohy needle is then carefully removed and the operative site is cleaned with chlorhexidine and alcohol.
- Next, the leads must be anchored externally. Lead migration is a common cause of an inadequate or unsuccessful trial. Most anchors consist of cylindrical sleeves that are designed to improve skin fixation and reduce lead migration. Newer anchor designs that reduce lead migration and breakage are being investigated [28, 29].
- The lead is passed through the anchor sleeve and attached to the skin using a figure-of-8 stitch or without an anchor using the drain stitch technique with non-absorbable sutures (Fig. 15.7). The leads and anchors can be further secured by carefully applying Steri-Strips to the lead or anchor.
- Fluoroscopic imaging can be used to confirm that the anchoring process did not result in any lead migration of the electrode tip.
- A tension loop is usually placed, and then a sterile occlusive dressing is applied.
- Each lead is attached to an extension wire, which connects the trial lead(s) to the pulse generator.
- After the procedure, the manufacturer's representative performs final programming. The patient is asked to minimize bending or squatting, as these might encourage lead migration.
- The trial length is determined by the physician's experience and practice. Trials usually last 3–8 days.
- During the trial, the manufacturer's representative should be available for continued programming and any emergencies that require physician involvement.

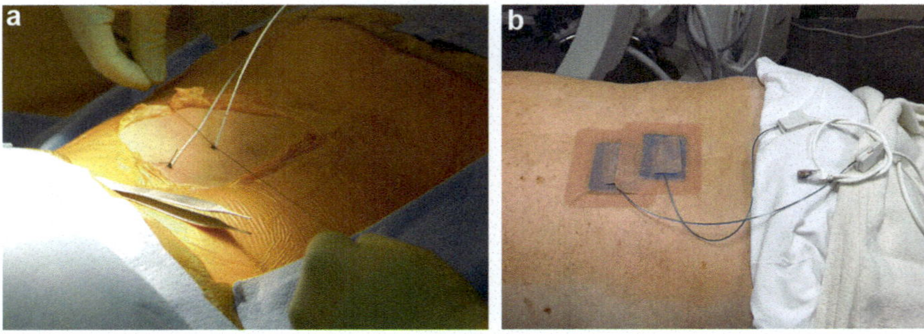

Fig. 15.7 (**a**) After the final positioning, leads are secured to the skin by method of choice. Here is an example of a drain stitch tie securing the lead to the skin. (**b**) Another method shown here is an adhesive catheter fixation bandage

- Patients are instructed to keep the incision site dry and to watch for symptoms of infection at the needle entry site such as increasing pain, erythema, purulent drainage, as well as symptoms of possible epidural hematoma, including increasing neck or back pain and progressive weakness or numbness of the legs (Fig. 15.7b).

15.3.1 SCS Trial Assessment

To determine the degree of pain relief and positive changes in quality of life, the patient is encouraged to perform activities that predictably cause their pain to manifest. Over the time of the trial, the patient should document pain scores, functional improvements, and any reduction of medication use. Current criteria used by insurance companies to approve permanent implantation of an SCS device requires documentation of at least 50% reduction in pain intensity. Documentation should also include any improvement in the patient's quality of life during the SCS trial. Before lead removal, physicians may choose to verify the position of the lead tips using fluoroscopy, and document their final positions if it is thought that any migration may have occurred.

15.4 Troubleshooting

Complications are inevitable when practicing neuromodulation. Close follow-up with patients undergoing trial and permanent implantation is paramount, and helps reduce the incidence and sequela of such complications. One retrospective study of 234 patients who underwent a temporary trial followed by implantation in an academic facility concluded that one-third developed some sort of complication, with hardware complications representing about 75% of those complications [30]. Despite hardware failure comprising the majority of possible complications, the most dangerous complications lead to permanent neurologic catastrophes or even death. It is thus imperative that physicians be cognizant and vigilant not only post-operatively, but that they also extensively educate patients about these risks during the initial discussion. We suggest incorporating the excellent review published by Yang for the ASRA Neuromodulation SIG website [31]. The most common complications are summarized here.

Complications requiring immediate attention and subsequent intervention are epidural hematomas and abscesses. Patients having associated sensory or motor deficits post-implantation should be immediately examined with imaging to evaluate and screen for the possibility of cord compression, which can lead to irreversible neurologic deficits. Neurosurgical intervention is necessary, within 8 h of cord compression symptomatology, for washout and possible explantation of the device.

Other complications that require urgent attention include infections at the surgical site, which may be elucidated by examination of the implantation site for erythema, edema, induration, tenderness. These findings warrant further examination of constitutional findings and collecting laboratory data with wound culture, blood cultures, erythrocyte sedimentation rate, and C-reactive protein levels. Debridement and washout of the implantation pocket, with or without associated explantation, is warranted, along with appropriate antibiotic therapy with the assistance of an infectious disease specialist [32].

While anchoring devices and techniques continue to improve, lead migration can still occur following implantation and may be associated with loss of stimulation in the affected area [33]. Other lead malfunctions associated with similar patient findings are fractures of the lead along implant and loss of connection with implanted pulse generator. Plain radiographs in comparison with immediate successful post-procedure images should be obtained to evaluate whether repositioning, replacement, or reconnection are necessary.

References

1. North RB, Kidd DH, Farrokhi F, Piantadosi SA. Spinal cord stimulation versus repeated lumbosacral spine surgery for chronic pain: a randomized, controlled trial. Neurosurgery. 2005;56:98–106.
2. Kemler MA, Barendse GA, van Kleef M, de Vet HC, Rijks CP, Furnée CA, van den Wildenberg FA. Spinal cord stimulation in patients with chronic reflex sympathetic dystrophy. N Engl J Med. 2000;343:618–24.
3. Kemler MA, de Vet HC, Barendse GA, van den Wildenberg FA, van Kleef M. Spinal cord stimulation for chronic reflex sympathetic dystrophy—five-year follow-up. N Engl J Med. 2006;354:2394–6.
4. North RB, Kumar K, Wallace MS, Henderson JM, Shipley J, Hernandez J, et al. Spinal cord stimulation versus re-operation in patients with failed back surgery syndrome: an international multicenter randomized controlled trial (EVIDENCE Study). Neuromodulation. 2011;14:330–6.

5. Kumar K, Taylor RS, Jacques L, Eldabe S, Meglio M, Molet J, et al. Spinal cord stimulation versus conventional medical management for neuropathic pain: a multicentre randomised controlled trial in patients with failed back surgery syndrome. Pain. 2007;132:179–88.
6. Kumar K, Taylor RS, Jacques L, Eldabe S, Meglio M, Molet J, et al. The effects of spinal cord stimulation in neuropathic pain are sustained: a 24-month follow-up of the prospective randomised controlled multicenter trial of the effectiveness of spinal cord stimulation. Neurosurgery. 2008;63(4):762–70.
7. Thomson S. Spinal cord stimulation for neuropathic pain. International Neuromodulation Society. http://www.neuromodulation.com/spinal-cord-stimulation-for-neuropathic-pain. Accessed 28 June 2017.
8. Melzack R, Wall PD. Pain mechanisms: a new theory. Science. 1965;150:971–9.
9. Linderoth B, Foreman RD. Mechanisms of spinal cord stimulation in painful syndromes: role of animal models. Pain Med. 2006;7(Suppl 1):S14–26.
10. Kumar K, Hunter G, Demeria D. Spinal cord stimulation in treatment of chronic benign pain: challenges in treatment planning and present status, a 22-year experience. Neurosurgery. 2006;58:481–96.
11. Deer TR, Mekhail N, Provenzano D, Pope J, Krames E, Thomson S, et al. The appropriate use of neurostimulation: avoidance and treatment of complications of neurostimulation therapies for the treatment of chronic pain. Neuromodulation. 2014;17:571–98.
12. Lee C-J, Lee S-C, Kim Y-C. Spinal cord stimulation. In: Kim DH, Kim Y-C, Kim K-H, editors. Minimally invasive percutaneous spinal techniques. Philadelphia: Saunders Elsevier; 2010. p. 221–38.
13. Raso LJ. Trials and their applicability. In: Arle JE, Shils JL, editors. Essential neuromodulation. London: Academic; 2011. p. 283–99.
14. Kumar K, Malik S, Demeria D. Treatment of chronic pain with spinal cord stimulation versus alternative therapies: cost-effectiveness analysis. Neurosurgery. 2002;51:106–15.
15. Bala MM, Riemsma RP, Nixon J, Kleijnen J. Systematic review of the (cost-) effectiveness of spinal cord stimulation for people with failed back surgery syndrome. Clin J Pain. 2008;24:741–56.
16. Kemler MA, Barendse GA, van Kleef M, Egbrink MG. Pain relief in complex regional pain syndrome due to spinal cord stimulation does not depend on vasodilation. Anesthesiology. 2000;92:1653–60.
17. Kemler MA, Reulen JP, Barendse GA, van Kleef M, de Vet HC, van den Wildenberg FA. Impact of spinal cord stimulation on sensory characteristics in complex regional pain syndrome type I: a randomized trial. Anesthesiology. 2001;95:72–80.
18. Kemler MA, de Vet HC, Barendse GA, van den Wildenberg FA, van Kleef M. Effect of spinal cord stimulation for chronic complex regional pain syndrome type I: five-year final follow-up of patients in a randomized controlled trial. J Neurosurg. 2008;108:292–8.
19. Kemler MA, De Vet HC, Barendse GA, Van Den Wildenberg FA, Van Kleef M. The effect of spinal cord stimulation in patients with chronic reflex sympathetic dystrophy: two years' follow-up of the randomized controlled trial. Ann Neurol. 2004;55:13–8.
20. Calvillo O, Racz G, Didie J, Smith K. Neuroaugmentation in the treatment of complex regional pain syndrome of the upper extremity. Acta Orthop Belg. 1998;64:57–63.
21. Augustinsson LE. Spinal cord electrical stimulation in severe angina pectoris: surgical technique, intraoperative physiology, complications, and side effects. Pacing Clin Electrophysiol. 1989;12:693–4.
22. Augustinsson LE. Spinal cord stimulation in peripheral vascular disease and angina pectoris. J Neurosurg Sci. 2003;47(1 Suppl 1):37–40.
23. Jacobs MJ, Jörning PJ, Joshi SR, Kitslaar PJ, Slaaf DW, Reneman RS. Epidural spinal cord electrical stimulation improves microvascular blood flow in severe limb ischemia. Ann Surg. 1998;207:179–83.
24. Stanton-Hicks M. Peripheral nerve stimulation for pain, peripheral neuralgia and complex regional pain syndrome. In: Krames ES, Peckham PH, Rezai AR, editors. Neuromodulation. London: Elsevier; 2009. p. 397.

25. Weiner RL, Alo KM. Occipital neurostimulation for treatment of intractable headache syndromes. In: Krames ES, Peckham PH, Rezai AR, editors. Neuromodulation. London: Elsevier; 2009. p. 409.
26. Kreis PG, Fishman S. Spinal cord stimulation: percutaneous implantation techniques. New York: Oxford University Press; 2009.
27. Deer T, Pope J, Hayek S, Narouze S, Patil P, Foreman R, et al. Neurostimulation for the treatment of axial back pain: a review of mechanisms, techniques, outcomes, and future advances. Neuromodulation. 2014;17(Suppl 2):52–68.
28. Shaw A, Sharma M, Deogaonkar M, Rezai A. Technological innovations in implants used for pain therapies. Neurosurg Clin N Am. 2014;25:833–42.
29. North RB, Recinos VR, Attenello FJ, Shipley J, Long DM. Prevention of percutaneous spinal cord stimulation electrode migration: a 15-year experience. Neuromodulation. 2014;17:670–6; discussion 676–7.
30. Hayek SM, Veizi E, Hanes M. Treatment-limiting complications of percutaneous spinal cord stimulator implants: a review of eight years of experience from an academic center database. Neuromodulation. 2015;18:603–9.
31. Yang M. Troubleshooting for spinal cord stimulation therapy. ASRA Pain Neuromodulation Special Interest Group Resources. https://www.asra.com/page/215/troubleshooting-for-spinal-cord-stimulation-therapy
32. Provenzano DP. Perioperative precautions for infection control. In: Deer TR, Pope JE, editors. Atlas of implantable therapies for pain management. New York: Springer; 2016.
33. Bendersky D, Yampolsky C. Is spinal cord stimulation safe? A review of its complications. World Neurosurg. 2014;82(6):1359–68.

Chapter 16
Spinal Cord Stimulation—Hybrid Lead Array: Epidural and Peripheral Nerve Field Stimulation Trial

Lucas W. Campos and Michael Yang

Spinal cord stimulation (SCS) is an advanced modality in contemporary pain management. It is commonly used to treat complex pain conditions of the lumbar spine and lower extremities. However, one of the shortcomings of this treatment is poor coverage of axial back pain. Despite recent advances in improving axial low back pain coverage, such as high-frequency spinal cord stimulation, it is still challenging to treat this type of pain distribution. One of the successful approaches to resolve this problem is the use of peripheral nerve field stimulation (PNFS). PNFS involves placement of cylindrical stimulation leads subcutaneously over the painful areas. PNFS evokes a sense of paresthesia, which should cover the painful region for adequate treatment to be delivered. This chapter discusses procedural details of trials involving PNFS, SCS, and both modalities to create a hybrid system to treat nociceptive and neuropathic low back pain. It also provides the scientific and clinical rationale for placing PNFS electrodes in isolation or with SCS placement. Results of published studies on the use of PNFS in the management of low back pain are summarized, and the criteria for proper patient selection are listed. The published studies provide evidence that PNFS is a safe and well-tolerated pain control option for intractable pain conditions, including chronic low back pain. Efficacious pain relief relies on correct patient selection and the optimal placement of the leads, ensuring a lead depth of 10–12 mm from the surface of the skin to maximize the target sensation of PNFS and provide effective pain relief.

L.W. Campos (✉) • M. Yang
Summit Pain Alliance, Santa Rosa, CA, USA
e-mail: lwcamposmdphd@gmail.com; Michael.i.yang@gmail.com

S. Diwan, T.R. Deer (eds.), *Advanced Procedures for Pain Management*,
https://doi.org/10.1007/978-3-319-68841-1_16

16.1 Introduction

Pharmacological management of chronic pain is widespread. The application of this therapeutic approach is associated with various barriers including side effects, drug interactions, drug abuse and dependence, problems with patient compliance, and unrealistic expectations of efficacy [1]. These problems have led to the investigation of other modes of treating chronic pain. Electrical stimulation is a powerful medical therapy that can restore biological functions such as vision, hearing, movement, tactile perception, and proprioception. For chronic pain, both central and peripheral electrical stimulation are used for advanced treatment. Historically, the first demonstrated electric shock-induced pain relief, by John Wesley, occurred in the eighteenth century [2]. Yet it was the nineteenth century that became the golden age of medical electricity. This age began with the discovery of the electrochemical battery in 1800 and the introduction of the electric generator in 1848 [3]. In those years, electrical machines could be found in every doctor's consulting room. Over the years, mechanisms related to the application of electricity for chronic pain treatment led to the discovery and implementation of dorsal column spinal cord stimulation.

Spinal cord stimulation (SCS) is now a widespread and popular method of treatment for intractable chronic low back and lower extremity pain. Recent developments have allowed improved coverage of axial back pain [4]. The recent advent of high-frequency SCS has given pain practitioners new mechanisms to provide relief from axial back and leg pain [5]. Nevertheless, this newly proven technological advance is not always successful in treating axial low back pain [6]. The most consistent application of electrical stimulation to treat axial low back pain has come from the use of subcutaneous lead placement. This approach involves the generation and application of an electric field through subcutaneous stimulation leads, which inhibits pain signal transmission from the surrounding peripheral nerves. This use of subcutaneous electrical stimulation to treat peripheral nerve pain is called peripheral nerve field stimulation (PNFS); it targets the most distal sensory fibers.

In PNFS, a cylindrical electrode, similar to the type used in SCS, is implanted subcutaneously in the painful area. This technique has been used to treat many different painful conditions related to neuropathic and nociceptive pain [7]. PNFS evokes a sense of paresthesia (preferably covering the painful region) and is thought to provide pain relief by activation of non-nociceptive Aβ fibers [8]. In contrast, activation of Aδ fibers will lead to increased pain perception and discomfort, and must therefore be minimized. In cases of occipital neuralgia, PNFS applied over the greater and lesser occipital nerves has been successfully used by many practitioners to treat migraine headaches, using the activation of these non-nociceptive Aβ fibers [9, 10]. PNFS also has been used successfully to treat thoracic neuralgia, postherpetic neuralgia, scapular pain, and facial pain [11–13], and over a decade of literature has demonstrated the success of PNFS in treating axial low back pain (Figs. 16.1 and 16.2) [14–19].

PNFS has a number of advantages over the traditional neuromodulation approach of SCS, especially that it does not carry the same neurological risks, which include epidural hemorrhage, paralysis, and meningitis. Given the low invasiveness of

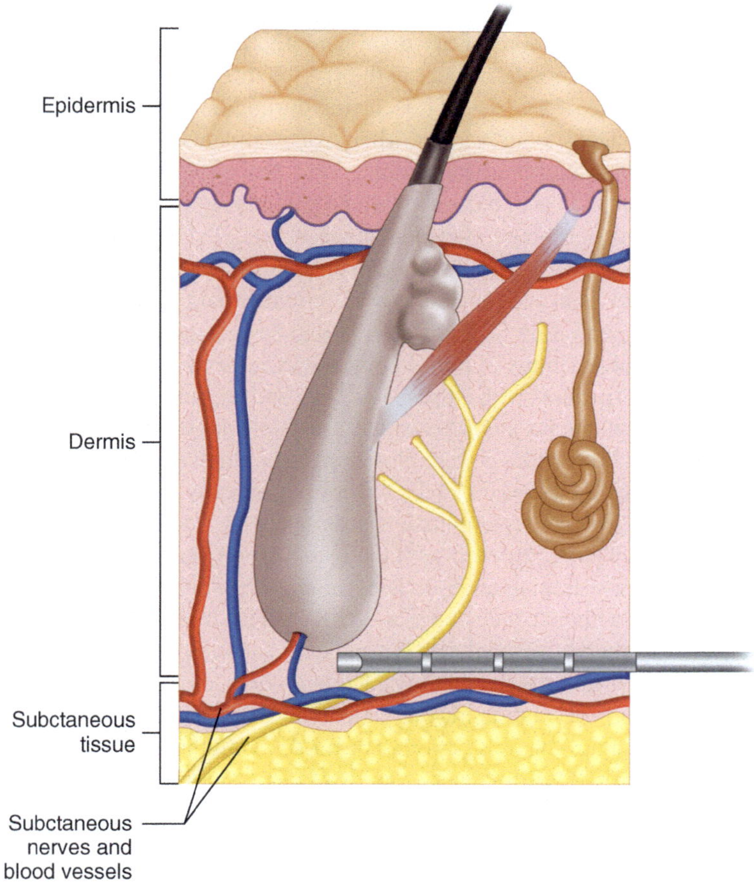

Fig. 16.1 Ideal placement for a peripheral nerve field stimulation (PNFS) lead

Fig. 16.2 Example of PNFS lead placement to treat axial low back pain. (*Reprinted from* Krutsch et al. [15]; *with permission*)

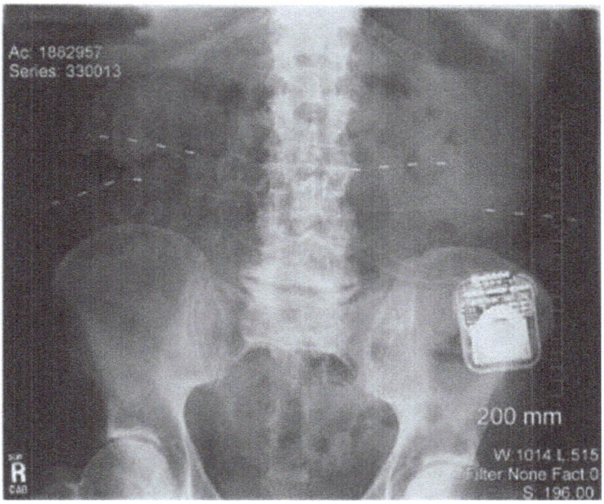

PNFS and its reversibility, testability, and adjustability, it is also a preferable option when compared with the more invasive surgical alternatives available. The main issue, as with any implantable device, is the risk of infection. Some practitioners report an infection rate of 6%, usually occurring during the first 2 weeks following implantation [18]. Other complications when using implantable electrical systems include lead migration and hardware failure. Two key publications have reported these occurrences in 5–13% of patients, with no patients reporting serious or severe adverse events. This combined evidence suggests that PNFS is a safe and well-tolerated pain control option for intractable pain conditions [18, 20].

Patients with both axial and radicular lower extremity pain could possibly benefit from an approach combining SCS and PNFS, and several studies have shown the superior efficacy and flexibility of the combined SCS and PNFS approach. Bernstein et al. [21] studied 20 patients with chronic low back and leg pain syndromes who had failed conventional therapies and who underwent implantation of a combination of traditional SCS and PNFS. Leads were placed in the epidural space as well as superficially in the subcutaneous tissues of the lower back, directly in the region of maximum pain. In some patients, a combination was used at the time of the initial trial. In other cases, the decision to proceed with the combination was made later, either at the time of permanent implantation or later, after SCS alone failed to adequately control pain. These authors concluded that PNFS used in combination with SCS is a safe and effective alternative treatment for patients with chronic low back and leg pain. They observed that the availability of this combined approach for a trial of stimulation prior to implantation allows patients to compare SCS with PNFS and indicate a preference for one over the other or for the combination (Fig. 16.3) [21].

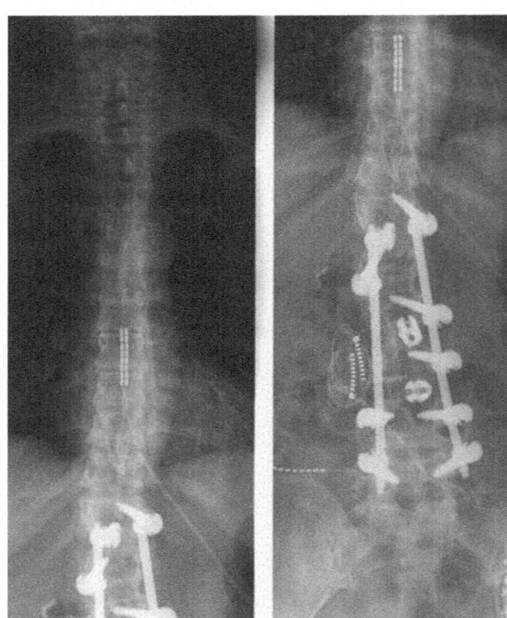

Fig. 16.3 Example of spinal cord stimulation (SCS) placement (*left*), which was converted to a hybrid system (*right*) to treat nociceptive and axial back pain. (*Reprinted from* Reverberi et al. [22]; *with permission*)

Mironer et al. [23] performed a prospective two-part study that included patients with low back pain because of failed back surgery syndrome (FBSS) and/or spinal stenosis. In the first part, 20 patients were implanted with SCS and PNFS, and the best program out of three (SCS alone, PNFS alone, or both together) was selected. In the second part, another 20 patients with the same implanted leads selected between three programs: SCS and PNFS separately, SCS as anode and PNFS as cathode, or the reverse. In the first part, 79% of the patients selected the simultaneous use of SCS and PNFS. The overall success of the trials in reducing pain scores on the visual analogue scale (VAS) by at least half was 85%. In the second part, communication between SCS and PNFS provided wider coverage of axial pain. The overall success of the trials in reducing VAS pain scores was 90%. The authors concluded that simultaneous use of SCS and PNFS increases the efficacy of both methods for axial back pain [23].

16.2 Pre-trial Preparation

A successful trial of neuromodulation devices is not an infallible indicator of a successful outcome. Very careful screening of potential candidates is necessary.

Screening for the PNFS trial should include several steps:

- Perform a thorough physical exam to clearly define the focal region of pain.
- Document the patient's failure to respond to conservative treatments, including medications and psychological and physical therapies.
- Screen for addiction, major depression, and other major psychological disorders. If present, these conditions should be treated and the patient re-evaluated for a PNFS trial.
- Get informed consent, with discussion of the benefits, alternatives, and risks such as lead migration requiring lead placement revisions, loss of therapy requiring revision, lead erosion, infection, and burning pain at the implanted pulse generator site.

Screening for the SCS trial also requires a number of steps:

- Examine the MRI for any anatomical anomalies and determine whether trial lead placement is possible without spinal cord compression.
- Examine the MRI for signs of instability of the spine, such as excessive anterolisthesis due to par interarticularis defects. A referral for a surgical consult should be done if any instability exists. Once any instability is treated, the patient may undergo an SCS trial.
- Perform a thorough physical exam to document the painful areas.
- Any signs of addiction, major depression, and other major psychological disorders should be treated and the patient re-evaluated for the SCS trial.
- Obtain informed consent, with discussion of the benefits, alternatives, and risks, including infection at surgical sites, bleeding that may cause an epidural hema-

toma requiring emergent decompressive surgery, and damage to surrounding nerves that could making the pain worse.

- Follow the guidelines of the American Society of Regional Anesthesia and Pain Medicine (ASRA) regarding stopping and restarting any anticoagulation medication. Consultation with the patient's cardiologist or neurologist may be necessary before stopping anticoagulation medication.

16.3 Trial Procedure for an SCS Lead in the Lumbar Spine

Following are the steps for implanting an SCS lead in the lumbar spine [24]:

- Airway equipment and resuscitation drugs must be maintained and be readily available.
- Patients can receive a preoperative weight-based dose of intravenous antibiotics, but they typically are not given for a trial.
- Oral or IV analgesic and antianxiety medications can be given preoperatively, but it is possible to perform a trial with local anesthetic only. Minimal sedation should be used during the procedure, as the patient must be alert and communicative during intraoperative stimulation, to ensure proper lead placement.
- The patient is placed in a prone position with the arms abducted and flexed at the elbow to ensure that they are outside the fluoroscopic field. A pillow is placed beneath the abdomen to reduce lumbar lordosis, facilitating needle entry into the epidural space.
- Following intradermal and subcutaneous injection of local anesthetic, make a small stab incision with a #11 blade over the insertion site, which is typically one level caudad to the target interlaminar space.
- A 14G Tuohy needle is inserted through the stab incision site at a 30°–45° angle to the skin. The needle is aimed toward the midline for optimal entry into the epidural space.
- The needle should contact the interlaminar bone just below the target interlaminar entry site. The needle stylet can be removed and a loss of resistance (LOR) syringe attached.
- The Tuohy should then be angled more steeply and walked down the bone to enter the epidural space. Once LOR occurs, the syringe is detached and a trial electrode lead is slowly advanced through the needle into the epidural space.
- Anteroposterior (AP) and lateral fluoroscopic guidance is used to verify the correct course of the lead cephalad in the dorsal epidural midline.
- If dual leads are going to be used during the trial, the second lead is usually placed on the opposite side or the same side as the entry point for the previous needle.
- Most patients with lower back and leg pain find adequate coverage with a lead placed midline between T8 and T10. Placing two leads, each slightly off the physiologic midline to the right and left, between T8 and T10, will also allow for both back and lower extremity stimulation [25]. Leads should be no more than

2–4 mm off the midline. During the procedure, and at the end, AP and lateral fluoroscopic images should be saved to document the level and the correct placement of the leads in the epidural space.

- When the electrodes are in place, the manufacturer's representative calibrates the SCS to achieve a strong yet comfortable paresthesia over the painful area(s). The lead stylets are then carefully removed and a fluoroscopic record of the final electrode placement is obtained.
- The Tuohy needle is then carefully removed and the operative site is cleaned with chlorhexidine and alcohol.
- Next, the leads must be anchored externally. Lead migration is a common cause of an inadequate or unsuccessful trial. Most anchors consist of cylindrical sleeves that are designed to improve skin fixation and reduce lead migration. Newer anchor designs that reduce lead migration and breakage are being investigated [26, 27].
- The lead is passed through the anchor sleeve and attached to the skin using a figure-of-8 stitch with nonabsorbable sutures. The leads and anchors can be further secured by carefully applying Steri-Strips to the lead or anchor.
- Fluoroscopic imaging can be used to confirm that the anchoring process did not result in any lead migration of the electrode tip.
- A tension loop is usually placed, and then a sterile occlusive dressing is applied.
- Each lead is attached to an extension wire, which connects the trial lead(s) to the pulse generator.
- After the procedure, the manufacturer's representative performs final programming. The patient is asked to minimize bending or squatting, as these might encourage lead migration.
- The trial length is determined by the physician's experience and practice. Trials usually last 3–8 days.
- During the trial, the manufacturer's representative should be available for continued programming and any emergencies that require physician involvement.
- Patients are told not to get the entry site wet and to watch for symptoms of infection at the needle entry site, such as chills, fever, or headache, as well as symptoms of possible epidural hematoma, including increasing neck or back pain and progressive weakness or numbness of the legs.

16.3.1 SCS Trial Assessment

The patient is told to do all the activities that normally cause pain, to determine the level of pain relief and positive changes in quality of life. Over the time of the trial, the patient should document pain scores, functional improvements, and any reduction of medication use. Current criteria used by insurance companies to proceed with permanent implantation of an SCS device require documentation of at least 50% reduction in pain intensity. Documentation should also include any improvement in the patient's quality of life during the SCS trial. Before lead removal, physicians can also verify the position of the lead tips using fluoroscopy and document their final position.

16.4 Trial Technique for Peripheral Nerve Field Stimulation (PNFS)

Following are the steps for trial implantation of PNFS leads [8, 20]:

- In the preoperative period, the area of pain is carefully outlined. If allodynia or hyperesthesia is noted, the leads are placed just outside of this region. Note that leads placed over bony protuberances may later cause lead erosion through the skin. The largest area of pain treated with a single lead is approximately 20 × 15 cm.
- Patients can receive a preoperative weight-based dose of intravenous antibiotics, but they typically are not given for a trial.
- The patient is placed in a prone position with the arms abducted and flexed at the elbow to ensure that they are outside the fluoroscopic field.
- Minimizing the amount of local anesthetic used avoids the spread of anesthetic, which may inhibit the patient's perception of paresthesia during intraoperative trial stimulation.
- After lidocaine 1% is delivered into the entry point, a stab incision is made over the entry side and a 14G Tuohy needle or angiocath is inserted.
- During tunneling, application of slight posterior pressure creates a tenting of the tissue as the distal portion of the needle enters below the skin surface.
- One hand advances the needle and the other is used to palpate the skin surface over the tented area of the skin. Minimal resistance should be present as the tip of the needle is advanced subcutaneously. Increased resistance during advancement of the needle or skin dimpling suggests that the lead is in the skin and should be redirected into a deeper plane. If the needle cannot be palpated, it is too deep and should be redirected more superficially.
- Leads that are placed too deep cause the patient to experience deep aching or muscle contraction. Leads that are placed too superficially cause the patient to experience painful dysesthesia in the form of burning and stinging at low sensory thresholds.
- Under fluoroscopy, the leads are tunneled to a site within 1 cm of the area of greatest pain.
- Studies have found that the optimal electrode depth is 10–15 mm below the skin surface [28]. The thickness of the adipose tissue affects the neural activation only when the layer is thin (<10 mm) [29].
- The needle is then withdrawn and stimulation of the leads is performed to ensure adequate paresthesia over the painful area(s).
- The lead or leads are then sutured to the skin and dressings are applied. The leads are connected to an external power source for the trial duration (3–8 days). Stimulation parameters are then reviewed and adjusted for further improvements.

16.5 The Role of Hybrid Trials of SCS and PNFS

There is no optimal treatment for failed back surgery syndrome (FBSS). Once triggered, the psychological and physical effects on patients contribute to a multifactorial and complex pain syndrome. The literature demonstrates that the outcomes of patients who have been subjected to multiple surgical procedures on the spine are worse than those who underwent SCS [30]. More spine surgeries often lead to a worse clinical picture owing to additional epidural fibrosis and segmental vertebral microinstability [31]. Thus, the sooner patients are exposed to therapies such as hybrid SCS and PNFS trial and implantation, the more likely they will experience the relief they have been seeking.

Hybrid system trials in which PNFS is used in combination with SCS (instead of spine surgery) as a treatment for chronic low back and leg pain present several advantages [21]:

- The hybrid system is easily reversible and has low morbidity.
- The percutaneous lead trial is minimally invasive, which avoids invasive surgical dissection.
- A hybrid system trial can examine coverage provided by SCS or PNFS alone or in combination, to assess which option works best for each individual, prior to the implantation of a permanent system.
- Hybrid systems cover the neuropathic and nociceptive components of lower back pain more adequately than each can do on its own.
- Complex programs can be used to rotate between different areas of involvement or can simultaneously stimulate the entire involved area.

One significant difference between PNFS and SCS is the potential for a greater distance between cathode and anode polarities with PNFS. Typical SCS contact distances between cathode and anode are less than 10 mm, whereas in PNFS, polarity distances of over 30 mm can be achieved, with dense paresthesia between contacts. This creates a longer flow of current than can be accomplished with traditional SCS therapy. With PNFS leads, patients often report the area between the electrodes as one solid area of paresthesia. This dense paresthesia is not perceived to be diluted as the area increases; increased power consumption is required, however, leading to shorter battery life [8].

Much work has been done to determine how much of a painful area can be covered by paresthesia from a subcutaneous cylindrical lead. By itself, one lead usually covers an area the size of a credit card. Other investigators have developed more sophisticated programming techniques that reduce energy consumption and provide a larger area of paresthesia, resulting in wider coverage and better pain relief [8]. Based on the area likely to be covered, careful consideration about how many leads will be placed must be factored into the trial plan [8, 32]. To cover most painful areas, the use of two to four leads is generally required [33]. It has been shown that the degree of stimulation coverage of the painful low back area during trial is an important predictor for the efficacy of lumbar PNFS [36].

Studies analyzing the effectiveness of hybrid systems using both SCS and PNFS have shown promising results. Navarro and Vercimak [34] analyzed retrospective data to evaluate patients treated for chronic intractable pain using these hybrid systems. The study included 40 patients with one lead placed epidurally at T8-9, and two PNFS leads placed in the painful axial lumbar area bilaterally. These three leads created a triangle and produced a paresthesia over the targeted painful area. Most of the patients experienced immediate pain relief and were able to reduce their oral pain medications with this lead configuration. Pain relief was maintained for most patients at 6 months.

Hamm-Faber et al. [35] studied 11 FBSS patients with chronic limb and/or low back pain who initially had leads placed in the epidural space for an SCS trial. The SCS trial reduced lower extremity pain by 50% in 75% of the patients at 12 months, but none of the SCS trial patients had sufficient pain relief of axial back pain, and they were offered PNFS lead placement at the time of SCS implantation. Nine patients proceeded with PNFS lead placement. If the lower back pain was on both sides of the lower back, two PNFS leads were placed on each side. Pain relief was measured using a 100-point VAS scale. The overall reduction of low back pain using PNFS was 48%, with four patients having more than 50% relief of axial low back pain. This relief was maintained up to 12 months following implantation of the hybrid system.

Despite the success of these hybrid systems during trial, along with stringent patient selection, practitioner expertise, and advanced technological knowledge, a small proportion of patients fail to show improvement after implantation—a frustrating but consistent trend reported in neuromodulation studies [36, 37]. Reasons for failure or loss of efficacy proposed in the literature include practitioner technique, mechanisms of the original injury, failure of the device, scarring, genetic predisposition to developing neuropathic pain, placebo effect during the trial, and undetected psychological or psychiatric disorder [14, 35, 38, 39]. Currently, we remain unable to identify this tiny proportion of patients who will proceed to implant after a positive trial but experience later failure of the therapy [40].

References

1. Bogduk N. Pharmacological alternatives for the alleviation of back pain. Expert Opin Pharmacother. 2004;5:2091–8.
2. Stillings D. A survey of the history of electrical stimulation for pain to 1900. Med Instrum. 1975;9:255–9.
3. Krabbenbos IP, van Dongen E, Nijhuis H, Liem AL. Mechanisms of spinal cord stimulation in neuropathic pain. In: Carillo-Ruiz J, editor. Topics in neuromodulation treatment. Intech; 2012. http://www.intechopen.com/books/topics-in-neuromodulationtreatment/mechanisms-of-action-of-spinal-cord-stimulation-in-neuropathic-pain
4. Mironer YE, Satterthwaite JR, Lewis EM, Haasis JC, Latourette PC, Skoloff EM, et al. Efficacy of a single, percutaneous, across midline, Octrode® lead using a "midline anchoring" technique in the treatment of chronic low back and/or lower extremity pain: a retrospective study. Neuromodulation. 2008;11:286–95.

5. Van Buyten J-P, Al-Kaisy A, Smet I, Palmisani S, Smith T. High-frequency spinal cord stimulation for the treatment of chronic back pain patients: results of a prospective multicenter European clinical study. Neuromodulation. 2013;16:59–65; discussion 65–6.
6. Oakley JC. Spinal cord stimulation in axial low back pain: solving the dilemma. Pain Med. 2006;7(Suppl 1):S58–63.
7. Deogaonkar M, Slavin KV. Peripheral nerve/field stimulation for neuropathic pain. Neurosurg Clin N Am. 2014;25:1–10.
8. Cairns KD, McRoberts WP, Deer T. Peripheral nerve stimulation for the treatment of truncal pain. Prog Neurol Surg. 2011;24:58–69.
9. Slavin KV, Nersesyan H, Wess C. Peripheral neurostimulation for treatment of intractable occipital neuralgia. Neurosurgery. 2006;58:112–9; discussion 112–9.
10. Weiner RL, Reed KL. Peripheral neurostimulation for control of intractable occipital neuralgia. Neuromodulation. 1999;2:217–21.
11. Theodosiadis P, Samoladas E, Grosomanidis V, Goroszeniuk T, Kothari S. A case of successful treatment of neuropathic pain after a scapular fracture using subcutaneous targeted neuromodulation. Neuromodulation. 2008;11:62–5.
12. Kouroukli I, Neofytos D, Panaretou V, Zompolas V, Papastergiou D, Sanidas G, et al. Peripheral subcutaneous stimulation for the treatment of intractable postherpetic neuralgia: two case reports and literature review. Pain Pract. 2009;9:225–9.
13. Reverberi C, Bonezzi C, Demartini L. Peripheral subcutaneous neurostimulation in the management of neuropathic pain: five case reports. Neuromodulation. 2009;12:146–55.
14. Paicius RM, Bernstein CA, Lempert-Cohen C. Peripheral nerve field stimulation for the treatment of chronic low back pain: preliminary results of long-term follow-up: a case series. Neuromodulation. 2007;10:279–90.
15. Krutsch JP, McCeney MH, Barolat G, Al Tamimi M, Smolenski A. A case report of subcutaneous peripheral nerve stimulation for the treatment of axial back pain associated with postlaminectomy syndrome. Neuromodulation. 2008;11:112–5.
16. Ordia J, Vaisman J. Subcutaneous peripheral nerve stimulation with paddle lead for treatment of low back pain: case report. Neuromodulation. 2009;12:205–9.
17. Land M, Hoederath P, Gautschi O, Fournier JY. Subcutaneous lead implantation and neurostimulation for the treatment of chronic low back pain following spinal fusion in the lumbar spine. Pain Pract. 2009;9:122. Ovid Insights: https://insights.ovid.com/pain-practice/painp/2009/03/001/subcutaneous-lead-implantation-neurostimulation/375/00134456.
18. Sator-Katzenschlager S, Fiala K, Kress HG, Kofler A, Neuhold J, Kloimstein H, et al. Subcutaneous target stimulation (STS) in chronic noncancer pain: a nationwide retrospective study. Pain Pract. 2010;10:279–86.
19. McRoberts WP, Wolkowitz R, Meyer DJ, Lipov E, Joshi J, Davis B, et al. Peripheral nerve field stimulation for the management of localized chronic intractable back pain: results from a randomized controlled study. Neuromodulation. 2013;16:565–74; discussion 574–5.
20. Verrills P, Vivian D, Mitchell B, Barnard A. Peripheral nerve field stimulation for chronic pain: 100 cases and review of the literature. Pain Med. 2011;12:1395–405.
21. Bernstein CA, Paicius RM, Barkow SH, Lempert-Cohen C. Spinal cord stimulation in conjunction with peripheral nerve field stimulation for the treatment of low back and leg pain: a case series. Neuromodulation. 2008;11:116–23.
22. Reverberi C, Dario A, Barolat G. Spinal cord stimulation (SCS) in conjunction with peripheral nerve field stimulation (PNFS) for the treatment of complex pain in failed back surgery syndrome (FBSS). Neuromodulation. 2013;16:78–82; discussion 83.
23. Mironer YE, Hutcheson JK, Satterthwaite JR, LaTourette PC. Prospective, two-part study of the interaction between spinal cord stimulation and peripheral nerve field stimulation in patients with low back pain: development of a new spinal-peripheral neurostimulation method. Neuromodulation. 2011;14:151–4; discussion 155.
24. Kreis PG, Fishman S. Spinal cord stimulation: percutaneous implantation techniques. New York: Oxford University Press; 2009.

25. Deer T, Pope J, Hayek S, Narouze S, Patil P, Foreman R, et al. Neurostimulation for the treatment of axial back pain: a review of mechanisms, techniques, outcomes, and future advances. Neuromodulation. 2014;17(Suppl 2):52–68.
26. Shaw A, Sharma M, Deogaonkar M, Rezai A. Technological innovations in implants used for pain therapies. Neurosurg Clin N Am. 2014;25:833–42.
27. North RB, Recinos VR, Attenello FJ, Shipley J, Long DM. Prevention of percutaneous spinal cord stimulation electrode migration: a 15-year experience. Neuromodulation. 2014;17:670–6; discussion 676–7.
28. Mørch CD, Nguyen GP, Wacnik PW, Andersen OK. Mathematical model of nerve fiber activation during low back peripheral nerve field stimulation: analysis of electrode implant depth. Neuromodulation. 2014;17:218–25; discussion 225.
29. Frahm KS, Hennings K, Vera-Portocarrero L, Wacnik PW, Mørch CD. Nerve fiber activation during peripheral nerve field stimulation: importance of electrode orientation and estimation of area of paresthesia. Neuromodulation. 2016;19:311–8.
30. North RB, Kidd DH, Farrokhi F, Piantadosi SA. Spinal cord stimulation versus repeated lumbosacral spine surgery for chronic pain: a randomized, controlled trial. Neurosurgery. 2005;56:98–106; discussion 106–7.
31. Talbot L. Failed back surgery syndrome. BMJ. 2003;327:985–6.
32. Baralot G. Peripheral subcutaneous stimulation: a photographic surgical atlas. Denver: The Barolat Institute; 2009.
33. Verrills P, Russo M. Peripheral nerve stimulation for back pain. Prog Neurol Surg. 2015;29:127–38.
34. Navarro RM, Vercimak DC. Triangular stimulation method utilizing combination spinal cord stimulation with peripheral subcutaneous field stimulation for chronic pain patients: a retrospective study. Neuromodulation. 2012;15:124–31.
35. Hamm-Faber TE, Aukes HA, de Loos F, Gültuna I. Subcutaneous stimulation as an additional therapy to spinal cord stimulation for the treatment of lower limb pain and/or back pain: a feasibility study. Neuromodulation. 2012;15:108–16; discussion 116–7.
36. Kloimstein H, Likar R, Kern M, Neuhold J, Cada M, Loinig N, et al. Peripheral nerve field stimulation (PNFS) in chronic low back pain: a prospective multicenter study. Neuromodulation. 2014;17:180–7.
37. Verrills P, Mitchell B, Vivian D, Sinclair C. Peripheral nerve stimulation: a treatment for chronic low back pain and failed back surgery syndrome? Neuromodulation. 2009;12:68–75.
38. Dominguez CA, Lidman O, Hao J-X, Diez M, Tuncel J, Olsson T, et al. Genetic analysis of neuropathic pain-like behavior following peripheral nerve injury suggests a role of the major histocompatibility complex in development of allodynia. Pain. 2008;136:313–9.
39. Song JJ, Popescu A, Bell RL. Present and potential use of spinal cord stimulation to control chronic pain. Pain Physician. 2014;17:235–46.
40. Mitchell B, Verrills P, Vivian D, DuToit N, Barnard A, Sinclair C. Peripheral nerve field stimulation therapy for patients with thoracic pain: a prospective study. Neuromodulation. 2016;19:752–9.

Chapter 17
Hybrid Neuromodulation

W. Porter McRoberts

Along with exciting new therapies such as high-frequency and dorsal root ganglion (DRG) stimulation, coming to the forefront of neuromodulation with great interest is the utilization of tonic stimulation using cross talk or "hybrid neuromodulation" (HN). Programming between leads confers a completely different electrical model of the depolarization of neural tissue. As such, it offers promise in many hard-to-treat conditions. This chapter examines and explains HN, reviews the current available literature for HN, evaluates specific indications that respond to HN, evaluates possible mechanisms of action, and attempts to give direction to the implanter regarding tips and pitfalls for the successful utilization of HN in chronic, intractable, neuropathic pain conditions.

Readers should keep in mind a number of key points:

- Exciting and new therapies such as HF10™ (Nevro; Redwood City, CA), DRG stimulation, and "burst" stimulation have limitations in treatment approaches, and many painful conditions may not be adequately treated by these new modalities.
- HN utilizes programming between leads, often at some distance to each other, sending current through tissue that may be very difficult to stimulate with traditional tonic approaches to spinal cord stimulation, or even with the newer approaches mentioned above.
- HN can generate large areas of paresthesia across areas that are difficult to stimulate.

W.P. McRoberts (✉)
Holy Cross Hospital, Anodyne Research, University of Miami, School of Medicine, Miami, USA
e-mail: portermcroberts@gmail.com

S. Diwan, T.R. Deer (eds.), *Advanced Procedures for Pain Management*,
https://doi.org/10.1007/978-3-319-68841-1_17

- Cranio-facial pain syndromes, headache, cervical and/or thoracic axial pain syndromes, focal pain in the trunk or extremity, and other pain may robustly respond to HN where other approaches fail.
- Many of the approaches may be "off-label."
- Despite great advancement, the morphology of the nervous system still eludes our scientific understanding, and we remain in the infancy of neuromodulation. The implanter who pairs a deep understanding of mechanisms and neuroanatomy of pain with a willingness to think beyond the borders of our current offerings may be many patients' best hope for amelioration of their hard-to-treat pain.

17.1 What Is Hybrid Neuromodulation?

Hybrid neuromodulation (HN) uses leads placed at a distance from each other to carry current through tissues, between the leads, for special and often surprisingly positive effect. Radicular pain, and many pain syndromes from failed back surgery, may be well treated with typical spinal cord stimulation approaches. But any neuromodulator reading this text knows many pain syndromes will simply not respond to tonic stimulation, high-frequency stimulation, dorsal root ganglion (DRG) stimulation or other approved approaches. What follows is a description of the methodology and rationale for an effective but controversial method for treating "hard to treat" syndromes that may fail traditional and newly approved approaches.

Peripheral nerve field stimulation (PNFS) was likely initially developed simultaneously by both Giancarlo Barolat [1] and Teo Goroszeniuk [2] in the early 2000s. The aim was to provide paresthetic coverage of difficult-to-treat areas such as the axial areas overlying the low back, the thoracic spine, and the neck. Traditional spinal cord stimulation (SCS) excels at the treatment of radicular, buttock, and neuropathic pain, but for several neurophysiologic reasons, it largely fails at the treatment of axial pain [3], focal pain of the trunk and limbs, and headache and cervico-occipital junction pain. The more central and more cephalad the pain, the more difficult it is to treat [4–6]. Similarly, the more focal or articular the pain is, the more difficult it is to treat.

Depolarization of neural tissue has been long argued to occur only within the direct vicinity of the electrodes [7]. This assumption, however, exists secondary to electrical modeling mathematics and does not address the possibility of depolarization across distant tissues between anodes and cathodes. Hypothetically, when current leaves an anode (for example, in the periphery from either a peripheral nerve stimulation [PNS] lead or a PNFS lead) and then returns either to the pulse generator or to another contact acting as the cathode, that current and those electrons have flowed through the body. Termed "cross talk" in his sentinel paper, Falco described and measured the effect [8]. What the patient reports, though, does not match the neurophysiologic understanding of neural depolarization. If one were to believe the modelers, the only depolarization would occur in the immediate sub-centimeter vicinity of the activated electrodes regardless of cross talk programming between the distant electrodes, or individual programming of those electrodes without cross talk. However, when the current is sent through the tissues between the leads, from PNS to PNS, SCS to PNS, or SCS to PNFS, a very different phenomenon occurs: the patient reports much, much larger maps of paresthesia. They describe paresthesia in the area of the body between the electrodes, in addition to paresthesia at the electrodes. This effect has been argued to be a function of temporal summation within the sensory hemisphere of the brain. Still, if this were true, simultaneous stimulation of the individual contacts without cross talk would have the same, large paresthesia effect, but it certainly does not: it has discrete paresthesia.

It is well established with a high degree of study correlation that human tissues vary in bioelectrical impedance and dielectric effect, thus presenting different resistances not only at different frequencies, but also in different tissues such as skin, bone, and fat, which have very high relative electrical resistance [9]. Nerve, in contrast, has lower electrical impedance than surrounding tissues [10]. It is then hypothesized that neural depolarization may occur over a great distance between active electrodes as a function of a path-of-least-resistance effect. Current entering the body at the cathode depolarizes at the electrode, then travels the path of least resistance to the electron sink—the anode depolarizing along the way.

17.2 Indications and Case Presentations

17.2.1 Facial Pain

Successful neuromodulation for facial pain has been ongoing for decades, with multiple case reports and publications [11–13]. Approaches include direct ganglion stimulation [14], motor cortex stimulation [15], high cervical cord stimulation of the nucleus caudalis [16], and many instances of PNFS [17]. Despite many examples of success, there remain cases that do not respond. This author is witness to multiple cases where high cervical stimulation fails to provide meaningful facial paresthesia, and facial PNS or PNFS also provide inadequate relief, even when combined. However, when current is cross talked between facial leads and high SCS leads, success follows. One such case report exists in the recent literature (Figs. 17.1, 17.2 and 17.3) [18]. With programming from the facial lead as the cathode with the anodal sink in the epidural space, the patient continued to report near 100% relief of his pain at about 40 months. It is surmised that in addition to the trigeminal peripheral sensory fibers, there is further depolarization occurring at the cord deep to the cathode, as entire left face stimulation was achieved with the cross talk programming. In a separate instance of facial pain from electrocution, cross talk between facial leads and SCS leads was again the key to success (Figs. 17.4, 17.5 and 17.6). Cross talking from multiple cathodes in the periphery to the central anodal sink in the spinal canal provided a deeper and more complete paresthesia than any intralead programming could match, even in parallel.

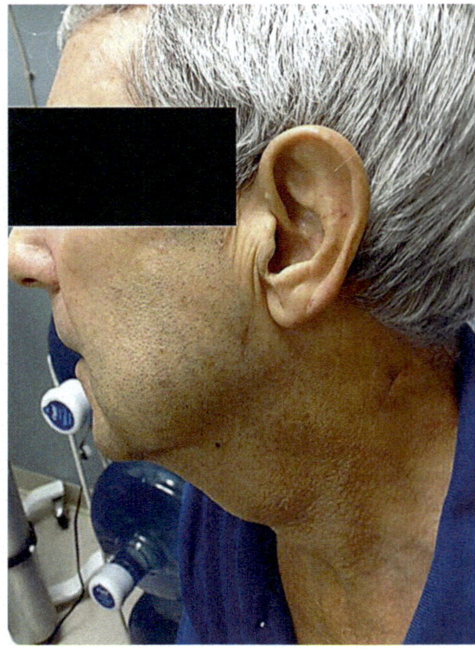

Fig. 17.1 Postoperative photograph showing incisions used in facial skin creases for cosmesis

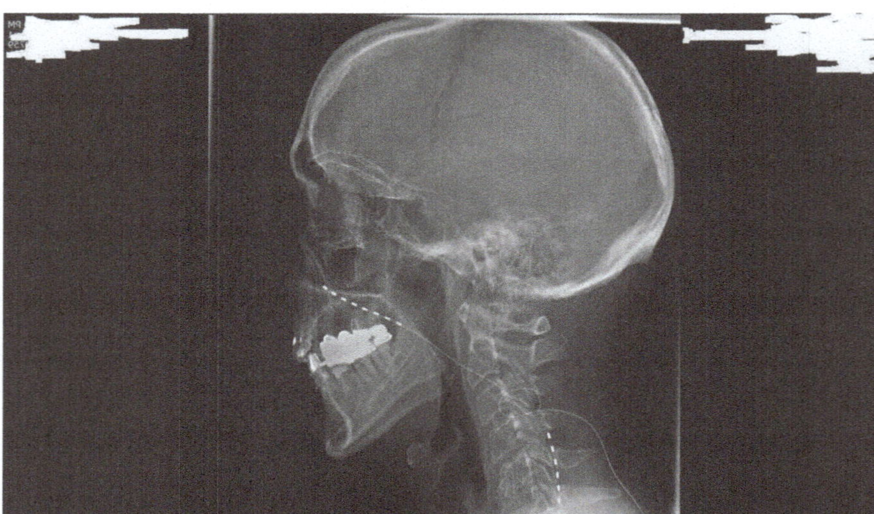

Fig. 17.2 Lateral radiograph revealing permanent lead position with 100% relief

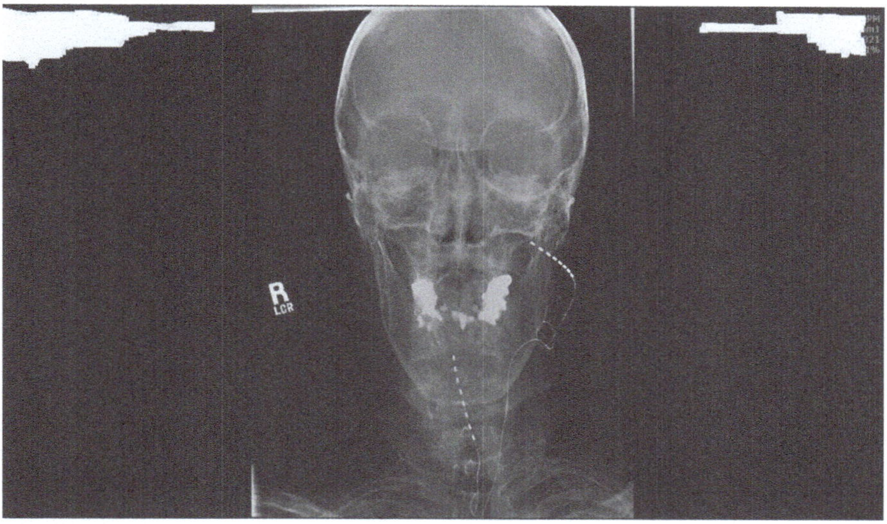

Fig. 17.3 Posteroanterior (PA) radiograph showing lead location

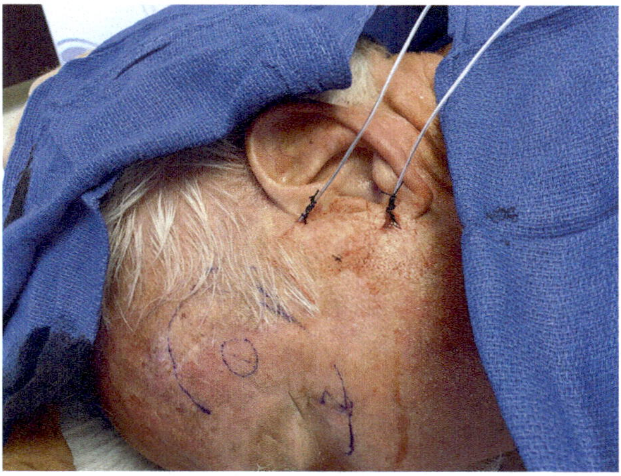

Fig. 17.4 Two facial leads with a cervical spinal cord stimulation (SCS) lead for periorbital pain

17.2.2 Axial Pain: Syndromes

Great promise has been shown in the treatment of axial low back pain with the recent HF10 trial, but there are few data regarding the success of spinal neuromodulation for axial thoracic or cervical pain, and with good reason: neurophysiologically, the targets are deep and elusive [4]. The more central and rostral the pain exists, the more difficult it is to treat with traditional dorsal column techniques

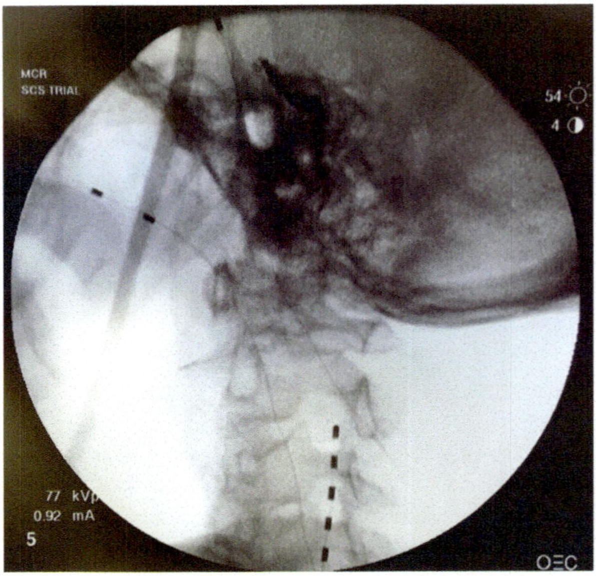

Fig. 17.5 Lateral radiograph showing the cervical lead with V1 and V2 leads partially visualized

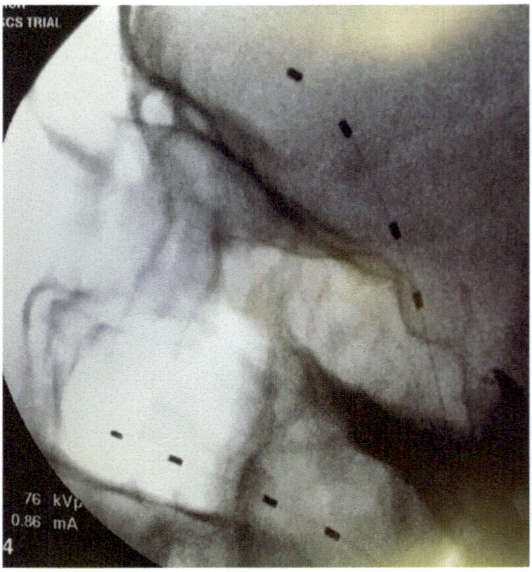

Fig. 17.6 Lateral radiograph of V1 and V2 leads

[5, 6, 19]. Frank, subcutaneous PNFS has been shown to be effective in multiple studies [20–23], but one retrospective review of 20 patients revealed that patients preferred hybrid stimulation to either SCS or PNFS alone [24]. Additionally, Mironer et al. [25] conducted a prospective two-part study evaluating individual SCS or PNFS compared with hybrid SCS and PNFS. Combination SCS/PNFS was preferred by 79% of patients over either modality alone, and hybrid communication between the SCS and PNFS leads increased treatment success to a 90% responder rate.

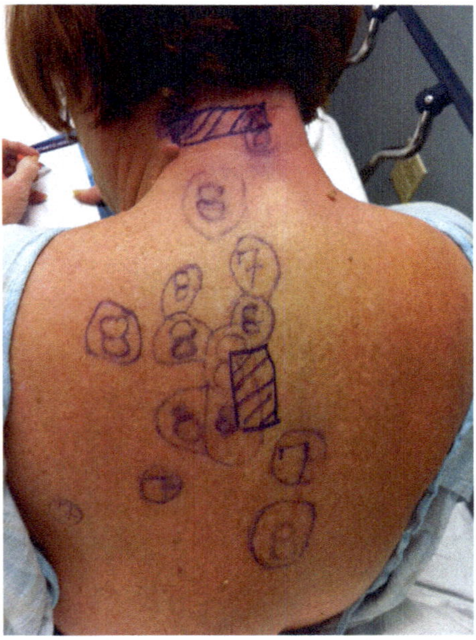

Fig. 17.7 Pain mapping of the thoracic spine

17.2.3 Axial Pain: Methodology

Understanding exactly where and how the patient hurts is extremely important to the success of the procedure. It is highly suggested to have the patient mark on the skin the pattern of the pain. The author suggests writing the visual analogue scale (VAS) score on the skin with indelible marker, in order to accurately and appropriately visualize what hurts and where it hurts (Figs. 17.7 and 17.8). The aim of the implanter should be to place the pain between the electrodes, both in the field as well as between the spinal electrode and the field electrode. The array may have a quite disparate placement, as shown in Fig. 17.8, or it may be very tight, as in focal axial pain syndromes (Figs. 17.9, 17.10, 17.11 and 17.12).

Programming is nearly as important as lead placement. Because neural recruitment takes three to seven times the energy with anodal stimulation [26] as opposed to cathodal stimulation, placing the anode over the dorsal column and cathode in the periphery results in a more focal stimulation pattern with paresthesia, more likely approximating the field stimulation array. The converse programming, with the cathode in the canal and the anode in the field, results in the paresthetic field more likely adhering to the expected dorsal column pattern of paresthesia. Adding cathodes and anodes can spread the patterns; blending interleavened programs can merge the spinal and peripheral patterns.

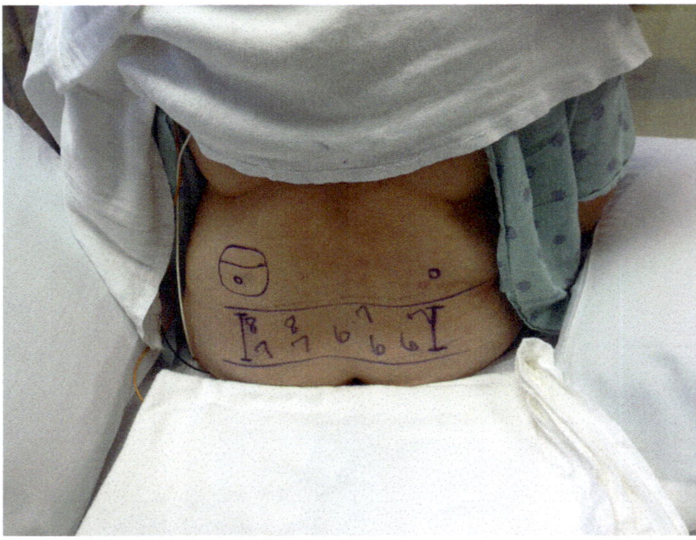

Fig. 17.8 Pain mapping for two peripheral nerve field stimulation (PNFS) leads for hybrid communication

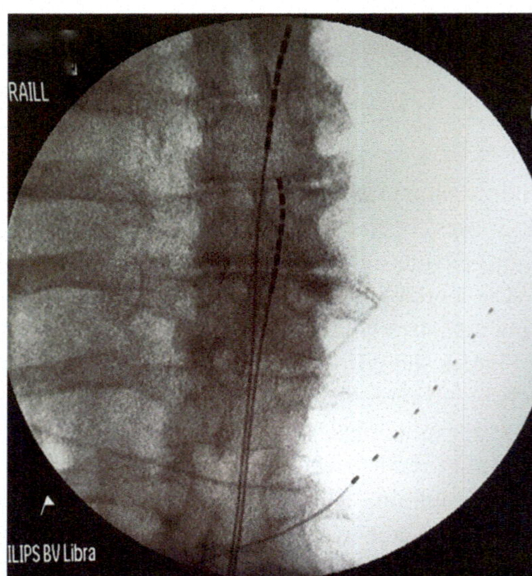

Fig. 17.9 Two SCS leads: one dorsal column, one lateral recess, entering dorsal root entry zone of the nerve root

17.2.4 Abdominal Pain: Methodology

When considering neuromodulation for the patient with chronic abdominal pain, it is again important to understand not only the pattern but also the etiology of the pain. Visceral pain responds well to anatomically higher cord stimulation [27] and

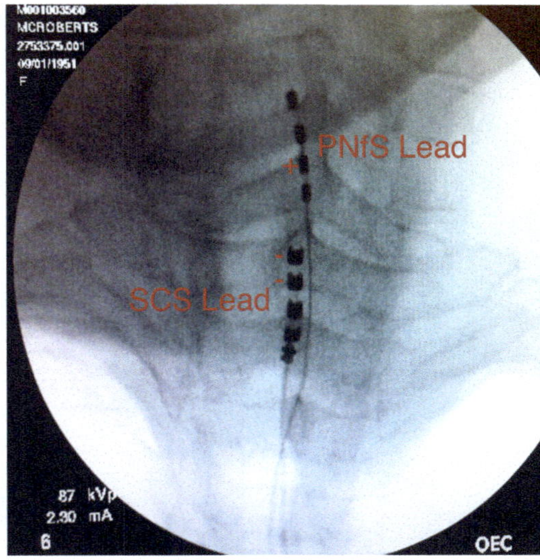

Fig. 17.10 Programming of overlying leads and cross-talk between SCS and PNFS

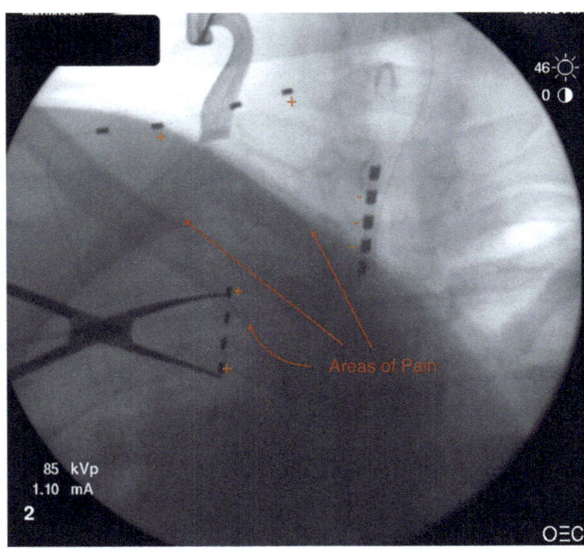

Fig. 17.11 Programming of stimulation with cross talk for left thoracic posterior wall pain

also has been shown to respond to PNFS [28]. Cross talking the two leads for visceral pain requires higher dorsal column lead placement, as described by Kapural et al. [27], and then cross talking to the PNFS ventrally. Somatic approaches are similar, but dorsal column placement focuses on dermatome placement; lateral recess placement focuses on entering nerve root areas. Both can additionally be cross talked to PNFS, as seen in Fig. 17.13.

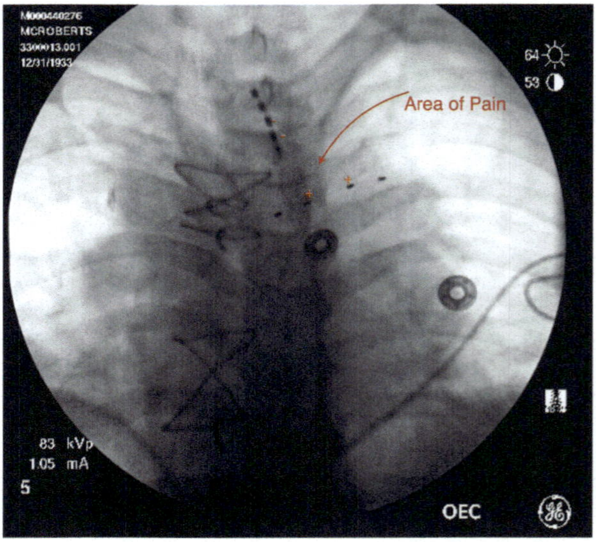

Fig. 17.12 Programming of stimulation for very focal thoracic pain, with an overlying PNFS lead in the horizontal position

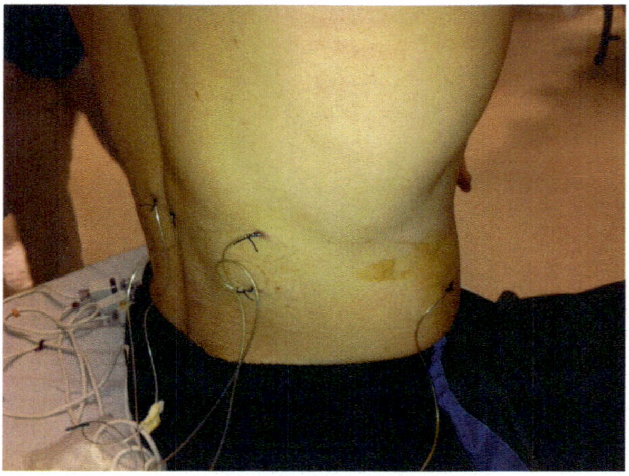

Fig. 17.13 Trialing various leads for renal pain. The patient responded robustly to cross talk of one ventral PNFS cross talked to a dorsal column lead and a lateral gutter lead

17.3 Implementation and Patient Selection

A familiarity with both SCS and PNFS is a necessity. It is essential to understand that success in pain relief with hybrid stimulation is predicated on an understanding of the usefulness of the neural target in mitigating pain, as well as the basic understanding of bioelectric impedance and programming. The optimum patient describes facial, truncal, or proximal neuropathic pain that has been longstanding and unchanging. Yet as the breadth of the surgeon's understanding of central and peripheral neuromodulation expands, other targets and syndromes may seem appropriate.

Planning is essential, and it is suggested to ask the patient to draw representations of the painful areas on his or her body. Understand the patient's areas of maximal pain and most meaningful pain. Palpate and prod and generate a concept of the depth and type of pain. Keep in mind that the patients who do well with HN are the same patients who do well with SCS; they understand the limitations of the therapy and have reasonable expectations and goals.

17.4 Conclusion

Though SCS and recently DRG stimulation continue to evolve, many pain syndromes remain challenging for patients, surgeons, and interventionists, for a variety of reasons. The sources of axial pain are often elusive, and even when identified, they often do not remit with newer approaches. Understanding these profound challenges, the concept of "hiding the pain from the brain" seems a reasonable alternative. Although long practiced by a few neuromodulators, hybrid stimulation remains in its infancy. Though to date it has been minimally studied, perhaps eclipsed by more robust evaluations, the evidence and case reports of success among the cognoscenti suggest that it remains a most effective approach to treating recalcitrant pain in those for whom traditional approaches have failed.

References

1. Krutsch JP, McCeney MH, Barolat G, Al Tamimi M, Smolenski A. A case report of subcutaneous peripheral nerve stimulation for the treatment of axial back pain associated with postlaminectomy syndrome. Neuromodulation. 2008;11:112–5.
2. Goroszeniuk T, Koothari S. Targeted external area stimulation. Reg Anesth Pain Med. 2004;29(Suppl 2):98.
3. Melzack R, Wall PD. Pain mechanisms: a new theory. Science. 1965;150:971–2.
4. Lipov EG. 'Hybrid neurostimulator': simultaneous use of spinal cord and peripheral nerve field stimulation to treat low back and leg pain. Prog Neurol Surg. 2011;24:147–55.
5. North RB. Spinal cord and peripheral nerve stimulation: technical aspects. In: Simpson BA, editor. Pain research and clinical management. Electrical stimulation and the relief of pain. Philadelphia: Elsevier; 2003. p. 183–96.
6. North RB, Ewend MG, Lawton MT, Piantadosi S. Spinal cord stimulation for chronic, intractable pain: superiority of "multi-channel" devices. Pain. 1991;44:119–30.
7. Holsheimer J, Wesselink W. Effect of anode-cathode configuration on paresthesia coverage in spinal cord stimulation. Neurosurgery. 1997;41:654–60.
8. Falco FJE, Berger J, Vrable A, Onyewu O, Zhu J. Cross talk: a new method for peripheral nerve stimulation. An observational report with cadaveric verification. Pain Physician. 2009;12:965–83.
9. Faes TJ, van der Meij HA, de Munck JC, Heethaar RM. The electric resistivity of human tissues (100 Hz-10 MHz): a meta-analysis of review studies. Physiol Meas. 1999;20:R1–10.
10. Vydyanathan A, Kosharskyy B, Nair S, Gritsenko K, Kim RS, Wang D, Shaparin N. The use of electrical impedance to identify intraneural needle placement in human peripheral nerves: a study on amputated human limbs. Anesth Analg. 2016;123:228–32.

11. Klein J, Sandi-Gahun S, Schackert G, Juratli TA. Peripheral nerve field stimulation for trigeminal neuralgia, trigeminal neuropathic pain, and persistent idiopathic facial pain. Cephalalgia. 2016;36:445–53.
12. Levi V, Messina G, Franzini A, Zanin L, Castelli N, Dones I. Peripheral nerve field stimulation (PNFS) as a treatment option for intractable radiation-induced facial neuropathic pain in a survivor of laryngeal cancer: a case report. World Neurosurg. 2016;91:671.
13. Jakobs M, Unterberg A, Treede RD, Schuh-Hofer S, Ahmadi R. Subcutaneous trigeminal nerve field stimulation for refractory trigeminal pain: a cohort analysis. Acta Neurochir (Wien). 2016;158:1767–74.
14. Elahi F, Reddy CG. Sphenopalatine ganglion electrical nerve stimulation implant for intractable facial pain. Pain Physician. 2015;18:E403–9.
15. Rasche D, Tronnier VM. Clinical significance of invasive motor cortex stimulation for trigeminal facial neuropathic pain syndromes. Neurosurgery. 2016;79:655–66.
16. Chivukula S, Tempel ZJ, Weiner GM, Gande AV, Chen CJ, Ding D, Moossy JJ. Cervical and cervicomedullary spinal cord stimulation for chronic pain: efficacy and outcomes. Clin Neurol Neurosurg. 2014;127:33–41.
17. Feletti A, Santi GZ, Sammartino F, Bevilacqua M, Cisotto P, Longatti P. Peripheral trigeminal nerve field stimulation: report of 6 cases. Neurosurg Focus. 2013;35:E10.
18. McRoberts WP. Optimizing stimulation in a case of facial pain through "cross-talk" of peripheral and central leads: a case report. Neuromodulation. 2016;19:885–8.
19. Sharan A, Cameron T, Barolat G. Evolving patterns of spinal cord stimulation in patients implanted for intractable low back and leg pain. Neuromodulation. 2002;5:167–79.
20. McRoberts WP, Wolkowitz R, Meyer DJ, Lipov E, Joshi J, Davis B, et al. Peripheral nerve field stimulation for the management of localized chronic intractable back pain: results from a randomized controlled study. Neuromodulation. 2013;16:565–75.
21. Kloimstein H, Likar R, Kern M, Neuhold J, Cada M, Loinig N, et al. Peripheral nerve field stimulation (PNFS) in chronic low back pain: a prospective multicenter study. Neuromodulation. 2014;17:180–7.
22. Sator-Katzenschlager SS, Fiala K, Kress HG, Kofler A, Neuhold J, Kloimstein H, et al. Subcutaneous target stimulation (STS) in chronic noncancer pain: a nationwide retrospective study. Pain Pract. 2010;10:279–86.
23. Verrills P, Vivian D, Mitchell B, Barnard A. Peripheral nerve field stimulation for chronic pain: 100 cases and review of the literature. Pain Med. 2011;12:1395–405.
24. Bernstein CA, Paicius RM, Barkow SH, Lempert-Cohen C. Spinal cord stimulation in conjunction with peripheral nerve field stimulation for the treatment of low back and leg pain: a case series. Neuromodulation. 2008;11:116–23.
25. Mironer YE, Hutcheson JK, Satterthwaite JR, LaTourette PC. Prospective, two-part study of the interaction between spinal cord stimulation and peripheral nerve field stimulation in patients with low back pain: development of a new spinal-peripheral neurostimulation method. Neuromodulation. 2011;14:151–4; discussion 155.
26. Nement SL, Ranck JB. A quantitative study of electrical stimulation of central myelinated fibers with monopolar electrodes. Exp Neurol. 1969;24:147–70.
27. Kapural L, Nagem H, Tlucek H, Sessler DI. Spinal cord stimulation for chronic visceral abdominal pain. Pain Med. 2010;11:347–55.
28. Barolat G. Peripheral subcutaneous stimulation for intractable abdominal pain. In: Slavin KV, editor. Peripheral nerve stimulation. Chicago: Karger; 2011. p. 70–6.

Chapter 18
Permanent Percutaneous Spinal Cord Stimulator Implantation: Cervical/Lumbar

Jonathan D. Carlson, Eric T. Lee, and Greg Zakas

Spinal cord stimulation (SCS) has been an effective therapeutic treatment for many years in a wide variety of chronic pain conditions. Though there is well-established evidence for treatment of several diseases, but most of the key indications have been in neuropathic pain states. A physician using this treatment option should be familiar with the surgical anatomy, preoperative considerations, and operative techniques, including the instruments and tools needed. To properly care for patients, physician performing such procedures also must be vigilant in monitoring for postoperative complications.

18.1 Relevant Anatomy

As with any interventional procedure, the surgeon must understand the anatomical structures surrounding the sites of implantation. Following are the structures and tissue planes (from superficial to deep) involving the spine:

- Skin
- Subcutaneous tissue (adipose, connective tissue, fascial layers)
- Paraspinous muscles (paramedian needle placement)

J.D. Carlson (✉)
Arizona Pain/Pain Doctor, Glendale, AZ, USA
e-mail: jcarlsonmd@gmail.com

E.T. Lee
Musculoskeletal Care and Regenerative Medicine, Summit Pain Alliance, Santa Rosa, CA, USA
e-mail: eric.lee@summitpainalliance.com

G. Zakas
The C.O.R.E. Institute, Mesa, AZ, USA
e-mail: greg.zakas@gmail.com

S. Diwan, T.R. Deer (eds.), *Advanced Procedures for Pain Management*,
https://doi.org/10.1007/978-3-319-68841-1_18

- Supraspinous ligament (midline)
- Interspinous ligament (midline)
- Ligamentum flavum
- Epidural space
- Dura mater
- Subdural space
- Arachnoid mater
- Subarachnoid space
- Pia mater
- Spinal cord

Anatomical landmarks of the spinal column should be identified on fluoroscopy before implantation:

- Vertebral body endplates (superior, inferior)
- Pedicles
- Spinous processes
- Laminae
- Interlaminar spaces

In planning the surgical pocket for the generator, certain anatomical landmarks are to be considered:

- 12th rib location
- Posterior superior iliac spine (PSIS)
- Iliac crest
- Cluneal nerves (if lower lateral lumbar placement)
- Iliohypogastric nerve (if abdominal placement)

18.2 Indications

Spinal cord stimulation (SCS) may be used as an effective therapeutic option to treat a wide variety of conditions. Though the list of potential targets is vast, we believe the following diagnoses and conditions may benefit most from SCS:

- Failed back surgery syndrome/Post-laminectomy pain [1]
- Complex regional pain syndrome [1, 2]
- Radiculopathy/plexopathy [3]
- Painful peripheral neuropathy [4]
- Other neuropathic pain disorders [5]
- Refractory angina pectoris [6]

Other factors also suggest that implantation of an SCS system is indicated:

- The patient has severe pain than can be interrupted via the dorsal column.
- The patient has failed conservative therapy.

- Significant psychologic issues have been ruled out.
- The patient does not have a surgically correctable lesion, or the patient likely will not tolerate more invasive surgery.
- The patient does not desire more invasive surgery.
- The patient had pain relief from the SCS trial.

18.3 Contraindications [7, 8]

18.3.1 Anatomic

- Critical central canal stenosis
- Pregnancy
- Serious neurological deficit or significant dynamic spine instability with surgically correctable pathology
- Anatomic spine instability at risk for progression

18.3.2 Medical

- Necessity for future serial MRIs (depending on device being implanted)
- Coagulopathy, immunosuppression, or other comorbidities that greatly increase surgical risk
- Need for therapeutic diathermy
- Active Infection

18.3.3 Psychosocial

- Severe cognitive impairment
- Active substance abuse
- Living environment that could be potentially hazardous
- Inability to provide informed consent
- Unrealistic patient expectations

18.4 Preoperative Considerations

18.4.1 Anatomic

- *Spinal stenosis:* MRI of the operative area should be obtained before implantation is considered, for evaluation of narrowing of the central canal where leads could be placed so as to not induce damage to the spinal cord.
- *Previous spine surgeries:* Previous lumbar fusions and hardware placement can make fluoroscopic visualization of anatomy more challenging. Fusions and laminectomies can lead to epidural scar formation, which can make obtaining epidural access more hazardous.
- *Spondylosis:* Severe degenerative changes including facet hypertrophy and osteophytes can make fluoroscopic identification of landmarks more difficult.
- *Spine abnormalities:* Severe scoliosis, kyphosis, and other abnormalities should be assessed with imaging before proceeding with implantation [9].

18.4.2 Medical

- *Anticoagulation:* The risks versus benefits of discontinuing anti-coagulants and/or anti-platelet medications should be discussed with the patient and prescribing physician before proceeding with implantation. Though there are no SCS specific guidelines, most interventional pain physicians adopt the epidural axis procedural anticoagulation guidelines issued by American Society of Regional Anesthesia (ASRA) in determining how long prior and post procedure to stop and resume such medications.
- *Immunosuppression:* Patients with illnesses or requiring medications that suppress their immune system are at a higher risk of post-operative infection [9].
- *Tobacco use:* Patient who use tobacco have a higher risk of post-operative infection and wound dehiscence compared to non-smokers [10].

18.4.3 Psychological

Patients should be assessed for the following psychiatric disorders that may affect outcomes of stimulator implantation. These conditions should be maximally optimized prior to deciding to proceed with SCS implantation [9]:

- Personality disorders
- Unstable or unsupportive family environment
- Suicidal tendencies
- Severe depression

- Severe sleep disturbances
- Somatization/somatoform disorder
- Active alcohol or drug use
- Marked cognitive impairment

18.5 Fluoroscopic Views

An anterior-posterior (AP) image is utilized first, with focus at the thoracolumbar junction for implantation of the percutaneous leads. The C-arm can be tilted cephalad or caudal in order to get the best view of the interlaminar space of T12-L1 or L1-L2, two common entry points, with squaring off the vertebral body endplates. The leads are typically advanced in this view. An AP view is also used to identify the border of the iliac crest for correct placement of the internal pulse generator (IPG).

A lateral view can be used to judge depth when the Tuohy needle is being advanced. This view should also be used intermittent with AP images as the leads are being advanced, to ensure that they are posterior in the epidural space. A contralateral oblique view may be helpful in advancing the needle between the lamina at the ideal angle.

18.6 Positioning of the Patient

The patient is placed prone for the entirety of the procedure. Pillows and cushioning can be used under the thorax and/or abdomen to help bring the spine into flexion and open up the interlaminar space (Fig. 18.1). Cushioning is also placed under any hard or bony pressure points of the patient's anatomy.

18.7 Equipment

Permanent SCS implantation must take place in a fully equipped operating room with a fluoroscopy table, C-arm, and full resuscitation equipment. The following are typically needed for successful implantation:

- Lead aprons with thyroid guards
- Surgeon scrubs with chlorhexidine, dries, then utilizes waterless surgical hand scrub such as Avagard™ to prevent rinse with city water from the hospital or surgery center
- Surgeon double gloves
- Sterile preparation with chlorhexidine scrub and then ChloraPrep™ paint

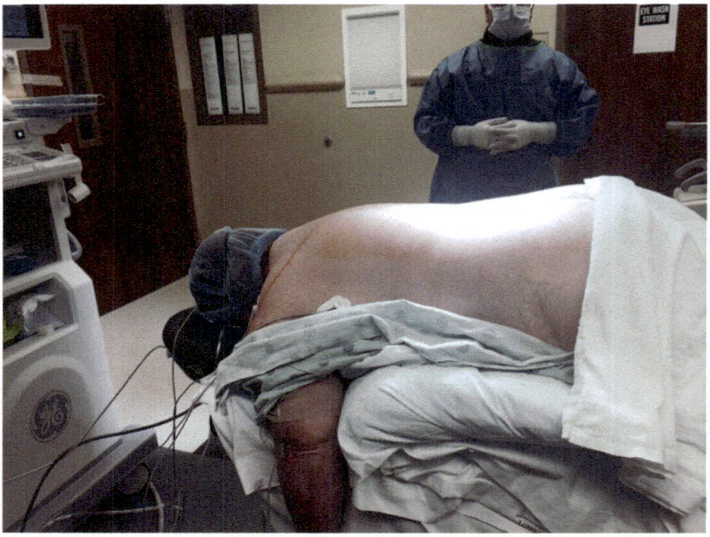

Fig. 18.1 Patient positioned to optimize "opening" of the thoracic/lumbar interspaces for needle placement. Noticed multiple pillows placed. This point cannot be stressed enough

- #11 and #15 scalpel blades
- Full surgical gowns/sterile gloves
- Bipolar electrosurgery unit and grounding pad
- Mayo stand/Metzenbaum/Suture scissors
- Retractors (of physician's preference)
- Forceps/clamps
- Tunneling tool
- Suction equipment
- Sponges
- Needle drivers/holders
- Sutures: absorbable (Vicryl, Monocryl) and nonabsorbable (Ethibond)
- Suture scissors
- Surgical needles
- Surgical adhesive
- Surgical drapes (lap drapes, half drapes, sterile drapes)
- Towels
- Pulsator/Loss-of-resistance (LOR) syringe
- Percutaneous leads
- Internal pulse generator (IPG)
- Needles
  - 14-gauge Tuohy
  - 18-gauge 1½ in.
  - 22-gauge 1½ in.
  - 25-gauge 1½ in.

- Medications
  - 1% lidocaine with epinephrine
  - NaCl irrigation with bacitracin
  - Tissue adhesive (Indermil®, Dermabond®)
  - Medications for sedation (fentanyl, midazolam [Versed], etc.)
  - Antibiotics

  Prior to implant surgery, the patient is to have a chlorhexidine bath twice daily for 3–5 days, with intranasal bactroban three times daily [1].

  Confirm that the patient has received preoperative antibiotics (cefazolin, 1–2 g based on weight; clindamycin; or vancomycin) 30 min prior to incision. This carries the strongest evidence for prevention of postoperative infection [1].

  Vancomycin powder [11]

18.8 Operative Technique: Lumbar Percutaneous Lead Placement

1. The patient is placed prone with pillows under the abdomen and chest to bring the spine into flexion.
2. Select level of entry (usually between T11-T12 and L2-3).
3. Align the vertebral endplates on the fluoroscope at the optimal level.
4. Identify the medial aspect of the ipsilateral pedicle at the level below the desired interlaminar entry level. This will be the skin entry point and may be marked with a sterile marker.
5. Anesthetize the skin and subcutaneous tissue at the skin entry point.
6. Some surgeons may do an initial incision with the scalpel and dissection down to the thoracolumbar fascial layer PRIOR to needle placement.
7. Using a 30-degree to 45-degree angle, enter with a styleted Tuohy needle (Fig. 18.2).
8. Advance the needle medially and cephalad with the bevel up or down until contact is made with lamina just lateral to the spinous process.
9. Walk the needle cephalad and medial to the edge of the lamina. Remove the stylet and attach a loss-of-resistance (LOR) syringe (Fig. 18.3). A combination of preservative-free saline and air may be used to evaluate for equivocal LOR and may avoid potential pneumocephalus with unintentional dural puncture.
10. Walk the needle off the edge of the lamina and engage the ligamentum flavum using ballottement or constant pressure on the LOR syringe.
11. A loss of resistance indicates entry into the epidural space.
12. Remove the LOR syringe and advance the percutaneous lead into the epidural space.

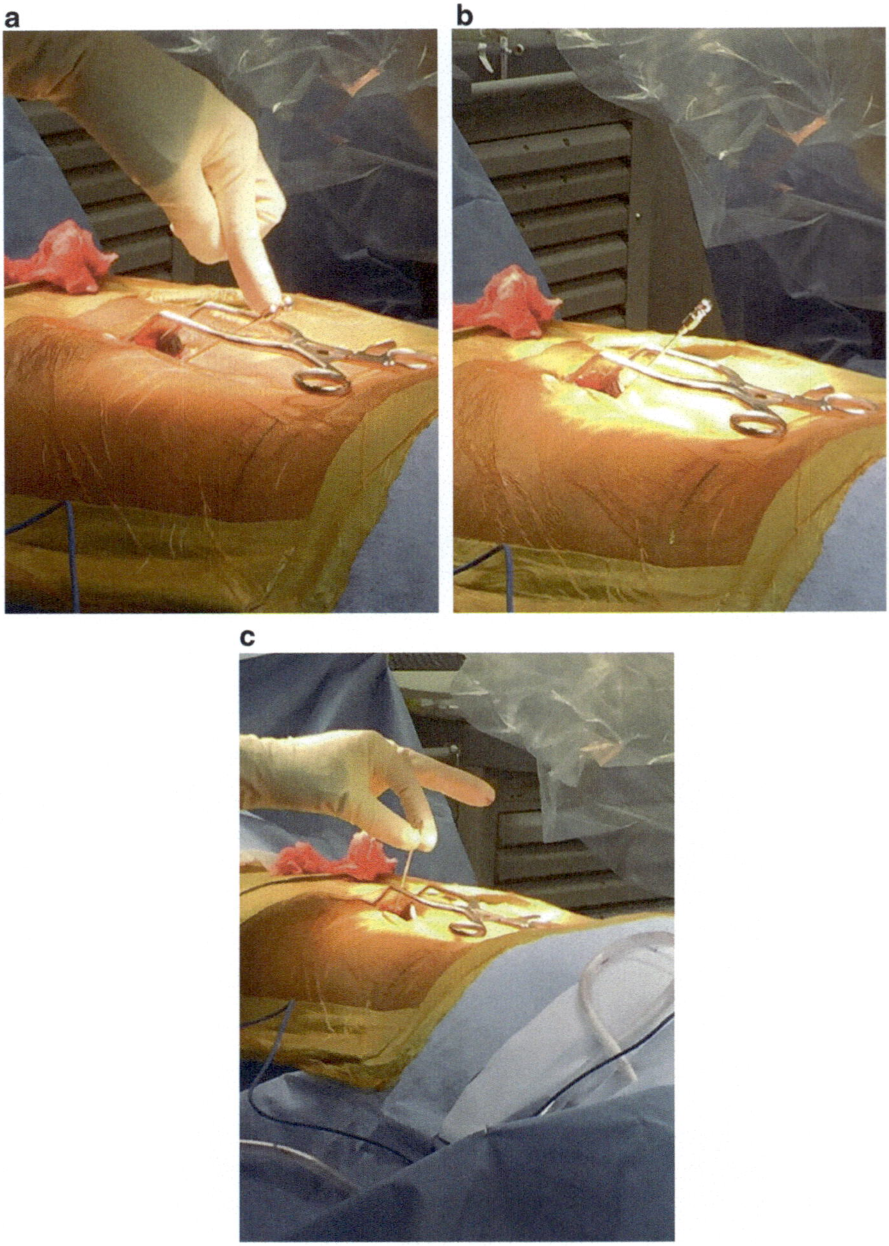

Fig. 18.2 (**a**) Needle entry angle 30°. (**b**) Needle entry angle 45°. (**c**) Needle entry too steep

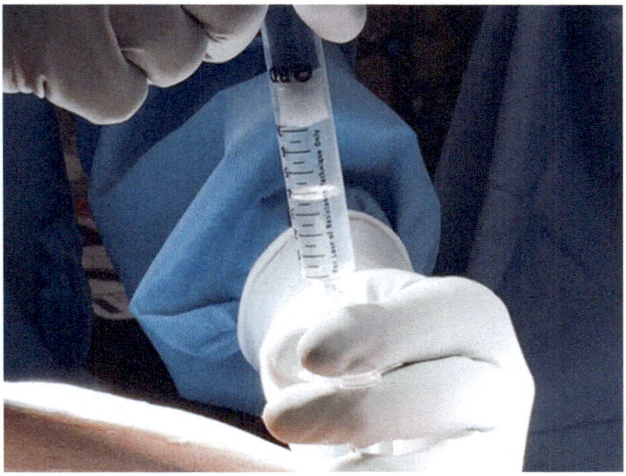

Fig. 18.3 Pulsator/loss-of-resistance (LOR) syringe with half saline and half air

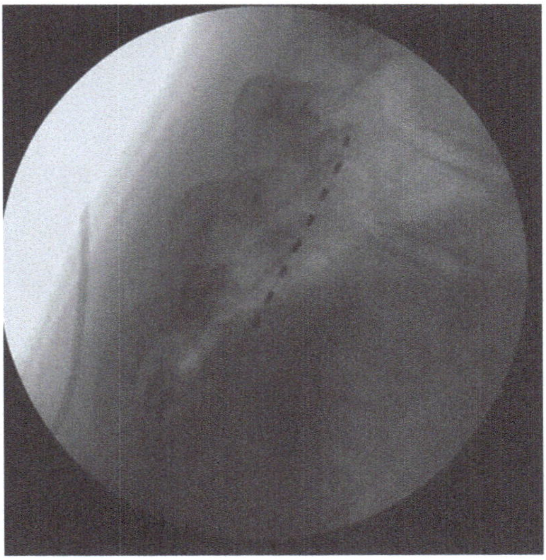

Fig. 18.4 Fluoroscopic image shows octrode lead in the posterior epidural space

13. A lateral fluoroscopic image may be obtained to confirm lead placement in the posterior epidural space (Fig. 18.4).
14. Under live fluoroscopy (low-dose and/or pulse setting preferred), steer the lead, using the hand most proximal to the needle for movements in the cephalad-caudal direction, and the distal hand to maneuver the tail of the lead in a lateral or medial direction by using a "rolling" motion as you advance or pull back the lead.
15. For low back and leg coverage, lead placement varies. Typically, T8 to T11 levels are desired, but it may be placed from T6 to L2 depending on the pain targets (Table 18.1).

Table 18.1 Barolat paresthesia mapping with anatomic lead placement [12][a]

Level	Typical paresthesia coverage
C2-C3	Occipital
C3-C4	Shoulder (SCS leads usually placed more lateral)
C4-C5	Radial
C5-C6	Median (SCS leads usually more mid-line)
C6-C7	Ulnar
T1-T4	Angina
T4-T6	Abdomen/Viscera (SCS leads usually lateral T8-T11)
T6-T8	Low back
T8-T11	Lower extremities
T10-L1	Foot
T5-S3	Pelvic pain (Tripole array/Paddle lead)

[a]Modified version of neurosurgeon Barolat's paresthesia mapping chart for typical SCS lead placement
SCS spinal cord stimulation

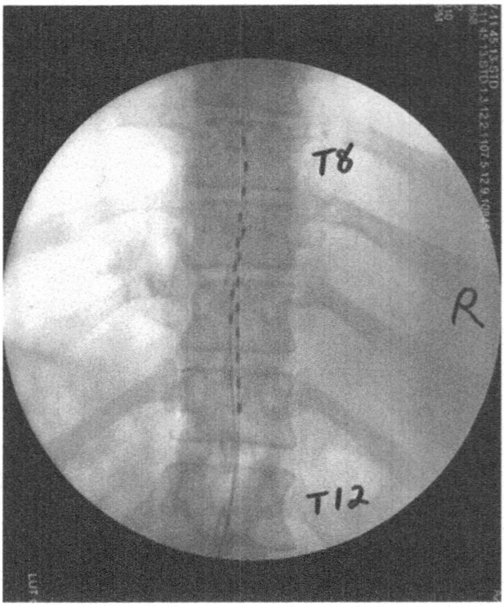

Fig. 18.5 Nevro SCS leads placed at T8 (cranially) staggered to T11 (caudally). Leads usually overlap at the T9-T10 interspace. High-frequency stimulation does not require paresthesia mapping because the system is typically free of paresthesia

16. A paresthesia-free system does not require mapping; two leads would classically be placed to intersect at the T9-T10 interspace for a high-frequency system with stimulation at 10 kHz (Fig. 18.5) [13].
17. If you are placing a second lead, repeat the procedure on the contralateral or ipsilateral side at the same level or the level above or below the initial entry level (Figs. 18.6 and 18.7).

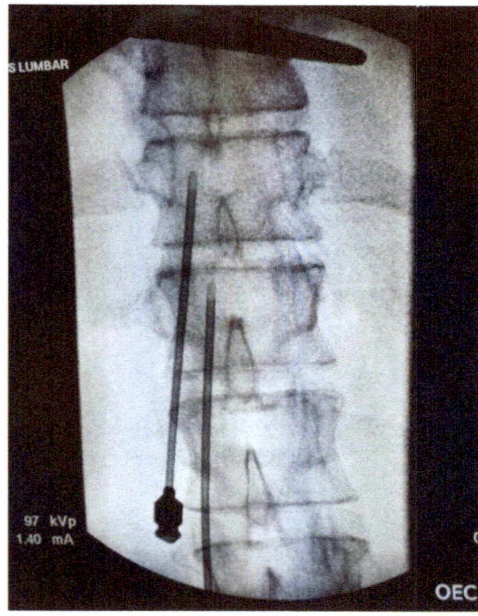

Fig. 18.6 Ipsilateral Tuohy needle placement at T11-12, T12-L1 for SCS lead placement for implant

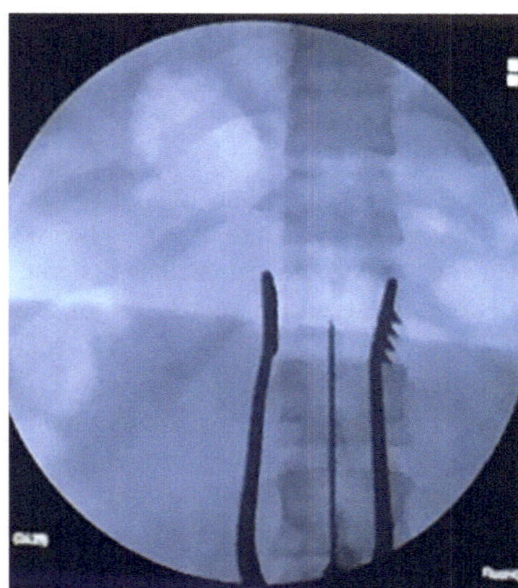

Fig. 18.7 Fluoroscopic Tuohy needle placement with access of epidural space at T12-L1

18.9 Operative Technique: Cervical Percutaneous Lead Placement

1. The patient is placed prone with pillows under the abdomen and chest to bring the spine into flexion.
2. Level of entry will vary (usually C7-T1 to L2-L3).
3. Align the vertebral endplates on the fluoroscope at the optimal level.

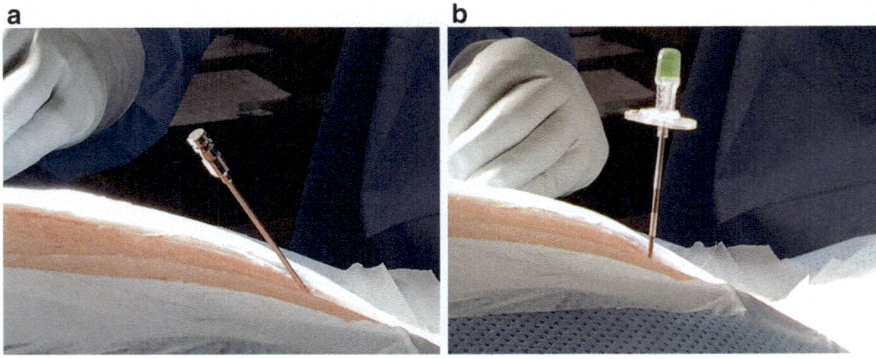

Fig. 18.8 (**a**) Classic shallow needle angle, typically at T2-T3 or T3-T4 interspaces with traditional SCS Tuohy needle. (**b**) Steeper needle angle, which can be done with the RX Coudé® needle, typically at the T1-T2 or C7-T1 levels

4. Identify the medial aspect of the ipsilateral pedicle at the level below the desired interlaminar entry level. This will be the skin entry point and may be marked with a sterile marker.
5. Anesthetize the skin and subcutaneous tissue at the skin entry point.
6. Some surgeons may do an initial incision with the scalpel and dissection down to the aponeurosis/fascial layer PRIOR to needle placement.
7. Using a 30-degree to 90-degree angle, enter with styleted Tuohy or RX Coudé® needle (Fig. 18.8)
8. Advance the needle medially with bevel up or down until contact is made with lamina just lateral to the spinous process.
9. Walk the needle cephalad and medial to the edge of the lamina.
10. Remove stylet and attach loss-of-resistance (LOR) syringe. A combination of preservative-free saline and air is may be used to evaluate for equivocal LOR and may avoid potential pneumocephalus with unintentional dural puncture.
11. Walk the needle off the edge of the lamina and engage the ligamentum flavum using ballottement or constant pressure on the LOR syringe.
12. A loss of resistance indicates entry into the epidural space.
13. Remove LOR syringe and advance the percutaneous lead into the epidural space.
14. Steer the lead under live fluoroscopy (low-dose and/or pulse setting preferred) using the hand most proximal to the needle for movements in the cephalad-caudal direction and the distal hand to maneuver the tail of the lead in a lateral or medial direction by using a "rolling" motion as you advance or pull back the lead.
15. For upper extremity, low back, and leg coverage, lead placement varies; anywhere from the C3 to C7 level is usually desired. Refer to Table 18.1.
16. If you are placing a second lead, repeat the procedure on the opposite side of the body or on the ipsilateral side one level below (Fig. 18.9).

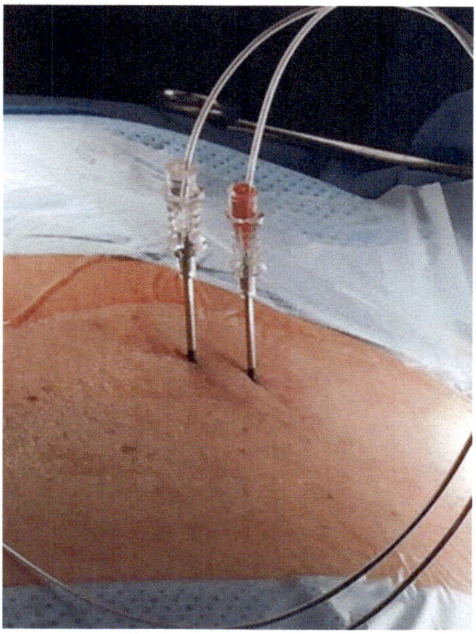

Fig. 18.9 RX Coudé® needle placed on ipsilateral side one level apart. (Minimal heme was not of significance in this case)

18.10 Incision and Implanting: Lumbar and Cervical

For percutaneous SCS implants, some implanters choose to make their incision PRIOR to needle and lead placement. They then dissect down to the pertinent fascial layer and place their needles. They feel that this increases efficiency with the implant. Other implanters choose to place needles and leads first, arguing that needle and lead placement may need to be changed because of potential adhesions resulting from the trial. There is no evidence to suggest that one technique is superior to the other.

1. Use a sterile marker to outline the incision site with interrupted marks to optimize approximation of the skin when closing (Fig. 18.10).
2. Topicalize the skin with local anesthetic (lidocaine 1% with epinephrine or bupivacaine 0.25%).
3. Make the incision with a #11 or #15 blade scalpel (Fig. 18.11).
4. Using sharp and blunt dissection, as well as careful bipole cautery, the fascial layer is exposed. The implanter must use extreme caution if cautery is utilized; touching the leads or needles with cautery could be detrimental to the patient. Weitlaner retractors can be utilized to optimize the incision site for anchoring (Fig. 18.12).
5. Nonabsorbing braided nylon suture such as Ethibond should be used to anchor the leads to the fascial connective tissue. This technique varies between implanters; some will tie the suture to the fascia first (Fig. 18.13), but others will suture the fascia and anchor at the same time.

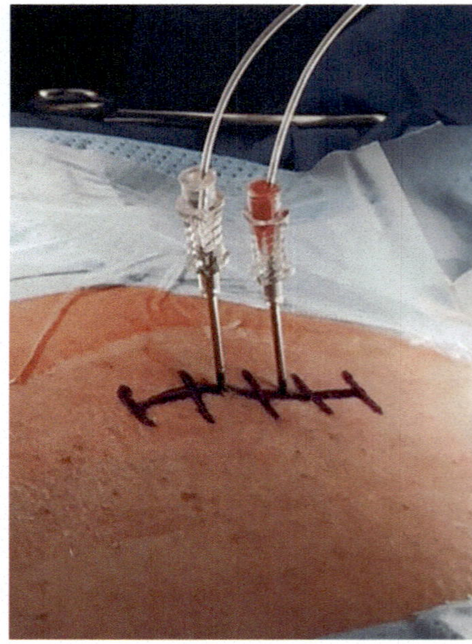

Fig. 18.10 Skin is marked at the incision site with interrupted markings to optimize approximating the skin with closure. (Minimal heme was not of significance in this case)

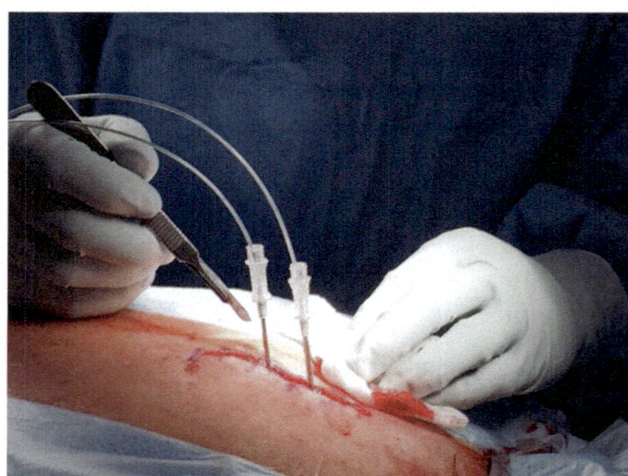

Fig. 18.11 RX Coudé® needles placed on the ipsilateral side for cervical placement

6. A gentle "pull test" confirms that the suture is strongly secured to the fascia (Fig. 18.14).
7. The needles are then removed. Some advocate removal under live fluoroscopy.
8. Anchors are placed and secured to the leads with nonabsorbable suture and the patented locking system, if one is available (varies with SCS vendor) (Fig. 18.15).
9. Using careful blunt dissection, undermine the adjacent tissue to optimize the placement of tension strain relief loops. Evidenced-based medicine notes that strain relief loops minimize migration significantly (Fig. 18.16) [1].

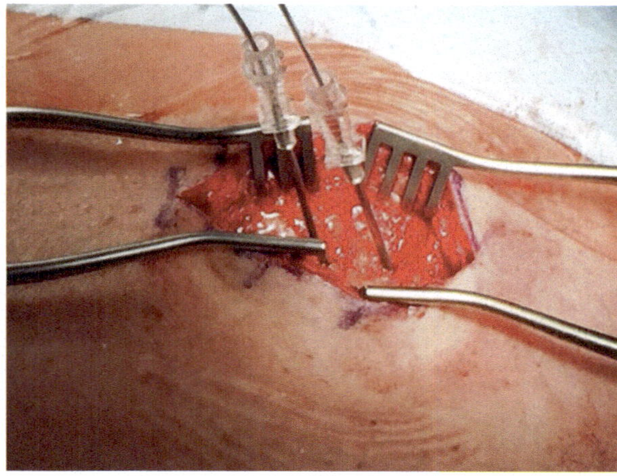

Fig. 18.12 Incision site with fascial plane exposed with Weitlaner retractors

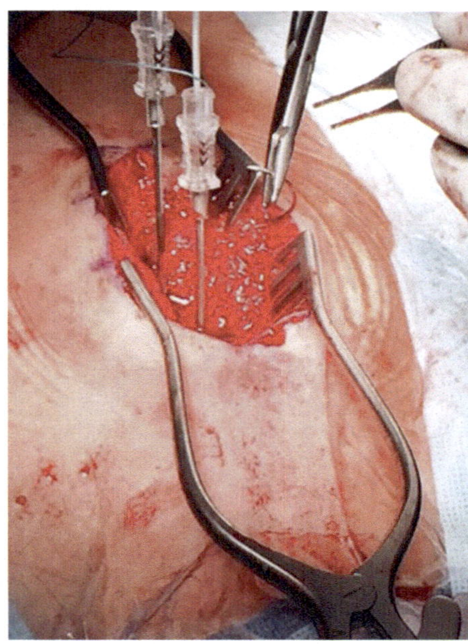

Fig. 18.13 Nonabsorbable Ethibond suture is first secured to the fascia

18.10.1 Tunneling

1. Once the leads have been placed and the pocket has been made, the tunneling to allow the leads to pass from the spine to the IPG should commence.
2. Starting from the spine and heading towards the pocket, a path is marked using a sterile surgical marker.
3. This trajectory skin and superficial soft tissues are infiltrated with local anesthetic.

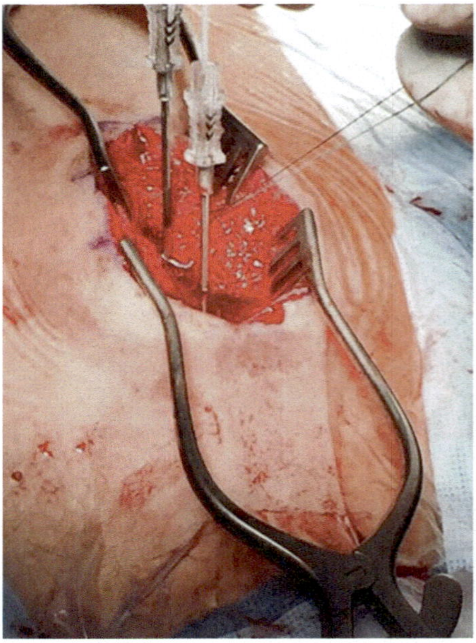

Fig. 18.14 A gentle pull to the suture confirms that it is securely tied to the fascia, thus minimizing the likelihood of migration

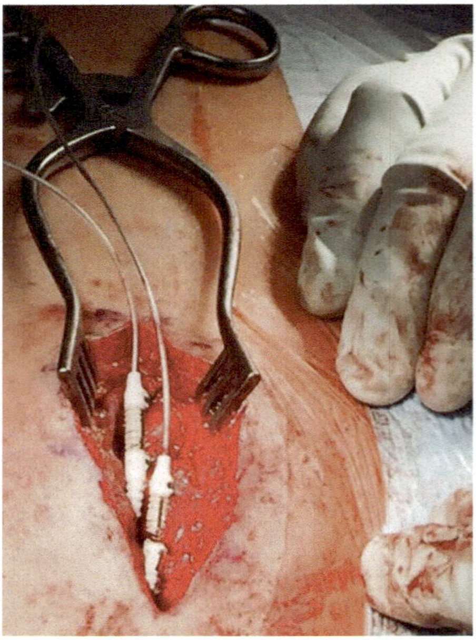

Fig. 18.15 Anchors locked and sutured to fascia

4. The tunneling device enters at the fascial plane deep to the superficial level but above the muscle tissue plane.
5. Advance the tunneling device toward the IPG pocket, being sure not to let the sharp end go too deep.

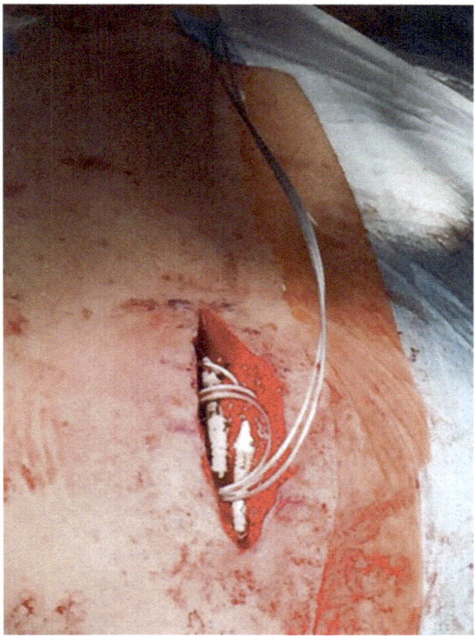

Fig. 18.16 Undermining adjacent tissue and placement of strain relief loops

6. Use a hemostat or forceps to grasp the sheath around the tunneling device.
7. Withdraw the tunneling device, leaving the sheath in place.
8. Place the electrode through the sheath and advance it into the IPG pocket.
9. Once there, attach it to the IPG per the manufacturer's instructions.

18.10.2 Implantable Pulse Generator Placement

Selection of the IPG location is an equally critical part of the procedure. Typical locations are usually the superior gluteal region or the low back, with the side determined by patient preference.

1. Mark the skin surface with a transverse line of the intended incision, using sterile surgical marker.
2. This line should be only slightly wider than the device to be implanted.
3. Use a sterile marker to outline the incision, and create interrupted marks to optimize skin approximation.
4. Using 1% lidocaine with epinephrine, the skin and pocket soft tissue are anesthetized.
5. Using a #15 scalpel blade, a continuous incision is made (Fig. 18.17).
6. Blunt dissection is recommended to extend the pocket along fascial planes parallel to the skin surface.
7. Hemostasis is achieved using a bipolar electrosurgical device.
8. The pocket should be deep enough to close over the IPG without tension.

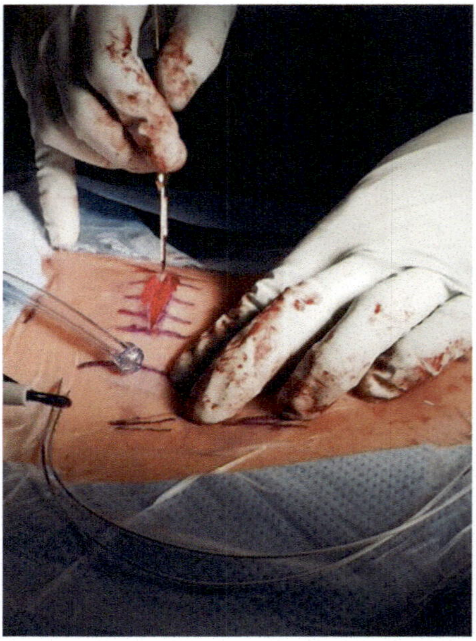

Fig. 18.17 The skin is marked and the IPG incision is made

9. A sizing device is used to ensure adequate size and depth of the pocket. A rechargeable IPG is usually placed at 1 cm depth beneath the skin surface to prevent erosion; placing it deeper may inhibit optimal recharging. A primary cell IPG or non-rechargeable IPG usually can be placed at a depth of 2–4 cm.
10. Clean the leads and place in the IPG, screw in the leads, and do a "pull test." After screwing the leads in the IPG until an audible click is appreciated, a "pull test" on each lead should be executed to confirm that the leads have been fully "tightened" within the IPG. Failure to do this confirmatory step may result in a disconnection of the leads from the IPG, despite tightening of the screws.
11. Copious irrigation of the pocket with saline and bacitracin should commence. Some physicians may consider applying 1 g vancomycin powder to the surgical sites after irrigation [9].
12. Implant the IPG with the leads connected and excess lead coiled in a loop posterior to the IPG (Fig. 18.18). Adequate anchoring and strain relief loops seem to be best at decreasing the likelihood of lead migration [1].
13. Closure of the pocket begins with suturing of the deep fascial layer (Fig. 18.19).
14. Closure of the pocket continues with suturing of the dermis layer.
15. Closure of the pocket concludes with either sutures or staples on the superficial layer.
16. Sterile dressing is applied over the wound site.

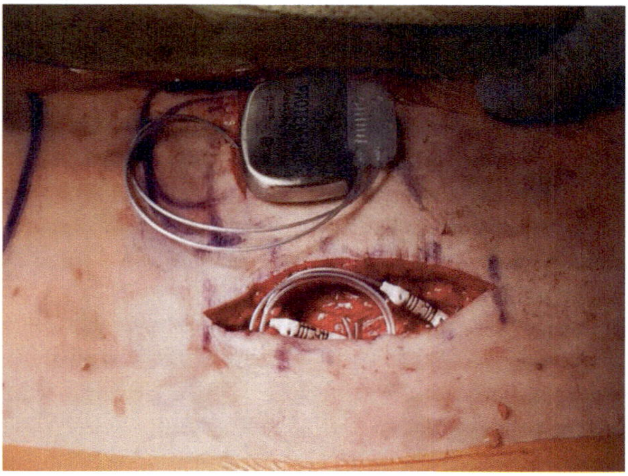

Fig. 18.18 Lumbar SCS placement with strain relief loops at the lead anchor site and the IPG site

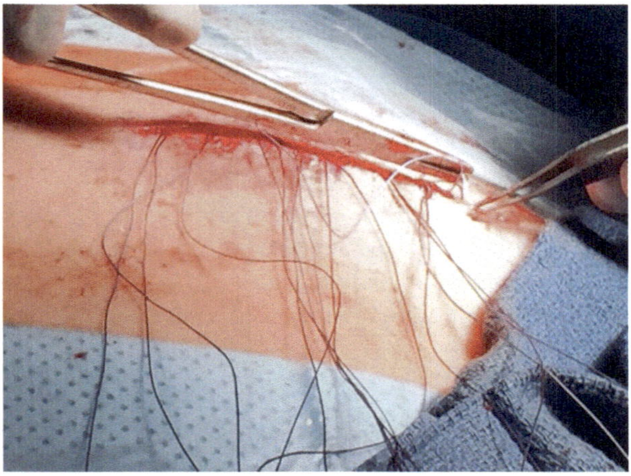

Fig. 18.19 Closure of deep fascial layer with Vicryl suture

18.11 Post-procedure Considerations

Upon discharge, patients should be instructed to begin taking their usual medications. Discussion on when anticoagulants and antiplatelet medication should be re-initiated varies among implanters. Regardless, coordination of patient care should be done during the preoperative planning, based on discussion with the patient and written consent of other managing physicians. Patients should avoid excessive physical exertion, but ambulation is recommended within the first 48 h after the surgery. Oral opioid medications may be used for pain control. The patient is advised to avoid sudden movements, bending, twisting, lifting, reaching, or pulling for 6 weeks. The patient is instructed to keep the wound completely clean and dry for at least the first 48 h, and to report any fevers, increasing areas of tenderness, or erythema.

The first postoperative appointment is typically on post-op day 3 or 4, when the wound is checked. Sutures or staples are usually removed at a postoperative visit 10–14 days after implantation. The patient can usually bathe or submerge after the wound has been checked at about 3 weeks.

18.12 Potential Complications and Pitfalls

Studies on spinal cord stimulation have shown complications in 14–43% of patients [14], with the incidence of a complication requiring a revision in 23–33%, with explantation required in 11% [14, 15]. Following are the known complications of spinal cord stimulation:

18.12.1 Technical Complications [16]

- Lead migration: the most common complication, occurring in an estimated 11–13% [17]
- Lead fracture: occurs 5–9% of the time [18]
- Hardware malfunction and battery failure: Battery failure rates are 1.6% [17]; other equipment fails at a rate of 6.5% [17].
- Misplacement of epidural lead
- Stimulation leading to unwanted paresthesia

18.12.2 Biologic Complications

- Pain over the IPG: 0.9–5.8% [18]
- Infection: superficial in approximately 5%, deep in 0.1% [19]
- Skin erosion
- Epidural abscess [20]
- Seroma
- Neuraxial hematoma
- Quadriparesis
- Headache
- CSF hygroma
- Immunologic reactions
- Epidural fibrosis
- Urologic complications: renal failure, micturition inhibition
- Gastrointestinal complications: nausea, diarrhea, worsening reflux, flatulence

18.12.3 Intraoperative Complications

- Local anesthetic toxicity
- Hemodynamic instability
- Inadvertent subarachnoid injection (total spinal block)
- Dural puncture
- Dehiscence
- Perforated viscus
- Spinal cord injury, nerve damage
- Excessive sedation

18.13 Clinical Pearls

- Proper patient selection is critical to successful outcomes.
- Preoperative planning includes medical optimization and recognition of contra-indications and psychological factors.
- A plan to stop and resume anticoagulation medications should be determined with the consent of the prescribing provider. Risk of an untoward event such as a cardiac event or stroke may actually be much higher than risk of an epidural bleed or hematoma. The risks versus benefits of withholding anticoagulants should be carefully weighed with the pertinent providers and the patient before moving forward with implantation.
- In the operating room, patient positioning is the first important step to optimize lead placement.
- Using fluoroscopy to set up optimal views of the spinal anatomy allows for easier lead placement.
- Vigilance with sterile technique and preoperative antibiotic precautions have the highest evidence in preventing postoperative infection.
- Two-handed technique allows for more efficient lead advancement.
- Adequate anchoring and strain relief loops have the highest likelihood of preventing lead migration.
- Hemostasis and copious irrigation in pocket creation reduces pocket complications.
- Pocket formation should be made in parallel to surface of the skin, not extending beyond the maximum depth.

References

1. Deer TR, Mekhail N, Provenzano D. The appropriate use of neurostimulation of the spinal cord and peripheral nervous system for the treatment of chronic pain and ischemic diseases: the Neuromodulation Appropriateness Consensus Committee (NACC). Neuromodulation. 2014;17:515–50.
2. Taylor RS, Van Buyten JP, Buchser E. Spinal cord stimulation for complex regional pain syndrome: a systematic review of clinical and cost-effectiveness literature and assessment of prognostic factors. Eur J Pain. 2006;10:91–101.
3. Chivukula S, Tempel ZJ, Weiner GM, Gande AV, Chen CJ, Ding D, Moossy JJ. Cervical and cervicomedullary spinal cord stimulation for chronic pain: efficacy and outcomes. Clin Neurol Neurosurg. 2014;127:33–41.
4. Kumar K, Toth C, Nath RK. Spinal cord stimulation for chronic pain in peripheral neuropathy. Surg Neurol. 1996;46:363–9.
5. Simpson EL, Duenas A, Holmes MW, Papaioannou D, Chilcott J. Spinal cord stimulation for chronic pain of neuropathic or ischaemic origin: systematic review and economic evaluation. Health Technol Assess. 2009;13:iii, ix–x, 1–154.
6. Augustinsson LE. Spinal cord electrical stimulation in severe angina pectoris: surgical technique, intraoperative physiology, complications and side effects. Pacing Clin Electrophysiol. 1989;12:693–4.
7. North R, Shipley J, Prager J, Barolat G, Barulich M, Bedder M, et al. Practice parameters for the use of spinal cord stimulation in the treatment of chronic neuropathic pain. Pain Med. 2007;8:S200–75.
8. North RB, Wetzel FT. Spinal cord stimulation for chronic pain of spinal origin: a valuable long-term solution. Spine. 2002;27:2584–92.
9. Kreis PG. SCS screening trial: patient selection and preparation. In: Kreis PG, editor. Spinal cord stimulation: percutaneous implantation techniques. New York: Oxford University Press; 2009. p. 11–34.
10. Peters MJ, Morgan LC, Gluch L. Smoking cessation and elective surgery: the cleanest cut. Med J Aust. 2004;180:317–8.
11. Amrani J. Intraoperative powdered vancomycin use with paddle lead placement. Neuromodulation. 2015;18:177–81.
12. Barolat G, Massaro F, He J, Zeme S, Ketcik B. Mapping of sensory responses to epidural stimulation of the intraspinal neural structures in man. J Neurosurg. 1993;78:233–9.
13. Kapural L, Yu C, Doust MW, Gliner BE, Vallejo R, Sitzman BT, et al. Novel 10-kHz high-frequency therapy (HF10 therapy) is superior to traditional low-frequency spinal cord stimulation for the treatment of chronic back and leg pain: the SENZA-RCT Randomized Controlled Trial. Anesthesiology. 2015;123:851–60.
14. Cameron T. Safety and efficacy of SCS for the treatment of chronic pain: a 20-year literature review. J Neurosurg. 2004;100:254–67.
15. Kumar K, Wilson IR, Taylor RS. Complications of spinal cord stimulation, suggestions to improve outcome, and financial impact. J Neurosurg. 2006;5:191–203.
16. Eldrige JS, Weingarten TN, Rho RH. Management of cerebral spinal fluid leak complicating spine cord stimulator implantation. Pain Pract. 2006;6:285–8.
17. Kumar K, Buchser E, Linderoth B, Meglio M, Van Buyten JP. Avoiding complications from spinal cord stimulation: practical management recommendations an international panel of experts. Neuromodulation. 2007;10:24–33.
18. Turner JA, Loeser JD, Deyo RA, Sanders SB. Spinal cord stimulation for patients with failed back surgery syndrome or complex regional pain syndrome: a systematic review of effectiveness and complications. Pain. 2004;108:137–47.
19. Pope JE. Complications of spinal cord stimulation. In: Ranson MT, Pope JE, Deer TR, editors. Reducing risks and complication of interventional pain procedures. Philadelphia: Saunders; 2012. p. 3–10.

20. Sarubbi F, Vasquez J. Spinal epidural abscess associated with use of temporary epidural catheters: report of two cases and review. Clin Infect Dis. 1997;25:1155–8.

Suggested Reading

Deer TR, Mekhail N, Provenzano D. The appropriate use of neurostimulation of the spinal cord and peripheral nervous system for the treatment of chronic pain and ischemic diseases: the Neuromodulation Appropriateness Consensus Committee (NACC). Neuromodulation. 2014;17:515–50.

Mazloomdoost D, Perez-Toro MR, Burton AW. Spinal cord stimulation. In: Waldman SD, editor. Pain management. 2nd ed. Philadelphia: Saunders; 2011. p. 1303–10.

Ranson MT, Pope JE, Deer TR. Reducing risks and complication of interventional pain procedures. Philadelphia: Saunders; 2012.

Rathmell JP. Spinal cord stimulation system placement. In:Atlas of image-guided intervention in regional anesthesia and pain medicine. 2nd ed. Philadelphia: Lippincott, Williams & Wilkins; 2012. p. 219–34.

Chapter 19
Spinal Cord Stimulation for Chronic Abdominal Pain

Arun Ganesh and Leonardo Kapural

19.1 Introduction

Abdominal pain prompts about 16 million visits a year to primary care offices in the United States and is a major source of morbidity, lost productivity, and healthcare costs. About two million patients continue on to visit a specialist, usually a gastroenterologist [1]. Chronic abdominal pain of visceral origin can be difficult to treat. Over the past few years, spinal cord stimulation (SCS) has emerged as a potential therapy for those patients who are refractory to medical therapies and less invasive interventional therapies.

Recent studies suggest that SCS may be a very useful therapeutic option when trialed in patients with various chronic abdominal pain conditions. To elucidate the mechanisms behind such modulatory effects, additional basic science research is required. In addition, prospective, randomized studies are needed to determine the long-term clinical efficacy of SCS. This chapter provides some detailed background and suggested reading, and describes implantation techniques.

19.2 Mechanism of SCS Relief for Visceral Pain

The mechanism by which SCS relieves visceral pain is not clearly understood, but many theories have been put forward, including these possible mechanisms of SCS-induced analgesia [2–12]:

A. Ganesh
Department of Anesthesiology, Duke University, Durham, NC, USA
e-mail: ag397@duke.edu

L. Kapural (✉)
Wake Forest School of Medicine, Carolinas Pain Institute, Winston-Salem, NC, USA
e-mail: lkapural@ccrpain.com

S. Diwan, T.R. Deer (eds.), *Advanced Procedures for Pain Management*,
https://doi.org/10.1007/978-3-319-68841-1_19

- Sympathectomy
- Suppression of the visceromotor reflex
- Stimulation of dorsal column visceral afferents
- Release of GABA or other inhibitory neurotransmitters
- Supraspinal modulatory pathway activation
- Blockade of afferent input via antidromic activation

19.3 Evidence for SCS Relief of Chronic Visceral Pain

To date, no randomized controlled trials have been performed to evaluate the efficacy of SCS for chronic visceral pain. As such, chronic visceral pain is not an indication for SCS that has been approved by the US Food and Drug Administration (FDA); SCS has been trialed in off-label use. Nevertheless, reports of a few dozen case reports and case series have documented long-term improvements in pain scores and reductions in opioid use (Table 19.1).

Table 19.1 Studies with successful outcomes from spinal cord stimulation for control of chronic abdominal pain[a]

Abdominal pain syndromes studied	Patients, *N*
Chronic pancreatitis, gastroparesis, adhesions [13]	70
Chronic pancreatitis, gastroparesis, adhesions, mesenteric ischemia, post–gastric bypass pain [14]	35
Chronic pancreatitis [15]	30
Chronic pancreatitis, post-traumatic splenectomies, post-laparotomy pain [16]	9
Endometriosis, pelvic adhesions, vulvodynia, vulvar vestibulitis, uterovaginal prolapse [3]	6
Familial Mediterranean Fever [17]	2
Gastroparesis [18]	2
Chronic pancreatitis [19]	1
Chronic pancreatitis [20]	1
Chronic pancreatitis [21]	1
Mesenteric ischemia [22]	1
Mesenteric ischemia [23]	1
Irritable bowel syndrome [24]	1
Irritable bowel syndrome [25]	1
Irritable bowel syndrome [26]	10
Esophageal dysmotility [27]	1
Chronic renal pain from ureteropelvic junction obstruction [28]	1
Bannayan-Riley-Ruvalcaba syndrome [29]	1

[a]These include case reports and case series

19.4 The Role of SCS in Chronic Visceral Pain

Though SCS has been successful in treating chronic visceral pain, it should not be considered the first-line treatment [30]. We advocate a multidisciplinary approach for the treatment of chronic abdominal pain, which includes gastroenterologists, pain specialists, surgeons, psychiatrists, and sometimes physical therapists. If medical management with nonopioid analgesics, physical therapy, or psychological counseling fails, and there is no defined source of the patient's pain, a differential epidural block may help to distinguish between visceral and nonvisceral chronic pain and frequently will point to a likely source [31]. For those with visceral pain, sympathetic blocks should be tried, with subsequent radiofrequency ablation (RFA) of splanchnic nerves, if successful, but frequently, sympathetic blocks and/or RFA do not provide long-lasting pain relief [32, 33]. In those instances, SCS or definitive surgical correction of an underlying problem (such as pancreatectomy for chronic pancreatitis) may be tried. Figure 19.1 shows our proposed treatment algorithm for chronic visceral pain. Note that this treatment algorithm has not been validated in evidence-based literature [34].

19.4.1 Contraindications and Precautions

Contraindications for SCS placement for visceral pain are the same as those for SCS placement for other indications [30]:

- Psychiatric comorbidities that are poorly controlled
- Anticipated poor compliance with SCS therapy
- Chronic infections
- Chronic immunosuppression
- Chronic antiplatelet or anticoagulation therapy that cannot be discontinued for the SCS trial or implantation
- High risk for mortality or morbidity with anesthesia

Additional contraindications may be considered relative or absolute:

- Active inflammatory bowel disease (especially advanced disease with a history of bowel perforation), ulcerous colitis, or Crohn's disease
- Active endometriosis
- Acute pancreatitis
- Other malignant or nonmalignant abdominal or truncal diseases in which SCS could conceal the acuteness or progression of disease

To evaluate whether psychiatric comorbidities are present, psychological screening is recommended [30]. Patients should have an anesthesia evaluation for preoperative clearance before permanent SCS implantation. MRI of the thoracic spine

Fig. 19.1 Proposed simplified algorithm for interventional management of chronic abdominal pain

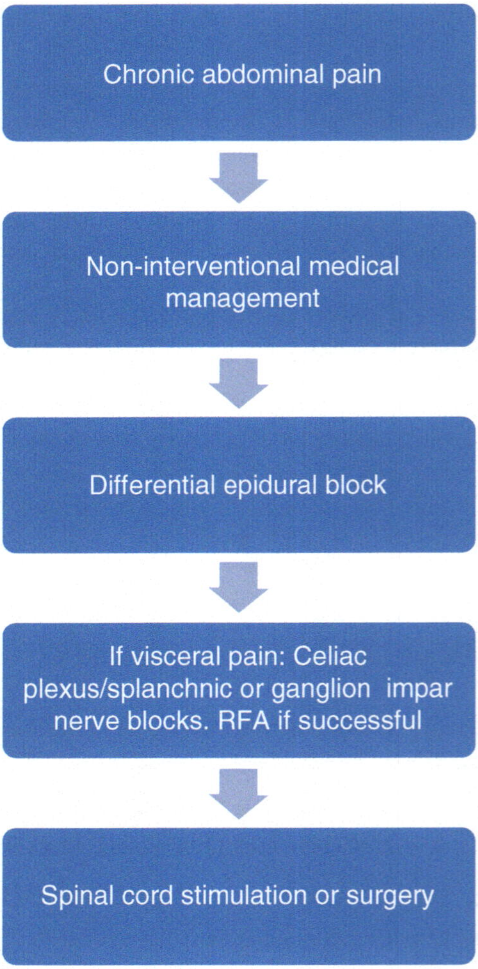

should be performed preoperatively to evaluate for critical spinal stenosis, which would make lead placement difficult or may cause spinal cord impingement by the leads [30].

19.4.2 Management of Anticoagulation

For patients on chronic anticoagulation, a proper plan for discontinuing therapy before the SCS trial needs to be established with the prescribing physician, and more elaborate anticoagulation plans are sometimes needed before the permanent implantation [30]. If anticoagulation can be discontinued, we recommend adherence to guidelines put forth by the Neuromodulation Appropriateness Consensus Committee (Table 19.2) [30].

Table 19.2 Recommendations from the Neuromodulation Appropriateness Consensus Committee for management of anticoagulation before spinal cord stimulation trial or permanent implantation [30]

Anticoagulant	Recommendation for trial	Recommendation for permanent implant
Warfarin	Discontinue 5–7 days before, INR < 1.5; if bridging required, refer to bridging medication; continue cessation during duration of trial, resume 24 h following trial lead removal	Discontinue 5–7 days before, INR < 1.5; if bridging required, refer to bridging medication; resume 24 h postoperatively
Enoxaparin (LMWH)	Hold therapeutic dose of LMWH 24 h before procedure; hold for duration of trial; resume 24 h following lead removal	Hold therapeutic dose of LMWH 24 h before procedure; resume 24 h following surgery
Clopidogrel (ADP receptor antagonists)	High-risk patients for cardiac events—discontinue at least 5 days before; low risk 7–10 days before; hold for duration of trial; resume 24 h following lead removal	High-risk patients for cardiac events-discontinue at least 5 days before; low risk 7–10 days before; resume 24 h following surgery
Effient (ADP receptor antagonist)	Discontinue 7–10 days prior to procedure, hold for duration of trial, resume 24 h following lead removal	Discontinue 7–10 days prior to procedure, hold for duration of trial, resume 24 h following lead removal
Ticlopidine (ADP receptor antagonists)	Discontinue 14 days prior to procedure, hold for duration of trial, resume 24 h following lead removal	Discontinue 14 days prior to procedure; resume 24 h following surgery
Abciximab, eptifibatide, tirofiban (platelet GPIIb/IIIa receptor)	Discontinue for 3 days prior to procedure, hold for duration of trial, restart 24 h following lead removal[a]	Discontinue for 3 days prior to procedure, hold for duration of trial, restart 24 h following the surgery[a]
Dipyridamole, aggrenox (aspirin/dipyridamole) (phosphodiesterase inhibitors)	Discontinue 7 days prior to procedure, hold for duration of trial, restart 24 h following lead removal[b]	Discontinue for 7 days prior to procedure, hold for duration of trial, restart 24 h following the surgery[b]
Naproxen, ketorolac, ibuprofen, etodolac, etc. (nonsteroidal anti-inflammatory drugs)[b]	Discontinue 7 days prior to procedure, hold for duration of trial, reinitiate 24 h following lead removal	Discontinue 7 days prior to procedure, hold for duration of trial, reinitiate 24 h following the surgery
Aspirin[b]	Discontinue 7 days prior to procedure, hold for duration of trial, reinitiate 24 h following lead removal	Discontinue 7 days prior to procedure, hold for duration of trial, reinitiate 24 h following surgery

(continued)

Table 19.2 (continued)

Anticoagulant	Recommendation for trial	Recommendation for permanent implant
Herbals (ginseng, ginkgo, garlic)	Discontinue 7 days prior to the procedure, hold for duration of trial, reinitiate 24 h following lead removal	Discontinue 7 days prior to the procedure, reinitiate 24 h following surgery
Pradaxa (dabigatran etexilate), Xarelto (rivaroxaban) (direct thrombin inhibitors)	Discontinue 5 days prior to procedure, hold for duration of trial, reinitiate 24 h following lead removal	Discontinue 5 days prior to procedure, hold for duration of trial, reinitiate 24 h following surgery
Heparin IV[c]	NA	NA
Heparin SQ[d]	NA	NA

[a]Typically contraindicated 4 weeks following surgery. If reinitiated, careful follow-up and vigilance is suggested (50)
[b]Current recommendations (50) suggest variable stoppage is necessary based on clinical context and on the specific half-life of the nonsteroidal anti-inflammatory drug in question. The half-life determines the time required for discontinuation in order to limit the drug's effect on platelet function. *INR* international normalized ratio, *ADP* adenosine diphosphate, *LMWH* low-molecular-weight heparin, *NA* not applicable
[c]Requires inpatient hospitalization and monitoring, suggesting a special need or indication for neurostimulation, and should be assessed on case-by-case basis
[d]Peaks at 2–4 h after administration; typically thrombotic prophylaxis as inpatient and may require platelet assessment if more than 4-day dosing. Please refer to American Society of Regional Anesthesia guidelines and determine on a case-by-case basis

19.4.3 Infection Prophylaxis

We recommend full precautions mentioned by the Neuromodulation Appropriateness Consensus Committee to minimize infectious complications from the SCS trial or permanent implantation (Table 19.3) [30]. Briefly, we recommend pre-incision antibiotics (a cephalosporin or clindamycin) before the trial and implantation, followed by a 7- to 10-day course of the same antibiotic orally. Additionally, diabetic patients should have HbA1c optimized, and patients should be advised to stop smoking. Standard aseptic surgical precautions and sterile technique should be undertaken for both the trial and permanent implantation [30].

19.4.4 Trial Duration and Measurements of Success

Patients with chronic visceral pain for whom SCS is deemed appropriate should undergo a trial before permanent implantation. A 2010 national survey of physicians who place SCS for visceral pain showed that the average trial duration was 4.7 days, with a median of 4 days [13]; we typically trial our patients for 7 or more days. Success is defined as >50% improvement in pain, stable or reduced use of the baseline opioid regimen, and stable or improved ability to perform activities of daily living [30].

Table 19.3 Recommendations from the Neuromodulation Appropriateness Consensus Committee for infection control measures for permanent SCS implantation [30]

Recommendations	Evidence rankings
Preoperative measures	
Optimize glucose control	IB
Discontinue tobacco use	IB
If hair is removed, use electric clippers immediately before surgery	IA
Use prophylactic antibiotic therapy	IA
Vancomycin should not be used routinely	IB
Intraoperative measures	
Use appropriate preparation technique and agent selection for skin antisepsis	IB
Maintain positive pressure ventilation in the operating room (OR)	IB
Keep the OR doors closed during procedure	IB
Limit OR traffic	II
Handle tissue gently and eradicate dead space	IB
Postoperative measures	
Use occlusive sterile dressing for 24–48 h postoperatively	IB
If a dressing change is required, use:	
Handwashing	IB
Sterile technique	II

19.5 Technical Considerations for a Trial of SCS for Visceral Pain

19.5.1 Positioning

- The patient is placed prone.
- A pillow is gently placed beneath the abdomen to minimize lumbar lordosis. A few abdominal pain patients (especially when allodynia is present) will need minimal IV analgesia in order to tolerate such a position. Keep in mind that your access to the epidural space is most likely in the lower thoracic area of the spine using a paramedian approach.

19.5.2 Anesthesia

- For SCS trials, the patient can be sedated with IV anesthetics but should be able to communicate during elicitation of paresthesias, to ensure proper coverage of the painful areas if traditional SCS is used. To minimize pain, local anesthetic should be applied subcutaneously at the Tuohy insertion sites and applied deeper

with a spinal needle along the intended trajectory of the Tuohy needle in the deeper fascia. Local anesthetic should also be applied subcutaneously at the suture sites for the lead anchors.
- Newer stimulation parameters such as the HF10™ (Nevro; Redwood City, CA) waveform of SCS may not elicit paresthesias, so the patient may not need to communicate during the trial, so deep sedation or general anesthesia may be employed. However, communication by the patient does allow for early detection of inadvertent spinal cord or nerve injury during the procedure.

19.5.3 Lead Placement

- Using anteroposterior (AP) fluoroscopy, the thoracic interlaminar space is visualized and the spinous processes are kept midline.
- The entry point for the 14G Tuohy needle (supplied by the manufacturer) is approximately at the right or left pedicle of T10. Using AP fluoroscopy, the Tuohy is advanced in a paramedian fashion towards the T8 or T9 lamina and kept as close to the T9 spinous process as possible.
- Using lateral fluoroscopy, the Tuohy is advanced into the epidural space using standard loss-of-resistance technique. The angle of the Tuohy needle may be more acute in the presence of thoracic kyphosis (Fig. 19.2).
- A 2010 national survey for physicians who place SCS for visceral pain showed that 50% of patients received two leads for their trial, with the other 50% receiving only one lead. By the end of the trial, there was no difference in outcomes if one, two, or three leads were used. Most leads had eight contacts (octrodes) [13].

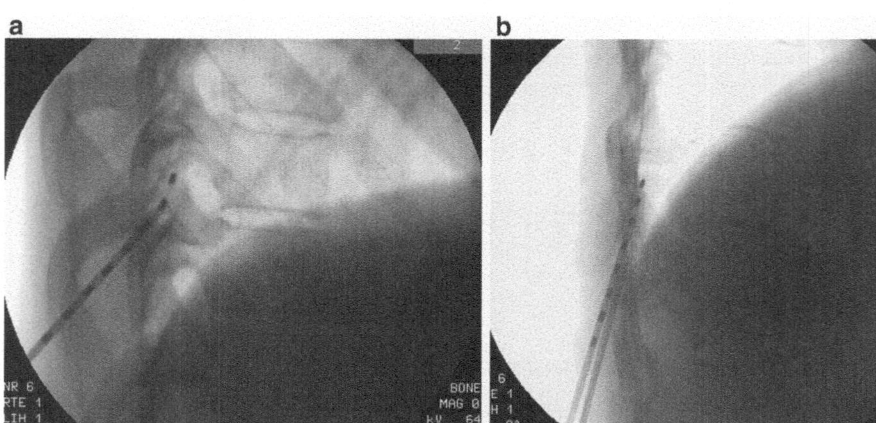

Fig. 19.2 (**a**, **b**) Lateral fluoroscopic view of needle and lead placement in the thoracic epidural space. Notice the various angle of Tuohy needles accessing the posterior epidural space. Such angle variation directly depends on the patient's spinal kyphosis in the lower thoracic area

Thus, the number of leads to place for a trial should be left to the provider's judgment. We typically place two leads.

- If two leads are desired, the second 14G Tuohy is then placed on the same or opposite side in similar fashion to the previously placed Tuohy.
- The leads are then placed through the Tuohy needles; their position in the posterior epidural space is confirmed via lateral fluoroscopy (Fig. 19.3).
- In the AP view under continuous fluoroscopy, the leads are moved cranially to the top of the T4 vertebral body and in a midline position and posterior epidural space (Fig. 19.4). If paresthesia-based, traditional stimulation is used, the leads should be trolled caudally under fluoroscopy and using detectable stimulation amplitude. The aforementioned survey from 2010 showed that most leads were placed in a midline position with their tips at the T5, T4, or T6 position with appropriate coverage of painful areas (Figs. 19.4 and 19.5) [13].
- For paresthesia-based stimulation, if the painful area is not covered, lead positions are adjusted until appropriate coverage is attained.
- The Tuohy needles and SCS lead stylets are cautiously removed under continuous live fluoroscopy in the AP view to ensure that there is no lead migration.

19.5.4 Lead Securing

- Lead anchors supplied by the device manufacturer are placed over the leads near the insertion site and sutured into the skin after application of local anesthetic.
- Other supporting strips and sterile covers can be applied.
- The leads are then connected to the SCS battery and programmed.

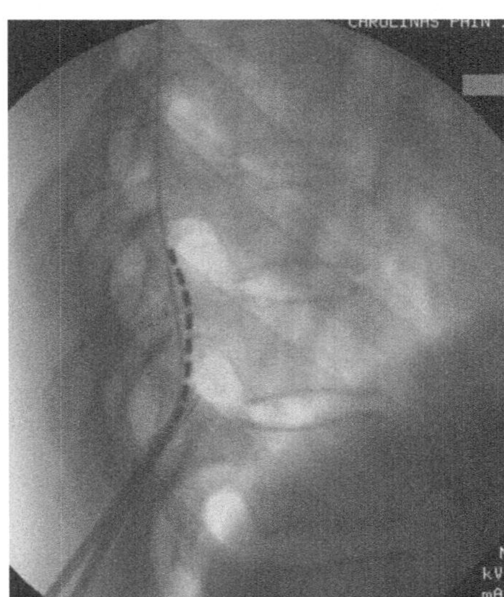

Fig. 19.3 Another lateral fluoroscopic view of a second lead advancing into the posterior epidural space. Frequently, two octrode leads are positioned in the epidural space to provide proper stimulation and therapeutic longevity

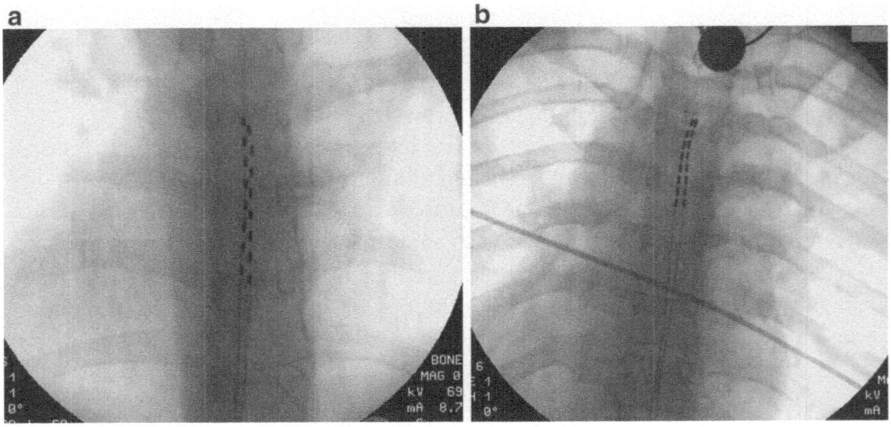

Fig. 19.4 (**a**, **b**) Final position of the stimulation leads. Such positioning may vary depending on captured paresthesias. (**a**) Stacked two octrodes at about the top of T5. (**b**) Two octrodes at the top of the T4 thoracic level, where optimal paresthesias were achieved within the abdominal area

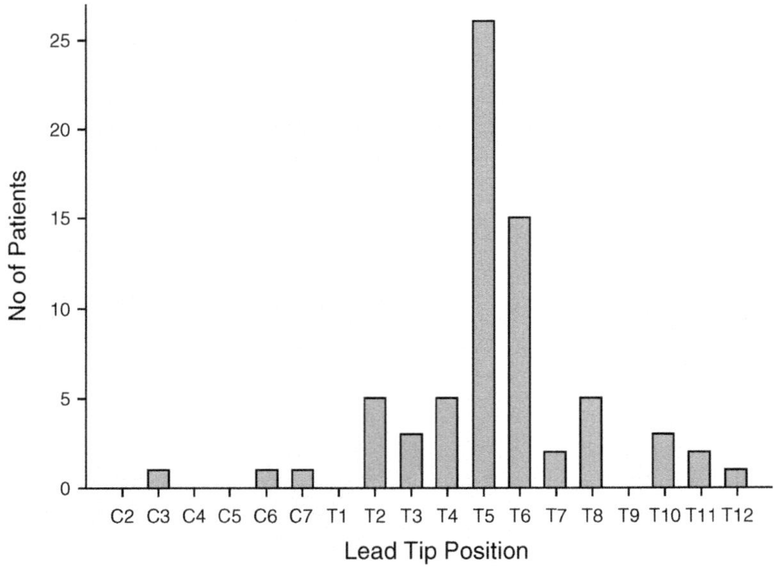

Fig. 19.5 Most frequently placed locations of lead(s) during SCS trials for chronic visceral pain, from a survey of physicians who place SCS for visceral pain. (*From* Kapural *et al.* [13], with permission)

19.6 Technical Considerations for Permanent SCS Implantation for Visceral Pain

19.6.1 Positioning and Anesthesia

- Positioning is the same as for the trial.
- Anesthesia for permanent SCS implantation may be provided using an algorithm similar to the trial, with added local anesthetic at the incision and lead tunneling sites to minimize pain. Patients are often kept at a deeper plane of anesthesia with IV agents (*eg*, propofol) during incision, tunneling of leads, and suturing of the implantable pulse generator (IPG) pocket. To enable communication, patients are emerged from anesthesia during elicitation of paresthesias. Close communication with the anesthesia provider is critical to success. HF10™ therapy does not require paresthesia mapping, so any type of anesthesia can be used.

19.6.2 Paraspinal and IPG Site Incisions

- The intended site for the SCS IPG should be marked preoperatively on the basis of a discussion with the patient for site preferences, such as avoiding the area of an underwear or belt line. It is usually marked in a sitting position because if the site is marked with the patient in prone position, the generator may be placed too low in the buttock.
- Many younger patients and women opt for generator placement under the iliac crest and below the belt line so it is not visible or bulging. We typically place the IPG in the right or left lower back below the iliac crest.
- After application of local anesthetic, a horizontal incision is made at the intended IPG site and blunt dissection of fascia is performed with fingers or cutting scissors, to open the site and create an appropriately sized pocket for the IPG. Electrocautery can be used to facilitate creation of the pocket and for hemostasis. A bacitracin-soaked wet lap is placed in the pocket while the rest of the procedure is continued.
- Using AP fluoroscopy, the T9/10 interlaminar space is visualized and the spinous processes are kept midline.
- The entry point for the Tuohy is approximately at the left (or right) T9 or T10 pedicle. A 3- to 4-cm paraspinal vertical incision is made, with this insertion site at the center of the incision.
- This incision site is then opened with retractors, and electrocautery is used to dissect the incision to the fascial layers overlying the spine.
- The 14G Touhey needle is then inserted at the level of the T10 pedicle under AP fluoroscopy and is advanced in a paramedian fashion towards the lamina, being kept as close to the spinous process as possible.

- Using lateral fluoroscopy, the Touhey is advanced into the epidural space using standard loss-of-resistance technique.
- In the previously mentioned 2010 survey [13], 55% of patients received two octrode leads for the permanent implantation. Thus, the number of leads to place for permanent implantation should be left to the provider's judgment. We typically place two leads.
- If two leads are desired, the second 14G Tuohy is then placed on the same side in similar fashion, with an entry point below the previously placed Tuohy.
- The leads are then placed through the Tuohy needles, and their position in the posterior epidural space is confirmed via lateral fluoroscopy.
- In the AP view under continuous fluoroscopy, just as in the trial, the leads are moved superiorly towards the T4/T5 vertebral body and in a midline position [13].
- The patient is emerged to a lighter plane of anesthesia and the SCS leads are then interrogated with elicitation of paresthesias. If the painful area is not covered, the lead positions are adjusted until appropriate coverage is attained when traditional is stimulation used.
- The Tuohy needles and SCS lead stylets are cautiously removed under continuous live fluoroscopy in the AP view to ensure that there is no lead migration.

19.6.3 Lead Securing

- The lead anchors supplied by the manufacturer are coursed over the leads and carefully placed into the deep fascia. These anchors are then sutured into the fascia.
- Another AP image is obtained to ensure that no lead migration occurred during the suturing.

19.6.4 Tunneling of Leads

- The manufacturer-supplied tunneling device is used to connect the paraspinal incision site with the previously formed IPG pocket. Tunneling should be done in subcutaneous tissue.
- Once the tunneling device connects the two sites, the leads are threaded through the device and the device is then removed. The leads are then connected to the IPG and impedance testing is performed by the manufacturer's representative.
- The IPG is then sutured to the fascia in the pocket.

19.6.5 Closing

- The paraspinal and IPG incision sites are irrigated with bacitracin solution, then closed with a three-layer closure.
- Steri-Strips are placed over the incision sites and a Tegaderm dressing is placed on top.

19.6.6 Postoperative Instructions

- The patient is asked to wear an abdominal binder until the first follow-up appointment on postoperative day 7
- To minimize lead migration, the patient should curtail any extension or flexion maneuvers, twisting, or lifting of objects for at least 2 weeks. We recommend careful bending over 4 months.

19.7 Complications of SCS for Visceral Pain

Potential complications from SCS placement for visceral pain are no different from complications seen with SCS placement for other indications. These include post–dural puncture headache, direct spinal cord or nerve injury, epidural hematoma, epidural abscess, meningitis, epidural fibrosis, lead migration or fracture, IPG failure, IPG seroma, and other infections of SCS implanted hardware [30]. Management of these complications is beyond the scope of this review, but is well discussed in previous guidelines put forth by the Neuromodulation Appropriateness Consensus Committee [30].

References

1. Peery AF, Dellon ES, Lund J, Crockett SD, McGowan CE, Bulsiewicz WJ, et al. Burden of gastrointestinal disease in the United States: 2012 update. Gastroenterology. 2012;143:1179–87.e1–3.
2. Greenwood-Van Meerveld B, Johnson AC, Foreman RD, Linderoth B. Attenuation by spinal cord stimulation of a nociceptive reflex generated by colorectal distention in a rat model. Auton Neurosci. 2003;104:17–24.
3. Kapural L, Narouze SN, Janicki TI, Mekhail N. Spinal cord stimulation is an effective treatment for the chronic intractable visceral pelvic pain. Pain Med. 2006;7:440–3.
4. Krames ES, Foreman R. Spinal cord stimulation modulates visceral nociception and hyperalgesia via the spinothalamic tracts and the postsynaptic dorsal column pathways: a literature review and hypothesis. Neuromodulation. 2007;10:224–37.

5. Linderoth B, Stiller CO, Gunasekera L, O'Connor WT, Ungerstedt U, Brodin E. Gamma-aminobutyric acid is released in the dorsal horn by electrical spinal cord stimulation: an in vivo microdialysis study in the rat. Neurosurgery. 1994;34:484–8; discussion 488–9.
6. Palecek J. The role of dorsal columns pathway in visceral pain. Physiol Res. 2004;53(Suppl 1):S125–30.
7. Palecek J, Willis WD. The dorsal column pathway facilitates visceromotor responses to colorectal distention after colon inflammation in rats. Pain. 2003;104:501–7.
8. Qin C, Lehew RT, Khan KA, Wienecke GM, Foreman RD. Spinal cord stimulation modulates intraspinal colorectal visceroreceptive transmission in rats. Neurosci Res. 2007;58:58–66.
9. Linderoth B. Mechanisms of spinal cord stimulation in painful syndromes: role of animal models. Pain Med. 2006;34:484–8.
10. Linderoth B. Spinal cord stimulation: mechanisms of action. In: Burchiel K, editor. Surgical management of pain. New York: Thieme Medical; 2002.
11. Cui JG, O'Connor WT, Ungerstedt U, Linderoth B, Meyerson BA. Spinal cord stimulation attenuates augmented dorsal horn release of excitatory amino acids in mononeuropathy via a GABAergic mechanism. Pain. 1997;73:87–95.
12. Kapural L. Spinal cord stimulation for visceral abdominal pain. In: Hayek SM, Levy R, Deer T, editors. Neurostimulation for the treatment of chronic pain, vol. 1. Philadelphia: Elsevier; 2011. p. 113–7.
13. Kapural L, Deer T, Yakovlev A, Bensitel T, Hayek S, Pyles S, et al. Technical aspects of spinal cord stimulation for managing chronic visceral abdominal pain: the results from the national survey. Pain Med. 2010;11:685–91.
14. Kapural L, Nagem H, Tlucek H, Sessler DI. Spinal cord stimulation for chronic visceral abdominal pain. Pain Med. 2010;11:347–55.
15. Kapural L, Cywinski JB, Sparks DA. Spinal cord stimulation for visceral pain from chronic pancreatitis. Neuromodulation. 2011;14:423–6; discussion 426–7.
16. Khan YN, Raza SS, Khan EA. Application of spinal cord stimulation for the treatment of abdominal visceral pain syndromes: case reports. Neuromodulation. 2005;8:14–27.
17. Kapur S, Mutagi H, Raphael J. Spinal cord stimulation for relief of abdominal pain in two patients with familial Mediterranean fever. Br J Anaesth. 2006;97:866–8.
18. Tiede JM, Ghazi SM, Lamer TJ, Obray JB. The use of spinal cord stimulation in refractory abdominal visceral pain: case reports and literature review. Pain Pract. 2006;6:197–202.
19. Kapural L, Rakic M. Spinal cord stimulation for chronic visceral pain secondary to chronic non-alcoholic pancreatitis. J Clin Gastroenterol. 2008;42:750–1.
20. Kim JK, Hong SH, Kim MH, Lee JK. Spinal cord stimulation for intractable visceral pain due to chronic pancreatitis. J Korean Neurosurg Soc. 2009;46:165–7.
21. Al-Mahrouqi H, Munro Z, Acland RH, MacFarlane MR. Spinal cord stimulation for intractable chronic upper abdominal pain: a case report of the first patient in New Zealand. N Z Med J. 2012;125:132–4.
22. Ceballos A, Cabezudo L, Bovaira M, Fenollosa P, Moro B. Spinal cord stimulation: a possible therapeutic alternative for chronic mesenteric ischaemia. Pain. 2000;87:99–101.
23. Caruso C, Lo Sapio D, Ragosa V, Lo Sapio S, Cafora C, Romano L. Abdominal angina due to obstruction of mesenteric artery treated with spinal cord stimulation: a clinical case. Neuromodulation. 2011;14:146–9; discussion 149–50.
24. Krames E, Mousad DG. Spinal cord stimulation reverses pain and diarrheal episodes of irritable bowel syndrome: a case report. Neuromodulation. 2004;7:82–8.
25. Rana MV, Knezevic NN. Tripolar spinal cord stimulation for the treatment of abdominal pain associated with irritable bowel syndrome. Neuromodulation. 2013;16:73–7; discussion 77.
26. Lind G, Winter J, Linderoth B, Hellstrom PM. Therapeutic value of spinal cord stimulation in irritable bowel syndrome: a randomized crossover pilot study. Am J Physiol Regul Integr Comp Physiol. 2015;308:R887–94.
27. Jackson M, Simpson KH. Spinal cord stimulation in a patient with persistent oesophageal pain. Pain. 2004;112:406–8.

28. Kim CH, Issa M. Spinal cord stimulation for the treatment of chronic renal pain secondary to uretero-pelvic junction obstruction. Pain Physician. 2011;14:55–9.
29. Yakovlev AE, Resch BE. Treatment of intractable abdominal pain patient with Bannayan-Riley-Ruvalcaba syndrome using spinal cord stimulation. WMJ. 2009;108:323–6.
30. Deer TR, Mekhail N, Provenzano D, Pope J, Krames E, Thomson S, et al. The appropriate use of neurostimulation: avoidance and treatment of complications of neurostimulation therapies for the treatment of chronic pain. Neuromodulation Appropriateness Consensus Committee. Neuromodulation. 2014;17:571–97; discussion 597–8.
31. Conwell DL, Vargo JJ, Zuccaro G, Dews TE, Mekhail N, Scheman J, et al. Role of differential neuroaxial blockade in the evaluation and management of pain in chronic pancreatitis. Am J Gastroenterol. 2001;96:431–6.
32. Garcea G, Thomasset S, Berry DP, Tordoff S. Percutaneous splanchnic nerve radiofrequency ablation for chronic abdominal pain. ANZ J Surg. 2005;75:640–4.
33. Raj PP, Sahinler B, Lowe M. Radiofrequency lesioning of splanchnic nerves. Pain Pract. 2002;2:241–7.
34. Kapural L. Spinal cord stimulation for chronic abdominal pain. In: Kapural L, editor. Chronic abdominal pain: an evidence-based comprehensive guide to clinical management. New York: Springer; 2015. p. 195–200.

Chapter 20
Spinal Cord Stimulation: Pelvic Pain

Grant H. Chen and Corey W. Hunter

20.1 Introduction

Pelvic pain is a lesser-known indication for spinal cord stimulation due to the difficulty in capturing the area of need. Typical lead arrays and positioning are seldom effective and thus require novel techniques. This chapter outlines how to effectively capture and treat this subset of patients.

20.2 Indications

Chronic pelvic pain (CPP) is defined as a "non-malignant pain perceived in the pelvis in either men or women. In the case of documented nociceptive pain that becomes chronic, the pain must have been chronic or continuous for at least 6 months" [1]. CPP is a complex, multifactorial pathology with social, psychological, economic, and even cultural influences. It presents more often in females and is commonly referred to as interstitial cystitis or painful bladder syndrome; in males, it is typically labeled chronic prostatitis. CPP is a crippling, even disabling syndrome that is considered to be a diagnosis of exclusion.

G.H. Chen
Department of Anesthesiology and Critical Care, Memorial Sloan Kettering Cancer Center, New York, NY, USA
e-mail: cheng@mskcc.org; granthchen@gmail.com

C.W. Hunter (✉)
Ainsworth Institute of Pain Management, New York, NY, USA

Department of Physical Medicine and Rehabilitation, Mount Sinai Hospital, New York, NY, USA
e-mail: corey.hunter@me.com

S. Diwan, T.R. Deer (eds.), *Advanced Procedures for Pain Management*, https://doi.org/10.1007/978-3-319-68841-1_20

For the pain physician, CPP is frustrating to treat, as it is often recalcitrant to traditional treatment methods. Medications may be mildly effective, but more aggressive therapy is almost always necessary. Interventions targeting the hypogastric plexus, the ganglion impar, and pudendal nerves have been shown to be modestly effective in treating malignant and non-malignant pelvic pain even when the exact etiology is not directly identifiable [2]. Perhaps the greatest challenge in treating CPP is that the pathophysiology is typically unknown. It appears to have a centralized, neuropathic component, leading some to suggest that CPP may in fact be a form of complex regional pain syndrome (CRPS), postulating that a "wind-up" phenomenon serves to hypersensitize neurons in a similar manner, but in the pelvic region [3].

Given CPP's pathophysiological similarities to disease states like CRPS and sympathetically driven pain, which are known to respond to spinal cord stimulation (SCS), neuromodulators began to utilize SCS as a treatment modality. Neuromodulators naturally focused on the sacral nerve roots as the target for stimulation in CPP, given that the predominance of innervation to the region is from the sacral spinal cord. Success rates were surprisingly low, however, as it was difficult to obtain consistent coverage over all of the painful areas. The dermatomal distribution of the pelvic area presents an obvious challenge, in that there are regions where T12 and L1 derived nerves are immediately adjacent to sacrally derived nerves.

Over time, neuromodulators have begun to explore novel targets of the spinal cord in an attempt to obtain more complete coverage over the pelvic region—including the conus and T5 through T7. The thought process has been to search for regions of the spinal cord where one could recruit as many fibers to the painful area as possible, all in one place.

Sacral stimulation is effective for pain syndromes with a purely sacral distribution and for the treatment of urinary disorders (InterStim™ neurostimulator from Medtronic) [4]. (*See* Chap. 28.) Sometimes the pain or other symptoms extend beyond the distribution of the sacral nerves, however:

- Interstitial cystitis/painful bladder syndrome
- Chronic prostatitis/prostadynia
- Vaginal pain
- Coccygodynia
- Vulvodynia/vestibulodynia
- Anorectal pain
- Chronic pelvic inflammatory disease
- Pelvic floor abnormalities/pelvic floor muscle pain syndrome
- Herpes simplex–caused dyspareunia
- Radiation vaginitis
- Scrotal/testicular/epididymal pain syndrome
- Penile pain syndrome
- Urethral pain syndrome

When these indications occur, other parts of the cord need to be targeted, which can recruit sacral, lumbar, and even thoracic fibers, depending on the anatomical location of the pain.

20.3 Relevant Anatomy

The pelvis is a complex region composed of visceral and somatic structures with innervation from the sympathetic, parasympathetic, and somatic nervous system. The region includes a number of organs:

- Bladder
- Urethra
- Rectum
- Anus
- Perineum
- Inguinal canal
- Female reproductive organs: uterus, vagina, labia, clitoris, ovaries, fallopian tubes
- Male reproductive organs: testes, penis, glans, scrotum, prostate, vas deferens, epididymis

The pelvic region is innervated by eight cutaneous nerves with thoracic, lumbar, and sacral cord contributions (Table 20.1, Fig. 20.1). The relevant dermatomes include L1, L2, L3, and S1 through S5 (Figs. 20.2 and 20.3). The external genitalia receive innervation from the local cutaneous nerves (pudendal, genitofemoral, and ilioinguinal), whereas the internal genitalia and organs of the pelvis are innervated by the sympathetic and parasympathetic nervous system:

- Sacral splanchnic nerves
- Pelvic splanchnic nerves
- Superior hypogastric plexus
- Inferior hypogastric plexus
- Ganglion impar

The pelvic viscera are innervated parasympathetically by the S2–S4 nerve roots and innervated sympathetically by the T12–L2 nerve roots. Exiting parasympathetics are transmitted by splanchnic nerves, which converge into the preganglionic pelvic splanchnic nerves. Sympathetic input to the pelvis arises from the thoracolumbar cord by way of the superior hypogastric plexus.

Table 20.1 Relevant nerves of the pelvic region and the spinal nerve segments from which they are derived

Nerve	T12	L1	L2	L3	L4	S1	S2	S3	S4	S5
Iliohypogastric	■	■								
Ilioinguinal		■								
Genitofemoral		■	■							
Obturator			■	■	■					
Posterior femoral cutaneous						■	■	■	■	
Inferior rectal							■	■	■	
Pudendal							■	■	■	
Coccygeal									■	■

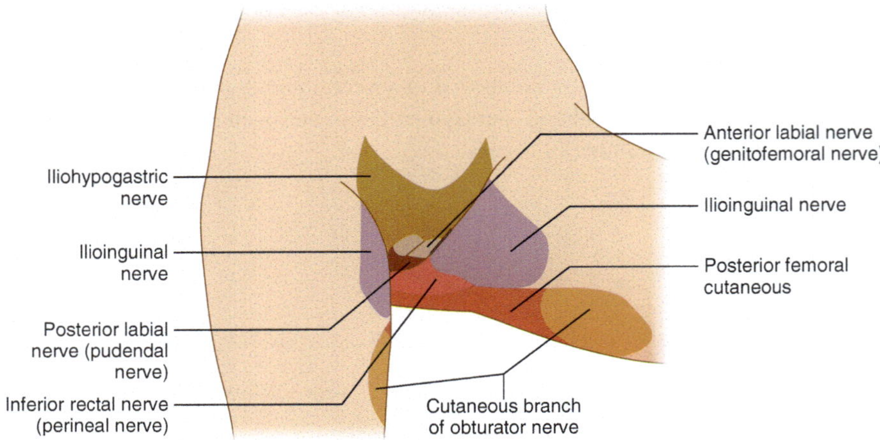

Fig. 20.1 The cutaneous innervation to the pelvic region in a female

Visceral pain fibers, or sympathetic nerve fibers, often travel with somatic fibers. Each spinal nerve receives sympathetic input in the form of unmyelinated, postganglionic fibers from the adjacent ganglion via gray rami communicans. White rami communicans, present from T1 to L1/2, allow this input to continue into the spinal cord, now as myelinated, preganglionic fibers. This suggests that information carried via sympathetic fibers originating caudal to L2 would enter the paravertebral chain at its respective level via a grey rami communicans and travel within the chain cephalad until at least L2 (or possibly several levels higher). It will now seek its corresponding white rami communicans, travel into the spinal cord, and continue within the central nervous system.

Sympathetic innervation into the pelvis may also travel via the lumbar splanchnics. These contain preganglionic sympathetic and visceral afferent fibers that travel directly between the sympathetic trunk and pelvic viscera via a local ganglion. These originate at L1/2, which obviously is much more cephalad than the sacral region.

20.4 Basic Concerns and Contraindications

As with any stimulator trial, some concerns should be considered before performing the procedure. Gaining access to the epidural space requires little more than an interlaminar injection, which is well tolerated by the average patient, but one must carefully consider each patient and his or her individual presentation of pain. CPP patients have a high degree of anxiety and may perseverate on every sensation they encounter in the area of their discomfort. All available information pertaining to the patient should be carefully considered before proceeding with a stimulator trial. Achieving a successful outcome requires selecting the right patient.

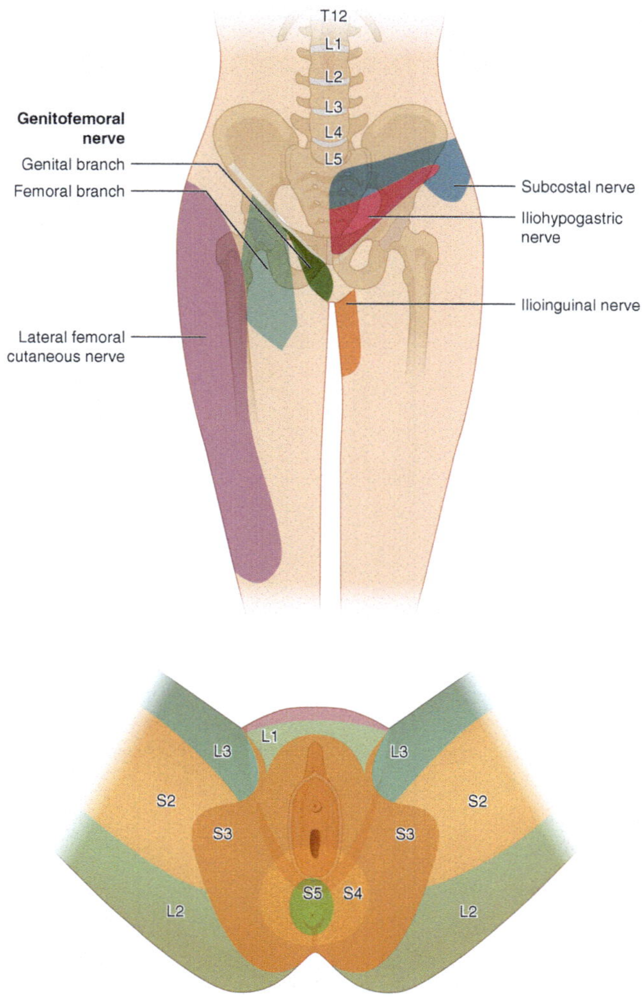

Fig. 20.2 The cutaneous innervation of the pelvic region in a woman and the corresponding dermatomes

There are a number of relative contraindications for an SCS trial for pelvic pain:

- Infection
- Anticoagulation therapy
- Psychiatric comorbidity and/or failed psychiatric clearance
- Metastatic cancer with local lesions/tumors in the vicinity of the intended procedure site
- Pacemaker or defibrillator
- Risk of falls

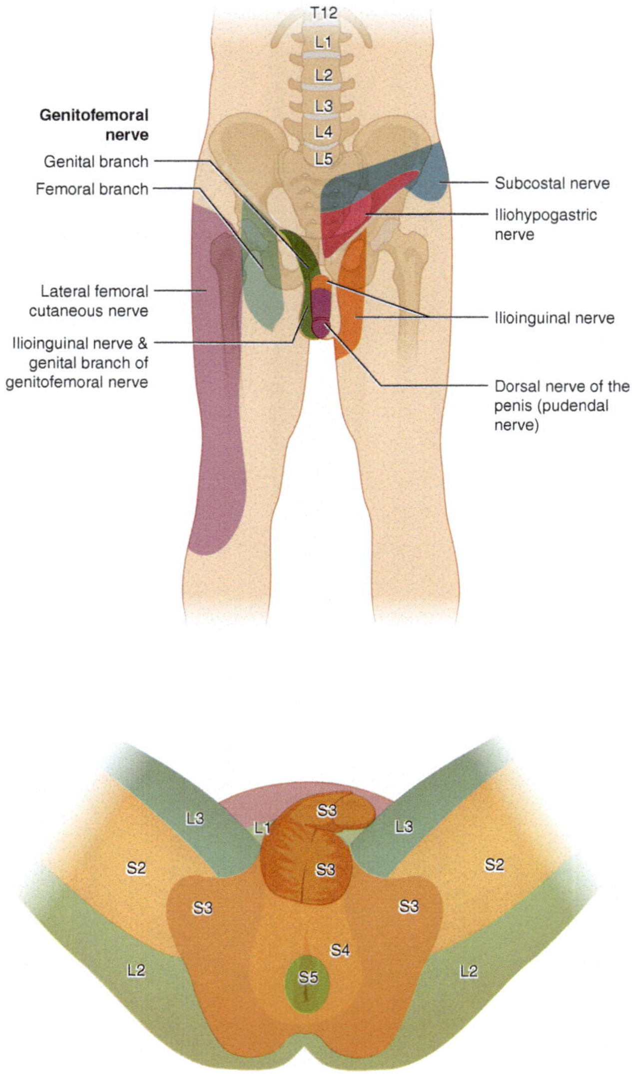

Fig. 20.3 The cutaneous innervation of the pelvic region in a man and the corresponding dermatomes

There are also some absolute contraindications:

- Pregnancy
- Patient refusal
- Spine instability
- Senility or inability to control/operate the device
- Not a surgical candidate or unacceptable surgical risk (coagulopathy or immunosuppression)

20.5 Preoperative Considerations

Preoperative steps and considerations are important:

- Informed consent and proper explanation of all potential complications
- Anticoagulation therapy and timeline: Patients should be cleared by their primary care physician to stop anticoagulation
- Physical examination of the area for infection, skin ulceration or necrosis, and extent of disease
- Patient's ability to lie prone for the intended length of the procedure
- Intravenous access for IV fluid and medications for sedation or hypotension
- Psychological screening; all major psychiatric comorbidity must be addressed.

Fluoroscopic views should include an anterior-posterior (AP) view, used for obtaining epidural access and steering the lead to the appropriate spinal level. A lateral view image is used to verify the posterior position of the lead over the dorsal column.

20.5.1 Equipment and Kits

- 25G 1.5-inch needle
- 10 mL syringe for local anesthetic
- 14-gauge Coudé or Touhy needle
- 15 blade on a scalpel handle
- Spinal cord stimulation kit with standard eight-contact leads

20.5.2 Medications

- 1% lidocaine with epinephrine (1:100,000)

20.6 Technique

Various regions of the spinal cord have been suggested as possible targets of neuromodulation to treat CPP:

- Sacrum
- Conus
- Mid-thoracic region (T5 through T7) [5]

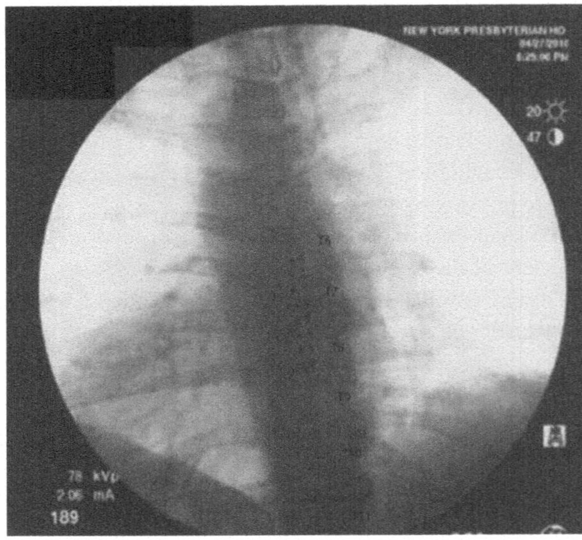

Fig. 20.4 Mid-thoracic lead placement

Though sacral stimulation is effective in treating urinary disorders and certain pain disorders with a strictly sacral distribution, it has shown inconsistent results when treating other types of pelvic pain with broader pain patterns representing extrasacral innervation. The complex web of sympathetic innervation to the area provides a seemingly countless number of routes for pain to travel and escape the sacral region.

Visceral pain fibers are theorized to travel a path via the corresponding sympathetic nerves of the region or organ in question, with their cell bodies in the thoracolumbar spinal ganglia and their central projections entering the spinal cord at L2 and as high as T2 [6]. This could explain why patients with described pain that appears sympathetically maintained are not always responsive to conventional blocks (*ie*, ganglion impar or hypogastric plexus). It is for this reason we feel that a lead placed sacrally could potentially leave a significant portion of pertinent fibers unrecruited. Once might create a dermatomally appropriate area and even capture a good share of the visceral and sympathetic fibers but still leave significant portion of those unaccounted for, leaving a patient with incomplete stimulation.

Neurostimulation for pelvic pain can be placed in the mid-thoracic region (Fig. 20.4) or conus (Fig. 20.5). Mid-thoracic leads placed at the T5-6 level have been shown to help decrease pain in patients with chronic pancreatitis. As mentioned previously, visceral pain fibers do not follow basic dermatomal distributions. The exact reason for the cephalad placement is not well known but may be due to the dorsal column. Sacral fibers lie more medially and should theoretically allow for stimulation of fibers at any point along the spinal cord.

Conus placement, on the other hand, is located from T12 to L2, where the termination of the spinal cord is located. Anatomy suggests that the conus can be the area of maximal pelvic innervation. Placement of the stimulator at the conus ideally

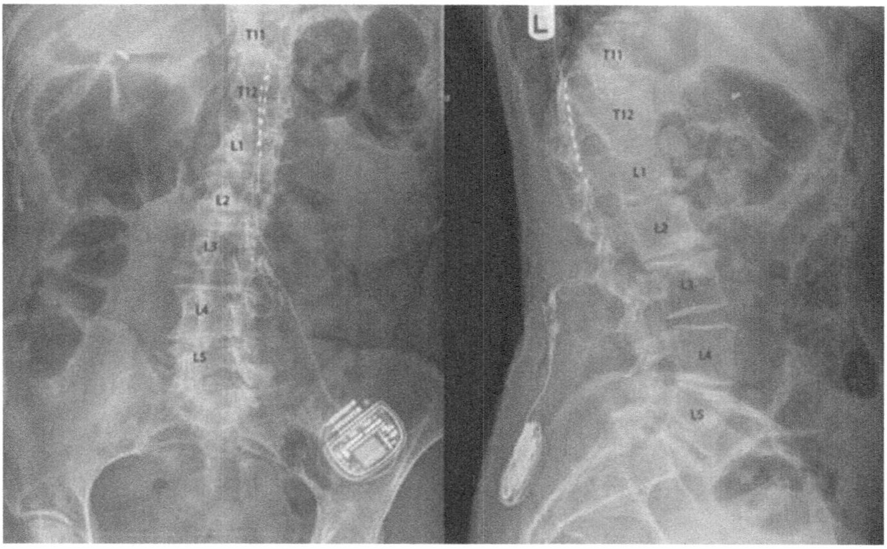

Fig. 20.5 Conus lead placement

should minimize the amount of nociceptive inputs that escape, but placement of leads at the conus provides inconsistent stimulation secondary to the increased mobility of the spinal cord within the cerebrospinal fluid at that level. Also, the increased volume of fluid at that level creates a greater distance between the epidural space and the actual tissue of the conus. This extra space requires a higher voltage from the stimulator to activate the dorsal column, which may inadvertently stimulate segmental roots and cause discomfort for the patient.

20.6.1 Our Preferred Technique: Mid-Thoracic or Conus Stimulation

Various levels may be selected as entry points for the stimulator electrodes. We recommend L2/L3 as the entrance site, to allow plenty of room for the tip of the electrode to range anywhere from T5 to the conus (T12/L1). Because of some of the drawbacks of conus stimulation (the high degree of mobility and the large volume of local CSF dispersing stimulation energy), mid-thoracic stimulation should be attempted first, before attempting conus stimulation.

- The patient is placed in a prone position with a pillow under the abdomen to reduce the lumbar lordotic curvature.
- The skin overlying the L2/L3 interspace is identified with an AP fluoroscopic image and marked.

- The skin entry site, one interspace below (L3/L4) and approximately 1–2 cm laterally, is also marked and prepped in a typical sterile fashion.
- 1% lidocaine with epinephrine is then used to infiltrate the skin using the 25-gauge 1.5″ needle to provide adequate skin analgesia.
- A 14-gauge Touhy needle is then advanced using a paramedian approach directed midline towards the L2/L3 interspace, using intermittent fluoroscopic guidance.
- A loss-of-resistance technique is used to locate the L2/L3 epidural space, with confirmation of location using fluoroscopy.
- Once the Touhy needle is in the proper location, the lead is inserted through the needle and into the epidural space.
- Using live/intermittent fluoroscopic guidance, the tip is steered up to T5.
- Once the tip is in the proper location, the electrode is connected to the external impulse generator and stimulation is activated.
- With the stimulation on, the lead is "trolled" caudally from T5 to T7 while asking the patient to look for activation in the pelvic region.
- Repeat with additional leads if desired.
- If the patient is unable to feel any stimulation in the pelvic region, pull the lead down to the region of the conus (approximately T12–L2 level) and attempt stimulation again.
- Upon completion of testing, when the leads are in satisfactory positions, the stylet(s) and needle(s) are removed, paying careful attention to preserve the intended position of the lead(s).
- For the trial, bacitracin ointment is then applied to the skin around the lead(s) and a StayFIX® dressing (Merit Medical) is then applied to secure the lead(s) in place, directing the leads toward the preferred side.

20.7 Post-procedure Considerations

The patient should be followed up by telephone the day after the trial placement to determine whether potential complications have occurred. The patient should also be queried regarding pain relief and whether the stimulation is too strong. The patient should be advised to contact the physician for any procedure-related complications or any unexpected neurologic deficit. The patient should be monitored closely for the following symptoms:

- Positional headache
- Weakness
- Urinary or bowel incontinence
- Inability to tolerate sensation
- Fever
- Bleeding
- Rectal bleeding
- Numbness
- Exacerbation of symptoms

20.8 Potential Complications and Pitfalls

- Lead migration
- Infection
- Bleeding and hematoma
- Intrathecal lead placement
- Cauda equina syndrome
- Dural puncture
- Spinal cord/nerve root injury
- Lead fracture
- Allergic reaction to implant
- Fibrosis around leads

20.9 Clinical Pearls

- The pelvic region is innervated by eight cutaneous nerves with thoracic, lumbar, and sacral cord contributions.
- The dermatomal distribution of the pelvis includes L1, L2, L3, and S1 through S5.
- The visceral pain fibers from the pelvis have been suggested to travel within the sympathetic pathways providing innervation to the region.
- There are three potential targets for SCS in treating CPP: sacral, conus, and mid-thoracic.

References

1. Kothari S. Neuromodulation approaches to chronic pelvic pain and coccydynia. Acta Neurochir Suppl. 2007;97:365–71.
2. De Leon Casasola OA, Kent E, Lema MJ. Neurolytic superior hypogastric plexus block for chronic pelvic pain associated with cancer. Pain. 1993;54:145–51.
3. Janicki TI. Chronic pelvic pain as a form of complex regional pain syndrome. Clin Obstet Gynecol. 2003;46:797–803.
4. Van Kerrebroeck PE. Advances in the role of sacral nerve neuromodulation in lower urinary tract symptoms. Int Urogynecol J. 2010;21:S467–74.
5. Hunter C, Davé N, Diwan S, Deer T. Neuromodulation of pelvic visceral pain: a review of the literature and case series of potential novel targets for treatment. Pain Pract. 2013;13:3–17.
6. Cervero F. Visceral pain: what's in the gut and what's in the brain. In: Tache Y, Wingate D, editors. Brain-gut interactions. Boca Raton: CRC Press; 1991. p. 339–46.

Suggested Reading

Alo KM, Yland MJ, Redko V, Feler C, Naumann C. Lumbar and sacral nerve root stimulation (NRS) in the treatment of chronic pain: a novel anatomic approach and neurostimulation technique. Neuromodulation. 1999;2:23–31.

Kapural L, Narouze SN, Janicki TI, Mekhail N. Spinal cord stimulation is an effective treatment for the chronic intractable visceral pelvic pain. Pain Med. 2006;7:440–3.

McDonald JS, Alo KM. Pain of urogenital origin. In: Loeser J, editor. Bonica's management of pain. 3rd ed. Philadelphia: Lippincott, Williams & Wilkins; 2001. p. 1448–61.

Chapter 21
Truncal Stimulation Trial and Implant

Javid Baksh

Neuromodulation practitioners to a greater extent are acknowledging the potential of peripheral nerve field stimulation (PNfS) to relieve truncal pain. Pain developed or begun in the trunk that traditionally responds well to PNfS includes (but is not limited to) postherpetic neuralgia, inguinal neurapraxia, lumbar and cervical postlaminectomy syndrome, and postthoracotomy pain. The inventive and diligent workings of Slavin, Weiner, and Kapural have reignited interest in stimulating sensory nerves in the periphery.

21.1 Mechanism of Action

The mechanism of action of peripheral nerve field stimulation (PNfS) likely occurs through the gate-control theory of Melzack and Wall [1]. It is likely, too, that stimulation of A-beta fibers in the subcutaneous layer and, subsequently, inhibition of A-delta and C fibers is what causes PNfS to alleviate pain. Perhaps the most notable difference between spinal cord stimulation (SCS) and PNfS is that with PNfS there is the possibility of more significant distance between polarities (cathode and anode)—sometimes more than 30 in. carrying dense paresthesia between contacts, compared with less than 10 mm with typical SCS [2]. Electronically stimulating the subcutaneous region may increase concentration of local endorphins, inhibit cell depolarization, alter neurotransmitters, and affect blood flow, thus inhibiting nociceptors in a manner similar to temporary percutaneous electrical nerve stimulation (PENS) and transcutaneous electrical nerve stimulation (TENS) [3]. Further examination of the mechanism of action is needed to better understand the localized changes and neurophysiology that occur once current is delivered to the

J. Baksh (✉)
Premier Pain Solutions, Asheville, NC, USA
e-mail: jbaksh34@yahoo.com

S. Diwan, T.R. Deer (eds.), *Advanced Procedures for Pain Management*,
https://doi.org/10.1007/978-3-319-68841-1_21

subcutaneous layer, but animal studies suggest that peripheral nerve stimulation may alter the excitation of the central pain processing system, thereby alleviating pain [4].

21.2 Patient Selection

Patients considered for PNfS trials typically have failed more traditional interventional spinal procedures, including medial branch blocks, sacroiliac (SI) injections, facet joint nerve ablations, and epidural steroid injections. Conditions most responsive to PNfS are axial cervical pain, postherpetic neuralgia (PHN), lumbar postlaminectomy syndrome, inguinal pain, postthoracotomy pain, and ilioinguinal neurapraxia [5–8]. Direct stimulation along the nerve roots and in the lateral recess has been described for PHN, ilioinguinal neurapraxia, and postthoracotomy pain. Lumbar postlaminectomy syndrome is perhaps the diagnosis most commonly treated with PNfS.

Patients with postsurgery truncal pain often have few interventional options that are not pharmacological. Paicius et al. [5] reported a series of six patients, including five who previously had undergone lumbar surgery. All patients noted greater than 50% pain relief. Krutsch et al. [9] reported a patient with lumbar failed back surgery syndrome (FBSS) who exhibited 90% improvement 1 year after implantation. Verrills et al. [10] observed that among 13 consecutively implanted patients, 85% noted greater than 50% pain relief with a 7-month average follow-up period. Improvement of discogenic pain has been reported in a single patient, with 100% relief at 9 months follow-up [6]. Anesthesia dolorosa, age, presence of hardware, and large-fiber sensation in the pain region are all general considerations when identifying patients for PNfS after lumbar surgery.

21.3 PNfS Technical Considerations

Lead depth and lead positioning in relation to the region of maximal pain are the two fundamental details in proper placement of PNfS leads. Placement in the subcutaneous layer is important for correct stimulation of the terminal sensory fibers. With superficial placement, patients often report a burning sensation at low sensory thresholds. Conversely, placing PNfS leads too deep may result in the lead being inserted either into muscle tissue or too far away from terminal sensory afferents to recruit at low energies, and patients note an absence of evoked paresthesia. The subcutaneous layer is cooperative as an electrical conduit to create long-distance circuits, likely allowing depolarization of terminal sensory afferents over larger areas [2].

To ensure correct depth with regard to the needle and to maintain a uniformity of depth, most practitioners implant percutaneous four-contact or eight-contact leads

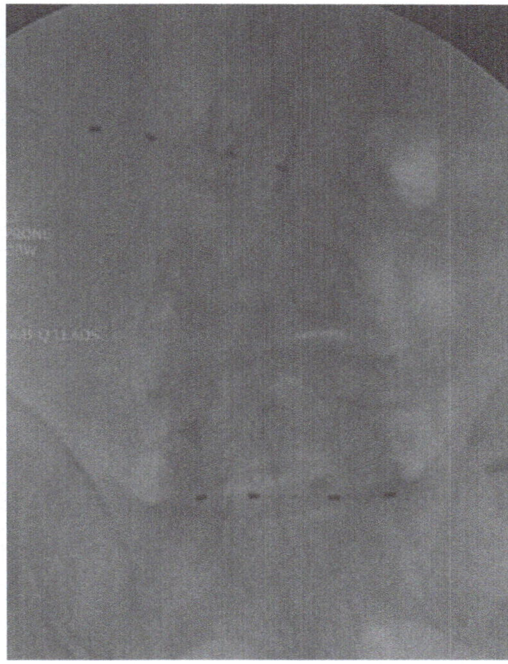

Fig. 21.1 Two quad leads placed subcutaneously across lumbar spine

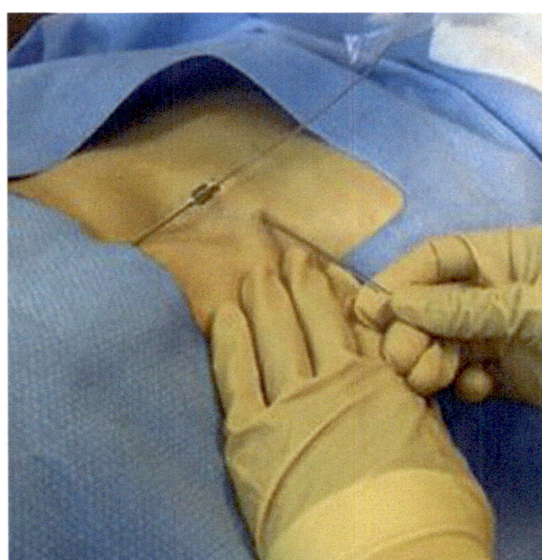

Fig. 21.2 Modified Tuohy needle inserted subcutaneously across the lower lumbar spine

by palpating the distal element of the Tuohy needle (Figs. 21.1, 21.2, 21.3 and 21.4). A careful approach should be taken to correctly judge the depth of the Tuohy needles within the fascial layers upon insertion. Percutaneous leads carry advantages over paddle leads, including circumferential stimulation allowing possible recruitment of additional terminal sensory fibers, ease of placement, and ability to minimize

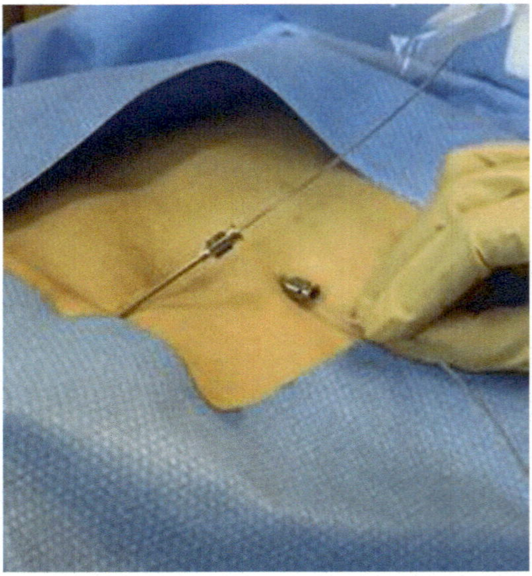

Fig. 21.3 Threading quad lead

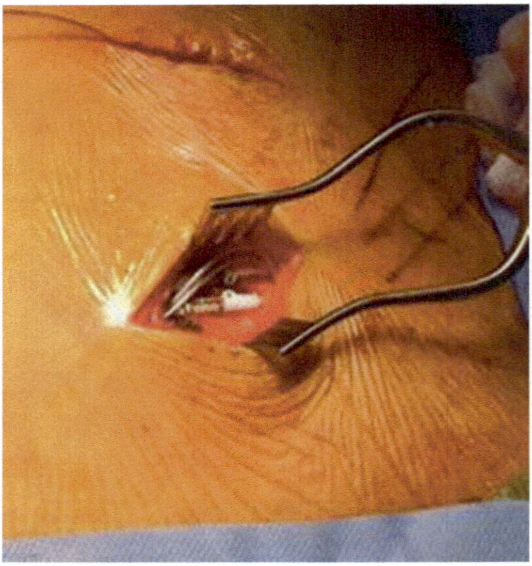

Fig. 21.4 Anchoring two peripheral leads with Swift-Lock™ anchoring devices (St. Jude Medical) with Ethibon Excel® sutures

local anesthetic inhibition of sensory fibers during intraoperative stimulation. The paddle leads can direct stimulation away from the skin, however, thus minimizing the stimulation of A-delta fibers that may cause dysesthesia.

21.4 PNfS Programming

Wide-spaced cross talk and triple-anode single-cathode (3A1C) stimulations are the two most common programming strategies. The former references an electrode array construct with significant distances between polarities (cathode and anode) on different leads. A group of 18 chronic pain patients who were all implanted with PNfS systems using wide-spaced cross talk programming noted significant reduction in pain medication and also significant pain relief [2].

Across the board, patients observed less burning and stinging sensation and a larger area of paresthesia with wide-spaced arrays. Triple-anode single-cathode programming strategy uses four-lead PNfS systems to create a large area of paresthesia. Each of the four, interleavened stimulation sets is comprised of a single cathode with three anodes; all active electrodes are on separate leads. Patients observe significant pain relief and less burning.

References

1. Melzack R, Wall PD. Pain mechanisms: a new theory. Science. 1965;150:971–9.
2. Falco F, Berger J, Vrable A, Onyweu O, Zhu J. Cross talk: a new method for peripheral nerve stimulation: an observational report with cadaveric verification. Pain Physician. 2009;12:965–83.
3. Campbell JN, Long DM. Peripheral nerve stimulation in the treatment of intractable pain. J Neurosurg. 1976;45:692–9.
4. Bartsch T, Goadsby PJ. Stimulation of the greater occipital nerve induces increased central excitability of dural afferent input. Brain. 2002;125:1496–509.
5. Paicius RM, Bernstein CA, Lempert-Cohen C. Peripheral nerve field stimulation for the treatment of chronic low back pain: preliminary results of long-term follow-up: a case series. Neuromodulation. 2007;10:279–90.
6. Lipov EF, Joshi JR, Sanders S, Slavin KV. Use of peripheral subcutaneous field stimulation for the treatment of axial neck pain: a case report. Neuromodulation. 2009;12:292–5.
7. Yakovlev A, Peterson A. Peripheral nerve stimulation in treatment of intractable postherpetic neuralgia. Neuromodulation. 2007;10:373–5.
8. Stinson LE, Roderer GT, Cross NE, Davis BE. Peripheral subcutaneous electrostimulation for control of intractable postoperative inguinal pain: a case report series. Neuromodulation. 2001;4:99–104.
9. Krutsch JP, McCeney MH, Barolat G, Al Tamimi M, Smolenski A. A case report of subcutaneous peripheral nerve stimulation for the treatment of axial back pain associated with postlaminectomy syndrome. Neuromodulation. 2008;11:112–5.
10. Verrills P, Mitchell B, Vivian D, Sinclair C. Peripheral nerve stimulation: a treatment for chronic low back pain and failed back surgery syndrome? Neuromodulation. 2009;12:68–75.

Chapter 22
Peripheral Nerve Stimulation for the Painful Extremity

Javid Baksh

In patients with extremity pain for whom conventional pain-control methods have failed and surgical treatment has been deemed unsuitable, an exceptional option for pain control is peripheral nerve stimulation (and, more recently, peripheral nerve field stimulation). Smaller generators, ultrasound guidance, task-specific neuromodulatory hardware and leads, and new techniques result in increasingly effective and safe treatment of pain in the extremity.

22.1 Mechanism of Action

In the 1960s, Melzack and Wall introduced their gate control theory of pain, which single-handedly altered the paradigm of pain epistemology, thus opening the door for new ways of thinking about pain modulation [1]. Said theory called for activation of A-beta fibers, which conduct the safe stimuli of position and vibration. They initiate inhibitory interneurons within the substantia gelatinosa in the peak of the posterior horn, in turn influencing the wide-dynamic-range neuron, onto which both small and large pain fibers synapse. In theory, when activated, the gate closes and hinders the cephalad conduction of pain. Though it is hypothesized that electrical stimulation of A-beta fiber afferents within the peripheral nervous system impedes transmission of A-delta and C fibers, application of this concept to stimulation continues to be somewhat controversial. Ellrich and Lamp [2], however, find that the lower sensory threshold of A-beta fibers permits selective activation of sensory nerve fibers without excitation of A-delta and C fibers.

J. Baksh (✉)
Premier Pain Solutions, Asheville, NC, USA
e-mail: jbaksh34@yahoo.com

S. Diwan, T.R. Deer (eds.), *Advanced Procedures for Pain Management*,
https://doi.org/10.1007/978-3-319-68841-1_22

22.2 Patient Selection

Historically, peripheral nerve lead deployment has placed patients at greater risk of complications than spinal cord stimulation (SCS). That being said, positioning of an SCS electrode over the dorsal column poses risk of infection and injury to the cord. Other concerns and limitations include reduced effect over time and lead migration. Moreover, central stimulation may also prove difficult in terms of covering the bases of some main target areas, including the feet and groin [3]. Although implantable pulse generators (IPGs) are becoming increasingly smaller, they are still relatively large and depend upon meticulous planning and placement. Weiner [4] devised the following criteria in selecting a patient for peripheral nerve stimulation (PNS):

- Direct injury/source of pain
- Failure of other therapies and treatments (at times including surgery)
- Absence of drug dependency
- Patient intelligence and motivation
- Patient education and subsequent understanding that PNS controls chronic pain but does not cure disease
- Successful trial stimulation
- Identification of the specific compromised nerve using selective nerve/root blocking techniques

22.3 Selection of Neuromodulation System

The availability and variety of generators continue to improve. Because every patient carries his or her own individual collections of pain, implanters increasingly merge various elements of the implanted system in order to meet the needs of each patient. The implanter's ultimate goal is to provide the safest method available via the densest concordant paresthesia possible. Though SCS is lauded as the safest modality in many cases, at times it lacks adequate coverage and general pain relief. At that point, PNS or peripheral nerve field stimulation (PNfS) becomes a more acceptable option for the painful extremity. PNfS may also provide a level of additional nociceptive pain relief, as opposed to the common neuropathic pain relief found in central neuromodulation [2, 5].

22.4 Neuromodulation Trial

The percutaneous trial affords the rare ability, in the surgical sphere, to reversibly test a proposed modality without significant risk for either patient or physician. The trial not only tests the modality and proposed montage but also tests the patient's

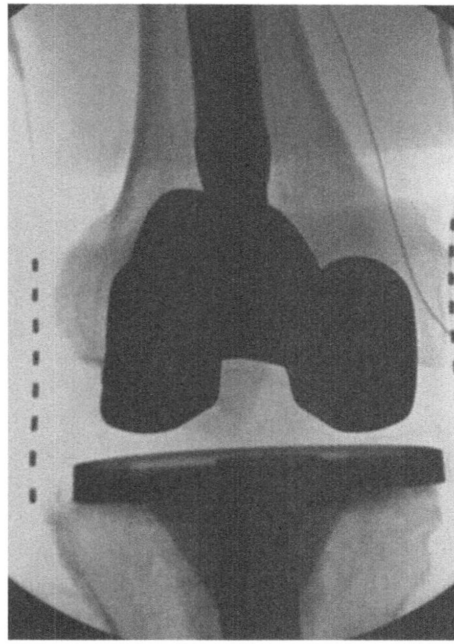

Fig. 22.1 Two Octrode® leads placed laterally for complex regional pain syndrome following three total knee replacements

willingness and understanding that pain may be chronic but can be adequately treated by electricity. Though the foremost goal in neuromodulatory trialing is to reasonably conclude therapy effectiveness, it is also imperative to consider both possible epidural abscess and fibrosis in longer trials. It is widely suggested that, for trialing a patient using both PNS and PNfS, it is useful for the patient to locate his or her pain areas on the skin with a permanent marker. Preoperative planning should include a mapping of skin entry along with the ultimate lead location. The size and shape of the pain area greatly inform placement of the lead. If the area is small—no larger than the size of a credit card—one lead may be ideal. The greater the pain area, the more leads one might need. Currently, four leads can be used per generator. Lead entry should utilize the entirety of the needle as available, and insertion will likely go through the long axis (and thus be outside the area of pain). The distance between the pain area and skin entry is important, as the incision may exacerbate the intensity of chronic pain. Traditionally, leads should be placed at the periphery of pain, especially when treating a larger area.

At the conclusion of planning, the patient is draped in sterile fashion. Most procedures require only light sedation and a small amount of local anesthesia at the planned incision. After the needle has been advanced, initial pain stimulation is handled by altering stimulation amplitude and electrical configuration. If pain becomes persistent, or lack of paresthesia exists, the location of the lead or leads must be revised. The brand of pain will likely inform the angle of correction—deeper or shallower. That being said, repeat deployments should be kept at a minimum, as they might increase tissue damage and compromise testing results. Figure 22.1 illustrates a peripheral stimulation trial over a joint space.

22.5 Permanent PNS/PNfS Implantation

Most lead deployment equipment was originally designed for placement in the central neuroaxis, where much less movement occurs than in the extremities, with their vast and repetitive movements. Body type and weight are used to help determine if and where the IPG can be implanted. The patient should be monitored, as often weight loss may accompany the pain relief. Peripheral implantation eliminates the need for a surgeon to cross the shoulder or hip, thus strengthening system stability over time. If little adipose is available, one must choose instead central implantation in the shoulder, clavicle, lower abdomen quadrant, or buttock. Here, surgeons must keep in mind range of motion. Allow for sufficient strain relief loop size so that there is incomplete loop closure with ranging movement of the extremity. Though these loops allow for freedom of movement, the electrode array must move as little as possible in relation to the neutral target. In terms of anchoring, most choose direct ligation-like suturing. Nurolon® (Ethicon) braided nylon is suggested for highest integrity and strength over time. Suturing should be done via the "drain stitch" method, similar to that used in securing a chest tube. Care must be taken to avoid tightening the suture too tight on the lead, as doing so may break or compromise the lead wires; the lead should be anchored to the proximal part of the array. After lead is secured, attend to tunneling over the joint and the lead flexion point. The combination of proper planning, preoperative pain identification and marking, and attention to detail will ensure efficacy and lasting benefit.

References

1. Melzack R, Wall PD. Pain mechanisms: a new theory. Science. 1965;150:971–9.
2. Ellrich J, Lamp S. Peripheral nerve stimulation inhibits nociceptive processing: an electrophysiological study in healthy volunteers. Neuromodulation. 2005;8:225–32.
3. Aló KM, Holsheimer J. New trends in neuromodulation for the management of neuropathic pain. Neurosurgery. 2002;50:690–703.
4. Weiner RL. Peripheral nerve neurostimulation. Neurosurg Clin N Am. 2003;14:401–8.
5. McRoberts WP, Roche M. Novel approach for peripheral subcutaneous field stimulation for the treatment of severe, chronic knee joint pain after total knee arthroplasty. Neuromodulation. 2010;13:131–6.

Chapter 23
Advanced Neuromodulation Techniques: Dorsal Root Ganglion Stimulation

Kasra Amirdelfan, Jeffrey Kramer, William F. Cusack, and Allen W. Burton

Objective: The dorsal root ganglion (DRG) houses the somata of primary sensory neurons and is located bilaterally along the posterior root at each spinal level. The DRG is involved in neuropathic pain and is therefore an attractive target for neuromodulation therapies. A specialized system now allows leads to be chronically implanted directly adjacent to DRGs. This report describes the procedures for implementing DRG stimulation. Practical problem-solving strategies from an experienced implanter are provided.

Patient Selection, Device, and Implantation Techniques: As with other neuromodulation interventions, DRG stimulation is for patients whose pain cannot be surgically remediated and is intractable (or intolerant of) using conventional pain management therapies. The DRG stimulation system resembles spinal cord stimulation (SCS) systems in that it uses up to four quadripolar leads powered by an implantable pulse generator (IPG). The leads are placed percutaneously in the epidural space with curved stylets under fluoroscopic guidance. Placement alongside DRGs in the vertebral foramen requires that the leads are extremely narrow and flexible; a removable stylet in the lumen stiffens the lead during implantation to enhance maneuverability. Long-term stability of the implanted leads is ensured by

K. Amirdelfan (✉)
IPM Medical Group, Inc., Walnut Creek, CA, USA
e-mail: DoctorA@ipmdoctors.com

J. Kramer
University of Illinois, College of Medicine, Chicago, USA
e-mail: JKramer@sjm.com

W.F. Cusack
Senior scientist, Abbott Laboratories, Plano, TX, USA
e-mail: WCusack@sjm.com

A.W. Burton
Divisional vice President and Medical Director, Neuromodulation, Abbott, Plano, TX, USA
e-mail: awburtonmd@gmail.com

S. Diwan, T.R. Deer (eds.), *Advanced Procedures for Pain Management*,
https://doi.org/10.1007/978-3-319-68841-1_23

creating S-shaped epidural slack and using lead anchors. The IPG is placed subcutaneously according to the patient's body shape, activities, and preferences.

Conclusions: DRG stimulation has emerged as an effective neuromodulation tool. Its putative benefits include coverage of focal pain locations that may not be amenable to treatment with conventional SCS. By employing good implantation techniques, patient outcomes with DRG stimulation can be optimized.

23.1 The Rationale for DRG Stimulation: Anatomy and Physiology

The dorsal root ganglion (DRG) is a bulbous structure located on the posterior spinal roots, at the interface of the central and peripheral nervous systems. On anterior-posterior (AP) fluoroscopic imaging, DRGs can be observed within or outside the foraminal space between the medial and lateral edges of the vertebral pedicles (Fig. 23.1) [1]; DRG anatomy is relatively consistent across healthy individuals [2]. DRGs are considered to be central nervous system (CNS) structures, as they are bathed in a thin layer of cerebrospinal fluid and covered in dura mater, similar to all other CNS neural structures [3, 4]. Surrounding each DRG is a narrow epidural space and an immobile bony encasement.

DRGs contain the somata of pseudo-unipolar primary sensory neurons. Each DRG receives peripheral input from dendritic mechanosensitive and chemosensitive sensory transducers on its neurons' distal processes. In general, non-noxious afferent stimuli are carried on large, myelinated fibers (Aα or Aβ), whereas noxious

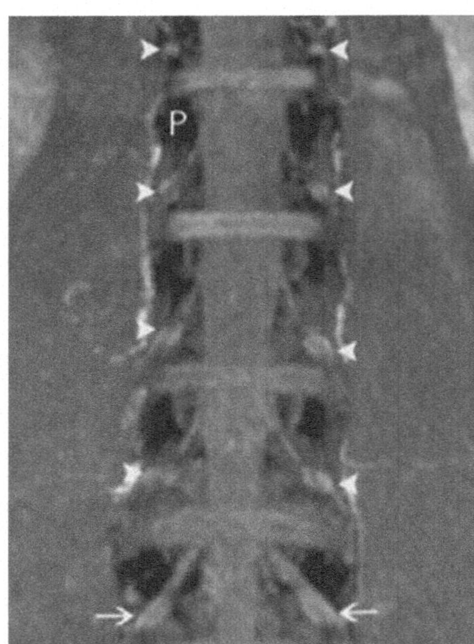

Fig. 23.1 Lumbar DRGs from coronal magnetic resonance imaging. The L1–L4 DRGs are indicated with *white arrowheads* and the L5 DRGs are indicated with *white arrows*. Of note is the uniform position of the DRGs relative to the dark-colored pedicles (*white P*). Most DRGs in healthy individuals lie between the medial and lateral borders of the pedicles (*Reproduced with permission from* Shen et al. [1])

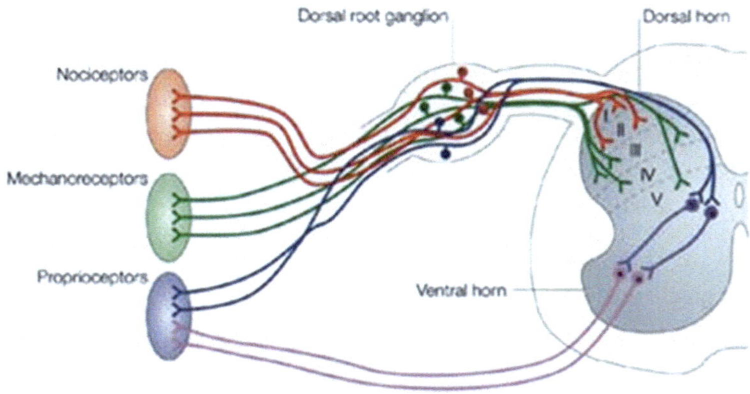

Fig. 23.2 The functional anatomy of the DRG: sensory afferent somata are contained within the bulbar structure just lateral to the spinal cord (*Reproduced with permission from* Caspary and Anderson [26])

signals, including pain, are carried on small-diameter, thinly myelinated (Aδ) fibers or non-myelinated fibers (C fibers) [5]. Considerable anatomic and physiologic cross-connection with the sympathetic nervous system also exists via the white rami communicantes [6]. Fibers of DRG neurons' proximal processes form synapses with neurons within the superficial layers of the spinal cord's gray matter (Fig. 23.2). These synapses include connections with the wide-dynamic-range (WDR) neurons that ultimately feed into the ascending fibers of the dorsal column, terminating in the thalamus and other supraspinal structures. Afferent signals transmitted by the DRG may be action potentials generated in the periphery and carried on the dendrites of the primary sensory neurons directly to the spinal cord. The action potentials may be transmitted along the unipolar dendrites to be modulated by the somata in the DRG [7], in addition to signaling the contribution of large populations of electrically active microglia and satellite glial cells, which envelop the primary sensory neurons [8, 9].

The DRG is involved in the generation and maintenance of the chronic pain signal. In animal models, experimental peripheral nerve constriction induces proinflammatory protein expression in the DRG. This triggers a number of pathological cascades involving changes in glial cell activity, ion channel conductance, ligand availability, receptor sensitivity, and ultimately membrane sensitivity [10]. In neuropathic pain conditions, the excitability of DRG neurons, whether induced or spontaneous, remains elevated long after the initiating injury has healed and its associated nociceptive pain has resolved [11, 12]. Pain-related neuropeptides in the spinal cord affect the genetic expression of receptor terminals in the dorsal horn and cause conformational changes in ion-channel expression at the DRG. Both of these actions modify the postsynaptic pain signals reaching the dorsal columns [13]. Additionally, intercommunication between glial cells and neurons in the DRG is adversely altered in chronic pain conditions [14]. Thus, the DRG may be the initiation site of spinal-mediated pain, particularly chronic pain.

Conventional spinal cord stimulation (SCS) involves placing electrodes in the epidural space over the dorsal columns of the spinal cord. In contrast, in DRG stimulation, the leads are maneuvered into the vertebral foramina and placed in the epidural space over the DRGs. Previously, this method was not pursued because of technical and anatomical barriers, but a new system with flexible, small-diameter leads with narrow intercontact spacing has made this technique possible and commonplace for the treatment of specific neuropathic pain conditions.

Although the availability of quantitative results from mechanistic and computer-stimulation studies is currently limited, in broad conceptual terms, DRG stimulation is differentiated from SCS in a number of ways:

- The electrical fields of DRG stimulation electrodes affect specific cell bodies, in contrast to neural fibers of passage through the dorsal column. Thus, DRG stimulation likely recruits a complex milieu of multiple interacting cell types and engages the underlying cellular machinery of the somata, which modulates production of neurotransmitters and neuropeptides. In contrast, SCS involves only the recruitment of isolated and functionally limited nodes of Ranvier in the neural fibers within the superficial dorsal column. In addition, because the electrodes are physically closer to their targets, DRG stimulation requires a fraction of the power of conventional SCS systems.
- DRGs contain intermingled populations of the small neurons responsible for nociception and the large neurons responsible for touch and proprioception in an approximately 2:1 ratio [15]. DRG stimulation would likely recruit a large portion of (if not all) such neurons. As such, it is possible that DRG stimulation is able to recruit a larger proportion of small-fiber neurons than dorsal column SCS, which preferentially recruits large, myelinated fibers [16].
- DRG somata project directly to the gray matter of the spinal cord. Orthodromic activation via DRG stimulation may therefore activate large numbers of spinal interneurons, wide-dynamic-range neurons, and projection neurons, which form the ascending fibers of the dorsal columns. The result may be a more equitable distribution of dorsal column activation, including deep medial fibers, than with conventional dorsal column stimulation.
- Peripheral afferent information converges and diverges across different spinal segments at the DRG level [17–19]. As a result, the anatomical regions innervated by any given DRG are non-dermatomal. Thus, DRG stimulation may give access to a more highly varied set of anatomical options for pain management applications. Depending on DRG lead placement and activation, it is possible to achieve pain control and paresthesia coverage across wide swaths of the body, as in SCS, or confined to very focal distributions.

23.2 Indications and Patient Selection

Neuromodulation techniques are reserved for chronic pain conditions that have failed to respond to more conservative care. Patients who would be appropriate candidates for SCS may also be considered for DRG stimulation, including those with radicular symptoms, peripheral neuropathies, postsurgical neuralgias, and peripheral vascular disease. The DRG stimulator's FDA-approved labeling states that it can be used for treating moderate to severe chronic intractable pain of the lower limbs in adult patients with complex regional pain syndrome (CRPS I and II) [20].

Relative and absolute contraindications for traditional SCS systems also apply to DRG stimulation technology. For example, for patients with psychological instability that may impede usage as prescribed, anatomical variances that prohibit proper lead placement (e.g., scar tissue), or limited life expectancy, both traditional SCS and DRG stimulation would be contraindicated. Similarly, patients with surgical contraindications or candidacy for surgical repair of the presenting pathology would be good candidates for neither DRG stimulation nor traditional SCS. Patient selection criteria have been described in detail elsewhere [21].

23.3 Device and Equipment Description

23.3.1 Surgical Tools

The technical tools required for DRG stimulation are essentially the same as other SCS devices. The manufacturer's kits for leads and IPGs (Axium™; St. Jude Medical, Minneapolis, MN) contain the necessary specialized tools for safe and efficient implantation [22, 23]. Any modern operating room is equipped with the basic surgical tools utilized in this procedure, such as a loss-of-resistance syringe. Fluoroscopic equipment and a radiolucent surgical table are essential components of the surgical suite utilized for DRG implantation. All implant kit components should be thoroughly evaluated by the physician prior to undertaking the first case, in order to ensure a safe and efficient implantation and operating room experience for the patient and all other team members.

23.3.2 Curved Delivery Sheath and Curved Stylet

The delivery sheath, along with the lead and stylet, is placed in the epidural space after achieving loss of resistance. This method allows the leads to be placed in the epidural space around the target DRG. The sheaths are currently available in two lengths (22 and 30 cm) and are structured with large (8 mm) and small (2 mm) curves at their distal ends. The choices of length and curvature of the sheaths allow the physician to steer the lead to its target site with precision. The stylet, a solid-core component 0.25 mm in diameter, is inserted into the hollow lumen of the lead in order to increase lead integrity during the steering and placement stage. It is intended to assist with precision positioning of the lead in the epidural space and is easily removed after appropriate lead placement. These components work in unison to allow safe and efficient steering of the lead into the lateral epidural space and dorsal to the DRG (Fig. 23.3).

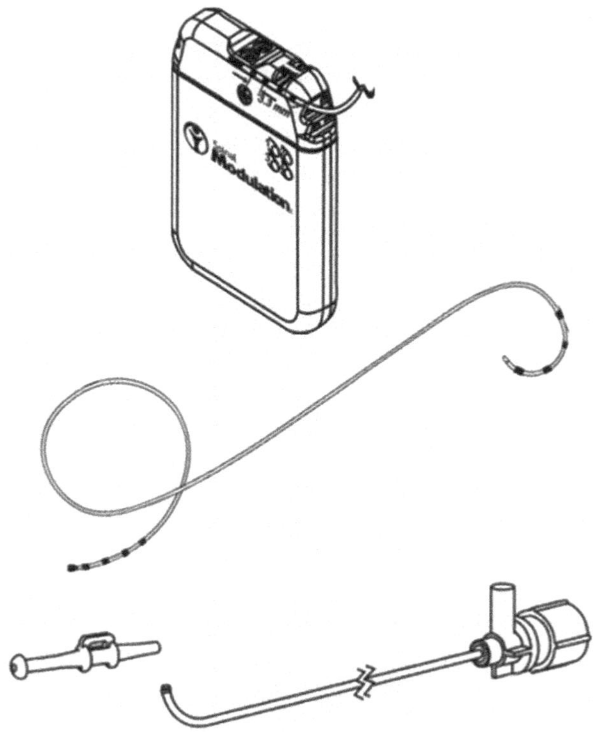

Fig. 23.3 Neurostimulator (*top*), lead (*middle*), and lead accessories (*bottom*) including a curved delivery sheath (*Reproduced with permission of* St. Jude Medical, ©2017)

23.3.3 Leads

The leads are 1 mm in diameter and are supplied in 50 and 90 cm lengths. The four electrodes on each lead are 1.25 mm long, with a 5-mm inter-spacing (*see* Fig. 23.3). The leads are flexible yet durable, as they are intended for long-term implantation. Lead extensions are also available if necessary. Silicone lead anchors are provided as a standard component in the kits.

23.3.4 External Power Generator

During the trial, the external power generator (EPG) is connected to verify lead placement via test pulses that generate perceptible paresthesia. The EPG can also be attached to the implanted leads via lead extensions and connector cables for up to 30-day trial periods. This type of 'permanent trial' is standard practice in European neuromodulation centers.

23.3.5 Internal Power Generator

The internal power generator (IPG) is a standard encasement which is 6.52 cm by 4.77 and 1.10 cm in thickness, with available ports for four leads (16 contacts) (*see* Fig. 23.3). It is designed to provide constant current stimulation with an available parameter range of 40–1000 μs (pulse width), 4–80 Hz (frequency), and 0–6000 μA (amplitude). It contains a non-rechargeable lithium carbon battery. The IPG is typically placed in a subcutaneous pocket in the flank or upper buttock, and subsequently is connected to the leads via a subcutaneous tunnel.

23.3.5.1 Pearls of Clinical Experience: Powering the DRG Stimulation System

The IPG shares attributes with existing SCS systems (adjustable frequency, waveform, pulse width, and range of amplitude). Its battery technology and size also resemble those of other available IPGs. Because there is minimal CSF around the DRG, however, the required amplitudes for optimal stimulation are far less for DRG stimulation than for comparable SCS systems. So the average primary-cell SCS system requires surgical replacement of the IPG approximately every 4 years [24], but the expected life of the DRG stimulator could extend to 5.3 years, depending on stimulation parameters [22].

23.3.6 Clinical Programmer

The Clinical Programmer is a hand-held tablet computer that remotely links to the implanted IPG to allow the setting of stimulation parameters for the utilization of the device. Each lead can be assigned to specific body regions, and multiple programs of stimulation settings can be created for each patient, thus configuring a patient-centered therapy. If required, the Clinical Programmer can also acquire identification, diagnostic, and historic information about the IPG's function and patient utilization, as well as electrode impedance values.

23.3.7 Patient Programmer

The Patient Programmer is a handheld device utilizing an intuitive touch-screen interface. It allows the patient to adjust the stimulation amplitude and to select from various programs defined by the Clinical Programmer.

23.4 Implantation Technique

23.4.1 History, Examination, and Comorbidities

As part of the determination of a patient's candidacy for DRG stimulation, a comprehensive review of the patient's presentation, history, and physical examination should be completed [22, 23]. Furthermore, advanced imaging techniques such as high-resolution MRI or CT scan must be considered as part of the evaluative process. As with any other implantable technology, the patient's comorbidities must also be taken into consideration for DRG stimulation. For example, the patient's coagulation status, diabetic control, and cardiovascular health all need to be assessed and appropriately addressed prior to undertaking a trial.

23.4.1.1 Pearls of Clinical Experience: Pre-implant Examinations

It is critical to conduct a detailed pre-implant assessment of the implant site, including imaging, as lead placement for DRG stimulation is more technically demanding and intricate than for dorsal column SCS. Anatomical variations at the index level (e.g., spinal or foraminal stenosis, epidural adhesions) could create a barrier to successful lead deployment and render the lead implantation at the target DRG challenging, if not impossible.

For example, if a patient has undergone a laminectomy and discectomy at the target level, as is commonly encountered in lumbar regions, the epidural space may have been compromised to such an extent as to prevent the implanting physician from safely placing the DRG lead at that location. Because of the interneuron-mediated communication across multiple spinal cord levels and the cross-talk of adjacent DRGs, it may be possible to place the lead at adjacent levels and obtain optimal outcomes with DRG stimulation.

In contrast, the conventional placement of epidural SCS leads is dependent only on the thoracic spine anatomy and the condition of the dorsal epidural space at the thoracic levels, regardless of the target anatomy, anatomical variant, or surgical intervention.

23.4.2 Identifying the Appropriate DRG Level(s)

The relevant level(s) for DRG lead placement can be determined by the patient's description of the anatomic location of the chronic pain. An understanding of the relationship between dermatomal distributions and which sensory afferents arrive at the spinal cord is key to successful DRG lead implantation. For example, for back pain, groin pain, and lower extremity pain, target DRGs are often found at T11-L4. Optimal lead placement will significantly increase the probability of successful pain relief, but if the target DRG is unavailable for any reason, adjacent sites may prove to be viable secondary targets because of the multi-level arborization of DRG afferents in the spinal cord.

23.4.3 Procedure Preparation

In the operating room, the patient should be positioned prone and lumbar lordosis reduced with pillows under the patient's abdomen in order to facilitate lead placement in the thoracolumbar epidural space. For cervico-thoracic placement, accentuating the kyphotic curvature of the thoracic spine with pillows under the patient's target insertion area may prove similarly helpful. Patients are then prepared and draped with a sterile technique according to physician and facility standards [22, 23]. Fluoroscopy should be positioned with the upper vertebral end plate of the target site sufficiently aligned with the fluoroscopic axis such that the surgeon will have the best route of access possible, along with a realistic image of the actual location of the lead in the transforaminal space.

23.4.4 Inserting the Epidural Needle

The implanter must make a shallow skin entry and shallow approach towards the epidural space, just as in conventional SCS. The angle of the needle will, however, need to be slightly larger to the midline than in conventional SCS during this approach [22, 23]. As it enters the epidural space, the needle's bevel should be aimed directly towards the contralateral pedicle of the target level. Ideally, in a contralateral placement, the needle tip should be positioned just across the anatomical midline at epidural entry, in order to facilitate lead placement at the target DRG on the side opposite to the needle entry, but ipsilateral placement of the leads is also possible, and the flexible epidural sheath allows for both types of entry with ease. For ipsilateral placement, the needle should be more medial and parallel to the anatomical midline. Multiple leads can be placed at adjacent spinal levels or multiple segments away from the same epidural access point with the help of the epidural sheaths and longer leads (Fig. 23.4).

23.4.4.1 Pearls of Clinical Experience: Needle Angle

If the epidural needle enters the epidural space with a wider angle of entry, the implanter risks dural puncture and may also have a more challenging lead implant procedure. The maneuvering capability of the DRG lead placement apparatus will be compromised in this position. A shallow skin and epidural entry angle, with the needle pointing toward the contralateral pedicle, maximizes the epidural volume available for lead steering.

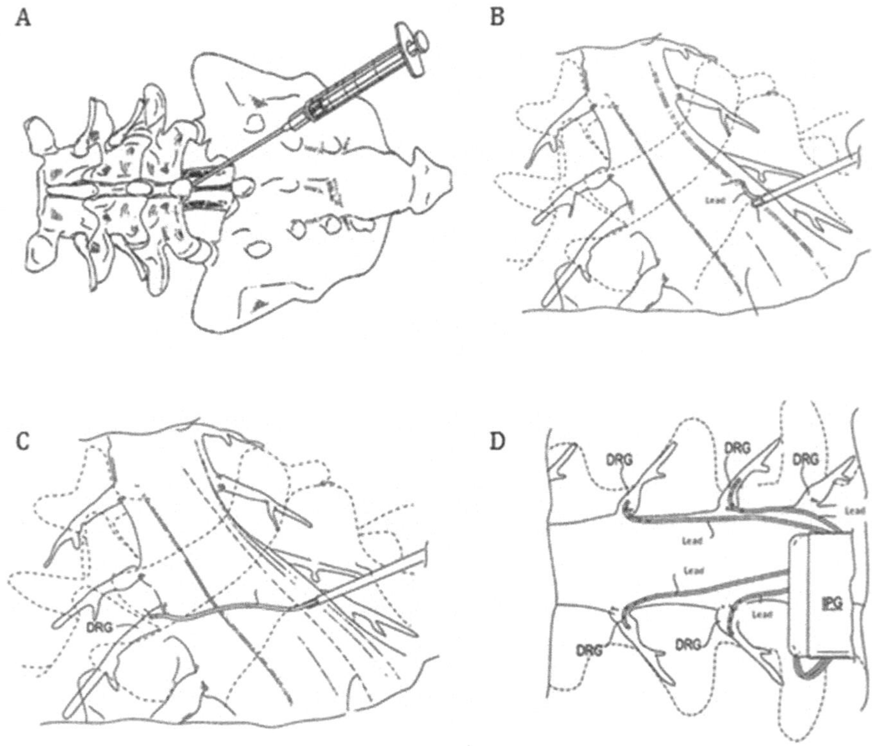

Fig. 23.4 Schematized DRG lead insertion procedure. (**a**) The epidural needle should make a shallow percutaneous entry. (**b**) The needle should be placed just past the anatomic midline of the spinal cord, and its bevel should be directed toward the contralateral target pedicle. (**c**) The lead can then be steered into the target vertebral foramen to be placed near the DRG. (**d**) From a single epidural entry point, up to four leads can be placed at multiple spinal levels (*Reproduced with permission of* St. Jude Medical, ©2017)

23.4.5 Steering the Leads to the DRG

Once the leads are delivered to the epidural space, caudal to the targeted DRG, the specialized stylet and delivery sheath then allow steering of the lead to its intended location. The styleted lead inside the delivery sheath is first delivered to the fenestration of the transforaminal space. Next, the lead and stylet apparatus is carefully deployed near the DRG under fluoroscopic guidance after the sheath is retracted back. The stylet is then retracted out of the lead to increase its flexibility, in order to conform to the dimensions of the intraforaminal space (Fig. 23.5).

The delivery sheath is pulled back closer to the needle bevel in the epidural space. Approximately 3–4 cm of slack lead is fed into the epidural space and formed into an 'S' shape with the delivery sheath. The lead slack delivered to the epidural space reduces the risk of lead migration. Experienced DRG stimulator implanters note that proper placement of the lead slack is a critical step to optimize the stabilized delivery of stimulation (Fig. 23.6).

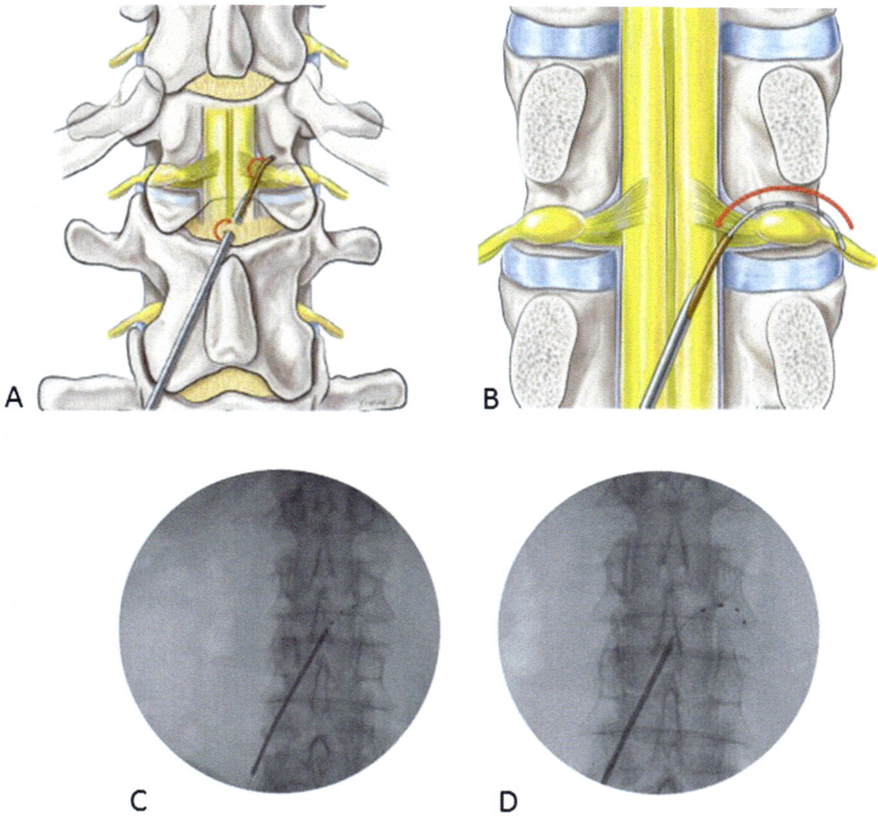

Fig. 23.5 Lead delivery for specialized DRG leads. (**a**) A styleted lead inside the delivery sheath is placed through an epidural needle. (**b**) The sheath-lead combination is then steered into the lateral epidural space, where the lead is delivered dorsal to the DRG. (**c**) The sheath should pass the target pedicle, foraminal ligaments, and epidural structures to enter the neural foramen. (**d**) When positioned, the lead should be in the cranial aspect of the foramen, with the contacts under the midpoint of the pedicle (*Reproduced with permission of* St. Jude Medical, ©2017)

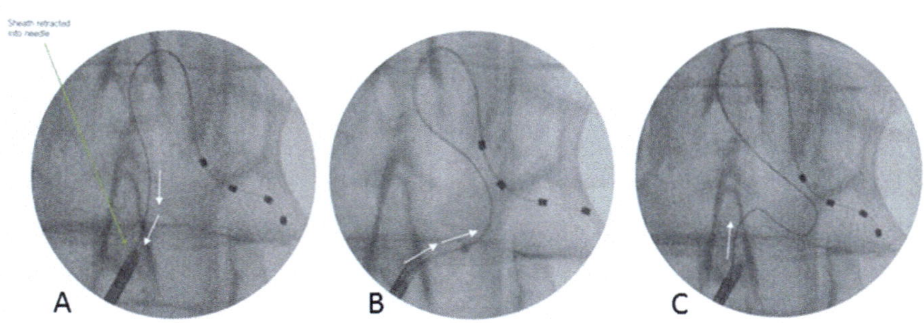

Fig. 23.6 'S'-shaped slack on each lead is deployed in the epidural space to reduce the risk of lead migration. It is formed by first retracting the sheath into the needle (**a**), advancing the sheath and lead together, laterally (**b**), and further retracting the sheath while advancing additional lead into the epidural space (**c**) (*Reproduced with permission of* St. Jude Medical, ©2017)

Once the leads are appropriately placed, the needle, delivery sheath, and stylet are removed. Fluoroscopic observation during this step will ensure the stability of the lead locations. For trial placements, the leads are anchored to the skin, dressed per the surgeon's preferences, and connected to the EPG. For permanent placements, a small pocket is made for anchoring the lead in the subcutaneous tissue.

23.4.5.1 Pearls of Clinical Experience: Proper Lead Placement

Poor placement of the leads can be identified by a visual inspection of the lead with fluoroscopic examination from AP and lateral angles. Expert implanters recommend that a lateral image is especially useful to confirm appropriate lead placement. Inadvertent ventral placement may not provide the optimal therapeutic effect and is particularly apparent at this angle.

23.4.6 Placing the IPG

The IPG is placed in a subcutaneous pocket in a location suitable for the patient's body type, preferences, and lead locations. The pocket should be no more than 2.5 cm deep, in order to allow adequate wireless communication with the Patient Programmer.

23.4.6.1 Pearls of Clinical Experience: Determining the Location for the IPG

An important step, often skipped by implanting physicians, is the determination of the location for the IPG prior to the transfer of the patient to the operating room. For this, communication with patients is key, as personal details and preferences should be considered:

- The side on which they prefer to sleep
- The shoulder and arm range of motion required to comfortably align the Patient Programmer with the IPG
- Clothing habits, such as their preferred belt line, as pressure on the subcutaneous IPG from clothing can be uncomfortable

The final determination of the IPG location should always defer to patient preference and comfort, with the location of the IPG recorded after the conversation. During the preoperative period, the implant site and an incision line need to be clearly marked with a surgical marker.

23.4.7 Wound Care

Procedural and post-procedural care is similar to standards typically utilized for fully implantable neurostimulator systems. As with implantation of any other SCS device, the standard of care for subcutaneous implantations and the physician preferences for prophylactic care of the implanted device should be implemented.

23.4.8 Potential Complications

As with any neuromodulation system, complications such as lead migration, infection, and unintended stimulation effects are possible. Early evidence indicates that the rates for these complications are similar to or less than rates for traditional SCS [25, 26]. As more published literature becomes available on this therapy, the specialized design and the placement of DRG leads inside immobile bony structures are expected to reduce the rate of lead migration and resulting changes to stimulation. All standard surgical precautions that apply to standard SCS are also valid for DRG stimulation, to ensure patient safety and optimal outcomes. The implanter is cautioned to proceed in the safest and most expeditious manner possible. The implantation plan established in the preoperative period should be maintained in order to prevent any risk to the patient and ensure the best outcome possible.

23.5 Conclusions

DRG stimulation has emerged as a robust method of neuromodulatory pain relief and has been successfully employed for a large number of intractable neuropathic pain indications. DRG stimulation offers advantages over conventional SCS, such as stimulation of specific areas and reduction in energy usage for optimal therapy. Appropriate candidates for DRG stimulation largely overlap with those for SCS, although a wider range of pain etiologies and locations may be amenable to treatment with DRG stimulation. More care must be taken in the preimplantation examination, however, including specific imaging of the target DRG sites, because of the relatively intricate lead implantation procedure. DRG stimulation leads are narrow and extremely flexible. They are placed dorsal to the DRGs using a standard percutaneous technique followed by precise epidural maneuvering with a stylet and curved delivery sheath for positioning support. The leads are stabilized with epidural lead slack and tissue anchors. Aside from these subtle differences, the implantation technique mirrors that of conventional SCS. The power requirements for DRG stimulation are much lower than for dorsal column SCS, due to the thin layer of CSF present between the dura and the DRG.

Acknowledgements Dr. Amirdelfan is a consultant of St. Jude Medical, Inc. Drs. Kramer, Cusack, and Burton are employees of St. Jude Medical, Inc. The authors thank Allison Foster, Ph.D., for medical writing assistance in drafting this chapter.

References

1. Shen J, Wang HY, Chen JY, Liang BL. Morphologic analysis of normal human lumbar dorsal root ganglion by 3D MR imaging. AJNR Am J Neuroradiol. 2006;27:2098–103.
2. Hasegawa T, Yoshihiro M, Ryo W, An HS. Morphometric analysis of the lumbosacral nerve roots and dorsal root ganglia by magnetic resonance imaging. Spine. 1996;21(9):1005.
3. Pope JE, Deer TR, Kramer J. A systematic review: current and future directions of dorsal root ganglion therapeutics to treat chronic pain. Pain Med. 2013;14:1477–96.
4. Liem L. Stimulation of the dorsal root ganglion. In: Slavin KV, editor. Stimulation of the peripheral nervous system. The neuromodulation frontier. Basel: Karger; 2016. p. 213–24.
5. Besson JM, Chaouch A. Peripheral and spinal mechanisms of nociception. Physiol Rev. 1987;67:67–186.
6. Devor M, Janig W, Michaelis M. Modulation of activity in dorsal root ganglion neurons by sympathetic activation in nerve-injured rats. J Neurophysiol. 1994;71:38–47.
7. Devor M. Unexplained peculiarities of the dorsal root ganglion. Pain Suppl. 1999;6:S27–35.
8. Hanani M. Satellite glial cells in sensory ganglia: from form to function. Brain Res Brain Res Rev. 2005;48:457–76.
9. Scholz J, Woolf CJ. The neuropathic pain triad: neurons, immune cells and glia. Nat Neurosci. 2007;10:1361–8.
10. Liem L, van Dongen E, Huygen FJ, Staats P, Kramer J. The dorsal root ganglion as a therapeutic target for chronic pain. Reg Anesth Pain Med. 2016;41:511–9.
11. Kajander KC, Wakisaka S, Bennett GJ. Spontaneous discharge originates in the dorsal root ganglion at the onset of a painful peripheral neuropathy in the rat. Neurosci Lett. 1992;138:225–8.
12. Ali Z, Ringkamp M, Hartke TV, Chien HF, Flavahan NA, Campbell JN, Meyer RA. Uninjured c-fiber nociceptors develop spontaneous activity and alpha-adrenergic sensitivity following L6 spinal nerve ligation in monkey. J Neurophysiol. 1999;81:455–66.
13. Xiao HS, Huang QH, Zhang FX, Bao L, Lu YJ, Guo C, et al. Identification of gene expression profile of dorsal root ganglion in the rat peripheral axotomy model of neuropathic pain. Proc Natl Acad Sci U S A. 2002;99:8360–5.
14. Gosselin RD, Suter MR, Ji RR, Decosterd I. Glial cells and chronic pain. Neuroscientist. 2010;16:519–31.
15. Kishi M, Tanabe J, Schmelzer JD, Low PA. Morphometry of dorsal root ganglion in chronic experimental diabetic neuropathy. Diabetes. 2002;51:819–24.
16. Holsheimer J. Which neuronal elements are activated directly by spinal cord stimulation. Neuromodulation. 2002;5:25–31.
17. Lee MW, McPhee RW, Stringer MD. An evidence-based approach to human dermatomes. Clin Anat. 2008;21:363–73.
18. Ohtori S, Takahashi Y, Takahashi K, Yamagata M, Chiba T, Tanaka K, et al. Sensory innervation of the dorsal portion of the lumbar intervertebral disc in rats. Spine (Phila Pa 1976). 1999;24:2295–9.
19. Malykhina AP, Qin C, Greenwood-Van Meerveld B, Foreman RC, Lupu F, Akbarali HI. Hyperexcitability of convergent colon and bladder dorsal root ganglion neurons after colonic inflammation: mechanism for pelvic organ cross-talk. Neurogastroenterol Motil. 2006;18:936–48.

20. Food and Drug Administration (FDA). Approval order statement: axium neurostimulator system. Premarket approval (PMA). 2016. http://www.accessdata.fda.gov/scripts/cdrh/cfdocs/cfpma/pma.cfm?id=P150004. Accessed 30 Jul 2016
21. Deer TR, Liem AL, Pope J, et al. Neurostimulation of the dorsal root ganglion (DRG) by spinal cord stimulation (SCS): a review of proper patient selection. In: Minimally invasive surgery for pain. New Orleans, LA: Southern Academic Press. p. 2015.
22. Medical SJ. Axium neurostimulator system physician implant manual. Menlo Park, CA: St. Jude Medical; 2016.
23. St. Jude Medical, Inc. Axium neurostimulator system procedure guide. St. Paul, MN: St. Jude Medical, Inc.; 2015.
24. Taylor RS, Ryan J, O'Donnell R, Eldabe S, Kumar K, North RB. The cost-effectiveness of spinal cord stimulation in the treatment of failed back surgery syndrome. Clin J Pain. 2010;26:463–9.
25. Liem L, Russo M, Huygen FJ, Van Buyten JP, Smet I, Verrills P, et al. One-year outcomes of spinal cord stimulation of the dorsal root ganglion in the treatment of chronic neuropathic pain. Neuromodulation. 2015;18:41–8.
26. Caspary T, Anderson KV. Patterning cell types in the dorsal spinal cord: what the mouse mutants say. Nat Rev Neurosci. 2003;4:289–97.

Chapter 24
High-Frequency Stimulation

Kasra Amirdelfan and Jasmine Silva

Spinal cord stimulation (SCS) has become an integral treatment option for many patients suffering from chronic, intractable neuropathic pain in the trunk and limbs. New iterations of SCS have been introduced, but the efficacy of such developments so far has been focused on providing more effective paresthesia coverage in the area of pain for appropriate patients. The advent of a new high-frequency SCS system, commercially available as HF10™ therapy, has created a new realm in neuromodulation where paresthesia coverage is no longer relevant. Moreover, HF10 therapy has been shown to be superior to traditional, paresthesia-based, low-frequency SCS in a large, level I randomized controlled study (The SENZA-RCT) [1]. In May of 2015, the evidence from the first of its kind RCT study in neuromodulation, along with strong evidence from the European and Australian experience, led to the approval of the SENZA® system, capable of HF10 SCS therapy, in the United States. HF10 therapy has since become increasingly popular among neuromodulators for the treatment of chronic low back and leg pain, among other indications commonly treated with SCS. The remarkable efficacy of HF10 therapy has helped this technology in finding itself among one of the most popular technologies in SCS in the United States and around the world. This chapter outlines some of the evidence supporting the safety and efficacy of SCS and HF10 therapy and provides a detailed, step-by-step guide for safe and efficient implementation of HF10 therapy SCS for appropriate patients.

K. Amirdelfan (✉) • J. Silva
IPM Medical Group, Inc., Walnut Creek, CA, USA
e-mail: doctorA@ipmdoctors.com; jasmines@ipmdoctors.com

S. Diwan, T.R. Deer (eds.), *Advanced Procedures for Pain Management*,
https://doi.org/10.1007/978-3-319-68841-1_24

24.1 Introduction

Interventional pain management physicians have increasingly utilized spinal cord stimulation (SCS) as a key treatment option for appropriate patients with chronic, intractable neuropathic pain in the trunk and the limbs. The recent exponential growth of this technology has largely been due to its low complication rate [2] and its high degree of efficacy [3]. The first spinal cord stimulator was described in 1971 [4]. Over the subsequent decades, SCS devices have undergone numerous technological advances in order to produce better outcomes with lower complication rates and to provide a more pleasant paresthesia experience for the pain patient. Paresthesia sensations caused by SCS therapy are commonly perceived as tingling, buzzing, or pins-and-needles, which some patients occasionally find uncomfortable. Paresthesia and its overlap of the painful areas continue to be the basis of all traditional, low-frequency SCS devices. Technological advances in SCS hardware have provided physicians with such benefits as multiple contacts on the same lead [5], rechargeable implantable pulse generators (IPGs) [6], and anchoring devices and techniques that mitigate the risk of migration [7]. More importantly, research and development (R&D) in this modality has been quite successful in improving the stimulation delivery by utilizing more efficacious waveforms, pulse widths, and frequencies, within a perceptible range, allowing improved delivery of paresthesia coverage to the patients' painful areas [8]. Until 2007, however, the focus of R&D in the SCS industry was limited to advancing hardware and software technologies towards an improved paresthesia experience for the patient. It was in that year when the newly formulated concept of high-frequency stimulation of the nervous system paved the way for what is now known as HF10 therapy.

The recent advent of high-frequency technology, HF10™ therapy (Nevro Corp., Redwood City, CA), has been one of the most remarkable technological advances in SCS treatment. HF10 therapy provides greater pain relief than traditional, low-frequency SCS, while being paresthesia-free [1]. As used here, "low-frequency SCS" refers to SCS at frequencies previously in use and approved by the FDA prior to 2015—frequencies below 1200 Hz, and typically on the order of 40–100 Hz. "High-frequency" stimulation is intended to refer to frequencies above 1200 Hz, which were not commercially available prior to 2015. HF10 therapy has a low complication rate similar to that of traditional low-frequency SCS [9]. The technology was the subject of a first-of-its-kind, head-to-head, randomized controlled trial (SENZA-RCT) [1], with long-term follow-up that clearly demonstrated superior pain control in low back and leg pain in the HF10 therapy subjects. The efficacy of this trial has also been demonstrated in other clinical trials [10]. The efficacy of HF10 therapy has been demonstrated for chronic low back and leg pain, and extensive research is currently under way to evaluate its outcome in other chronic pain indications typically treated with traditional SCS.

The May 2015 FDA approval of Nevro's HF10 therapy and Senza® system (Fig. 24.1) has ushered in a new era of more effective therapies for various chronic pain indications. Aside from providing a new realm in SCS therapy, the impressive

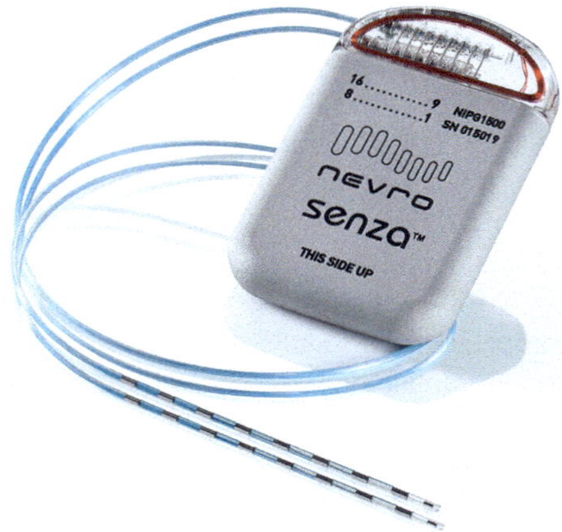

Fig. 24.1 Nevro's Senza® HF10™ therapy system leads and implantable pulse generator (IPG)

efficacy of HF10 therapy has motivated other SCS companies and scientists to develop new SCS features, which may provide better pain relief for chronic pain patients. Current research is under way by all SCS manufacturers to further improve the efficacy of their upcoming SCS technologies. The true victors are the chronic pain patients, who will benefit from advanced SCS devices with improved pain relief. For the foreseeable future, however, HF10 therapy is increasingly established as the superior standard for the treatment of chronic low back and leg pain, among other indications.

This chapter presents a step-by-step guide that encompasses appropriate patient selection and the safe and effective implementation of HF10 therapy in the identified candidates.

24.2 Materials and Methods

In the preparation for this chapter, an extensive literature search was performed utilizing PubMed, ScienceDirect, and Academic Search Complete for English-language publications on human subjects and SCS therapy. Relevant peer-reviewed publications from 1970 to April of 2016 were referenced for information cited in this chapter. Dr. Amirdelfan also provided his personal input as an investigator for HF10 therapy from the early stages of R&D up to the SENZA-RCT study, in addition to his clinical experience since the FDA's approval of the Senza system in the United States.

24.3 Evidence

Over the past decade, the evidence for high-frequency SCS at 10 kHz, commercially available as HF10 therapy, has rapidly accumulated. Tiede and colleagues published the first human study on HF10 therapy in 2013 [11]. The study demonstrated that subjects with chronic low back and leg pain preferred HF10 therapy to traditional, low-frequency SCS. Approximately 88% of the study subjects preferred HF10 therapy, versus 12% who preferred traditional SCS. The encouraging results of this feasibility project led to a single-arm, prospective long-term study for low back and leg pain in Europe [10]. This study demonstrated remarkable efficacy in the subjects who underwent implantation of the HF10 therapy device. In the 2013 European study, published by Van Buyten and colleagues, a mean reduction of back pain from a VAS of 8.4–2.7 was reported at 6 months. Similar results in reduction of leg pain demonstrated an improvement from a mean VAS of 5.4–1.4 for the same time period. Improvements in overall function and sleep patterns, and a reduction in pain medications were also reported [10].

The results from the abovementioned studies became the foundation for the SENZA-RCT study, a multicenter RCT comparing commercially available, traditional, low-frequency SCS versus HF10-therapy SCS in the United States. This study demonstrated the superiority of HF10 therapy over traditional SCS in all primary, secondary, and tertiary endpoints in patients with chronic low back and leg pain [1]. This study also led to the FDA approval of HF10 therapy and the Senza® system in the United States for the treatment of chronic, intractable trunk and limb pain, with superior labeling. Because of its paresthesia-free nature, the FDA did not pose restrictions on driving or operating heavy machinery with HF10 therapy, unlike traditional low-frequency SCS [12].

24.4 Indications

HF10 SCS therapy is indicated for all chronic pain conditions currently being treated with traditional SCS. As such, HF10 SCS therapy is indicated for chronic intractable pain in the trunk and limbs, including low back pain, based on the evidence and FDA labeling. Diagnoses most commonly treated with SCS therapy (traditional or otherwise) include but are not limited to multilevel lumbar degenerative disc disease where surgical repair is not clearly indicated, lumbar post-laminectomy syndrome with or without radiculopathy, and complex regional pain syndrome type I and II [2].

Similar to traditional SCS, contraindications of HF10 therapy include infection, history of drug abuse, coagulopathies, anatomical variations pronounced enough to hinder or prevent an optimal outcome, and psychological issues that are deemed risky or inappropriate for SCS therapy, as determined by a psychological professional [13].

It must be emphasized that the implanting physician should continue to be diligent in the identification and evaluation of the appropriate SCS and HF10 therapy candidate. A thorough history and physical examination will help elicit any relative or absolute contraindications for implantable technology. The preoperative assessment must include a psychological evaluation by an expert in pain psychology, in order to rule out any potential psychological concerns or barriers prior to undertaking SCS as a therapeutic option. The medical and psychological evaluation for HF10 SCS therapy is quite similar to an evaluation for traditional, low-frequency SCS. As such, experienced implanting physicians need not alter their routine SCS preoperative evaluation for HF10 therapy. The only exception is that the physician may consider patients with isolated axial back pain with a neuropathic component (failed back surgery syndrome, lumbar disc disease, etc.) as potential candidates for HF10 therapy, because of its proven efficacy in this patient population [1].

24.5 Trial Procedure

24.5.1 HF10 Therapy Pre-trial Considerations

Although the fundamentals of an HF10 therapy trial are quite similar to trials for traditional SCS, the most significant difference is the required length of the trial for this type of SCS. HF10 therapy is paresthesia-free. Thus, the patients will need additional time to acclimate to each alteration in programming and subsequently report their outcomes. The manufacturer has developed an efficient algorithm to test the various programs in order to optimize the patient's pain control in a timely manner. However, in order to thoroughly test the various parameters, a minimum of 5–7 days is strongly recommended for the trial period. Although most patients respond to HF10 therapy within the first 3–4 days, a prolonged trial will allow the system to be tested on patients with more complex pain patterns. Moreover, a prolonged trial will allow both the physician and the patient to thoroughly evaluate HF10 therapy as the right therapy for the patient. The ratio of trial to permanent conversion in the low back and leg pain population, utilizing this method, was shown to be approximately 88% in the SENZA-RCT [1] and in the European study [10].

Preoperative and postoperative antibiotics should be considered for the HF10 therapy trial as a prophylactic measure, similar to traditional SCS. The authors prefer one dose of IV antibiotics approximately 30 min prior to initiating the procedure, followed by at least 3 days of oral antibiotics. As is standard practice with surgical prophylaxis, the prophylaxis should target commonly anticipated organisms in a surgical infection [14]. Some centers may not use any antibiotics in the preoperative and postoperative period, however, based on their individual preferences, policies, and procedures.

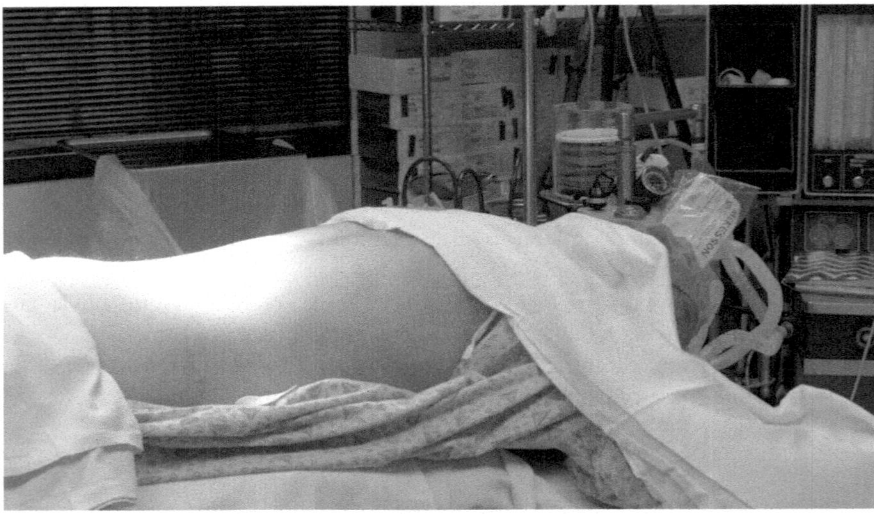

Fig. 24.2 Ideal position with reduction in lumbar lordosis

During the preoperative interview, the authors recommend that the implanting physician determine which side is the preferred side for sleep in any particular patient. The leads should be directed to the contralateral side after placement, based on the patient's preference, to maximize comfort during the trial period and to reduce the chances of mechanical interruption due to untoward manipulation of connections to the leads.

24.5.2 Patient Positioning

Position the patient prone on the operating table with at least one pillow below the patient's abdomen in order to reverse lumbar lordosis (Fig. 24.2). This helps to facilitate needle entry into the epidural space at the necessary angle. Prepare and drape the patient in the standard sterile fashion, based on physician's standards and the facility's requirements.

24.5.3 Sedation

Patients may or may not be sedated, based on the surgeon's preference. Anesthesia can be administered using oral or IV sedation. Since HF10 therapy is paresthesia-free, no paresthesia mapping is required in the operating theater. In fact, paresthesia mapping is not recommended, as HF10 therapy is more effective when the leads are simply placed at the anatomical midline. As such, the patient need not be awake during an HF10 therapy trial or respond to questions regarding paresthesia coverage. However, the surgeon may choose to keep the patient alert in order to reduce the risk of nerve root or spinal cord damage. A local anesthetic should be used through a small-gauge needle in the skin and over the intended trajectory of the 14-G Tuohy needle in the deeper tissue, in order to minimize soft tissue discomfort during and after the procedure. The authors prefer 1% lidocaine with epinephrine for this purpose.

24.5.4 Identification of Landmarks

Position the fluoroscopy arm over the patient to identify the needle epidural entry level and final lead destination of the leads. Tilt the image intensifier of the fluoroscope toward the patient's feet in order to line up the upper end plate of the epidural entry target vertebrae. Epidural entry typically occurs at L1, T12, or L2 (in order of preference). However, the lead placement targets for HF10 therapy are the top of the T8 endplate and the middle of the T9 vertebral bodies, both at the anatomical midline. The anatomical midline placement is a unique characteristic of HF10 therapy. The evidence, accumulated from various research studies, has demonstrated that the optimal results are achieved with such a placement (Fig. 24.3). This varies from the placement goals of traditional, low-frequency SCS, which is adjacent, and lateral to, the anatomical midline.

24.5.5 Needle Entry

After the administration of the local anesthetic to the skin and soft tissue, the entry point for the manufacturer-supplied 14-gauge Tuohy needle is medial to the pedicle at the level below the target interlaminar space (Fig. 24.4). The needle should be introduced at a shallow angle to the skin surface (≤30 degrees), with an equally

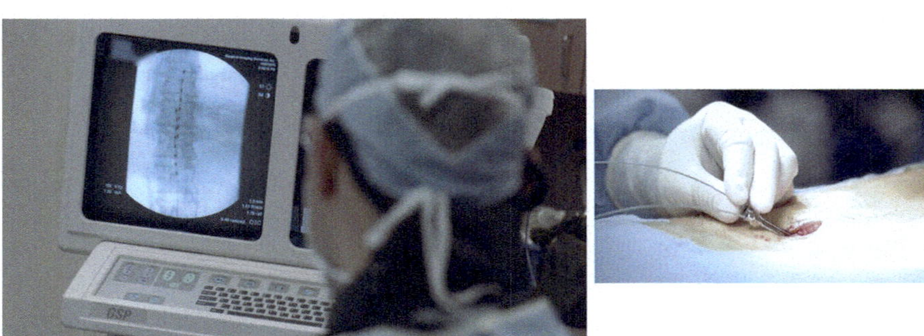

Fig. 24.3 HF10 therapy method for lead placement at anatomical midline

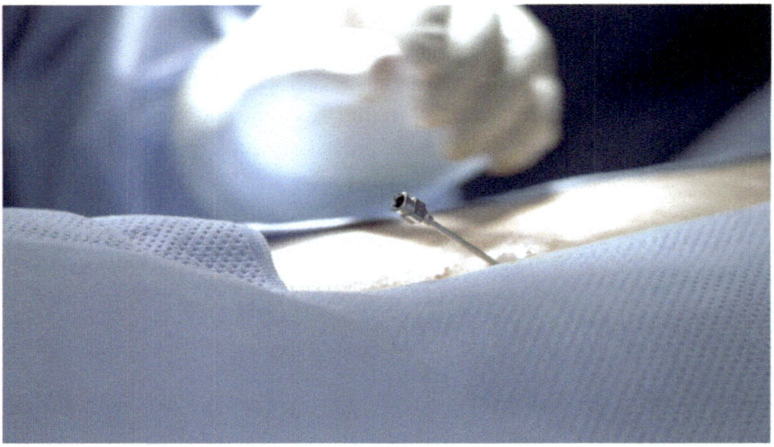

Fig. 24.4 Needle placement for epidural entry

shallow trajectory angle towards the interlaminar target (Fig. 24.5). The shallow angle of approach will allow the appropriate trajectory for facilitated lead advancement into the epidural space. The needle is then advanced in a paramedian fashion towards the anatomical midline of the target lamina. The Tuohy needle is introduced slowly into the epidural space using a standard loss-of-resistance technique.

24.5.6 Lead Placement

Prior to lead placement, the appropriate stylet should be loaded into the lead. The authors prefer the 14-G curved stylet for the initial thoracolumbar entry. Gently advance the lead into the epidural space under live fluoroscopy. Advance the first lead to the top of the superior T8 endplate, while maintaining a position at the anatomical midline, using fluoroscopic guidance (Fig. 24.6).

24.5.7 Placement of the Second Needle and Lead

Place the second needle in either an ipsilateral or contralateral manner to the first needle with respect to the spinous process, utilizing the same shallow angle of approach (Fig. 24.5). Once loss of resistance has been achieved, advance the second lead towards the target at the mid-body of T9 at the anatomical midline.

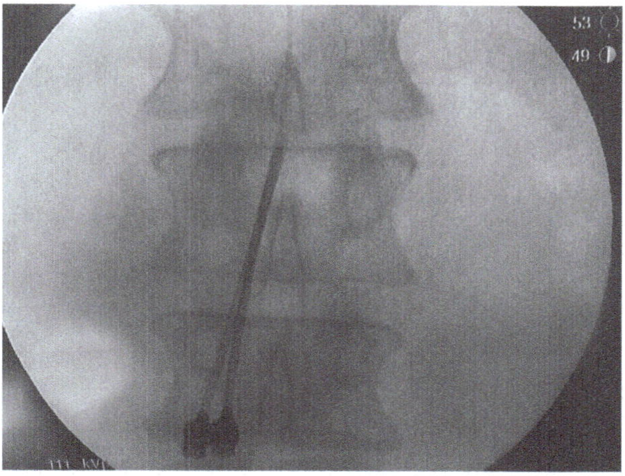

Fig. 24.5 Shallow angle of entry for ipsilateral needle placement

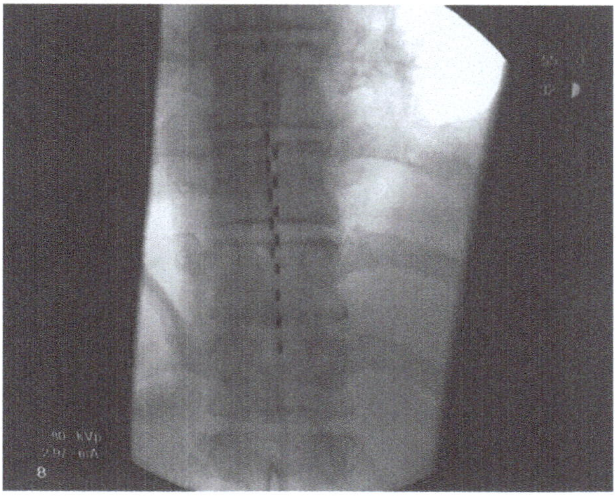

Fig. 24.6 Midline lead placement at T8 upper end plate and T9 mid body

24.5.8 Finalizing Placement

It is important to stagger the electrodes on the two adjacent leads in the final position in order to reduce the risk of contact between the leads. Most importantly, a lateral fluoroscopic view of the leads to ascertain their location in the dorsal epidural space is imperative. As HF10 therapy is paresthesia-free, an accidental ventral placement will render the trial a failure. As such, a lateral view to confirm dorsal placement is an absolute requirement with HF10 therapy (Fig. 24.7).

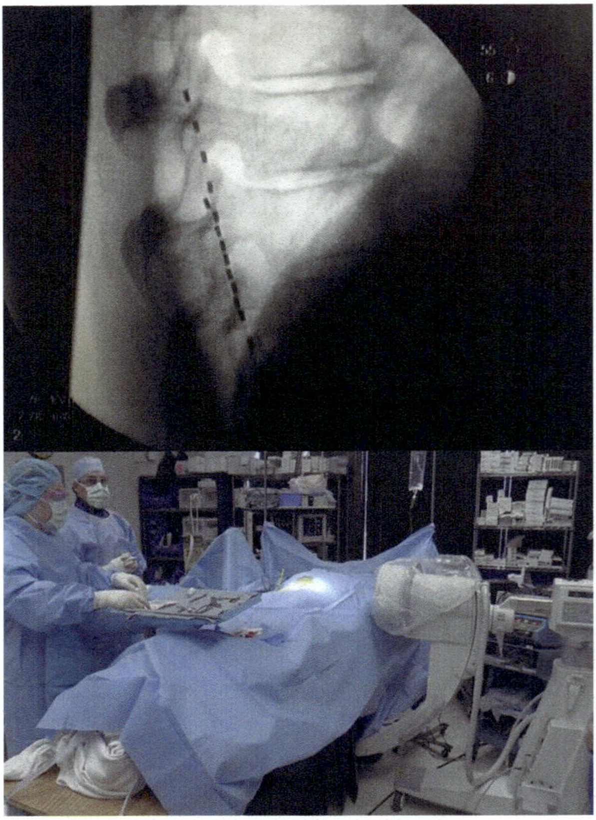

Fig. 24.7 Lateral confirmation of dorsal lead placement

24.5.9 Programming the System

Connect the leads to the testing cables provided by the manufacturer's representative. The representative will subsequently check the impedance and auto-align the leads and contacts for future programming (Fig. 24.8). This process does not require patient participation or paresthesia mapping, and takes less than 10 s to complete. This is another remarkable benefit of HF10 SCS therapy when compared with traditional SCS, which involves unpredictable intraoperative paresthesia mapping.

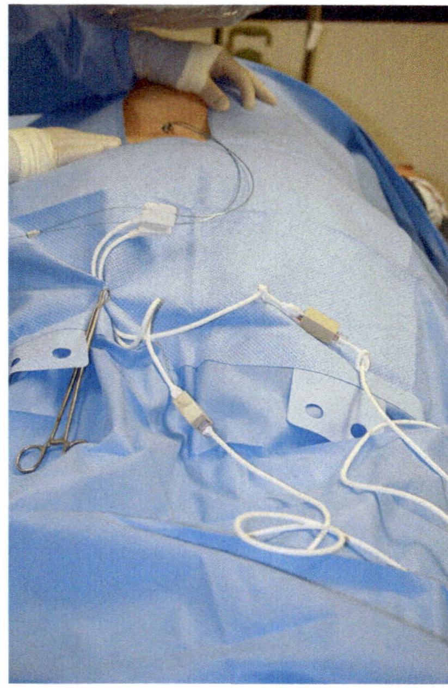

Fig. 24.8 Connected leads for impedance check

24.5.10 Lead Anchoring

Once the impedance check is completed, the needles and the stylets are carefully removed using a "twist and pull" technique for the needle, while stabilizing the lead with the opposite hand. The stylet can then be slowly removed, along with the needle, while holding the lead in place close to its skin entry site. Fluoroscopic imaging should be performed to ensure lack of lead migration during this process. The leads may be anchored using a woven suture such as 0–0 silk with a chest tube tie to the underlying skin and directly to the lead. Alternatively, the surgeon can use anchors provided with the SCS kit and a similar suture of his or her preference.

24.5.11 Application of Dressing

Coil the leads for a relief loop in an organized fashion and adhere the coils to the skin with sterile covers before connecting the ends of the leads to the cables. Apply a waterproof dressing over the entirety of the lead apparatus, as well as the cable connections, in order to secure the leads in place for the 5- to 7-day trial period (Fig. 24.9).

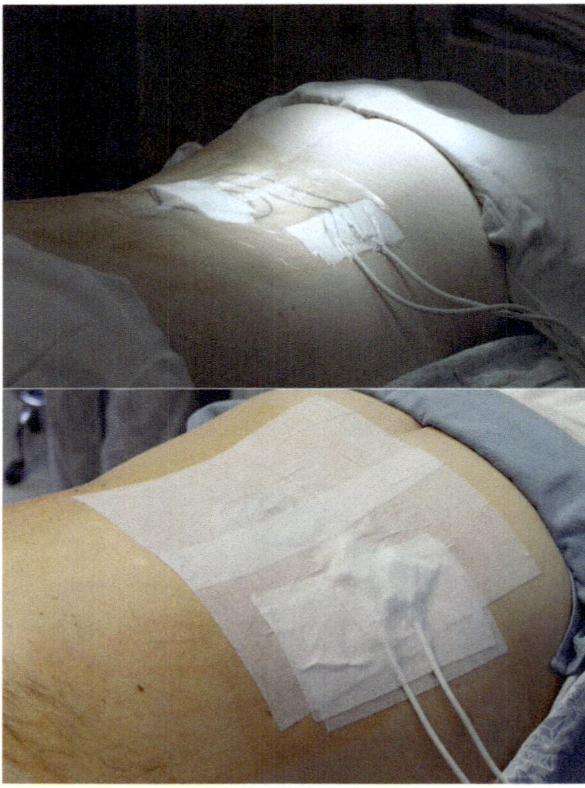

Fig. 24.9 Application of waterproof dressing (note connectors under the dressing for maximum security)

24.6 Permanent Procedure

The permanent procedure follows the same flow of an SCS trial, after the appropriate soft tissue pocket dissections have been completed. Preoperative and postoperative antibiotics are strongly recommended for this stage, as an infection of any degree at either the lead or IPG site would warrant immediate removal of the entire system, in order to mitigate the risk of epidural infection. Because HF10 therapy is paresthesia-free, full sedation for the permanent implantation is possible, similar to the trial stage, per the surgeon's preference, as patient response in the intraoperative period is not necessary.

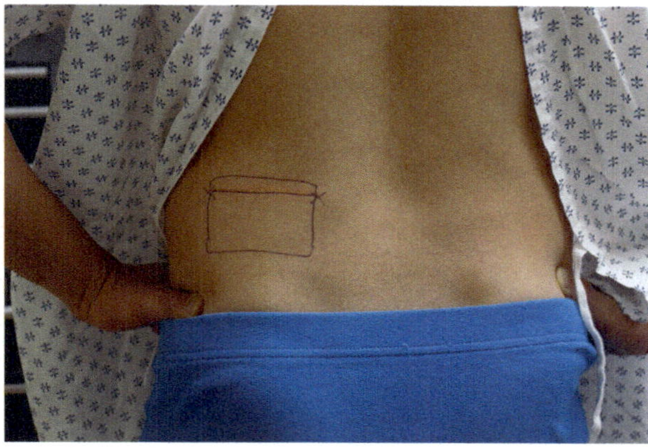

Fig. 24.10 Pocket template drawn with the patient in a standing position (horizontal placement)

24.6.1 IPG Pocket Placement

Mark the IPG implant site before the patient is on the OR table. Have the patient sit or stand with his or her hands indicating his or her preferred beltline level. Mark the implant site in the flank or buttock area (above or below the beltline), depending on patient and physician preference. Draw the outline of a pocket to the size and shape of the IPG. It is recommended that the incision line be placed in the upper third of the pocket, in order to facilitate the implantation and closure process (Fig. 24.10). The authors prefer a horizontal placement of the Senza® IPG in order to place the antenna, located in the header, as far lateral as possible for the patient's charging convenience, but a vertical placement is equally acceptable, based on the implanting physician's preference.

24.6.2 Patient Positioning

Positioning is identical to the trial procedure, in order to facilitate dissection and epidural access.

24.6.3 Sedation

Based on patient and physician preferences, any conventional level of anesthesia is appropriate, as patient participation and paresthesia mapping is not required. The usual safety precautions regarding sedation and anesthesia are always the main consideration, as well as the primary goal of the physician, anesthesiologist, and OR team.

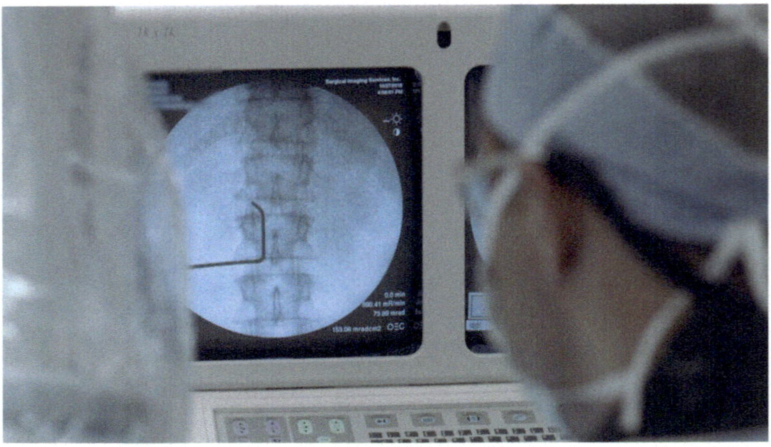

Fig. 24.11 Incision line below target level for ipsilateral double needle placement

24.6.4 Landmark Identification

The target lead and skin entry sites are once again identified under fluoroscopic guidance, similar to the trial procedure.

24.6.5 Lead Pocket Formation

Line up the superior endplate of the selected vertebra for epidural entry. Use a radio-opaque pointing tool to mark the area over that vertebra on the patient by using a sterile marker. The mid-portion of the incision line should be the needle insertion point into the soft tissue for the best needle trajectory.

If an ipsilateral needle approach is desired for the second needle placement, the mid-point of the incision line will be medial to the pedicle at the level below, in a patient of average weight and height. If a contralateral approach is desired, the incision will be at midline with the mid-portion between the pedicles along the spinous process, at the level below the epidural target (Fig. 24.11). The typical incision is about 3–4 cm in length. Using a scalpel, make the incision along the designated incision line, after local anesthetic has been administered in the surgical area. Dissection should be continued slowly and carefully until the thoracodorsal fascia is identified. Electrocautery or blunt dissection may be used to undermine the subcutaneous pocket along the fascial plane.

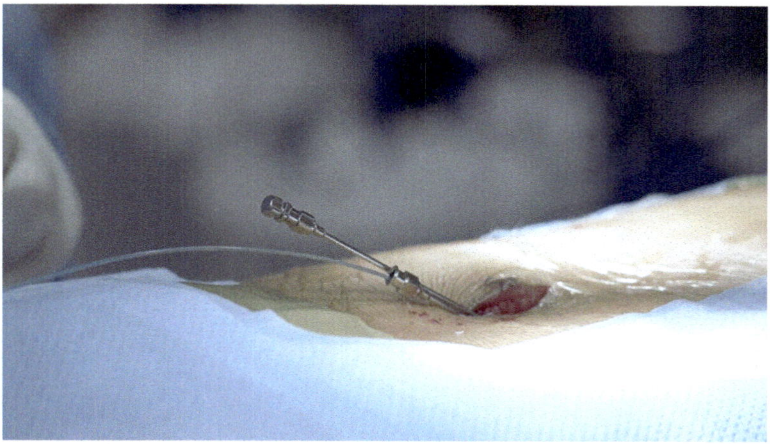

Fig. 24.12 Ipsilateral double needle placement

24.6.6 Needle Entry

Use a similar approach to that outlined in the trial procedure to achieve the required shallow angle for the needle trajectory towards the interlaminar target. The goal is an approach angle of 30° or less into the soft tissue, toward the midline, for the best results in lead placement (Fig. 24.12).

24.6.7 Lead Placement

Load the preferred stylet into each lead and steer the leads to the target sites (upper end plate of T8 for the first lead and mid-body of T9 for the second lead for low back and leg targeting) at the anatomical midline. Midline placement is strongly recommended, based on extensive research, regardless of the laterality of the painful area for low back and leg pain on any individual patient (*see* Fig. 24.6).

Check a lateral fluoroscopic image to confirm dorsal epidural placement (*see* Fig. 24.7). This is a crucial step in HF10 therapy because the therapy is paresthesia-free and a ventral placement will not be recognized with typical paresthesia testing. Each needle and lead placement should be completed in a consecutive manner in order to allow the physician to change the necessary approach if any barriers (such as scar tissue or bone spurs) or suboptimal interlaminar epidural placement is encountered.

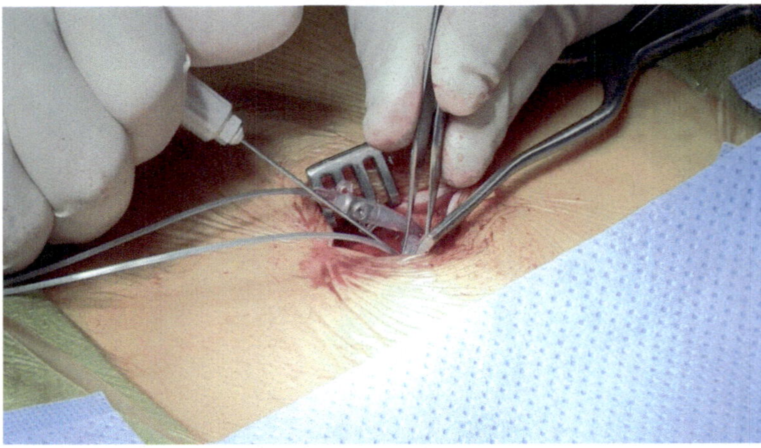

Fig. 24.13 Lead anchors securing lead placement

24.6.8 *Lead Anchoring*

Once the leads are appropriately placed, using the techniques outlined in the trial procedure to assure correct placement, the needles and the stylets can be removed. The anchors provided by the manufacturer greatly reduce the risk of lead fracture and/or migration, so their use for the permanent implant is imperative. Place the anchors slowly over the lead and move them to the lead insertion site without causing any untoward lead movement.

The tip of the anchor will need to penetrate the thoracodorsal fascia to mitigate the risk of lead migration and buckling at that site. Once the anchors are in place, the setscrew may be engaged with the supplied torque screwdriver. Tighten the setscrews until at least one or two clicks of the screwdriver are heard. Suture the anchors to adjacent ligamentous tissue. The authors prefer 0–0 silk suture for this process. Care must be taken at all times to refrain from unintentional movement of the leads from their target site (Fig. 24.13). Once the anchoring has been completed, a final AP fluoroscopic image is required for location confirmation and documentation.

24.6.9 *IPG Implantation*

Anesthetize the previously marked IPG implant site. Use a scalpel to incise the skin at the already-marked incision line. After the incision, use electrocautery to dissect down to Scarpa's fascia, which is 10–15 mm deep to the epidermis in most patients. Dissect to the fascial plane and begin undermining using electrocautery or blunt

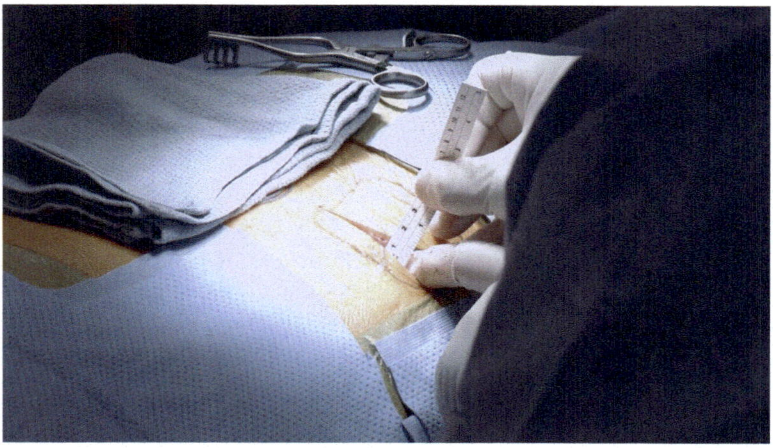

Fig. 24.14 Pocket depth should be 1.5 cm or less

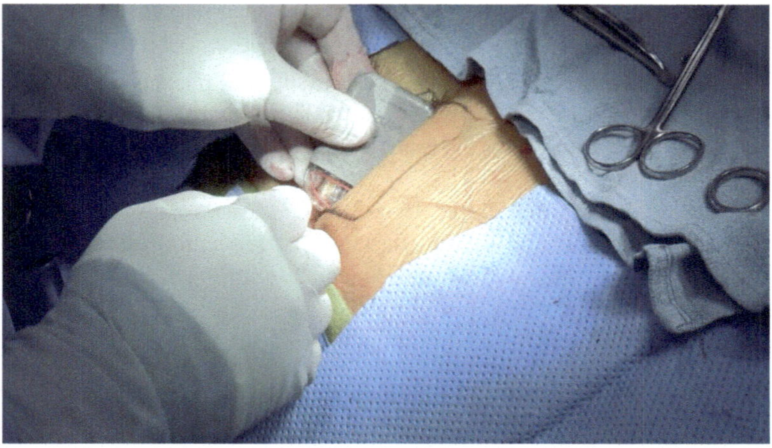

Fig. 24.15 Lateral header placement of the IPG in the pocket

dissection to the IPG outline already marked on the patient's skin. The IPG should not be implanted deeper than 1.5 cm, to ensure full communication between the remote control, the charging device, and the IPG (Fig. 24.14). An IPG sizer, a plastic model of the device available as an accessory, may be used to accurately size the pocket if necessary. A pocket that is too tight will hinder appropriate closure, whereas a pocket that is too loose may allow unwanted movement of the leads and the IPG, including potential inversion of the IPG, which would require a surgical revision (Fig. 24.15).

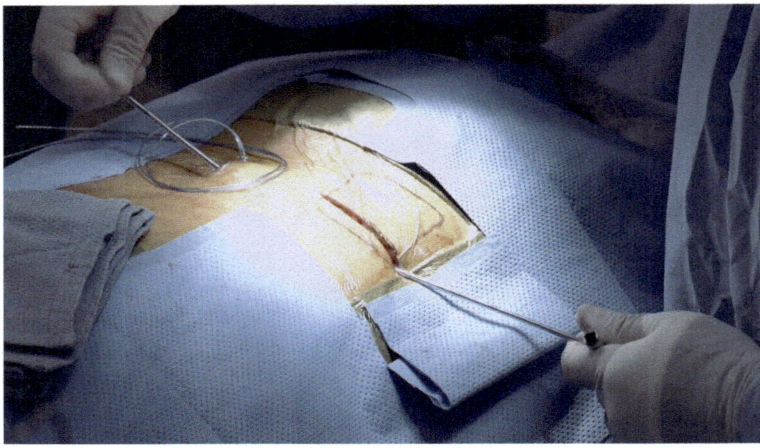

Fig. 24.16 Tunneling of the leads to the IPG pocket

24.6.10 Tunneling of the Leads

Utilize the tunneling tool to connect the IPG and the lead pockets through the subcutaneous tissue. Once the tunneling tool has passed along the desired path, remove the trocar tip to allow removal of the tunneling device, leaving the overlying plastic straw in place (Fig. 24.16).

Pass the leads through the plastic straw. Leave at least 3 cm of the leads in the midline pocket, in order to allow for the formation of a relief loop at the lead pocket. This loop will mitigate the risk of lead strain and migration.

24.6.11 Connecting the IPG and Leads

Insert the lead ends into the IPG ports. The representative will subsequently confirm impedance and auto-alignment of the leads, as well as the integrity of the new IPG. Place the cephalad (T8) lead into the bottom IPG port, which is labeled 1–8. The caudad lead will subsequently be placed into the upper IPG port, labeled 9–16. The Nevro representative can always check the placement remotely and, if necessary, ask the surgeon to switch the ports. Once the connections are fully confirmed, use the torque screwdriver to secure the leads to the IPG. Tighten the screw until at least one or two clicks are heard (Fig. 24.17).

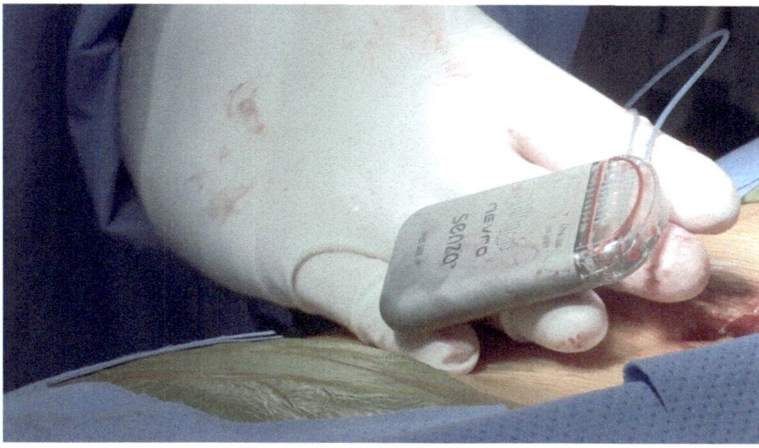

Fig. 24.17 Connecting the leads and IPG

24.6.12 IPG Placement

Place the IPG in the pocket with the logo side up. Coil any redundancy in the leads flat and place them behind the IPG. Although any orientation of the header is acceptable, the authors recommend a lateral header position in a horizontal placement, and a top header position in the case of a vertical placement, in order to facilitate charging for the patient (Fig. 24.18).

24.6.13 Closure

Irrigate both pockets with copious irrigation fluid of choice. Confirm the relief loops and the position of the IPG, with the logo up, prior to closure. Moreover, ensure that the leads are not kinked at any position. Utilize a subcutaneous deep closure followed by a running subcuticular closure of the skin edge. The manufacturer does not recommend using staples, as metal artifact may interfere with communication and charging of the device. Dress using a standard sterile postsurgical dressing.

24.7 Programming

The manufacturer has developed a sophisticated programming algorithm that is universally applied for all patients in the postoperative period, in order to provide every patient with the optimal pain relief possible. The algorithm will first implement the

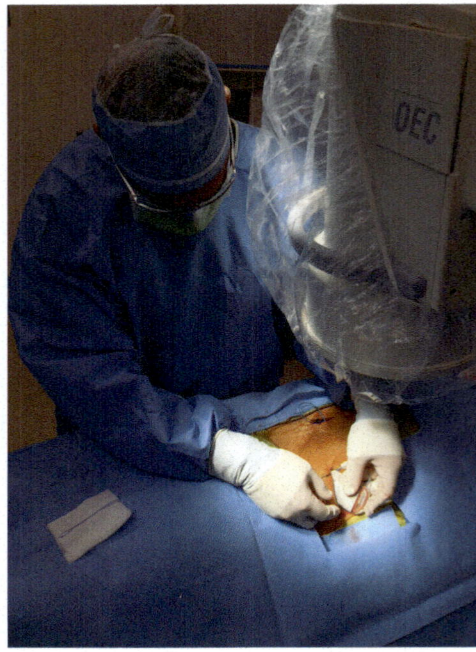

Fig. 24.18 IPG implantation

programs that are likely to provide the best relief, followed by subsequent programs with the next highest probability of success. Thus, all patients will have multiple programs to choose from at the onset of their trial or permanent implantation, regardless of the trial or the permanent stage of the procedure.

Additionally, programming changes may be applied by the patient, using the remote control, once they have conferred with a representative over the phone. This reduces or even eliminates the need for repeated office visits for reprogramming in order to optimize coverage. Patients are fully trained on autonomous utilization of their remote control device, in case a program or amplitude change is indicated.

24.8 Recharging the Device

The charging process for the Senza® system is also designed fora minimal amount of burden on the patient. So that the patient can develop a consistent charging habit, the manufacturer recommends daily charging of the device, which can be done within 30 to 45 minutes using a wireless recharging accessory. Patients may charge the device at any time throughout the day, and they are not limited with their function during the charging process. Therefore, there are no restrictions on charging while driving or operating machinery.

24.9 Conclusion

HF10 therapy has accumulated strong evidence to support its efficacious and long-term pain relief for chronic, intractable low back and leg pain, among other chronic neuropathic pain syndromes in the trunk and limbs. The FDA granted a superior labeling to HF10 therapy based on the evidence from the SENZA-RCT study. In addition to such attributes, the implementation of HF10 therapy is similar and familiar to all physicians proficient in the field of neuromodulation. Moreover, the lack of need for paresthesia mapping in the operating room renders a more predictable and consistent experience for the implanting physician and the OR team. Anatomical midline placement not only facilitates a more consistent and reproducible surgical experience, but also (and most importantly) HF10 SCS therapy allows for increased comfort due to lack of need for patient participation and paresthesia mapping. The overall skill set required for a traditional, low-frequency SCS trial or permanent implant compared with an HF10 SCS trial or implant is identical, rendering this technology readily available to the entire surgical team already familiar with the process of neuromodulation and its implementation. However the most notable attribute of HF10 therapy and the Senza® system is indeed its superior efficacy, providing patients with unprecedented relief of neuropathic pain in the trunk and limbs, based on level I evidence and clinical outcomes.

References

1. Kapural L, Yu C, Doust MW, Gliner BE, Vallejo R, Sitzman BT, et al. Novel 10-kHz high-frequency therapy (HF10 therapy) is superior to traditional low-frequency spinal cord stimulation for the treatment of chronic back and leg pain: the SENZA-RCT randomized controlled trial. Anesthesiology. 2015;123:851–60.
2. Mekhail NA, Mathews M, Nageeb F, Guirguis M, Mekhail MN, Cheng J. Retrospective review of 707 cases of spinal cord stimulation: indications and complications. Pain Pract. 2011;11:148–53.
3. Sears NC, Machado AG, Nagel SJ, Deogaonkar M, Stanton-Hicks M, Rezai AR, Henderson JM. Long-term outcomes of spinal cord stimulation with paddle leads in the treatment of complex regional pain syndrome and failed back surgery syndrome. Neuromodulation. 2011;14:312–8. discussion 318
4. Shimoji K, Higashi H, Kano T, Asai S, Morioka T. Electrical management of intractable pain. Masui. 1971;20:444–7. Japanese
5. North RB, Kidd DH, Olin JC, Sieracki JM. Spinal cord stimulation electrode design: prospective, randomized, controlled trial comparing percutaneous and laminectomy electrodes-part I: technical outcomes. Neurosurgery. 2002;51:381–9. discussion 389–90
6. Hornberger J, Kumar K, Verhulst E, Clark MA, Hernandez J. Rechargeable spinal cord stimulation versus non-rechargeable system for patients with failed back surgery syndrome: a cost-consequences analysis. Clin J Pain. 2008;24:244–52.
7. Mironer YE, Brown C, Satterthwaite JR, Cohen M, Tonder LM, Grumman S. A new technique of "midline anchoring" in spinal cord stimulation dramatically reduces lead migration. Neuromodulation. 2004;7:32–7.

8. Holsheimer J, Nuttin B, King GW, Wesselink WA, Gybels JM, de Sutter P. Clinical evaluation of paresthesia steering with a new system for spinal cord stimulation. Neurosurgery. 1998;42:541–547.; discussion 547–9.
9. Al-Kaisy A, Van Buyten J-P, Smet I, Palmisani S, Pang D, Smith T. Sustained effectiveness of 10 kHz high-frequency spinal cord stimulation for patients with chronic, low back pain: 24-month results of a prospective multicenter study. Pain Med. 2014;15:347–54.
10. Van Buyten JP, Al-Kaisy A, Smet I, Palmisani S, Smith T. High-frequency spinal cord stimulation for the treatment of chronic back pain patients: results of a prospective multicenter European clinical study. Neuromodulation 2013;16:59–65.; discussion 65–6.
11. Tiede J, Brown L, Gekht G, Vallejo R, Yearwood T, Morgan D. Novel spinal cord stimulation parameters in patients with predominant back pain. Neuromodulation. 2013;16:370–5.
12. Nevro Corporation. Patient manual revision B, 11052. Redwood City, CA: Nevro Corporation; 2015.
13. Campbell CM, Jamison RN, Edwards RR. Psychological screening/phenotyping as predictors for spinal cord stimulation. Curr Pain Headache Rep. 2013;17:307.
14. Shah KJ, Verghese A, Reddy MP, Sarfraz BK, Doddayya H. A study on prescribing pattern of antibiotics for surgical prophylaxis in a tertiary care teaching hospital. World J Pharmacy Pharmaceut Sci. 2016;5:1749–58.

Chapter 25
Burst Stimulation: An Innovative Waveform Strategy for Spinal Cord Stimulation

Jason E. Pope, Timothy R. Deer, and Navdeep Singh Jassal

25.1 Introduction

Since the advent of spinal cord stimulation (SCS) or traditional spinal cord stimulation (tSCS) by Norman Shealy in 1967, the evolution of dorsal column stimulation has continued, primarily focused on lead innovations. Disadvantages to current spinal cord stimulation strategies are inherent to how it works: it requires perceived congruent therapeutic paresthesia overlying the typical painful area. Challenges include the ability to place the paresthesia in congruent areas, the positionality associated with the required perception, and the need for the patient to consider the paresthesia therapeutic. New innovations in waveform strategies are moving away from the need to create a perceived paresthesia to achieve analgesia. This chapter explores one known as Burst Stimulation (Burst-SCS). It is important to appreciate that Burst-SCS was under investigation in the United States and required an Investigational Device Exemption (IDE). Because of the success of the trial, it was deemed superior to tSCS for back and leg pain treatment and is now FDA approved and available for use in the United States.

J.E. Pope (✉)
Summit Pain Alliance, Santa Rosa, CA, USA
e-mail: popeje@me.com

T.R. Deer
The Center for Pain Relief, Charleston, WV, USA
e-mail: doctdeer@aol.com; tdeermd@centerforpainrelief.com

N.S. Jassal
Florida Pain Medicine, Department of Neurology/Pain, University of South Florida, Wesley Chapel, FL, USA
e-mail: navdeepjassal@gmail.com; NJassal@floridapainmedicine.com

S. Diwan, T.R. Deer (eds.), *Advanced Procedures for Pain Management*,
https://doi.org/10.1007/978-3-319-68841-1_25

25.2 Technical Overview

Current tSCS strategies rely on the delivery of energy to the spinal cord through activation of a cathode, either by alternating the current (constant voltage system) or the voltage (constant current system). These systems typically deliver a frequency from 40 to 150 Hz. Burst-SCS delivers a cluster of five pulses at 500 Hz in 40-Hz intervals, where the pulse width is typically 1 microsecond (Fig. 25.1). The amplitude is adjusted to the individual patient, as it is for tSCS. Importantly, the energy required to deliver Burst-SCS is the same as for tSCS, in terms of battery life and recharging interval.

It is important to briefly comment on the mechanism of action, as Burst-SCS appears to work differently than tSCS. It is hypothesized that burst-SCS works by stimulating not only the lateral pathway typically activated in tSCS but also the medial pathway, responsible for the affective component of pain (Fig. 25.2). This difference may have implications in reducing the overall pain perception, which has been reported both anecdotally and in literature.

It is important to note that although the Burst-SCS creates analgesia without the need for the perceived paresthesia, it requires placement within the epidural space

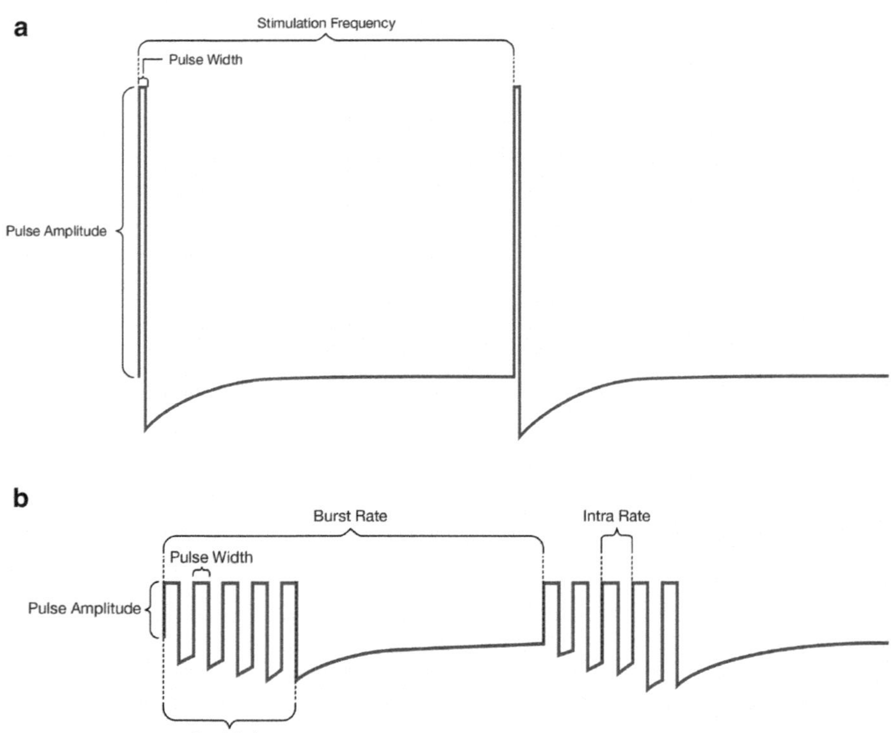

Fig. 25.1 Stimulation strategies. (**a**) Tonic stimulation, 40 Hz. (**b**) Burst stimulation

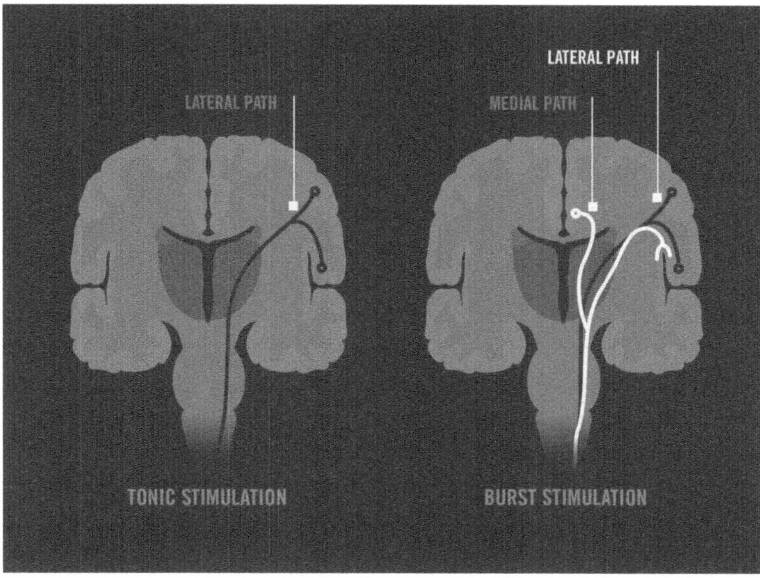

Fig. 25.2 The activation of the lateral pathway in tonic spinal cord stimulation (tSCS) and activation of the lateral and the medial pathways in Burst-SCS (*Courtesy of* St. Jude Medical, Plano, TX)

Table 25.1 Published burst stimulation investigations

Study	Participants	Conclusions	Complications
de Vos et al. (2014)	100 patients randomized to receive tSCS prior to Burst-SCS or vice versa. Analysis of the first 85 patients over 6 months.	69.4% preferred Burst-SCS vs tSCS. Burst-SCS patients received superior pain relief vs tSCS	None reported
De Ridder et al. (2013)	15 consecutive patients in limb and axial back pain; given Burst-SCS, tSCS, and placebo	Burst-SCS was better than tSCS or placebo in the treatment of back and leg pain	None reported
De Ridder et al. (2010)	12 patients with tSCS with paddle to treat neuropathic pain; given burst-SCS	Burst-SCS may be better than tSCS in the treatment of neuropathic pain	None reported

FBSS failed back surgery syndrome, *FBSS-PR* failed back surgery syndrome, poor responders, *PDN* painful diabetic neuropathy, *SCS* spinal cord stimulation, *tSCS* tonic spinal cord stimulation

in the same anatomic location as tSCS, namely relying on placement based on the Barolot mapping.

There is robust literature supporting Burst-SCS, as listed in Table 25.1. The double-blind, placebo-controlled trial performed by de Ridder et al. described that Burst-SCS was better than tSCS or placebo in improving back, limb, and general pain. The group led by de Vos found that Burst-SCS was more effective than tSCS in patient populations that are typically poorly treated, including those with painful diabetic neuropathy (PDN) or failed back surgery syndrome (FBSS), and FBSS patients that were poor responders to tSCS (FBSS-PR). Further, a prospective, randomized, multi-center study performed by Deer and Staats [1] described that patients preferred Burst-SCS over tSCS and also achieved superior pain relief with greater treatment success over tSCS.

25.3 Risk Assessment

Physicians considering the use of burst stimulation should be aware of the potential for risk:

- The procedure for employing burst stimulation relies on hardware similar to the hardware for traditional tonic stimulation, and consequently similar risks are expected. (*See* SCS lead placement in Chap. 12.)
- Burst stimulation may decrease battery life of the equipment and increase the recharging frequency.
- Prospective published research on burst stimulation has reported no complications, but it may have been accompanied by effects that included dizziness, headache, and the sensation of "heavy legs."
- Further prospective data are required to discern the unique challenges, if any, that may accompany burst stimulation.

25.4 Risk Avoidance

The clinician should use the same risk mitigation techniques as for traditional spinal cord stimulation (*See* Chap. 13). Vigilance is paramount, as Burst-SCS may stimulate the perceptive and affective components of the pain experience. Further prospective study is needed to determine its role in the neuromodulation armamentarium.

25.5 Conclusion and Future Directions

Interest in expanding the indications for SCS and nonpharmacologic, sustainable strategies push innovation towards new technology and indications. Burst-SCS may improve upon the challenges inherent in tSCS:

- Positionality of stimulation
- Presence of nonresponders
- Need for perceived therapeutic paresthesia and areas of coverage
- Development of therapeutic tolerance

The placement of Burst-SCS in the pain care algorithm (as salvage therapy or potentially as first-line therapy) will evolve with evidence of its potential advantages:

- Reduced paresthesia stimulation
- Possible function as salvage therapy after tSCS
- Possible elimination of the need for discrete stimulation
- Reduced or eliminated positionality challenges
- Possible stimulation of affective and perceptive pathways

Since non-inferiority and superiority was concluded as a result of the SUNBURST study, DR is now available both internationally and domestically. It has the potential to dramatically change the landscape of SCS as we know it today.

Reference

1. Deer TR, Staats P. A result of the SUNBURST study: a prospective randomized controlled trial assessing burst stimulation for the treatment of chronic pain. Presented at the 19th annual meeting of the North American Neuromodulation Society (NANS) in Las Vegas, NV, 10–13 Dec 2015

Suggested Reading

de Ridder D, Plazier M, Kamerling N, Menovsky T, Vanneste S. Burst spinal cord stimulation for limb and back pain. World Neurosurg. 2013;80:642–9.

de Ridder D, Vanneste S, Plaizer M, van der Loo E, Menovsky T. Burst spinal cord stimulation: toward paresthesia-free pain suppression. Neurosurgery. 2010;66:986–90.

de Vos CC, Bom MJ, Vanneste S, Lenders MW, de Ridder D. Burst spinal cord stimulation evaluated in patients with failed back surgery syndrome and painful diabetic neuropathy. Neuromodulation. 2014;17:152–9.

Pope JE, Deer TR, Amirdelfan K, Kapural L, Verrills P. New concepts for waveform and current delivery for spinal cord stimulation: burst and high frequency. Minimally invasive surgery for pain; 2015.

Pope JE, Falowski S, Deer TR. Advanced waveforms and frequency with spinal cord stimulation: burst and high-frequency energy delivery. Expert Rev Med Devices. 2015;12:431–7.

Schade CM, Sasaki J, Schultz DM, Tamayo N, King G, Johanek LM. Assessment of patient preference for constant voltage and constant current spinal cord stimulation. Neuromodulation. 2010;13:210–7.

Washburn S, Catlin R, Bethel K, Canlas B. Patient-perceived differences between constant current and constant voltage spinal cord stimulation systems. Neuromodulation. 2014;17:28–35.

Chapter 26
Novel Waveforms

W. Porter McRoberts

Since 2010, we have witnessed a great increase in the clinical availability of the expressions of waveform research. Though the benefits of traditional, tonic stimulation are well proven, significant interest is arising in alternative waveforms and frequencies such as burst, high-frequency, and high-energy/high-density. Additional attention has focused on the impact of energy delivery, specifically the concepts around charge delivery and associated neurophysiologic changes in the spinal cord. The aim of modulating unconventional neural targets such as the dorsal root ganglion will likely uncover mechanisms that could lead to improved responses to pain. This chapter seeks to familiarize the reader with new waveform modalities, their proposed mechanism of action, and the relevant literature.

26.1 Introduction

Spinal cord stimulation (SCS) has enjoyed both a relatively long history of use and burgeoning supportive literature. Recently there has been an explosion of research and multiple publications of level-one data arguing for its use. Some of the new data have focused on novel targets like the dorsal root ganglion, and additional large studies are examining how differing electrical pulse train rate (high frequency) and differing morphology and timing of trains (burst mode) can affect pain.

Additional attention has focused on the impact of energy delivery, specifically the concepts around charge delivery and associated neurophysiologic changes in the spinal cord. This chapter seeks to familiarize the reader with these modalities, their proposed

W.P. McRoberts (✉)
Holy Cross Hospital, Anodyne Research, University of Miami, School of Medicine, Miami, USA
e-mail: portermcroberts@gmail.com

S. Diwan, T.R. Deer (eds.), *Advanced Procedures for Pain Management*,
https://doi.org/10.1007/978-3-319-68841-1_26

mechanism of action, and with relevant literature. For purposes of brevity, the reader is assumed to be familiar with common monikers and abbreviations surrounding the topic.

SCS is becoming an increasingly popular and effective treatment of chronic, intractable pain. Traditional "tonic" SCS (constant and morphologically identical pulse trains at lower frequencies of 21–1200 Hz) has been used successfully to treat a variety of pain conditions including diabetic neuropathy [1], failed back surgery syndrome [2–5], complex regional pain syndrome [6–8], phantom limb pain [9], ischemic limb pain [10], refractory unilateral limb pain syndrome [11], postherpetic neuralgia, and acute herpes zoster pain [12] and angina pectoris. Existing benefits of neurostimulation treatment for SCS patients include reduced pain, improved quality of life, reduced analgesic use, ability for some patients to return to work, and potential significant cost savings over time, all while having minimally significant adverse events [3, 5, 13].

Though the benefits of traditional tonic stimulation are well proven, in the late 2000s significant interest in alternative waveforms and frequencies arose with an aim of modulating unconventional neural targets and uncovering mechanisms that could lead to improved responses to pain. At present, those efforts fall under distinct monikers known as "burst," "HF-10" and "high density". Additional efforts to study 50-kHz peripheral nerve stimulation and waveforms known as "chaos", "pink noise", and "white noise" are not supported by the US Food and Drug Administration (FDA) and are not discussed in this chapter.

26.2 Commonly Hypothesized Mechanisms

After testing the response of frequency on fiber recruitment, Arle et al. hypothesized in a 2013 poster [14] that higher frequencies recruited a much higher population of smaller-diameter nerve fibers and at levels of firing below the typical threshold level, while excluding the very large fibers that low-frequency stimulation relies upon. This phenomenon is hypothesized to allow for sub-perception stimulation while achieving wide dynamic range (WDR) inhibition at lower amplitudes across areas seen in both high-frequency (HF-10) and burst programming.

26.2.1 Burst Stimulation

Dirk De Ridder, who first conceptualized and then tested the applications of burst stimulation in the spinal cord, initially hypothesized that burst activates a "medial path" from the dorsal cord cephalad to the thalamus and subsequently from the thalamus projecting to the anterior cingulate gyrus and the rostral insula, thus having effects on the affective and attentive systems that modulate pain. De Ridder reports that the burst waveform more closely approximates the endogenous pattern of thalamic activation and propagation of signal to the neocortex [De Ridder, personal communication].

In contrast to burst stimulation, tonic stimulation consists of a continuous pulse train delivered at the same amplitude, frequency, and pulse width, typically producing paresthesia over the patient's area of pain. The only modifiable parameters in traditional tonic stimulation are the pulse frequency, width, and amplitude.

Burst stimulation is structurally different from tonic stimulation. The amplitudes used for burst programming are reported to be significantly lower than those traditionally used for tonic stimulation; the result is paresthesia-free therapy with continued pain suppression. Though burst stimulation features a group of pulses that are repeated in an on/off pattern, it is unlike an "on-off" cycle mode because it mimics the natural signaling of burst neurons utilizing closely spaced stimuli. Its programmable parameters include the burst train, the burst rate, and the intra-burst rate (Fig. 26.1).

Although many SCS manufacturers claim an ability to perform "burst," subtle differences exist in pulse trains among manufacturers concerning the timing of re-polarization and charge balancing (either after each individual pulse or delayed until the conclusion of the pulse train) that may or may not have significant therapeutic consequence. The parameters used for burst stimulation are all within the ranges that are currently available in commercial devices. More specifically, each individual parameter in burst is limited to a value that is equal to or less than what is commercially available today (Table 26.1).

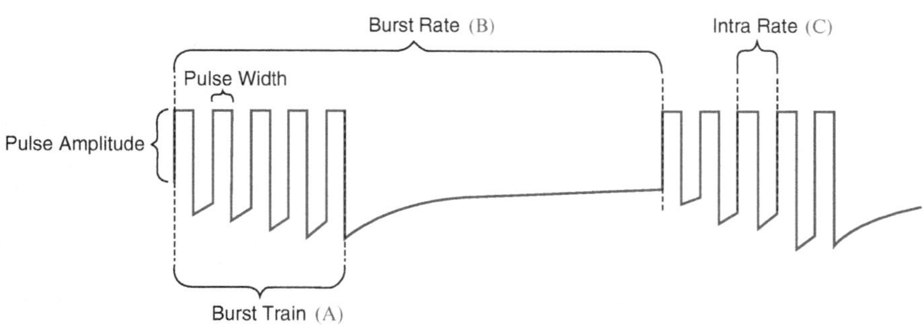

Fig. 26.1 Burst stimulation mode, showing the programmable parameters: the burst train (**a**), the time from the onset of the burst train to the time of onset of the next burst train (burst rate, **b**), and the rate of pulses within each train (intra-burst rate, **c**)

Table 26.1 Comparison of individual burst parameters with commercially available devices

Parameter	Burst stimulation	Tonic stimulation	SJM Renew®	Medtronic RestoreUltra®	Boston Scientific Precision™
Pulse amplitude	0–12.75 mA	0–25.5 mA	0–15 V	0–10.5 V	0–20.0 mA
Frequency	250–1000 Hz	2–1200 Hz	10–1500 Hz	2–1200 Hz	2–1200 Hz
Pulse width	50–1000 μs	50–500 μs	10–500 μs	60–1000 μs	20–1000 μs

SJM St. Jude Medical

26.2.2 Burst Stimulation Physiology and Justification for Use

Burst mode was initially incorporated into transcutaneous electrical nerve stimulation (TENS) devices in order to prevent habituation of the nervous system to tonic stimulation [15]. A few studies have shown improved pain relief with burst mode during TENS [15, 16], but others have failed to show any differences in efficacy. The neurological basis for the advantages of burst over tonic stimulation modes in TENS in an individual patient is not fully elucidated. Although both tonic and burst patterns of neuronal firing are inherent in the nervous system, burst stimulation may more closely mimic sensory signaling. Animal and in vitro studies have shown that both tonic and burst neuronal firing are used to transmit stimulus features within the nervous system [17, 18]. It has been posited that signal detection occurs through burst firing of neurons [18, 19], an observation that may be explained by the brain's ability to differentiate bursts from single spike inputs [20]. The thalamus also uses both tonic and burst firing patterns when projecting sensory information to cortical areas [21].

The reasons for using burst stimulation in TENS also apply to SCS. Specifically, processing of pain signals within the spinal cord and brain also appears to be dependent on both tonic and burst signals. For example, in a neuropathic pain model provided by experiments with mice, GABAergic neurons in the spinal lamina III were shown to exhibit tonic, burst, gap firing, and single spike firing [22]. The inflammatory response and endogenous opioids released in response to SCS appear to depend on the frequency and pattern of firing in the spinal cord [23–26]. This finding indicates that endogenous pain-response systems are sensitive not only to the frequency of firing of sensory afferents but also to their pattern. This could be interpreted to mean that firing patterns provide some low-level, spinal sensory information. Differential responses of endogenous pain responses, in combination with the fact that burst firing appears to be important for signal detection, may indicate that burst stimulation of the spinal cord could offer additional pain-reducing benefits when compared with conventional tonic stimulation. A systematic review of SCS showed that there is considerable variability in the efficacy of tonic stimulation [27]. Therefore, devices imitating the neural coding in the brain and spinal cord could prove to be more powerful in pain reduction while using less energy (Table 26.2) [19, 21, 28].

26.3 High-Frequency Stimulation

High-frequency stimulation, commonly understood as HF-10 therapy, is briefly described as tonic stimulation of the dorsal column of the spinal cord but at 10,000 Hz, much higher than the traditional settings of 1–1200 Hz. Following a European prospective study, the therapy gained a CE mark (Conformité Européene) and has been approved in the European Union. A prospective parallel-arm randomized controlled trial is completed in the United States [41].

Table 26.2 Summary of the burst stimulation literature

Study	Year	Description of the study	Summary of findings
De Ridder et al. [29]	2010	Prospective RCT: 12 patients during trial SCS randomly received 4 × 1-h. sessions of random tonic 500-Hz vs burst SCS. All pts. chose burst for remainder of trial	Burst stimulation was significantly better for pain suppression by both the VAS score and SF-MPQ. Paresthesia was present in 92% of patients during tonic stimulation, and in only 17% during burst stimulation. Average follow-up was 20.5 months
De Ridder et al. [30]	2010	Five patients with tinnitus, with auditory cortical stimulation with tonic vs burst programming	For pure tone tinnitus, tonic stimulation yielded 95% reduction in Sx, vs 97% for burst. For narrowband tinnitus, tonic had no effect; burst reduced Sx 62%
De Ridder et al. [31]	2013	Prospective placebo RCT of 15 trial patients to a week of sham, tonic, and burst SCS with ITT analysis	Primary outcome VAS for LBP, limb pain, and general pain: reduced from 7.4, 7.5, 8.3 respectively to 3.6, 3.6, 3.8. Burst > tonic for LBP but not for limb pain. All patients preferred burst
de Vos et al. [32]	2014	48 tonically implanted patients. Divided into 3 groups: PDN ($n = 12$), FBSS ($n = 24$), and FBSS patients who had become poor responders to SCS ($n = 12$). All reprogrammed to burst for 2 weeks	1. PDN Tonic to burst: 77% VAS decrement 2. Responder FBSS: 57% decrement 3. Non-responder FBSS: 23% decrement
Schu et al. [33]	2014	Twenty tonically implanted patients with FBSS then randomized to 3 groups: placebo, burst, and 500-Hz tonic	Results revealed: burst NRS 4.7 vs NRS 7.1 for 500-Hz, 8.3 for placebo. ODI was lowest in burst; 80% preferred burst, 10% chose 500-Hz tonic, 10% pre-study tonic
Courtney et al. [34]	2015	Multicenter 22-patient study of existing tonic, implanted patients converted to burst for 14 days. VAS studied in contrast	Tonic VAS of 54 mm dropped to 28 mm with burst, a 46% decrement. Pain catastrophizing dropped from 17.9 to 10.3 with burst. 91% preferred burst to tonic
De Ridder et al. [35]	2015	Two-center retrospective study included 102 patients with pre-existing SCS systems (either responder or non-responders) reprogrammed with burst SCS	Overall burst improved LBP by 29.82% and limb pain by 31.84% compared with tonic stimulation. 62.5% of tonic nonresponders were converted to responders after being reprogrammed with burst stimulation. In 76.5% of tonic responders, 94.9% reported improved pain relief during burst stimulation vs tonic stimulation
Van Havenbergh et al. [36]	2014	Evaluate whether 500-Hz burst or 1000-Hz burst had an impact in pain suppression	No difference in pain intensity, paresthesia, or any of the secondary outcome measures between the two groups. Frequency not related to effect

(continued)

Table 26.2 (continued)

Study	Year	Description of the study	Summary of findings
De Ridder et al. [37]	2014	Forty-nine patients: Does preoperative pain duration affect SCS effectiveness?	Pain duration, age, and SCS duration not correlated with the effects of either tonic or burst stimulation. For patients with both short and long periods of pain prior to SCS, burst stimulation was statistically superior to tonic stimulation. This study suggests that there is no reason to exclude patients with longstanding pain from SCS
Tang et al. [38]	2014	Explored possible differences in mechanisms of burst and tonic SCS on nociceptive spinal networks and/or gracile nucleus supraspinal relay	Low-intensity burst significantly decreased the nociceptive somatic response. Burst did not increase spontaneous activity of WDR and low-threshold neurons in the gracile nucleus, but tonic SCS significantly increased activity. The reason that paresthesia may be reduced or abolished in patients may be in part because burst SCS does not increase activity of neurons in the gracile nucleus
Crosby et al. [39]	2015	Rat study assessed burst and tonic SCS for the attenuation of WDR neuronal hyperexcitability in 8 rats before and after each mode of stimulation, 7 days post-cervical nerve root compression	The study suggests that despite similarities in its attenuation of spinal hyperexcitability and allodynia, burst SCS does not act via spinal GABAergic mechanisms
Crosby et al. [40]	2015	Rat study assessed how different parameters that define burst SCS modulate its efficacy, using a rat model of cervical radiculopathy, testing the effectiveness of burst SCS in reducing neuronal responses to noxious stimuli by altering stimulation parameters	Three parameters—pulses per burst, duration of pulses, and amplitude—were significantly correlated with the changes in neuronal response after burst. Pulse frequency and amplitude significantly affected the percentage of responsive neurons and charge per burst was correlated to a reduction of WDR neuronal firing and also had a nonlinear effect on the percentage of neurons responding to burst SCS. The results show that the action of burst SCS is dependent on the charge per burst

FBSS failed back surgery syndrome, *GABA* gamma aminobutyric acid, *ITT* intention to treat, *LBP* low back pain, *NRS* numeric rating scale, *ODI* Oswestry Low Back Disability Index, *PDN* painful diabetic neuropathy, *RCT* randomized controlled trial, *SCS* spinal cord stimulation, *SF-MPQ* Short-Form McGill Pain Questionnaire, *Sx* symptoms, *VAS* Visual Analogue Scale, *WDR* wide dynamic range

26.3.1 HF-10 Mode of Action

Gate control theory (GCT), proposed by Melzack and Wall, was the driver behind the first clinical application of SCS [42, 43]. GCT hypothesized that spinal pain processing is modified by increased activity of large, myelinated afferent fibers presynaptically inhibiting input to pain-transmitting projection neurons through two mechanisms: via inhibitory interneurons [43] and through activation of supraspinal circuits [43]. However, the detailed mechanisms of action of traditional, dorsal column–mediated, paresthesia-based SCS are still not completely understood [44]. Much progress has been made in advancing the understanding of paresthesia-based SCS. Preclinical studies proposed additional neural interactions (e.g., postsynaptic modulation), as well as key neurotransmitters and neuropeptides that may be involved in pain relief from stimulation [45–49]. Indeed, attempts to model and understand these circuits beyond the original GCT are still emerging [50, 51]. Early, preclinical work seems to indicate that HF-10 therapy may also modulate these same neural structures, as elucidated in rodent and caprine models by Cuellar et al. [51] demonstrating that high-frequency stimulation resulted in suppression or inhibition of evoked activity in wide dynamic range (WDR) neurons. WDR neurons are believed to play an integral role in pain perception at higher centers of the brain, namely the thalamus [52, 53]. It is also possible that HF-10 therapy may directly modulate structures in the spinal dorsal horn in a way that yields a more robust clinical outcome without requiring dorsal column activation [54]. Efforts are under way to further understand the direct spinal effects of HF-10 therapy.

26.3.2 HF-10 Studies

HF-10 therapy has emerged as a safe, effective, paresthesia-free treatment for chronic pain. Table 26.3 lists relevant publications and summarizes their findings.

26.4 High-Energy/High-Density Stimulation

High-energy/high-density (HD) stimulation is a term used to describe a higher than conventional amount of electric charge delivered per unit time to a neural substrate. Initially conceptualized and based on Dirk De Ridder's work [29, 31], HD stimulation refers to high-frequency bursting. De Ridder's 2010 work [29] focused on the concept of increased charge per time as a means for pain suppression. The main concept of interest in HD is charge delivery per unit time. Charge is understood as the area under the curve in an amplitude-pulse—in short, the stimulus strength times the stimulus duration. That multiple is then multiplied by the frequency per unit time to determine the "concentration of current" [62].

Table 26.3 Summary of HF-10 literature

Study	Year	Description of the study	Summary of findings
Cuellar et al. [51]	2012	Preclinical mechanism of action	HF stimulation results in suppression or complete blockade (depending on stimulation amplitude) of nociceptive afferent inputs
Van Buyten et al. [55]	2012	European prospective study in chronic back pain subjects	In 72 subjects with successful trial stimulation, HF-10 therapy reduced back pain from 8.4 cm at baseline to 2.7 cm at 6 months (median decrease, 78%). Leg pain decreased from 5.4 to 1.4 cm (median decrease, 83%)
Tiede et al. [56]	2013	United States prospective study in predominant back pain subjects	In 24 subjects, trial phase pain scores decreased from 8.7 cm at baseline to 3.9 cm (55% decrease, 58% responder rate) with conventional SCS, and to 2.0 cm with HF-10 therapy (77% decrease, 83% responder rate)
Al-Kaisy et al. [57]	2014	European prospective study in chronic neuropathic limb pain	Data from 11 of the 15 subjects who responded to HF-10 therapy was reported. Pain score decreased from 8.2 at baseline to 3.3 at 6 months (59% decrease, 73% responder rate)
Al-Kaisy et al. [58]	2013	2-year follow-up of European prospective back pain study	In 65 subjects, back pain decreased from 8.4 to 3.3 cm at 24 months (60% responder rate) and leg pain decreased from 5.4 to 2.3 cm (71% responder rate)
Annemans et al. [59]	2014	Cost-effectiveness of HF-10 therapy	HF-10 therapy demonstrated favorable incremental cost-effectiveness ratio of £3153 per quality-adjusted life year vs conventional medical management. This therapy also established dominance over traditional SCS (non-rechargeable, £8802; rechargeable, £5101)
Arcioni et al. [60]	2015	Chronic migraine	Of the 17 subjects who underwent a cervical HF-10 SCS trial, 14 were still implanted at 6 months (1 each, trial failure, trial infection, implant site infection). Of the 14, 7 had >30% reduction in headache days. The average reduction in headache days was 6.9 in the overall population and 12.9 in responders. Significant improvements were captured in Headache Impact Test (HIT-6) and Migraine Disability Assessment Scale (MIDAS)

(continued)

Table 26.3 (continued)

Study	Year	Description of the study	Summary of findings
Kapural et al. [61]	2015	SENZA-RCT: HF-10 vs traditional SCS in chronic back and leg pain subjects	Of the 198 randomized subjects with both back and leg pain, 171 passed a temporary trial and were implanted with an SCS system. At 12 months, 78.7% of implanted HF-10 therapy subjects were responders for back pain, and 78.7% for leg pain; 51.3% of traditional SCS subjects were responders for back pain, and 51.3% for leg pain ($P < 0.001$ for both back and leg pain). At 12 months, 62.9% of HF-10 therapy subjects had minimal or moderate disability, compared with 45.7% of traditional SCS subjects ($P = 0.03$). Functionally, 70.8% of subjects receiving HF-10 therapy had no symptoms to transient symptoms on the Global Assessment of Functioning at 12 months, compared with 59.3% of traditional SCS subjects ($P = 0.15$)

HF high frequency, *RCT* randomized controlled trial, *SCS* spinal cord stimulation

Low-frequency stimulation nerve depolarization occurs secondary to the product of amplitude and pulse width. Depolarization of nerve tissue is a function of the product of both amplitude and pulse width. To maintain depolarization, the degree of variance in one variable must be balanced by variance in the other so that the product remains the same. Each individual axon has its own strength duration curve based on the axon diameter and distance from the stimulation source [63]. Increase in either amplitude or pulse width therefore amplifies total charge and results in increased recruitment.

26.5 Alternative Stimulation Methods/Parameters in Spinal Cord Stimulation

For a number of years, physicians and basic researchers have assessed different ways to modulate stimulation output in order to optimize therapy with conventional SCS. The different stimulation methods that have been tried include the use of cycle mode (periods of stimulation followed by periods without stimulation) [64, 65], varying pulse width [66], constant current stimulation [67], and subthreshold stimulation (stimulation below the level of perception) [68, 69]. Newer methods of alternative stimulation output are emerging, such as the use of high-frequency stimulation [55, 56] and accelerometers to adjust stimulation in response to body position [70, 71]. Despite this progress, the understanding of therapy optimization by adjusting stimulation output remains in its infancy. At present, additional interest exists in testing white noise, pink noise, and chaotic or random burst patterns.

26.6 Future Directions for Investigation

Future research regarding HF-10 therapy is expected to focus on other chronic pain indications such as arm and neck pain, relative cost-effectiveness [Jeyakumar Subbaroyan, personal communication, May 2016], and a better understanding of the mechanism of action. Dirk De Ridder proposes further exploration of waveform in two distinct directions [Personal communication, August 2014]. The first direction is toward generating even more physiologically parallel—and thus biologically compatible—waveform patterns. His second interest is in constructing increasingly nonadaptable patterns, which then disrupt the neuro-adaptive loops that predict electrical neuromodulatory failure.

26.7 Summary

The United States has enjoyed a great increase in the clinical availability of the expressions of waveform research that began in the early 2000s. The aims of current approaches can most likely be categorized into two narrowing directions: variable waveforms for local, peri-electrode neural effects with resultant changes on local action and neurotransmission and projected effects at distant neural targets with rostral summation. Many options now exist, and it seems as if many more are coming. Selection choice may be complicated by noise from commercial interests, unproven claims, and the roar of scientific revolution. Practitioners would be wise to approach this topic with a demand for scientific evidence and a recognition that in order to evaluate the claims made, a deeper understanding of neurophysiology is needed. An ability to look through the miasma of pseudostatistics and commercial bias is required. The implanter must be first a skeptic and then an advocate for the patient. We likely stand at the edge of great forthcoming progress, but our enthusiasm must be tempered with a never-wavering demand for scientific clarity. Without it, we will lose our way.

References

1. de Vos CC, Rajan V, Steenbergen W, van der Aa HE, Buschman HP. Effect and safety of spinal cord stimulation for treatment of chronic pain caused by diabetic neuropathy. J Diabetes Complicat. 2009;23:40–5.
2. Duyvendak W. Spinal cord stimulation with a dual quadripolar surgical lead placed in general anesthesia is effective in treating intractable low back pain and leg pain. Neuromodulation. 2007;10:113–9.
3. Kumar K, Taylor RS, Jacques L, Eldabe S, Meglio M, Molet J, et al. Spinal cord stimulation versus conventional medical management for neuropathic pain: a multicentre randomised controlled trial in patients with failed back surgery syndrome. Pain. 2007;132:179–88.
4. Leveque JC, Villavicencio AT, Bulsara K, Rubin L, Gorecki J. Spinal cord stimulation for failed back surgery syndrome. Neuromodulation. 2001;4:1–9.
5. North RB, Kidd DH, Olin J, Sieracki JM, Farrokhi F, Petrucci L, et al. Spinal cord stimulation for axial low back pain: a prospective, controlled trial comparing dual with single percutaneous electrodes. Spine. 2005;30:1412–8.
6. Forouzanfar T, Kemler MA, Weber WE, Kessels AG, van Kleef M. Spinal cord stimulation in complex regional pain syndrome: cervical and lumbar devices are comparably effective. Br J Anaesth. 2004;92:348–53.
7. Harke H, Gretenkort P, Ladleif HU, Rahman S. Spinal cord stimulation in sympathetically maintained complex regional pain syndrome type I with severe disability. A prospective clinical study. Eur J Pain. 2005;9:363–73.
8. Kemler MA, de Vet HC, Barendse GA, van den Wildenberg FA, van Kleef M. Effect of spinal cord stimulation for chronic complex regional pain syndrome type I: five-year final follow-up of patients in a randomized controlled trial. J Neurosurg. 2008;108:292–8.
9. Katayama Y, Yamamoto T, Kobayashi K, Kasai M, Oshima H, Fukaya C. Motor cortex stimulation for phantom limb pain: comprehensive therapy with spinal cord and thalamic stimulation. Stereotact Funct Neurosurg. 2001;77:159–62.
10. Amann W, Berg P, Gersbach P, Gamain J, Raphael JH, Ubbink DT. Spinal cord stimulation in the treatment of non-reconstructable stable critical leg ischaemia: results of the European Peripheral Vascular Disease Outcome Study (SCS-EPOS). Eur J Vasc Endovasc Surg. 2003;26:280–6.
11. Kumar A, Felderhof C, Eljamel MS. Spinal cord stimulation for the treatment of refractory unilateral limb pain syndromes. Stereotact Funct Neurosurg. 2003;81:70–4.
12. Harke H, Gretenkort P, Ladleif HU, Koester P, Rahman S. Spinal cord stimulation in postherpetic neuralgia and in acute herpes zoster pain. Anesth Analg. 2002;94:694–700.
13. Taylor RS. Spinal cord stimulation in complex regional pain syndrome and refractory neuropathic back and leg pain/failed back surgery syndrome: results of a systematic review and meta-analysis. J Pain Symptom Manag. 2006;31:S13–9.
14. Arle J, Carlson K, Mei L, Shils J. Potential mechanisms of high-frequency and burst sub-perceptual threshold stimulation: differential fiber recruitment. Poster presented at the 17th National Annual Meeting of the North American Neuromodulation Society, Las Vegas, NV, 5–8 Dec 2013.
15. Tulgar M, McGlone F, Bowsher D, Miles JB. Comparative effectiveness of different stimulation modes in relieving pain. Part II. A double-blind controlled long-term clinical trial. Pain. 1991;47:157–62.
16. Tulgar M, McGlone F, Bowsher D, Miles JB. Comparative effectiveness of different stimulation modes in relieving pain. Part I. A pilot study. Pain. 1991;47:151–5.
17. Oswald AM, Chacron MJ, Doiron B, Bastian J, Maler L. Parallel processing of sensory input by bursts and isolated spikes. J Neurosci. 2004;24:4351–62.

18. Chacron MJ, Longtin A, Maler L. To burst or not to burst? J Comput Neurosci. 2004;17:127–36.
19. Sherman SM. Tonic and burst firing: dual modes of thalamocortical relay. Trends Neurosci. 2001;24:122–6.
20. Lisman JE. Bursts as a unit of neural information: making unreliable synapses reliable. Trends Neurosci. 1997;20:38–43.
21. Sherman SM. A wake-up call from the thalamus. Nat Neurosci. 2001;4:344–6.
22. Gassner M, Leitner J, Gruber-Schoffnegger D, Forsthuber L, Sandkühler J. Properties of spinal lamina III GABAergic neurons in naïve and in neuropathic mice. Eur J Pain. 2013;17:1168–79.
23. Go VL, Yaksh TL. Release of substance P from the cat spinal cord. J Physiol. 1987; 391:141–67.
24. Marvizon JCG, Adelson DW, Mayer EA. Frequency-dependence of neurokinin release measured by NK1 receptor internalization. Soc Neurosci Abstr. 2000;26:246.16.
25. Lever IJ, Bradbury EJ, Cunningham JR, Adelson DW, Jones MG, McMahon SB, et al. Brain-derived neurotrophic factor is released in the dorsal horn by distinctive patterns of afferent fiber stimulation. J Neurosci. 2001;21:4469–77.
26. Song B, Marvizón JC. Dorsal horn neurons firing at high frequency, but not primary afferents, release opioid peptides that produce micro-opioid receptor internalization in the rat spinal cord. J Neurosci. 2003;23:9171–84.
27. Frey ME, Manchikanti L, Benyamin RM, Schultz DM, Smith HS, Cohen SP. Spinal cord stimulation for patients with failed back surgery syndrome: a systematic review. Pain Physician. 2008;12:379–97.
28. Swadlow HA, Gusev AG. The impact of 'bursting' thalamic impulses at a neocortical synapse. Nat Neurosci. 2001;4:402–8.
29. De Ridder D, Vanneste S, Plazier M, van der Loo E, Menovsky T. Burst spinal cord stimulation: toward paresthesia-free pain suppression. Neurosurgery. 2010;66:986–90.
30. De Ridder D, Vanneste S, van der Loo E, Plazier M, Menovsky T, van de Heyning P. Burst stimulation of the auditory cortex: a new form of neurostimulation for noise-like tinnitus suppression. J Neurosurg. 2010;112:1289–94.
31. De Ridder D, Plazier M, Kamerling N, Menovsky T, Vanneste S. Burst spinal cord stimulation for limb and back pain. World Neurosurg. 2013;80:642–9.
32. de Vos CC, Bom MJ, Vanneste S, Lenders MW, De Ridder D. Burst spinal cord stimulation evaluated in patients with failed back surgery syndrome and painful diabetic neuropathy. Neuromodulation. 2014;17:152–9.
33. Schu S, Slotty PJ, Bara G, von Knop M, Edgar D, Vesper J. A prospective, randomized, double-blind, placebo-controlled study to examine the effectiveness of burst spinal cord stimulation patterns for the treatment of failed back surgery syndrome. Neuromodulation. 2014;17:443–50.
34. Courtney P, Espinet A, Mitchell B, Russo M, Muir A, Verrills P, Davis K. Improved pain relief with burst spinal cord simulation for two weeks in patients using tonic stimulation: results from a small clinical study. Neuromodulation. 2015;18:361–6.
35. De Ridder D, Lenders MW, de Vos CC, Dijkstra-Scholten C, Wolters R, Vancamp T, et al. A 2-center comparative study on tonic versus burst spinal cord stimulation: amount of responders and amount of pain suppression. Clin J Pain. 2015;31:433–7.
36. Van Havenbergh T, Vancamp T, Van Looy P, Vanneste S, De Ridder D. Spinal cord stimulation for the treatment of chronic back pain patients: 500-Hz vs. 1000-Hz burst stimulation. Neuromodulation. 2015;18:9–12. discussion 12
37. De Ridder D, Vancamp T, Lenders MWPM, de Vos CC, Vanneste S. Is preoperative pain duration important in spinal cord stimulation? A comparison between tonic and burst stimulation. Neuromodulation. 2014;18:13–7.

38. Tang R, Martinez M, Goodman-Keiser M, Farber J, Qin C, Foreman R. Comparisons of burst and tonic spinal cord stimulation on spinal neural processing in an animal model. Neuromodulation. 2014;17:143–51.
39. Crosby N, Weisshaar C, Smith J, Zeeman M, Goodman-Keiser M, Winkelstein B. Burst and tonic spinal cord stimulation differentially activate GABAergic mechanisms to attenuate pain in a rat model of cervical radiculopathy. IEEE Trans Biomed Eng. 2015;62:1604–13.
40. Crosby ND, Goodman-Keiser M, Smith JR, Seeman ME, Winkelstein BA. Stimulation parameters define the effectiveness of burst spinal cord stimulation in a rat model of neuropathic pain. Neuromodulation. 2015;18:1–8.
41. Clinical trial of the Senza™ SCS system in the treatment of chronic upper limb and neck pain (SENZA-ULN). 2015. ClinicalTrials.gov Identifier: NCT02385201. https://clinicaltrials.gov/show/NCT02385201.
42. Melzack R, Wall PD. Pain mechanisms: a new theory. Science. 1965;150:971–9.
43. Shealy CN, Mortimer JT, Reswick JB. Electrical inhibition of pain by stimulation of the dorsal columns. Anesth Analg. 1967;16:489–91.
44. Mendell LM. Constructing and deconstructing the gate theory of pain. Pain. 2014;155:210–6.
45. Linderoth B, Bertil G, Johan F, Ernst B. Dorsal column stimulation induces release of serotonin and substance P in the cat dorsal horn. Neurosurgery. 1992;31:289–97.
46. Cui JG, Meyerson BA, Sollevi A, Linderoth B. Effect of spinal cord stimulation on tactile hypersensitivity in mononeuropathic rats is potentiated by simultaneous GABAB and adenosine receptor activation. Neurosci Lett. 1998;247:183–6.
47. Schechtmann G, Song Z, Meyerson BA, Linderoth B. Cholinergic mechanisms involved in the pain relieving effect of spinal cord stimulation in a model of neuropathy. Pain. 2008;139:136–45.
48. Song Z, Meyerson BA, Linderoth B. Spinal 5-HT receptors that contribute to the pain-relieving effects of spinal cord stimulation in a rat model of neuropathy. Pain. 2011;152:1666–73.
49. Yang F, Zhang C, Xu Q, Tiwari V, He SQ, Wang Y, et al. Electrical stimulation of dorsal root entry zone attenuates wide-dynamic-range neuronal activity in rats. Neuromodulation. 2015;18:33–40.
50. Schneider SP. Local circuit connections between hamster laminae III and IV dorsal horn neurons. J Neurophysiol. 2008;99:1306–18.
51. Cuellar JM, Alataris K, Walker A, Yeomans DC, Antognini JF. Effect of high-frequency alternating current on spinal afferent nociceptive transmission. Neuromodulation. 2013;16:318–27. discussion 327
52. Price DD, Dubner R. Neurons that subserve the sensory-discriminative aspects of pain. Pain. 1977;3:307–38.
53. Price DD, Hayes RL, Ruda M, Dubner R. Spatial and temporal transformations of input to spinothalamic tract neurons and their relation to somatic sensations. J Neurophysiol. 1978;41:933–47.
54. Lee D. Comparison of four SCS stimulation strategies using a CNS interneuron model. Presented at the 19th annual North American neuromodulation society meeting, Las Vegas, NV, Dec 2015.
55. Van Buyten JP, Al-Kaisy A, Smet I, Palmisani S, Smith T. High-frequency spinal cord stimulation for the treatment of chronic back pain patients: results of a prospective multicenter European clinical study. Neuromodulation. 2013;16:59–65. discussion 65–6
56. Tiede J, Brown L, Gekht G, Vallejo R, Yearwood T, Morgan D. Novel spinal cord stimulation parameters in patients with predominant back pain. Neuromodulation. 2013;16:370–5.
57. Al-Kaisy A, Palmisani S, Smith T, Harris S, Pang D. The use of 10-kilohertz spinal cord stimulation in a cohort of patients with chronic neuropathic limb pain refractory to medical management. Neuromodulation. 2015;18:18–23. discussion 23

58. Al-Kaisy A, Van Buyten JP, Smet I, Palmisani S, Pang D, Smith T. Sustained effectiveness of 10 kHz high-frequency spinal cord stimulation for patients with chronic, low back pain: 24-month results of a prospective multicenter study. Pain Med. 2014;15:347–54.
59. Annemans L, Van Buyten JP, Smith T, Al-Kaisy A. Cost effectiveness of a novel 10 kHz high-frequency spinal cord stimulation system in patients with failed back surgery syndrome (FBSS). J Long term Effect Med Implants. 2014;24:173–83.
60. Arcioni R, Palmisani S, Mercieri M, Vano V, Tigano S, Smith T, et al. Cervical 10 kHz spinal cord stimulation in the management of chronic, medically refractory migraine: A prospective, open-label, exploratory study. Eur J Pain. 2016;20:70–8.
61. Kapural L, Yu C, Doust MW, Gliner BE, Vallejo R, Sitzman BT, et al. Novel 10-kHz high-frequency therapy (HF10 therapy) is superior to traditional low-frequency spinal cord stimulation for the treatment of chronic back and leg pain: the SENZA-RCT randomized controlled trial. Anesthesiology. 2015;123:851–60.
62. Miller JP, Eldabe S, Buchser E, Johanek LM, Guan Y, Linderoth B. Parameters of spinal cord stimulation and their role in electrical charge delivery: a review. Neuromodulation. 2016;19:373–84.
63. West DC, Wolstencroft JH. Strength-duration characteristics of myelinated and non- myelinated bulbospinal axons in the cat spinal cord. J Physiol. 1983;337:37–50.
64. Kumar K, Wilson JR. Factors affecting spinal cord stimulation outcome in chronic benign pain with suggestions to improve success rate. Acta Neurochir Suppl. 2007;97:91–9.
65. Kumar K, Buchser E, Linderoth B, Meglio M, Van Buyten JP. Avoiding complications from spinal cord stimulation: practical recommendations from an international panel of experts. Neuromodulation. 2007;10:24–33.
66. Yearwood TL, Hershey B, Bradley K, Lee D. Pulse width programming in spinal cord stimulation: a clinical study. Pain Physician. 2010;13:321–35.
67. Washburn SN, Catlin R, Bethel K, Canlas B. Patient perceived differences between constant current and constant voltage spinal cord stimulation systems. Neuromodulation. 2014;17:28–35. discussion 35–6
68. Benyamin R, Kramer J, Vallejo R. A case of spinal cord stimulation in Raynaud's phenomenon: can subthreshold sensory stimulation have an effect? Pain Physician. 2007;10:473–8.
69. McRoberts WP, Wolkowitz R, Meyer DJ, Lipov E, Joshi J, Davis B, et al. Peripheral nerve field stimulation for the management of localized chronic intractable back pain: Results from a randomized controlled study. Neuromodulation. 2013;16:565–74. discussion 574–5
70. Schade CM, Schultz DM, Tamayo N, Iyer S, Panken E. Automatic adaptation of neurostimulation therapy in response to changes in patient position: results of the posture responsive spinal cord stimulation (PRS) research study. Pain Physician. 2011;14:407–17.
71. Schultz DM, Webster L, Kosek P, Dar U, Tan Y, Sun M. Sensor-driven position-adaptive spinal cord stimulation for chronic pain. Pain Physician. 2012;15:1–12.

Suggested Reading

Deer TR, Mekhail N, Provenzano D, Pope J, Krames E, Thomson S, Raso L, et al. The appropriate use of neurostimulation: avoidance and treatment of complications of neurostimulation therapies for the treatment of chronic pain. Neuromodulation appropriateness consensus committee. Neuromodulation. 2014;17:571–97. discussion 597–8

Dworkin RH, Turk DC, Wyrwich KW, Beaton D, Cleeland CS, Farrar JT, et al. Interpreting the clinical importance of treatment outcomes in chronic pain clinical trials: IMMPACT recommendations. J Pain. 2008;9:105–21.

Hjermstad MJ, Fayers PM, Haugen DF, Caraceni A, Hanks GW, Loge JH, et al. European Palliative Care Research Collaborative (EPCRC). Studies comparing numerical rating scales, verbal rating scales, and visual analogue scales for assessment of pain intensity in adults: a systematic literature review. J Pain Symptom Manag. 2011;41:1073–93.
Holsheimer J. Which neuronal elements are activated directly by spinal cord stimulation? Neuromodulation. 2002;5:25–31.
Linderoth B, Meyerson BA. Dorsal column stimulation: modulation of somatosensory and autonomic function. Semin Neurosci. 1995;7:263–77.
Meyerson BA, Linderoth B. Mode of action of spinal cord stimulation in neuropathic pain. J Pain Symptom Manag. 2006;31:S6–12.
Ostelo RW, Deyo RA, Stratford P, Waddell G, Croft P, Von Korff M, et al. Interpreting change scores for pain and functional status in low back pain: towards international consensus regarding minimal important change. Spine (Phila PA 1976). 2008;33:90–4.
Shatin D, Mullett K, Hults G. Totally implantable spinal cord stimulation for chronic pain: design and efficacy. Pacing Clin Electrophysiol. 1986;9:577–83.

Chapter 27
Transcutaneous Vagus Nerve Stimulation: Novel Treatment Strategies

Jared M. Huston, Jason R. Fritz, and Christopher J. Czura

27.1 Introduction

Electrical vagus nerve stimulation (VNS) was initially clinically approved for the adjunctive treatment of medically refractory seizures in 1997. In 2005, the FDA expanded its approval of VNS for treatment of chronic recurrent depression. Both therapeutic indications require surgical implantation of an electrical pulse generator. Obvious disadvantages to this approach include the high cost and invasive nature of surgery with potential risks of pain, bleeding, and infection. Moreover, replacement of the pulse generator battery is necessary approximately every 5–10 years. Recent innovations in electrical nerve stimulation, however, may facilitate introduction of novel approaches that avoid these limitations. In this chapter, we explore the role of non-invasive, transcutaneous vagus nerve stimulation (tVNS). It is important to note that non-invasive or tVNS is currently under investigation in the United States and is not FDA approved.

J.M. Huston (✉)
Surgery and Science Education, Hofstra Northwell School of Medicine, Center for Bioelectronic Medicine, The Feinstein Institute for Medical Research, Manhasset, NY, USA
e-mail: JHuston@northwell.edu

J.R. Fritz
Center for Bioelectronic Medicine, The Feinstein Institute for Medical Research, Manhasset, NY, USA
e-mail: jfritz@northwell.edu

C.J. Czura
The Feinstein Institute for Medical Research, Northwell Health, Manhasset, NY, USA
e-mail: cczura@northwell.edu

S. Diwan, T.R. Deer (eds.), *Advanced Procedures for Pain Management*,
https://doi.org/10.1007/978-3-319-68841-1_27

27.2 Technical Overview

Current VNS strategies employ an implantable pulse generator (Cyberonics, Houston, TX, USA) placed in the left upper chest, with the stimulation leads tunneled into the neck and the bipolar helical electrodes placed around the left cervical vagus nerve (Fig. 27.1). The pulse generator is programmed through the skin using a wand and external computer. Programmable stimulation parameters include the amplitude, pulse width, frequency, and on and off times. Typical settings include amplitudes of 1.0–3.5 mA (milliamperes), pulse widths of 130–500 μs (microseconds), frequencies of 20–30 Hz (hertz) and on and off times of 30 s and 5 min, respectively. Adjustment of these parameters is patient-specific, with the goal to both reduce disease symptoms and minimize side effects, which can include hoarseness, throat pain, cough, and voice alteration.

The overall mechanism of action of VNS on seizure prevention and alleviation of the symptoms of depression remains unknown. Theories include disrupting abnormal electrical activity underlying seizure formation, altering cerebral blood flow, and modulating release of neurotransmitters in the brain that reduce seizure activity and/or modulate depressive symptoms.

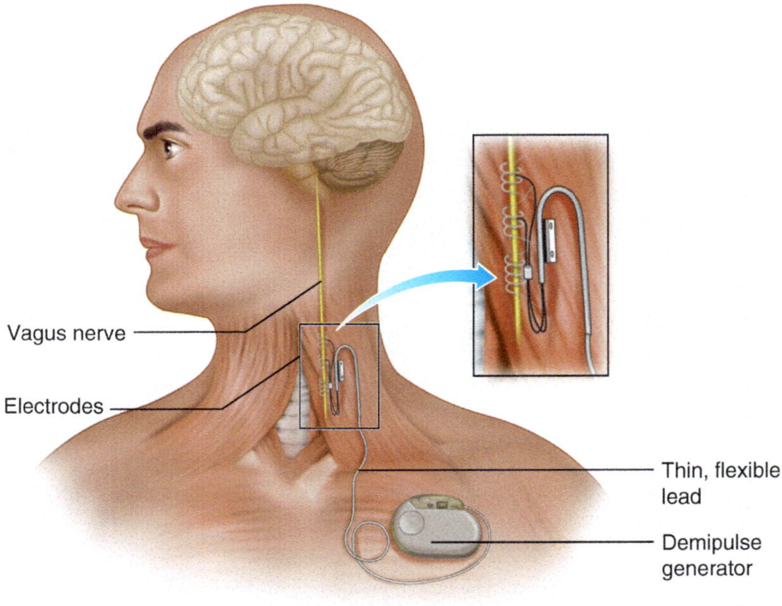

Fig. 27.1 Invasive electrical vagus nerve stimulation using implantable pulse generator. Surgically implanted pulse generator in the chest controls helical electrodes surrounding left cervical vagus nerve

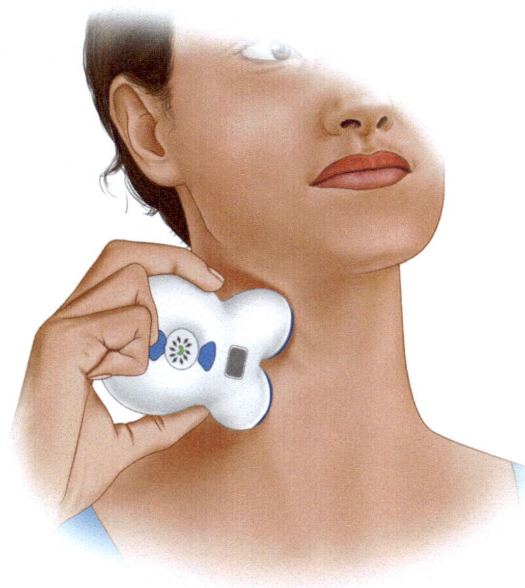

Fig. 27.2 Transcutaneous electrical vagus nerve stimulation. Handheld device positioned overlying carotid pulse to deliver electricity non-invasively to cervical vagus nerve

27.3 Transcutaneous Vagus Nerve Stimulation

An alternative to direct placement of electrodes on the vagus nerve is delivery of electricity through the skin overlying the cervical vagus nerve. One such device (GammaCore; ElectroCore LLC; Basking Ridge, NJ, USA) has received European approval for acute and prophylactic treatment of cluster and migraine headaches. The device has two disc electrodes that the patient presses against the anterior neck inferior to the mandibular angle, medial to the sternocleidomastoid muscle, and lateral to the larynx in the vicinity of the carotid pulse (Fig. 27.2). The device utilizes a voltage-driven electrical pulse with an intensity range of 0–24 V and a peak output current of 60 mA. The signal consists of a 1 ms (millisecond) burst of 5 kHz (kilohertz) sine waves repeating at a frequency of 25 Hz. Patients can control the overall stimulation intensity, and typical treatment protocols last for 90 s, several times per day.

27.4 Transauricular Vagus Nerve Stimulation

The auricular branch of the vagus nerve (ABVN), eponymously referred to as Arnold's nerve, is a sensory nerve that innervates specific portions of skin overlying the ear, including the external auditory meatus, cymba and cavum conchae, and

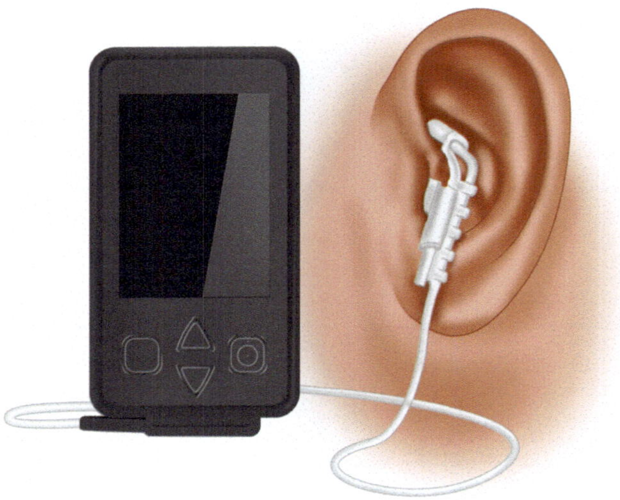

Fig. 27.3 Arnold's (ear-cough) reflex. Mechanical stimulation of the outer ear activates the auricular branch of the vagus nerve (Arnold's nerve), which travels to the brain stem and activates the efferent vagus nerve, resulting in a reflexive cough

antihelix. Afferent nerve fibers project to nuclei in the brainstem, including the nucleus of the solitary tract (NTS). Classically, this nerve has been implicated in an ear-cough reflex, where mechanical stimulation of the external auditory meatus evokes a cough through hypersensitivity of Arnold's nerve (Fig. 27.3).

More recently, transcutaneous electrical stimulation of the cymba conchae of the ear has demonstrated anticonvulsive effects similar to that of direct, invasive vagus nerve stimulation (Fig. 27.4). Currently available tVNS devices consist of an external ear electrode attached to a handheld stimulation unit (NEMOS; Cerbomed GmbH; Erlangen, Germany). This particular device received European clearance for the treatment of epilepsy and depression in 2010 and for the treatment of pain in 2012. The device delivers a series of 250 μs pulses at a frequency of 1 or 25 Hz, with a 30-seconds-on and 30-seconds-off duty cycle. Stimulation intensity is adjusted to elicit a tingling but not painful sensation, which optimizes activation of myelinated Aβ fibers of the ABVN. Patients self-administer treatment, which usually consists of 3–4 sessions per day, each one lasting one hour to several hours.

27.5 Conclusion and Future Directions

Non-invasive technologies will revolutionize nerve stimulation therapy through greater applicability, improved safety profiles, and lower overall costs. At this time, tVNS is available in the United States only in clinical trials, and in other nations as

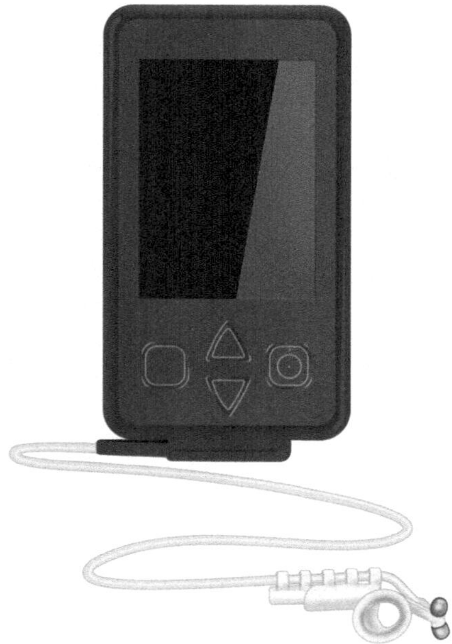

Fig. 27.4 Transauricular electrical vagus nerve stimulation. Handheld stimulation device delivers electricity non-invasively via electrode positioned over cymba conchae of ear

noted above. As the list of diseases responsive to vagus nerve stimulation continues to expand, non-invasive technologies may thrust this therapeutic approach to the forefront of clinical medicine.

Suggested Reading

Amar AP, Levy ML, Liu CY, Apuzzo MLJ. Vagus nerve stimulation. In: Krames ES, Peckham PH, Rezai AR, editors. Neuromodulation. London: Academic; 2009. p. 625–37.

Beekwilder JP, Beems T. Overview of the clinical applications of vagus nerve stimulation. J Clin Neurophysiol. 2010;27:130–8.

Grazzi L, Egeo G, Calhoun AH, McClure CK, Liebler E, Barbanti P. Non-invasive vagus nerve stimulation (nVNS) as mini-prophylaxis for menstrual/menstrually related migraine: an open-label study. J Headache Pain. 2016;17(1):91.

Kinfe TM, Pintea B, Muhammad S, Zaremba S, Roeske S, Simon BJ, et al. Cervical non-invasive vagus nerve stimulation (nVNS) for preventive and acute treatment of episodic and chronic migraine and migraine-associated sleep disturbance: preliminary findings from a prospective observational cohort study. J Headache Pain. 2015;16:101.

Ryvlin P, Gilliam FG, Nguyen DK, Colicchio G, Iudice A, Tinuper P, et al. The long-term effect of vagus nerve stimulation on quality of life in patients with pharmacoresistant focal epilepsy: the PuLsE (open prospective randomized long-term effectiveness) trial. Epilepsia. 2014;55(6):893–900.

Straube A, Ellrich J, Eren O, Blum B, Ruscheweyh R. Treatment of chronic migraine with transcutaneous stimulation of the auricular branch of the vagus nerve (auricular t-VNS): a randomized, monocentric clinical trial. J Headache Pain. 2015;16:63.

Vonck K, Boon P, Van Roost D. Anatomical and physiological basis and mechanism of action of neurostimulation for epilepsy. Acta Neurochir Suppl. 2007;97:321–8.

Chapter 28
Sacral Stimulation for Pelvic Pain

Corey W. Hunter and Grant H. Chen

28.1 Introduction

Pelvic pain is a poorly understood phenomenon that is notoriously difficult to treat. The exact pathophysiology is largely unknown, though it bears a striking resemblance to other neuropathic pain syndromes that are known to respond to neuromodulation, such as complex regional pain syndrome and sympathetically driven pain [1]. The use of spinal cord stimulation (SCS) to treat pelvic pain has been met with frustration, as neuromodulators have experienced extreme difficulty in obtaining coverage over the areas of pain. Patients with pelvic pain have an explantation rate of 33.3% (5 out of 15), which is the highest amongst diagnoses; the most commonly reported reason is loss of therapeutic effect (39%) [2]. This difficulty in obtaining coverage of the painful areas is likely due to the complexity of innervation of the pelvic region and its structures.

The pelvic viscera draw innervation from the lumbar and sacral regions of the spine, making it difficult to capture all areas of pain simultaneously. In a patient complaining of pain over the bladder/inguinal region and the perineum, one would need to obtain coverage over the ilioinguinal, iliohypogastric, genitofemoral, pudendal, and inferior rectal nerves, among others. As shown on Table 20.1, the dermatomal distribution of this area includes T12, L1 and L2, and then skips to S2 and S3.

C.W. Hunter (✉)
Ainsworth Institute of Pain Management, New York, NY, USA

Department of Physical Medicine and Rehabilitation, Mount Sinai Hospital, New York, NY, USA
e-mail: corey.hunter@me.com

G.H. Chen
Department of Anesthesiology and Critical Care, Memorial Sloan Kettering Cancer Center, New York, NY, USA
e-mail: cheng@mskcc.org; granthchen@gmail.com

S. Diwan, T.R. Deer (eds.), *Advanced Procedures for Pain Management*,
https://doi.org/10.1007/978-3-319-68841-1_28

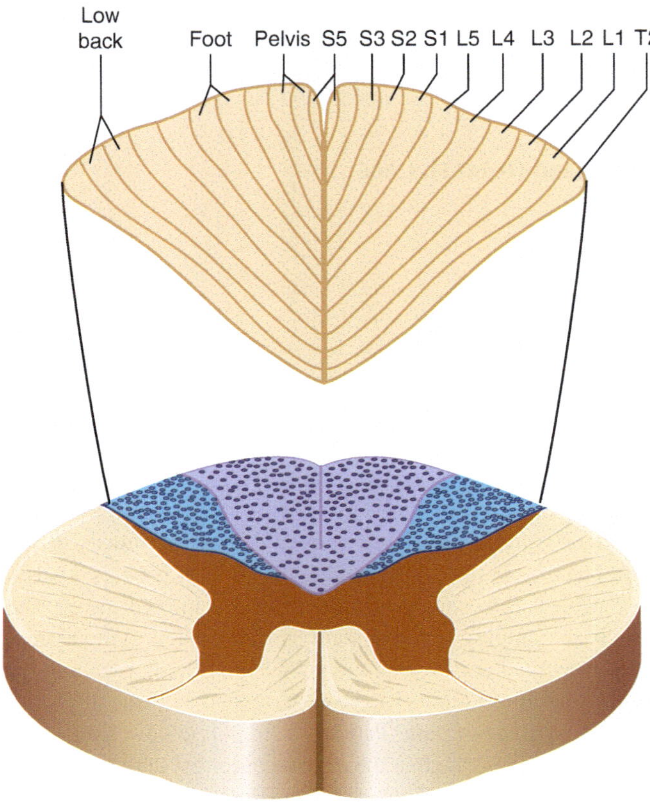

Fig. 28.1 Cross-section illustration of the dorsal columns showing the position of the sacral fibers with respect to the spinal cord

This distribution presents an obvious challenge when attempting to choose an appropriate target for lead placement.

Many of the early publications supporting the use of neuromodulation for pelvic pain have focused on the sacral region as the target for stimulation. In cases such as pudendal neuralgia, vulvodynia, or genital pain, the predominance of innervation is sacral, so stimulating the sacral nerve roots intuitively made the most sense. Although these fibers are obviously represented throughout the length of the spinal cord (especially in the thoracic spine, the most commonly targeted area for SCS), they are notoriously difficult to recruit with traditional stimulation because of their size and position (Fig. 28.1):

- **Sacral fibers are smaller than lumbar fibers**, and they require more energy to stimulate. As the pulse width and amplitude are increased to recruit these fibers, other unwanted areas will feel paresthesias and the intensity will start to become uncomfortable.

- **Sacral fibers are positioned over the anatomical midline**. In the thoracic spine, the low back fibers are the most lateral, the lumbar fibers for the lower extremities are just medial to them, and the sacral fibers are the most medial. A lead would need to be placed directly over the anatomical midline with unidirectional energy flow, straight down into the sacral fibers.

Thus the logical solution is to place the lead(s) within the sacrum, directly over the sacral nerve roots, to stimulate those fibers directly and avoid unwanted stimulation in other areas.

28.2 Indications

Indications for sacral stimulation include pain syndromes with an exclusively sacral pain distribution:

- Pudendal neuralgia
- Vulvitis
- Vulvodynia [1]
- Prostadynia [1]
- Perianal pain
- Rectal/anal pain (proctitis)
- Distal urethral pain
- Scrotal pain
- Penile pain
- Coccygodynia [1]
- Female pelvic/vaginal pain (distal one third)
- Sympathetically maintained pain to the region (complex regional pain syndrome)
- Endometriosis
- Pelvic floor dysfunction [1]
- Chronic prostatitis
- Proctalgia fugax
- Radiation proctitis
- Postherpetic neuralgia
- Burning and localized perineal pain associated with urgency

Sacral stimulation can also be employed for other uses:

- Urinary/urge incontinence [3]
- Fecal incontinence [4]
- Increased urinary frequency
- Urinary retention
- Chronic anal fissures [5]
- Spinal cord infarction [1]

28.3 Relevant Anatomy

The sacral portion of the spinal cord consists of five pairs of spinal nerves, which exit the sacrum via the sacral foramen at the lower end of the vertebral column. The sacral nerve roots begin at the L1/2 region, below the conus medullaris, where the cauda equina is formed. These nerve roots then descend into the sacral canal, a continuation of the vertebral canal that runs through the posterior portion of the sacrum. The rostral aspect of the canal is triangular and well formed, whereas the caudal aspect is oblong and has an incomplete posterior wall (Fig. 28.2). The sacral canal terminates at the sacral hiatus—the incomplete fusion of the lamina at L5, or occasionally L4.

There are four to five pairs of sacral foramina on both the anterior and posterior aspects of the sacrum, through which the sacral nerves exit the canal (Fig. 28.2). Those exiting anteriorly join with the sacral plexus to form larger nerves like the sciatic nerve and the pudendal nerve (Fig. 28.3). The other half of the sacral nerves emerge posteriorly to provide innervation to the sacroiliac joint.

The sacral nerves have both afferent and efferent fibers that coordinate sensory and motor information to and from the organs of the pelvis. Parasympathetic fibers arise from the S2, S3, and S4 nerves, which communicate with the inferior hypogastric plexus via the pelvic splanchnic nerves. The sacral nerves are responsible for

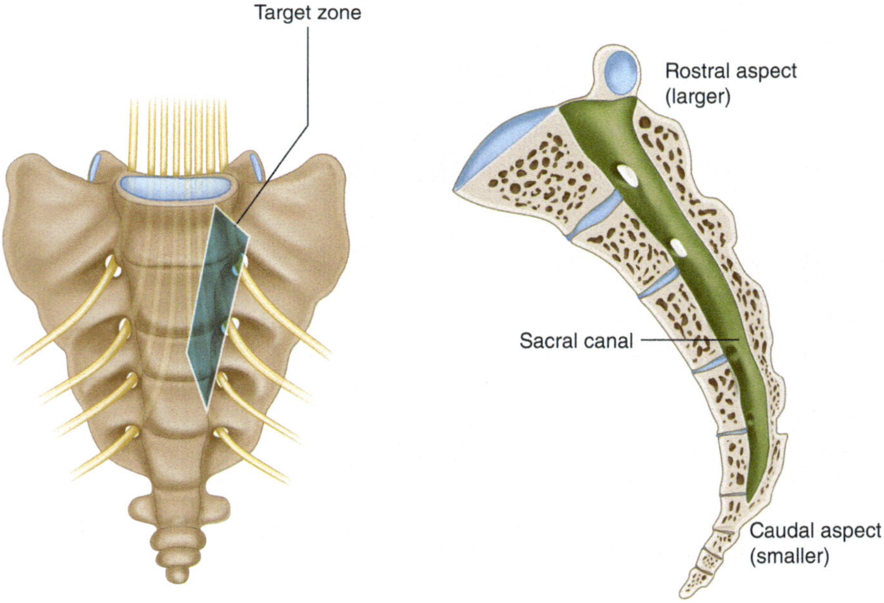

Fig. 28.2 **Left**, The sacral nerves within the sacrum and their paths of exit; the "Target Zone" illustrates where the lead should be placed to ensure that the nerve is still present within the canal and has not exited. **Right**, The shape of the sacral canal and its variation at the rostral *versus* the caudal aspects

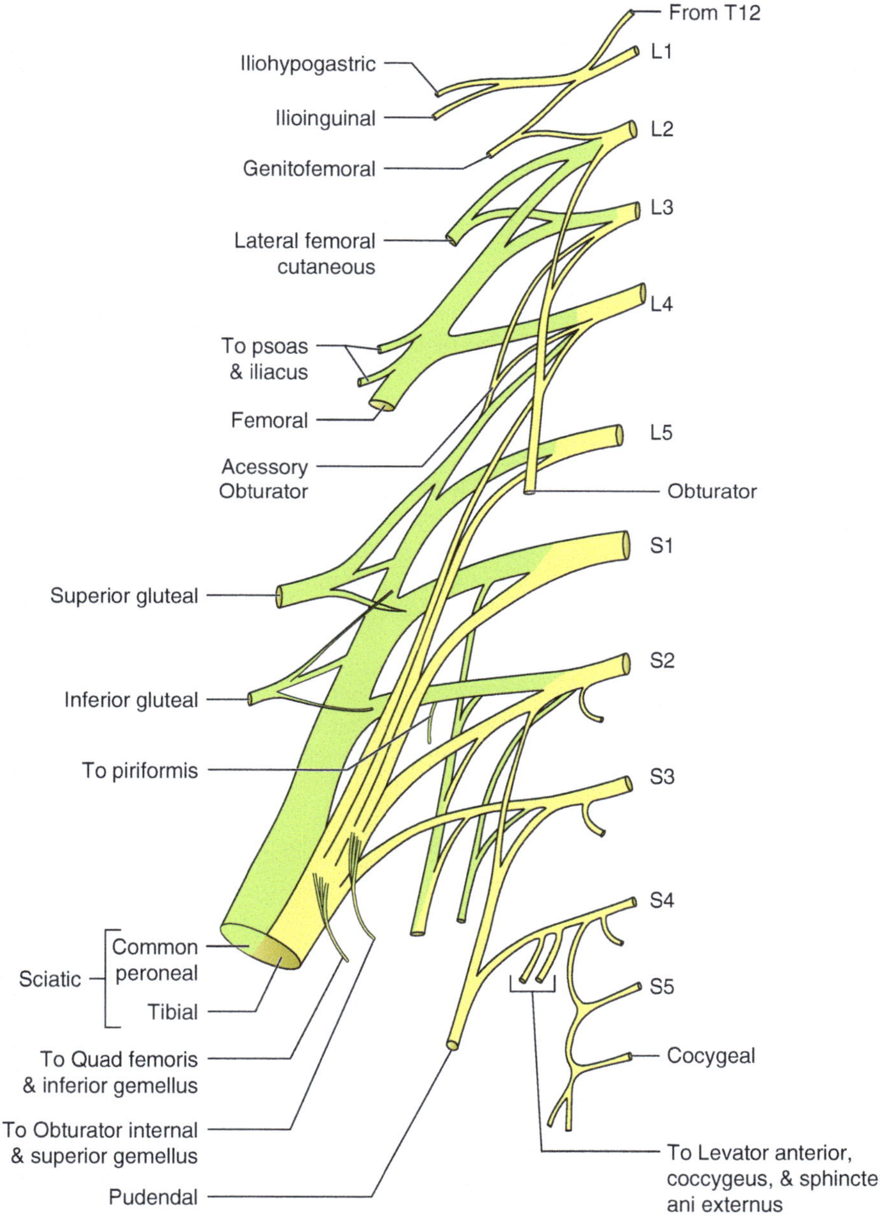

Fig. 28.3 The lumbosacral plexus

providing communication to the descending colon, rectum, urinary bladder, and genitalia.

The simplest technique for accessing the sacral canal is via the sacral hiatus, placing the leads anterograde. The key to successfully locating the sacral hiatus lies in identifying the following structures:

- Sacral cornua (the "roof" of the hiatus)
- Coccyx
- Sacral canal
- Sacrococcygeal junction (SCJ)
- The four to five bilateral sacral foramina (on the anterior and posterior aspects of the sacrum), for correct assessment of the anteroposterior (AP) image under fluoroscopy
- Sacral and coccygeal cornua—manually palpated to assess the surface anatomy, and compared with the image

The hiatus is more clearly identified with lateral fluoroscopic imaging than with AP imaging. The sacral cornua is easily palpated by placing an index finger over the intergluteal cleft, with the tip of the digit aligned with the distal-most edge of the coccyx. The cornua will typically lie under the proximal interphalangeal joint.

Other relevant anatomy also should be considered when performing this injection:

- Rectum, which lies just anterior to the sacrum and coccyx and is separated from them by a layer of extraperitoneal fat and connective tissue
- Exiting nerve roots from the sacral foramen anteriorly and posteriorly
- Coccygeal nerve, traveling within the sacral canal
- Erector spinae muscles
- Lateral and posterior sacrococcygeal ligaments (If calcified, these ligaments can produce resistance while the needle is advancing.)

28.4 Basic Concerns and Contraindications

As with any stimulator trial, basic concerns should be considered before performing the procedure. If the chosen method of gaining entry into the sacral canal is via the hiatus, the procedure is little more than a caudal epidural injection. Though this method is relatively well tolerated in the average patient and is considered to be a safer way of obtaining access to the epidural space than the interlaminar technique, one must carefully consider each patient and their presentation of pain individually. For example, a patient suffering from pudendal neuralgia may also complain of anorectal pain, so a needle placed through the hiatus may pass directly through an already painful area and could make this patient's pain even worse.

A number of basic concerns must be considered:

- Skin integrity, especially over the intergluteal cleft
- The amount of subcutaneous tissue around the sacral hiatus: Elderly or extremely thin patients may have inadequate subcutaneous tissue between the skin and the sacral periosteum, leading to skin erosion and breakdown.
- Anchoring/securing the leads with caudal access: Leads placed via traditional lumbar access are easily secured during a trial by taping or even using an anchor and a drain stitch. In an implant, an anchor is threaded over the lead down to the ligamentum flavum and then secured to the surrounding tissue. For this reason, many will consider the retrograde approach over the caudal approach, despite its extreme difficulty. Securing a trial lead placed through the sacral hiatus presents a challenge, as the intergluteal cleft can be an obstacle. During an implant, there may be little to no tissue to which the anchor can be secured, making migration a serious concern.
- Infection: As with any stimulator trial, there is always a concern for infection, but when a lead is placed through the sacral hiatus, the risk for infection is increased because of the proximity to the anus. One must consider the patient's hygiene and his or her ability to maintain cleanliness in the region, especially during the implant. Immunocompromised patients are potentially at high risk for infection.
- Retrograde lead placement, even by the most experienced neuromodulator, carries an extremely high incidence of dural puncture.
- Though patients with allodynia could benefit, they may also have pain in the very area where the lead is to be placed, which may complicate their ability to tolerate the procedure.
- Prone position may be difficult if patient has abdominal distension.
- Rectal perforation is possible if the needle is not advanced properly into the hiatus.
- Patients with pelvic pain often have a strong psychological component to their condition. A patient with considerable anxiety may not be able to tolerate the procedure, let alone differentiate the procedural pain from potential pain relief, thus complicating the ability to perceive success.

Several factors should be considered contraindications:

- Infection, systemic or localized
- Coagulopathy
- Distorted or complicated anatomy
- Patient refusal
- Failed psychiatric or psychological clearance

28.5 Preoperative Considerations

- Informed consent and proper explanation of all potential complications
- Anticoagulation

- Physical examination of the proposed skin entry point for infection, skin ulceration or necrosis, and extent of disease
- Ability of the patient to lie prone for the intended length of the procedure
- Intravenous access for IV fluid and medications for sedation or hypotension if the patient experiences a vasovagal reaction

28.6 Fluoroscopic Views

Start with an anteroposterior (AP) image of the sacrum with the coccyx in view (Fig. 28.4). A slight caudal tilt will allow for proper visualization of the sacral hiatus, given the curvature of the sacrum and coccyx. Mark the borders of the hiatus to ensure that the initial approach is sufficiently lateral to allow for a second needle if necessary, making sure the sacral foramina are equidistant from the spinous processes of the sacrum. When advancing the lead(s), an AP view will allow one to maintain sufficient laterality of the lead(s).

A lateral view is the most essential, as it will allow the physician to provide the proper shallow angle on approach into the hiatus (Fig. 28.5). Most importantly, it allows one to monitor the depth and subsequent entry into the hiatus, as there is no loss of resistance necessary. When advancing a lead, a lateral view is crucial to ensure that the tip of the lead has reached the appropriate level. The curvature of the sacrum will distort the AP view.

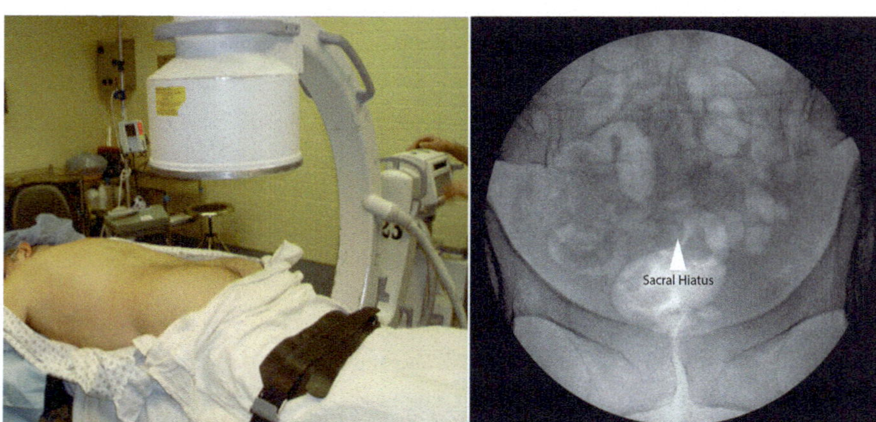

Fig. 28.4 **Left**, The initial positioning of the C-arm over the patient for an anteroposterior (AP) view. **Right**, The corresponding AP fluoroscopic view

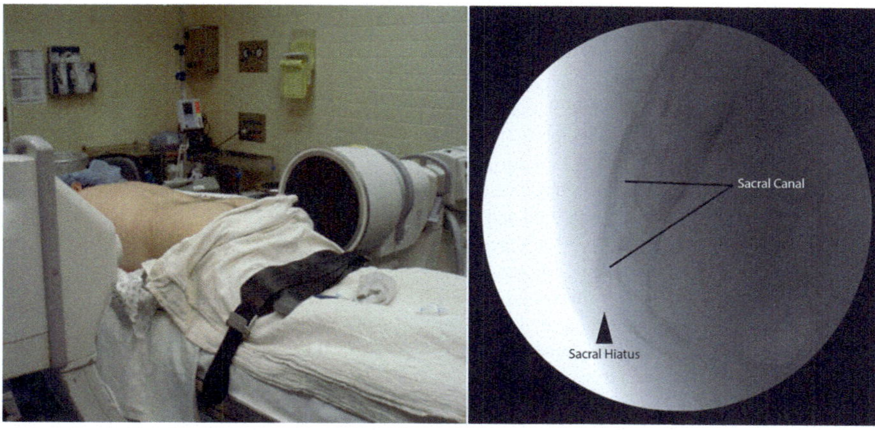

Fig. 28.5 **Left**, The C-arm positioned next to the patient for a lateral view. **Right**, The corresponding fluoroscopic view

28.7 Equipment

- 25-G 1.5-inch needle
- 10-mL syringe for local anesthetic
- 14-G Coudé or Touhy needle
- #15 blade on a scalpel handle
- Medication: 1% lidocaine with epinephrine (1:100,000)

28.8 Technique

Several techniques for sacral stimulation have been described in the literature:

- *Retrograde (cephalocaudal) technique*: The needle accesses the epidural space of the lumbar spine and the lead is advanced caudally.
- *Anterograde trans-hiatus technique*: The needle is placed through the sacral hiatus and advanced rostrally.
- *Transforaminal approach*: The needle is placed through the posterior sacral foramen and the lead is advanced anteriorly (utilized when placing an InterStim™ neurostimulator from Medtronic).
- *Epidural technique with laminotomy*
- *Percutaneous cephalocaudal/retrograde peripheral nerve stimulation*

The retrograde approach is technically more challenging and carries higher risk of dural puncture, but it tends to be considered more often by neuromodulators than the anterograde trans-hiatus technique [6], probably (at least in part) because the procedure as a whole is viewed as somewhat similar to traditional dorsal column

Table 28.1 Pros and cons of anterograde *versus* retrograde techniques for sacral stimulation

Technique	Advantages	Disadvantages
Retrograde (cephalocaudal)	• Steerability comparable to traditional dorsal column lead placement • Securing lead during trial same as a traditional trial • Tunneling lead and anchoring same as in traditional implant • Lower migration risk • Decreased dehiscence risk with implant • Avoids painful pelvic region or coccyx	• Technically more challenging • Increased risk of dural puncture • Increased risk of intrathecal lead placement
Anterograde trans-hiatus	• Technically less challenging procedure (same as a caudal epidural injection) • Decreased risk of dural puncture or intrathecal lead placement • Shorter distance to steer leads	• Increased risk of infection during trial due to proximity of lead to rectum • Increased difficulty in securing lead trial and maintaining site integrity during trial due to location in the intergluteal cleft • Increased challenge with anchoring due to lack of tissue surrounding hiatus • More challenging lead tunneling due to increased distance and having to navigate around the buttock • Increased risk of skin erosion due to proximity of implanted leads to skin • Limited steerability of leads

placements. The obvious difference is that the lead is advanced in reverse, but the starting point is still the lumbar spine and the lead is secured/anchored in the same fashion. A high rate of dural puncture and subsequent possibility of intrathecal lead placement has plagued practitioners when doing this procedure. In an attempt to decrease the potential for complication, Alò and colleagues described a variation of the retrograde approach whereby the needle was inserted laterally into the epidural space [7, 8].

28.8.1 Anterograde Trans-Hiatus Technique

For a sacral stimulation trial, we advocate the most direct approach to the sacral nerve roots with the lowest possibility of dural puncture (Table 28.1). If the trial succeeds and the patient is recommended for an implant, one should consider whether the trans-hiatus technique would be the best approach. This technique minimizes the risk of dural puncture and intrathecal lead placement, compared with the retrograde approach.

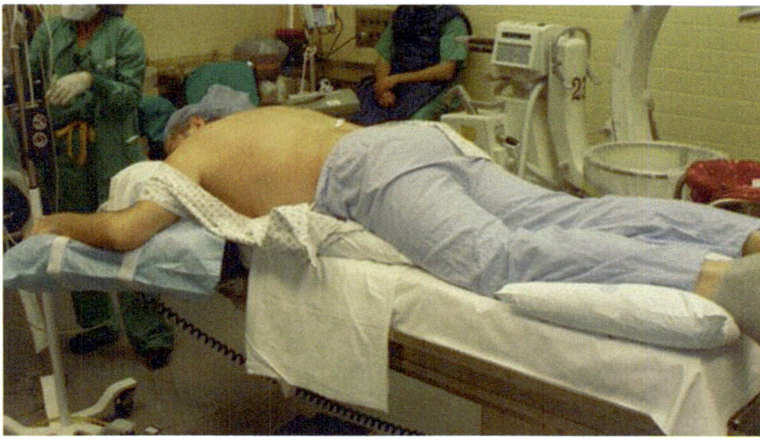

Fig. 28.6 Patient positioned in the prone position with pillow under the abdomen

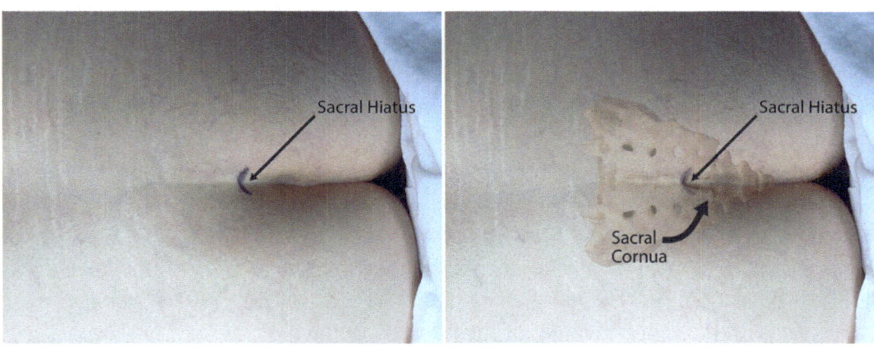

Fig. 28.7 **Left**, The skin marked for injection. **Right**, A representation of the underlying bony anatomy

Following are the steps for this technique:

- The patient is placed in a prone position with a pillow under the abdomen to reduce the lumbar lordotic curvature (Fig. 28.6).
- The sacral cornua are identified by palpation, and the skin is marked to outline the hiatus.
- The sacral hiatus is identified with a lateral fluoroscopic image (*see* Fig. 28.5). The intended skin entry point is verified and prepared in a typical sterile fashion (Fig. 28.7)
- 1% lidocaine with epinephrine is then used to infiltrate the skin using the 25-G 1.5-in. needle to provide adequate skin analgesia.
- #15 blade on a scalpel handle is used to make a small "stab" incision to one side of the hiatus, ipsilateral to the side of the sacral canal that the lead is to target, leaving enough room to place another needle beside this one.

- A 14-G Coudé needle (Touhy can also be used) is inserted into the sacral hiatus under lateral fluoroscopic imaging.
- Entry into the sacrum can be confirmed with the injection of 0.5 mL of nonionic contrast, but this may disrupt the clarity of the image when advancing the lead, especially if a second needle is to be introduced.
- The hub of the needle is then rotated to the ipsilateral side of the sacrum where the lead is to end up; this will correspond to the bend of the Coudé.
- The lead should be placed using the curved stylet in place. As the lead is introduced into the needle lumen, attention should be paid to ensure that the bend due to the curved stylet is in the direction of the bend of the needle and the side of the sacrum where the lead is intended to end up.
- The lead should be inserted through the needle in lateral view until 1–2 contacts are seen to have emerged from the needle, to ensure that the lead is within the sacral canal.
- The C-arm is now repositioned for the AP view.
- The lead is then steered to the ipsilateral side of the sacral canal, ensuring that it is lateral to the sacral foramen, preferably with the lead at the medial aspect of the foramen (Fig. 28.8). (Sacral nerves exit the canal via the foramen, so placement of a lead lateral to the foramen may be too far.)
- A lateral image (Fig. 28.9) is then taken to ensure that the tip has reached the proper distance. (Table 28.2 suggests appropriate targets depending on the patient's condition.) The tip's location can be verified by counting the sacral foramina. A lateral view is used because the curvature of the sacrum may distort perception of the position of the tip in an AP image.
- If a second lead is to be placed, the procedure is repeated on the opposite side.
- Once the leads have reached their intended targets, intraoperative testing is performed with the representative of the chosen company.

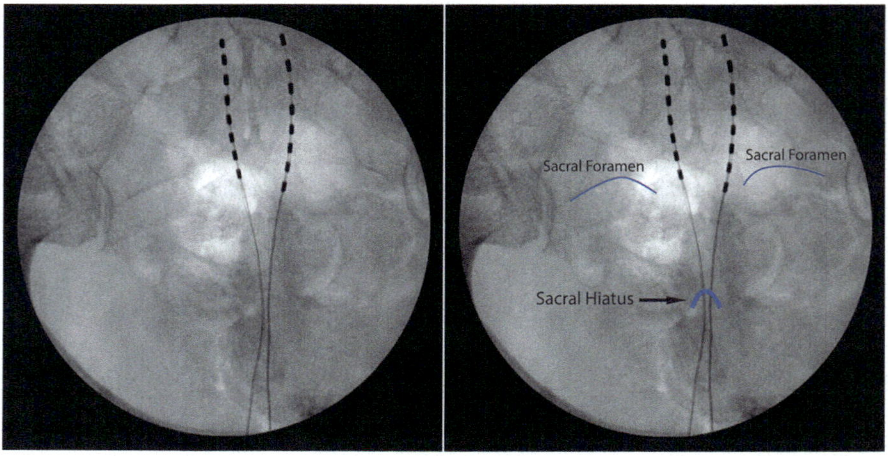

Fig. 28.8 AP fluoroscopic image of bilateral 8-contact leads within the sacral canal; each lead is placed medial to the sacral foramen

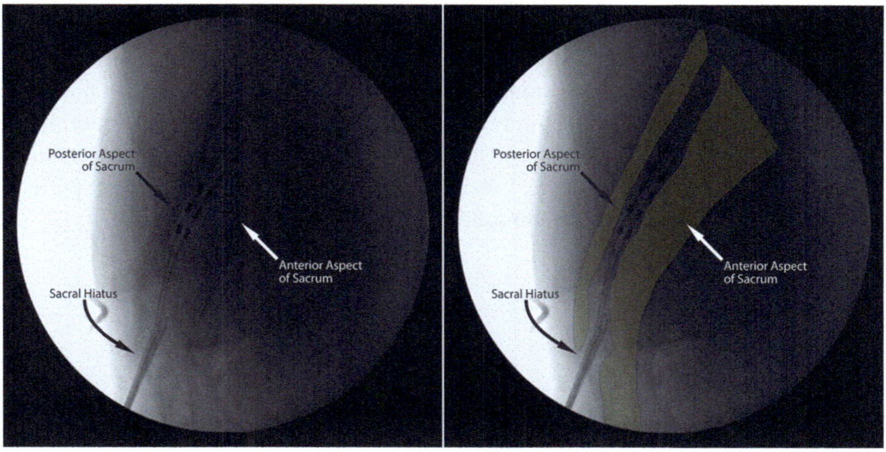

Fig. 28.9 Lateral fluoroscopic image, with the tips of the leads approximately at S1

Table 28.2 Potential sacral targets for conditions known to benefit from sacral stimulation

Condition	Sacral targets
Urge incontinence	S3
Fecal incontinence	S4
Urgency-frequency disorders	S2/3
Vulvodynia	S2 and S3
Pudendal neuralgia	S2 and S3
Interstitial cystitis	S2 and S3
Coccydynia	S4 and S5

- Upon completion of testing, when the leads are in satisfactory positions, the stylet(s) and needle(s) are removed, being careful to preserve the intended position of the lead(s).
- For the trial, bacitracin ointment is then applied to the skin around the lead(s) and a StayFIX® dressing (Merit Medical; South Jordan, UT) is then applied to secure the lead(s) in place, directing the leads in a rostral direction, up the low back.

28.9 Potential Complications and Post-procedure Follow-Up

Several complications are possible:

- Dural puncture
- Infection
- Intrathecal lead placement
- Bleeding

- Cauda equina syndrome
- Hematoma

As with any patient getting a spinal cord stimulator, follow-up is a must, not only to ensure proper coverage and pain relief, but also to assess for possible complications. The patient should be advised to call the pain service for any procedure-related complications and/or any unexpected neurological deficit. The patient should be monitored closely for the following symptoms:

- Positional headache
- Weakness
- Urinary or bowel incontinence
- Fever
- Bleeding
- Rectal bleeding
- Numbness
- Exacerbation of symptoms

28.10 Clinical Pearls

- Sacral fibers are smaller than lumbar fibers and are located in the midline of the cord, making them more difficult to recruit in the lumbar and thoracic spine.
- Sacral stimulation allows for direct stimulation of the sacral fibers without unwanted stimulation in the legs.
- There are two basic approaches for placing a lead in the sacrum: anterograde through the hiatus, and retrograde via the lumbar spine and driving the lead caudal.
- The retrograde approach is technically more challenging and has greater potential for dural puncture, but it is easier to secure the lead during the trial (and the anchor for the implant) than it is to secure the lead through the hiatus.
- The anterograde approach is easier to perform and has less risk of procedural complications.

References

1. Hunter C, Davé N, Diwan S, Deer T. Neuromodulation of pelvic visceral pain: a review of the literature and case series of potential novel targets for treatment. Pain Pract. 2013;13:3–17.
2. Hayek SM, Veizi E, Hanes M. Treatment-limiting complications of percutaneous spinal cord stimulator implants: a review of eight years of experience from an academic center database. Neuromodulation. 2015;18:603–8.
3. Hubsher CP, Jansen R, Riggs DR, Jackson BJ, Zaslau S. Sacral nerve stimulation for neuromodulation of the lower urinary tract. Can J Urol. 2012;19:6480–4.

4. Pascual I, González-Gómez CC, Ortega R, Jiménez-Toscano M, Marijuán JL, Lomas-Espadas M, et al. Sacral nerve stimulation for fecal incontinence. Rev Esp Enferm Dig. 2011;103:355–9.
5. Yakovlev A, Karasev SA, Dolgich OY. Sacral nerve stimulation: a novel treatment of chronic anal fissure. Dis Colon Rectum. 2011;54:324–7.
6. Alò KM, Yland MJ, Redko V, Feler C, Naumann C. Lumbar and sacral nerve root stimulation (NRS) in the treatment of chronic pain: a novel anatomic approach and neurostimulation technique. Neuromodulation. 1999;2:23–31.
7. Alò KM. Select nerve root stimulation: Facilitating the cephalocaudal "retrograde" method of electrode insertion. In: Deer TR, editor. Atlas of implantable therapies for pain management. New York, NY: Springer; 2011. p. 107–14.
8. Richter EO, Abramova MV, Alò KM. Percutaneous cephalocaudal implantation of epidural stimulation over sacral nerve roots – a technical note on the importance of the lateral approach. Neuromodulation. 2011;14:62–7.

Suggested Reading

Alò KM, McKay E. Selective nerve root stimulation (SNRS) for the treatment of intractable pelvic pain and motor dysfunction: a case report. Neuromodulation. 2001;4:19–23.

McDonald JS, Alò KM. Pain of urogenital origin. In: Loeser JD, editor. Bonica's management of pain. 3rd ed. Philadelphia, PA: Lippincott Williams & Wilkins; 2001. p. 1448–61.

Feler CA, Whitworth LA, Brookoff D, Powell R. Recent advances: sacral nerve root stimulation using a retrograde method of lead insertion for the treatment of pelvic pain due to interstitial cystitis. Neuromodulation. 1999;2:211–6.

Chapter 29
Intrathecal Drug Delivery: Pharmacokinetics and Dynamics

Kenneth Sunghoon Choi and Salim M. Hayek

29.1 Introduction

Implantation of an intrathecal drug delivery system (IDDS) requires a comprehensive knowledge of the process, including selection of appropriate patients and indications for implantation, the method of performing a trial, the surgical procedure of implantation, and the choice of pharmacologic agents. Additionally, knowledge of cerebrospinal fluid (CSF) dynamics plays an important role in determining IDDS success. This chapter addresses the pharmacologic fundamentals of the intrathecal agents that are typically used in an IDDS.

Three drugs have been approved by the U.S. Food and Drug Administration for intrathecal drug delivery: morphine and ziconotide for pain, and baclofen for spasticity. However, other medications such as hydromorphone, fentanyl, clonidine, and the local anesthetic bupivacaine are used off-label and are considered standard-of-care medications. This chapter focuses on the most commonly used agents for chronic pain in clinical practice today.

K.S. Choi (✉)
Olympus Pain and Orthopedics, Dallas, TX, USA
e-mail: kennethsunghoonchoi@gmail.com

S.M. Hayek
Department of Anesthesiology and Pain Management,
University Hospitals Cleveland Medical Center, Cleveland, OH, USA
e-mail: Salim.Hayek@UHhospitals.org

S. Diwan, T.R. Deer (eds.), *Advanced Procedures for Pain Management*,
https://doi.org/10.1007/978-3-319-68841-1_29

29.2 Cerebrospinal Fluid Dynamics

The classic bulk flow concept of CSF dynamics suggests that fluid circulates in a craniocaudal fashion from the choroid plexus of the ventricles to the spinal cord; it is then resorbed by the arachnoid villi in the dural sinuses. This one-dimensional, bulk flow concept has been debunked with the use of modern imaging techniques such as phase contrast magnetic resonance spectroscopy. Contemporary research shows that CSF moves in a pulsatile fashion, with oscillations occurring bi-directionally, both rostral and caudal. CSF flow is influenced by multiple factors, and different regions of the spinal cord are impacted by these factors to different degrees. Cardiac action is the main driver of pulsations in the upper to mid spinal canal. The flow of CSF in that region is subject to the Monro-Kellie doctrine: CSF flows cranially during diastole and caudally during systole, owing to the respective decrease and increase in blood volume in the cranial vault. Respiratory effects have a significant influence on the thoracolumbar region, where the systolic flow is elevated during late expiration and the diastolic upward movement is pronounced in early expiration [1–3]. Curvatures in the spine and other structures including nerve rootlets, venous plexuses, and epidural fat create points of turbulence that cause complex local mixing [4].

The result is that CSF undergoes poor and variable mixing in different areas. This has been shown for naturally occurring metabolites of the brain, infused medications in animal models, and radiographic studies [4–8]. As a result, a very low-volume, continuous infusions of medications (such as from an IDDS) do not disperse very much from the catheter tip. It should be noted that increases in movement or physical activity do increase spinal fluid mixing, so there would be a resultant increase in the spread of the drug delivered by an IDDS.

29.3 Opioids

The discovery of opiate receptors in the spinal cord first led to the recognition that opioids have a spinal action in addition to a supraspinal mechanism of action [9]. Subsequent research elucidated spinal cord pain pathways that inhibit or modulate nociceptive transmission to the brain [10]. Multiple studies trialing direct administration of opioids epidurally and intrathecally to treat cancer pain showed successful results [11–13].

All opioids have a common molecular mechanism of action that includes hyperpolarization of the nerve cell, which decreases its excitability. This effect occurs when endogenous opioid agonists (e.g., endorphin) or exogenous agonists (e.g., morphine, fentanyl) bind to the G-protein-coupled opioid receptor, which activates inhibitory G proteins. The G alpha and G beta/gamma subunits dissociate from one another and subsequently act on various intracellular effector pathways:

- The G alpha protein inhibits adenylyl cyclase, resulting in reduced intracellular cyclic adenosine monophosphate (cAMP) and downstream phosphorylation.
- The G beta/gamma subunit acts on two pathways:

Table 29.1 Organ system effects of morphine and all other clinically available opioid agonists [16]

Organ systems	Effects
Central nervous system	↑ Analgesia ↑Euphoria[a] ↑ Sedation ↓ Rate of respiration ↓ Cough reflex[b] ↑ Miosis (constriction of the pupils) ↑ Truncal rigidity[c] ↑ Nausea and vomiting
Gastrointestinal system	↑ Constipation ↓ Gastric motility ↓ Digestion in the small intestine ↓ Peristaltic waves in the colon ↑ Constriction of biliary smooth muscle ↑ Esophageal reflux
Other smooth muscle	↑ Depression of renal function ↓ Uterine tone ↑ Urinary retention
Skin	↑ Itching and sweating ↑ Flushing of the face, neck, and thorax
Cardiovascular system	↓ Blood pressure and heart rate if cardiovascular system is stressed
Immune system	↓ Formation of rosettes by human lymphocytes ↓ Cytotoxic activity of natural killer cells
Other	Behavioral restlessness

[a]Leading to risk of addiction and abuse
[b]Codeine used for treatment of pathologic cough
[c]Most apparent when using fentanyl, sufentanil, alfentanil

- It binds to the inward rectifying potassium channel, causing channel activation, hyperpolarizing the cell, and preventing signal propagation.
- It also binds to the N-type calcium channel, deactivating it and inhibiting further depolarization of the cell [14, 15].

The clinical effects of opioids are summarized in Table 29.1, and the physiological effects of different subtypes of opioid receptors are listed in Table 29.2.

Opioid potency is dictated primarily by the duration of exposure of the opioid agonist to the receptor site [18]. Therefore, pharmacodynamic interactions play a primary role in the potency of the opioid being administered. Different medications mimic certain endogenous opioids more than others, and these endogenous opioids have different receptor affinities. However, the common G-protein coupled pathway, outlined above, remains the predominant mechanism of opioid function in pain control.

The lipid solubility of a given opioid is a very important factor in determining the bioavailability at the spinal cord level [18]. Hydrophilic drugs such as morphine and hydromorphone have much greater bioavailability at the level of the dorsal horn of the spinal cord than more lipophilic opioids such as fentanyl and sufentanil [19]. The lipid solubility and potency properties of various intrathecal opioids are listed in Table 29.3. Lipophilic opioids have a larger volume of distribution due to their

Table 29.2 Opioid receptors involved with modulation of pain [17]

Receptor	Subtypes	Function
delta (δ) DOR OP_1	δ_1, δ_2	• Analgesia • Antidepressant effects • Convulsant effects • Physical dependence • May modulate μ-opioid receptor-mediated respiratory depression
kappa (κ) KOR OP_2	κ_1, κ_2, κ_3	• Analgesia • Anticonvulsant effects • Depression • Dissociative/hallucinogenic effects • Diuresis • Dysphoria • Miosis • Neuroprotection • Sedation • Stress
mu (μ) MOR OP_3	μ_1, μ_2, μ_3	μ_1: • Analgesia • Physical dependence μ_2: • Respiratory depression • Miosis • Euphoria • Reduced GI motility • Physical dependence μ_3: • Possible vasodilation

Table 29.3 Opioid intrathecal pharmacokinetics related to lipid solubility

	Duration of action, h	Lipid solubility (octanol:buffer distribution coefficient)	Protein binding, %	Potency (relative to morphine)
Morphine	12–24	1.4	20–40	1
Hydromorphone	7–15	1.3	8–19	5–7
Fentanyl	3–5	820	84	100
Sufentanil	2–4	1750	93	500–4000

more rapid diffusion out of the CSF and uptake into epidural fat and the systemic circulation, whereas hydrophilic opioids will remain in the CSF longer and have greater penetrance into the more hydrophilic gray matter of the dorsal horn (summarized in Table 29.4) [20]. Intrathecal opioids including morphine, hydromorphone, and fentanyl are cleared from the CSF by simple diffusion into the plasma. Once in the plasma, they are metabolized in the liver and their metabolites are renally excreted.

To justify the use of neuraxially administered opioids, the agents must demonstrate higher efficacy in the treatment of pain or a reduction in the side effect profile compared with opioids given by a less invasive route [21]. The principal target of

Table 29.4 Pharmacokinetic outcomes comparing lipophilic and hydrophilic intrathecal agents

Type of agent	Outcome
Hydrophilic	Slower to clear from CSF, resulting in longer duration of effect and more rostral spread, which may result in delayed respiratory depression, nausea
Lipophilic	Greater uptake into epidural fat and subsequent vascular uptake; shorter duration of action, significant blood levels

opioid agonists is the Rexed lamina II or substantia gelatinosa, located in the gray matter of the dorsal horn of the spinal cord [9, 22]. Intrathecal administration bypasses the blood–brain barrier and the hepatic "first pass effect," or drug metabolism that occurs after oral intake and prior to systemic circulation. The clinical result is the need for a much lower dose to provide equianalgesic effects compared with oral or intravenous administration, and decreased adverse events typically seen with opioids.

29.4 Local Anesthetics

An added benefit of direct delivery to the intrathecal space is the ability to use agents other than opioids to improve pain control. Multiple nonnarcotic agents have been investigated as different receptor systems involved with nociception and modulation of pain were considered. The local anesthetic bupivacaine is the adjunct agent most commonly used with opioids in intrathecal drug delivery systems [23].

Local anesthetics act on sodium ion (Na^+) channels in neuronal cell membranes. They bind a specific region of the α_1 subunit of the voltage-gated sodium channel intracellularly, inhibiting sodium influx and thus preventing action potential. Local anesthetics preferentially bind to open or inactivated channels, after depolarization has occurred.

Though Na^+ channels are found ubiquitously in the nervous system, local anesthetics, when administered intrathecally, preferentially act on fila radicularia, the rootlets that branch from the nerve root in a fanlike fashion before converging into the dorsal horn of the spinal cord, probably because of their large surface-to-volume ratio relative to the spinal cord [24].

Other factors that determine the sensitivity of nerve fibers to local anesthetics include anatomic location of the local anesthetic being injected, physiologic factors, axonal diameter, and myelination. Various factors play a role in the sensitivity of a nerve to local anesthetics. In vitro, unmyelinated fibers are more resistant to local anesthetics than myelinated fibers, and larger diameter fibers are more resistant to local anesthetics than myelinated fibers [25]. However, in clinical observation, sympathetic fibers are blocked by the lowest concentration of local anesthetics, then pain, touch, and motor being the most resistant. There is no clear explanation for this phenomenon, but is likely due to several reasons, such as length of each nerve in the thecal space, depth of the nerve fiber, or distribution of Na and K channels on each nerve [26–28].

Administration of local anesthetic directly into the intrathecal space would require less local anesthetic than epidural administration. In an epidural injection, the local anesthetic must cross the dura to act on neural structures. There is also extraneural absorption of the medication such as by epidural fat, as well as systemic distribution via the venous system in the epidural space [29]. Thus, epidural administration of local anesthetics requires a larger dose to produce an effect similar to intrathecal administration.

Distribution of medication in the intrathecal space in the classic daily volumes (<1 mL/day) delivered by a drug delivery device is very limited. One study in pigs suggested that when the spinal catheter tip was located posterior to the cord in the intrathecal space, the spread of the delivered medication was as small as 1 cm from the tip of the catheter, and it remained on the posterior aspect of the spinal cord [6]. Careful consideration of the catheter tip placement can have significant influence on the location of action, which in turn can impact the effectiveness of the therapy.

Potency is defined as the minimal amount of local anesthetic required to produce neural blockade. Lipophilicity, expressed as the octanol:water or buffer partition coefficient, is the primary component of the degree of potency of local anesthetics, and to some degree, of the duration of action. The p*K*a defines the pH, where half of the drug is ionized, or positively charged form, and half is nonionized. The p*K*a of each local anesthetic is unique and is the tendency of the molecule to accept a proton in the base form or to donate a proton in the acid form. The nonionized form penetrates the nerve membrane, whereas the ionized form binds to proteins on the intracellular side of the sodium channel [30]. The pharmacokinetic properties of common local anesthetics are summarized in Table 29.5.

Local anesthetics used as an adjunct to intrathecal opioids have been shown to have synergism in animal models and in acute pain [32]. These benefits also translate clinically as benefits in decreasing both opioid-induced adverse effects and the need to escalate the dosing of opioids [33]. However, one study suggests that there is no added analgesic efficacy with the co-administration of local anesthetics [34]. The maximal daily dose of bupivacaine in that study (8 mg) was lower than doses in other studies that have shown efficacy (~10 mg) [33, 35]. A recent study in patients with failed back surgery syndrome showed efficacy of a combination of hydromorphone and bupivacaine that was initiated from trial and maintained chronically. The authors followed the patients for 2 years, and analgesia persisted throughout the follow-up period. The patients in that study were all equipped with a patient-activated intrathecal bolus device for use for breakthrough pain. Given the presence of bupivacaine in the pump, patients experienced immediate relief and used the device 3–4

Table 29.5 Local anesthetic pharmacokinetics [31]

Local anesthetic	$t½$, h	Lipid solubility (octanol/buffer partition coefficient)	p*K*a	Protein binding, %	Partition coefficient
Bupivacaine	2.7	8.2	8.1	96	346
Ropivacaine	1.8	8.0	8.1	94	115
Lidocaine	1.6	2.9	7.72	64	2.4

times a day on average [36]. At current dosage recommendations, there are no reports of local anesthetic-induced neurotoxicity in the literature, suggesting an apparently favorable benefit-risk ratio for the use of bupivacaine as an adjunct with intrathecal opioids.

Ziconotide is a synthetic peptide analog to the original toxin derived from the venom of the *Conus magus* (cone snail). It is a 25 amino acid molecule and the synthetic form of the ω-conotoxin MVIIA. Ziconotide can only be administered intrathecally, because of its limited ability to cross the blood–brain barrier and its rapid metabolism by enzymes of the body [37]. Ziconotide possesses linear pharmacokinetics within the CSF and is cleared by diffusion into the systemic circulation, where it is metabolized by peptidases and proteases [38]. Yaksh et al. [39] reported on the pharmacokinetics of ziconotide:

Molecular weight	2500 Da
Half-life (t½) in CSF	4.6 ± 0.9 h (Animal models suggest 1.5-h t½ for bolus)
Peak concentrations in CSF after bolus	3 min
Ziconotide peak concentrations in plasma after intrathecal bolus	20 min
CSF:plasma ratio at peak plasma concentration	30,000:1
CSF:plasma ratio 8 h after peak plasma concentration	30:1
1 μg/h intrathecal infusion, time to peak CSF concentrations	8 h
5 μg/h intrathecal infusion, time to peak CSF concentrations	8 h
Ratio of ziconotide in lumbar CSF versus plasma	2400:1 (8 h); 1200:1 (24 h); 600:1 (48 h)
Terminal elimination t½ after 5 μg/h intrathecal infusion	2.35 h
Lumbar CSF:cisternal CSF ratio at 48 h	1:0.017 (1 μg/h); 1:0.015 (5 μg/h)

Various subtypes of voltage-activated calcium ion channels, including L-type, N-type, P/Q-type, and T-type channels, have been identified in the mammalian nervous system, but ziconotide acts primarily on the α1B subunit of the N-type calcium channels. Ziconotide, unlike other drugs, causes a complete N-type Ca^{2+} channel block at the pmoL range [37]. Immunocytochemical studies have revealed that N-type and P/Q-type calcium channels are localized predominantly on presynaptic nerve terminals throughout the nervous system, where they associate with and are regulated by other biochemical mechanisms involved in synaptic transmission [40]. N-type channels are evenly distributed throughout all the laminae of the dorsal horn and are the predominant subtype in the dorsal horn laminae I and II, consistent with the location of the synapses of most afferent pain fibers. Ziconotide is also associated with the inhibition of the release of glutamate, calcitonin gene-related peptide, and substance P in the dorsal horn of the spinal cord, further inhibiting transmission of pain signals [37].

Table 29.6 Actions of clonidine

Receptor	Physiologic action
α_1	Constriction of vascular smooth muscle
	Contraction of radial muscle of the eye
	Contraction of vas deferens
α_2	Inhibition of norepinephrine release from presynaptic neuron
	Centrally induced sedation (via locus ceruleus)
	Centrally mediated pain modulation via dorsal horn
	Inhibition of insulin release from pancreatic beta cells

The clinical efficacy of ziconotide remains constrained by its limited analgesic effect, its narrow therapeutic window, and its significant adverse events, which may occur acutely or after prolonged administration [41].

Clonidine acts on α-adrenergic receptors. These G-coupled proteins exist in two types, α_1 and α_2 adrenergic receptors, which have different physiologic actions (Table 29.6). The pharmacokinetics of clonidine include a half-life in CSF (intrathecal bolus) of 1.7–2.1 min, a partition coefficient of 7.1, and a lumbar:cistern ratio of 4.1.

Clonidine is an imidazoline derivative with predominantly α_2-adrenergic agonist activity, with an affinity for α_2 to α_1 receptors of 200:1. It was first used as a nasal decongestant, but is now used for the management of hypertension, spinal and regional anesthesia, control of opioid withdrawal symptoms, and ADHD and sleep disturbances in children.

Clonidine is a lipid soluble and readily penetrates the blood–brain barrier and the placenta. It activates inhibitory neurons of the rostral ventrolateral medulla in the brainstem, the final common pathway for sympathetic outflow, decreasing overall sympathetic activity. There is also evidence that much of clonidine's antihypertensive action occurs via binding to a nonadrenergic (imidazoline) receptor. In contrast, its analgesic effects are primarily located in the spinal cord, binding to presynaptic and postsynaptic α_2-adrenergic receptors that inhibit nociceptive transmission.

There are three subtypes of α_2 receptors: α_{2A}, α_{2B}, and α_{2C}. The α_{2B} receptors are found more frequently on vascular smooth muscle and mostly mediate vasopressor effects. All three subtypes are G protein-coupled receptors that inhibit adenylyl cyclase, in turn reducing the levels of cAMP. As cAMP levels are reduced, calcium-activated channels prevent calcium ions from entering the nerve terminal, leading to a suppression of vesicle release of norepinephrine. Stimulation of α_2 receptors in the dorsal horn of the spinal column inhibits nociceptive neurons and reduces the release of substance P. Although there is some evidence for supraspinal and peripheral sites of action, it is thought that the spinal mechanism produces most of the analgesic action of α_2 agonist drugs [42]. Other research suggests that clonidine exerts some of its antinociceptive effects by inhibiting the activation of NF-κB and p38 in glial cells, resulting in the inhibition of several proinflammatory cytokines that have been associated with neuropathic pain states [43].

Depression, insomnia, night terrors, and severe dry mouth have been reported as adverse effects of intrathecal clonidine administration in humans. Intrathecal clonidine can cause bradycardia and hypotension, particularly as a bolus dose. Sudden withdrawal of clonidine after chronic administration has been associated with rebound hypertension, which may occur up to 20 hours after cessation of the drug [44]. Clonidine is believed to be more effective in neuropathic pain states, and the effective dosage can be as high as 400 to 800 μg/day [45, 46]. If it is ineffective, the patient must be weaned off the drug slowly to avert serious withdrawal-related adverse events.

29.5 Choosing Intrathecal Analgesics

This chapter discusses the pharmacokinetics and pharmacodynamics of common medications currently used in intrathecal targeted drug delivery. As there are limited studies on the efficacy of different intrathecal analgesics, especially in admixtures, consensus statements have been developed to address gaps in studies, including maximum daily doses and concentrations (Table 29.7) [47]. A comprehensive understanding of the intrathecal drugs used is essential for safe and effective patient care. The choice of pharmacologic agents used in the control of pain is evolving, however, as reflected in recent changes in guidelines and recommendations. Remaining up to date on best practices in the selection of medication is as important as understanding the basics of pharmacology. This subject is covered in detail in subsequent chapters.

Table 29.7 Maximum daily concentrations and doses of intrathecal agents[a]

Drug	Maximum concentration	Maximum dose per day
Morphine	20 mg/mL	15 mg
Hydromorphone	15 mg/mL	10 mg
Fentanyl	10 mg/mL	1000 μg
Sufentanil	5 mg/mL	500 μg
Bupivacaine[†]	30 mg/mL	10 mg
Ziconotide	100 μg/mL	19.2 μg
Clonidine	1000 μg/mL	600 μg

[a]According to the 2012 and 2016 polyanalgesic consensus statements [47]

[b]Maximum daily dose of bupivacaine is significantly less than that recommended in 2007 (30 mg/day); some authors of the consensus statement had reservations about the lower recommended dose

References

1. Henry-Feugeas MC, Idy-Peretti I, Baledent O, Poncelet-Didon A, Zannoli G, Bittoun J, et al. Origin of subarachnoid cerebrospinal fluid pulsations: a phase-contrast MR analysis. Magn Reson Imaging. 2000;18:387–95.
2. Friese S, Hamhaber U, Erb M, Kueker W, Klose U. The influence of pulse and respiration on spinal cerebrospinal fluid pulsation. Investig Radiol. 2004;39:120–30.
3. Alperin N, Vikingstad EM, Gomez-Anson B, Levin DN. Hemodynamically independent analysis of cerebrospinal fluid and brain motion observed with dynamic phase contrast MRI. Magn Reson Med. 1996;35:741–54.
4. Stockman HW. Effect of anatomical fine structure on the flow of cerebrospinal fluid in the spinal subarachnoid space. J Biochem Eng. 2006;128:106–14.
5. Degrell I, Nagy E. Concentration gradients for HVA, 5-HIAA, ascorbic acid, and uric acid in cerebrospinal fluid. Biol Psychiatry. 1990;27:891–6.
6. Bernards CM. Cerebrospinal fluid and spinal cord distribution of baclofen and bupivacaine during slow intrathecal infusion in pigs. Anesthesiology. 2006;105:169–78.
7. Hettiarachchi HD, Hsu Y, Harris TJ Jr, Penn R, Linninger AA. The effect of pulsatile flow on intrathecal drug delivery in the spinal canal. Ann Biomed Eng. 2011;39:2592–602.
8. Weisner B, Bernhardt W. Protein fractions of lumbar, cisternal, and ventricular cerebrospinal fluid: separate areas of reference. J Neurol Sci. 1978;37:205–14.
9. Yaksh TL, Rudy TA. Analgesia mediated by a direct spinal action of narcotics. Science. 1976;192:1357–8.
10. Basbaum AI, Clanton CH, Fields HL. Opiate and stimulus-produced analgesia: functional anatomy of a medullospinal pathway. Proc Natl Acad Sci. 1976;73:4685–8.
11. Behar M, Magora F, Olshwang D, Davidson JT. Epidural morphine in treatment of pain. Lancet. 1979;1(8115):527–9.
12. Wang JK, Nauss LE, Thomas JE. Pain relief by intrathecally applied morphine in man. Anesthesiology. 1979;50:149–51.
13. Matsuki A. Nothing new under the sun – a Japanese pioneer in the clinical use of intrathecal morphine [editorial]. Anesthesiology. 1983;58:289–90.
14. Childers SR, Snyder SH. Guanine nucleotides differentiate agonist and antagonist interactions with opiate receptors. Life Sci. 1978;23:759–61.
15. Childers SR, Creese I, Snowman AM, Synder SH. Opiate receptor binding affected differentially by opiates and opioid peptides. Eur J Pharmacol. 1979;55:11–8.
16. Al-Hasani R, Bruchas MR. Molecular mechanisms of opioid receptor-dependent signaling and behavior. Anesthesiology. 2011;115:1363–81.
17. Kroin JS. Intrathecal drug administration: present use and future trends. Clin Pharmacokinet. 1992;22:319–26.
18. McQuay HJ, Sullivan AF, Smallman K, Dickenson AH. Intrathecal opioids, potency and lipophilicity. Pain. 1989;36:111–5.
19. Ummenhofer WC, Arends RH, Shen D, Bernards CM. Comparative spinal distribution and clearance kinetics of intrathecally administered morphine, fentanyl, alfentanil, and sufentanil. Anesthesiology. 2000;92:739–53.
20. Bernards CM, Shen DD, Sterling ES, Adkins JE, Risler L, Phillips B, Ummenhofer W. Epidural, cerebrospinal fluid, and plasma pharmacokinetics of epidural opioids (part 1). Anesthesiology. 2003;99:455–65.
21. Bernards CM. Understanding the physiology and pharmacology of epidural and intrathecal opioids. Best Pract Res Clin Anaesthesiol. 2002;16:489–505.
22. Kroin JS, Ali A, York M, Penn RD. The distribution of medication along the spinal canal after chronic intrathecal administration. Neurosurgery. 1993;33:226–30; discussion 230.

23. Staats P, Whitworth M, Barakat M, Anderson W, Lilienfeld S. The use of implanted programmable infusion pumps in the management of nonmalignant, chronic low-back pain. Neuromodulation. 2007;10:376–80.
24. Boswell MV, Iacono RP, Guthkelch AN. Sites of action of subarachnoid lidocaine and tetracaine: observations with evoked potential monitoring during spinal cord stimulator implantation. Reg Anesth. 1992;17:37–42.
25. Jaffe RA, Rowe MA. Differential nerve block. Direct measurements on individual myelinated and unmyelinated dorsal root axons. Anesthesiology. 1996;84:1455–64.
26. Fink BR. Mechanisms of differential axial blockade in epidural and subarachnoid anesthesia. Anesthesiology. 1989;70:851–8.
27. Raymond SA. Subblocking concentrations of local anesthetics: effects on impulse generation and conduction in single myelinated sciatic nerve axons in frog. Anesth Analg. 1992;75:906–21.
28. Jaffe RA, Rowe MA. Subanesthetic concentrations of lidocaine selectively inhibit a nociceptive response in the isolated rat spinal cord. Pain. 1995;60:167–74.
29. Burm AG. Clinical pharmacokinetics of epidural and spinal anaesthesia. Clin Pharmacokinet. 1989;16:283–311.
30. Covino BG, Scott DB, Lambert DH. Handbook of spinal anesthesia and analgesia. Philadelphia, PA: WB Saunders; 1994.
31. Datta S, Kodali BS, Segal S. Obstetric anesthesia handbook. 5th ed. New York, NY: Springer; 2010.
32. Hayek SM, Hanes MC. Intrathecal therapy for chronic pain: current trends and future needs. Curr Pain Headache Rep. 2014;18:388.
33. Veizi IE, Hayek SM, Narouze S, Pope JE, Mekhail N. Combination of intrathecal opioids with bupivacaine attenuates opioid dose escalation in chronic noncancer pain patients. Pain Med. 2011;12:1481–9.
34. Mironer YE, Haasis JC, Chapple I, Brown C, Satterthwaite JR. Efficacy and safety of intrathecal opioid/bupivacaine mixture in chronic nonmalignant pain: a double blind, randomized, crossover, multicenter study by the National Forum of Independent Pain Clinicians (NFIPC). Neuromodulation. 2002;5:208–13.
35. Deer TR, Caraway DL, Kim CK, Dempsey CD, Stewart CD, McNeil KF. Clinical experience with intrathecal bupivacaine in combination with opioid for the treatment of chronic pain related to failed back surgery syndrome and metastatic cancer pain of the spine. Spine J. 2002;2:274–8.
36. Hayek SM, Veizi E, Hanes M. Intrathecal hydromorphone and bupivacaine combination therapy for post-laminectomy syndrome optimized with patient-activated bolus device. Pain Med. 2015;17(3):561–71.
37. McGivern JG. Ziconotide: a review of its pharmacology and use in the treatment of pain. Neuropsychiatr Dis Treat. 2007;3:69–85.
38. Wermeling D, Drass M, Ellis D, Mayo M, McGuire D, O'Connell D, et al. Pharmacokinetics and pharmacodynamics of intrathecal ziconotide in chronic pain patients. J Clin Pharmacol. 2003;43:624–36.
39. Yaksh TL, de Kater A, Dean R, Best BM, Miljanich GP. Pharmacokinetic analysis of ziconotide (SNX-111), an intrathecal N-type calcium channel blocking analgesic, delivered by bolus and infusion in the dog. Neuromodulation. 2012;15:508–19; discussion 519.
40. Westenbroek RE, Hoskins L, Catterall WA. Localization of Ca2+ channel subtypes on rat spinal motor neurons, interneurons, and nerve terminals. J Neurosci. 1998;18:6319–30.
41. Hayek SM, Hanes MC, Wang C, Veizi IE. Ziconotide combination intrathecal therapy for noncancer pain is limited secondary to delayed adverse effects: a case series with a 24-month follow-up. Neuromodulation. 2015;18:397–403.
42. Sierralta F, Naquira D, Pinardi G, Miranda HF. α-Adrenoceptor and opioid receptor modulation of clonidine-induced antinociception. Br J Pharmacol. 1996;119:551–4.

43. Feng X, Zhang F, Dong R, Li W, Liu J, Zhao X, et al. Intrathecal administration of clonidine attenuates spinal neuroimmune activation in a rat model of neuropathic pain with existing hyperalgesia. Eur J Pharmacol. 2009;614:38–43.
44. Hassenbusch SJ, Gunes S, Wachsman S, Willis KD. Intrathecal clonidine in the treatment of intractable pain: a phase I/II study. Pain Med. 2002;3:85–91.
45. Rauck RL, North J, Eisenach JC. Intrathecal clonidine and adenosine: effects on pain and sensory processing in patients with chronic regional pain syndrome. Pain. 2015;156:88–95.
46. Hayek SM, Mekhail NA. Complex regional pain syndrome: redefining reflex sympathetic dystrophy and causalgia. Phys Sportsmed. 2004;32:18–25.
47. Deer TR, Pope JE, Hayek SM, Lamer TJ, Veizi IE, Erdek M, et al. The polyanalgesic consensus conference (PACC): recommendations for intrathecal drug delivery: guidance for improving safety and mitigating risks. Neuromodulation. 2017;20:155–76.

Chapter 30
Patient Selection for Drug Delivery System Implantation

Maged Hamza

30.1 Introduction

Pain currently affects approximately 100 million adults in the United States. Pain has been significant in terms of healthcare impact and the economic impact of direct and indirect costs, including a loss of productivity estimated to be between $560 billion and $635 billion annually.

Chronic pain is a complex condition with multiple physical, physiological, psychological, emotional, and social components. It is usually associated with significant impairment of well-being and limitations on relationships between the affected individual and his or her family and friends, though the impact of chronic pain varies greatly among affected individuals.

Over the past few decades, the understanding of chronic pain and the available management options have vastly improved, but many limitations, challenges, and opportunities for improvement persist. For example, many patients report positive impact from the increased use of opioid medications, but there has been growing concern and alarm about an epidemic of misuse and abuse. A lack of documented long-term efficacy and significant adverse events affecting 30–40% of patients are a few of the other concerns. The interventional techniques, on the other hand, have shown efficacy in a subset of patients, though many continue to suffer from intractable, severe pain despite the use of all currently available treatments.

Intrathecal drug delivery systems (IDDS), known as pain pumps, offer an alternative treatment option in the management of chronic, severe pain for those patients who have not responded well to less invasive, more commonly used lines of treatment [1–3]. Recently published reports have presented an algorithmic protocol utilizing IDDS in the management of chronic, severe pain that is not responsive to other treatment, showing good success in terms of pain relief and functional

M. Hamza (✉)
Virginia Innovative Pain and Spine Center, Richmond, VA, USA
e-mail: maged.hamza@gmail.com

S. Diwan, T.R. Deer (eds.), *Advanced Procedures for Pain Management*,
https://doi.org/10.1007/978-3-319-68841-1_30

improvement. It is very clear that patient selection is a crucial element in achieving good outcomes from the use of a drug delivery system for chronic, severe pain. The important point is matching the right patient with the right therapy at the right time [4, 5]. Selecting a suitable patient and ensuring that the patient is ready and optimized for the proposed therapy will positively impact outcomes. The clinician cannot change other aspects of the disease process, such as the previous occurrence of an injury, the predisposition to disease progression, or how the patient has dealt with the pain in the past, but patient selection that matches the right patient with the right therapy at the right time can have the greatest impact in producing positive outcomes.

30.2 Overview of the Evaluation and Assessment

It is important for the evaluating clinician to consider all previous therapies that the patient has undergone, including (but not limited to) the use of medications, with their dosages and response in terms of improvement and/or adverse effects. Also to be reviewed are minimally invasive interventions such as nerve blocks, physical therapy, previous surgeries, and nonmedicinal modalities such as massage and topical applications.

The evaluation of medical history and previous therapy should not be taken as a rigid check-box system in which all other treatments must be exhausted before implantation of a drug delivery system. The goal is to achieve a balance to determine the patient's appropriateness. For instance, if a patient had a trial of a specific medication with significant adverse events, there is no indication to continue it longer just to have done it. The fine balance of analyzing the risk-benefit ratio based on the response to medical and interventional modalities, including any adverse events or side effects, and assessing what expectations are realistic or obtainable for the proposed therapy is most important factor affecting outcomes [6–10].

The highest priority should be preparing the patient, family, and caregivers with an adequate understanding of the whole process, not merely the procedure of pump implantation. This process includes ensuring adequate explanation and understanding of patient selection, trialing, and implantation. In our practice, patients are provided with reading material that includes the protocols that will be followed in the implantation follow-up and post-implant surveillance. The patient and family are then returned to the clinic for discussion of the patient's expectations and goals. It is advisable to document those expectations so that the patient and clinician have a reference point during discussions after implantation regarding how well those expectations have been met [4, 5].

30.3 Type of Pain

The type of pain and presenting symptoms may have an impact on outcome, as usually patients with nociceptive somatic pain and occasionally visceral-type pain have responded well to an IDDS [7]. There is also evidence that neuropathic pain conditions may respond well and have been responsive to drug delivery system implantation [9], but more evidence and anecdotal experience support the perception that nociceptive somatic pain does respond more favorably to intraspinal delivery of medications.

30.4 Psychological Considerations

It has been estimated that 35% of chronic pain patients have some form of coexistent psychological and or psychiatric abnormalities. Psychological evaluation prior to implantation of a pain pump is essential. The goal of the psychological evaluation is to detect any underlying untreated or unaddressed psychological disorders; to re-emphasize adequate, realistic, achievable goals and expectations; and to give the patient and the family or caregiver an opportunity to discuss the whole process with a psychologist who is a member of the care team, allowing questions and ensuring adequate understanding of the process.

The goal is not to have all psychiatric disorders and concerns "treated" prior to implementation; we believe it is more appropriate to consider it a process of "optimization" rather than a treatment. It is not uncommon for some psychological concerns or diagnoses to coexist in chronic pain patients, but evaluation and optimization have been shown to greatly enhance the outcome following implantation. The psychological evaluation should also be able to shed some light on any cognitive impairment such as early dementia, early Alzheimer's disease, or chronic brain injury conditions. Any impairment or difficulties with comprehending educational material should also be pointed out in the psychological evaluation.

It is important to prepare the patient for the psychological evaluation. We clearly indicate to each patient that the rationale behind the psychological evaluation is not to imply in any way that the pain is not real. We suggest that seeing the psychologist is like seeing a physical therapist, but for the brain: Just as a physical therapist can teach techniques to improve physical functioning and conditioning status, the psychologist similarly can show the patient how to utilize nonmedicinal approaches to impact their pain behavior and coping skills. In this manner, the patient is more open-minded and less anxious in approaching the psych screen and is more of an active participant in the whole process [4, 5].

Within our practice, psychological evaluation involves a face-to-face interview over at least 50 min to an hour with a psychologist, followed by the administration of multiple questionnaires that are scored and evaluated by the psychologist before preparation of a final report. This report is then reviewed with the patient by the clinician prior to the implantation, and any concerns brought up by the psychologist are thoroughly addressed. These may include the need to initiate a regimen of relaxation techniques, or the need for more explanation and discussion of the therapy and its goals and expectations. The goal of psychological evaluation is to optimize the patient for the implantation process, to achieve optimal outcomes [11–15].

30.5 Medical Comorbidities

Patients with chronic pain usually suffer from multiple coexisting medical disorders. Understanding the nature, severity, and complexity of those disorders is of great importance in determining the nature and timing of the proposed intervention, a pump implant, and in maintaining optimal outcomes following implantation. The most common medical comorbidities of chronic pain patients are diabetes mellitus, hypertension, obesity, and sleep disorders.

The interplay between chronic deconditioning, obesity, and diabetes cannot be overemphasized, as lack of activity with deconditioning fosters the onset and progression of obesity. There is no clear evidence that pain pumps are especially useful in treating diabetic neuropathy per se, but the impact of diabetes on wound infection and wound healing has been documented in multiple clinical scenarios. Patients with diabetes should be thoroughly counseled regarding the increased risk of wound infection and delayed wound healing. It has been documented that achieving glycemic control and normal hemoglobin A1c immediately prior to surgery does not lower the incidence of infection or delayed wound healing, but long-standing, chronic management and maintenance of adequate glycemic control for a length of time before surgery may lower the incidence of infection associated with diabetes mellitus [16–22].

In the United States, the prevalence of obesity has been on the rise over the past few decades. Obesity is usually associated with some form of disturbed sleep pattern, particularly obstructive sleep apnea or hypo-apnea. Chronic pain patients usually suffer from some sort of sleep apnea or sleep disturbance, especially in conjunction with chronic opioid treatment. It is worth noting that the current guidelines for the American Society of Anesthesiologists call for special attention in observation and close monitoring of patients with any element of sleep apnea following the administration of neuraxial opioids; this attention would be significantly relevant in the setting of trialing and or implementation of pain pumps. The proper and careful assessment of obesity in chronic pain patients is also essential as it pertains to pump implantation, as it will have an impact on the closeness and the frequency of post-procedure monitoring [23–26].

Antiplatelet and anticoagulant agents have been used recently for multiple disorders such as coronary artery disease, history of transient ischemic attack (TIA), lupus, and hypercoagulable states. Use of these agents will affect many aspects of patient selection and care, including performing a trial, the type of anesthesia to use on the patient who is chronically anticoagulated, and the choice of postoperative anticoagulation for prevention of deep venous thrombosis (DVT), as currently recommended. Special emphasis should be placed on discussing the patient's preoperative use of nonconventional blood thinners such as garlic and other herbal supplements, or locally known anticoagulants such as BC Powder and Goody's Powder. In one report, a patient suffered post-implantation bleeding due to the use of BC Powder. When the patient was asked whether he was using blood thinners, he adamantly denied it, but he was using BC Powder for headaches, which were so frequent that he was using the powder almost daily. The patient did not know that BC Powder is a blood thinner, and the clinician also was not aware of its nature. Thus it is important to list all known and unconventional anticoagulants, including herbal supplements. The use of anticoagulants (blood thinners) should be thoroughly evaluated prior to considering implantation of a drug delivery system [27, 28].

The physician maintaining the patient's anticoagulation therapy should be consulted prior to considering trial and/or implantation. In some cases, for example, the cardiologist may indicate that it should be safe to withhold anticoagulants temporarily prior to interventions; this change should be thoroughly discussed with the patient and documented. Occasionally, when anticoagulation may need to be stopped, the clinician might want to consider the use of low-molecular-weight heparin subcutaneously as the intervention is performed in a closely monitored setting.

Acute, active infections are generally viewed as a contraindication for the implantation of a pain pump, and the patient selection process should be deferred or postponed until all such infections have been thoroughly treated. However, patients who are known as chronic carriers or who have chronic infection such as MRSA or those with an indwelling urinary catheter should be thoroughly evaluated, with surveillance nasal swabs and/or recent cultures. C-reactive protein levels should be normalized and treated. A consultation with an infectious disease specialist is worth consideration when the patient is being considered for pump implantation [29, 30].

Immune status should be reviewed, evaluated, and discussed with the patient. It is not uncommon for patients with chronic pain to have diabetes, chronic opioid use, or other conditions associated with decreased immune response. Examples of immune-compromised states include HIV infection with low cell count, chronic uncontrolled diabetes, chronic steroid use, and chemotherapy. In the absence of active HIV infection, infection rates for immune-compromised patients reportedly have been similar to those of the general population, but it is logical to thoroughly discuss this issue with patients with an immune-compromised state, as the patient and family or caregiver should be aware of the higher risk of infection or delayed wound healing following the procedure [27, 28].

Other chronic medical disorders such as coronary artery disease, chronic renal insufficiency, chronic lung disease (COPD), and chronic cardiac disease should also be sought out and assessed. Their impact on drug clearance will affect the anesthetic to be used, and they also may be associated with hypertensive adverse events.

30.6 Economic and Social Factors

Economic and social factors should also be considered in the process of patient selection. Obtaining proper authorization from the patient's insurance for coverage and of the trial, implantation, and post-implant surveillance and refills is extremely important. A consultation with office staff and review of the patient's insurance policy should be performed to clearly delineate copayments and all other out-of-pocket expenses so that patients are not surprised by any hidden or unexpected costs [7, 31].

Close attention to social history and social circumstances is also important. For example, does the patient have adequate transportation and adequate care when being discharged home following implantation? Will there be support and assistance in the initial healing phase [31]? Smoking status also should be reviewed during the patient selection process, as it has been clearly shown that the cessation of smoking for 6–8 weeks prior to any surgical intervention is associated with improved wound healing and decreased wound infection [32].

Inviting the patient to participate in a support group has been shown to be extremely helpful. Allowing patients to be a part of a peer group of other patients with implants or those who are being evaluated for implantation will allow patients to have a dialogue. Careful attention must be paid to all Health Insurance Portability and Accountability Act (HIPAA) regulations and guidelines [4, 5].

30.7 Summary

Table 30.1 outlines the characteristics to be considered in choosing which patients are likely to be optimal candidates for implantation of a drug delivery system.

Table 30.1 Characteristics of optimal candidates for drug delivery systems

• Chronic, severe, intractable pain that has not been responsive to less invasive forms of therapy
• No identifiable pathology accounting for the chronicity of the pain that is amenable to surgical intervention
• Ability to understand the process of implanting the intrathecal drug delivery system and to provide adequate consent
• Adequate expectations of the possible outcomes of the procedure, including risk-benefit analysis, after thorough and repeated discussion and presentation to the patient and caregivers
• No significant untreated psychological disorder following a formal psychological evaluation
• Ability to comply with office visits and evaluations required for post-implantation maintenance and surveillance
• Family or caregivers engaged in and supportive of the therapy process
• No active substance abuse or substance dependence
• Absence of any relative or absolute contraindications that would prohibit the implantation, such as local sepsis or chronic anticoagulation
• Considered a good candidate after medical and surgical review of the magnitude and complexity of comorbidities
• Appropriate economic and social support system to offer the patient the optimal possible outcome following the process

References

1. Manchikanti L, Singh V, Helm S, Schultz DM, Datta S, Hirsch J. An introduction to an evidence-based approach to interventional techniques in the management of chronic spinal pain. Pain Physician. 2009;12:E1–33.
2. Freburger J, Holmes G, Agans R, Jackman A, Darter J, Wallace A, et al. The rising prevalence of chronic low back pain. Arch Intern Med. 2009;169:251–8.
3. IOM (Institute of Medicine). Relieving pain in America: a blueprint for transforming prevention, care, education, and research. Washington, DC: The National Academies Press; 2011.
4. Hamza M, Doleys D, Wells M, Weisbein J, Hoff J, Martin M, et al. Prospective study of 3-year follow-up of low-dose intrathecal opioids in the management of chronic nonmalignant pain. Pain Med. 2012;13:1304–13.
5. Hamza M, Doleys DM, Saleh IA, Medvedovsky A, Verdolin MH, Hamza M. a prospective, randomized, single-blinded, head-to-head long-term outcome study, comparing intrathecal (IT) boluses with continuous infusion trialing techniques prior to implantation of drug delivery systems (DDS) for the treatment of severe intractable chronic nonmalignant pain. Neuromodulation. 2015;18:636–48.
6. Krames ES. Intraspinal opioid therapy for chronic nonmalignant pain: current practice and clinical guidelines. J Pain Symptom Manag. 1996;11:333–52.
7. Deer T, Winkelmuller W, Erdine S, Bedder M, Burchiel K. Intrathecal therapy for cancer and nonmalignant pain: patient selection and patient management. Neuromodulation. 1999;2:55–66.
8. Ghafoor VL, Epshteyn M, Carlson GH, Terhaar DM, Charry O, Phelps PK. Intrathecal drug therapy for long-term pain management. Am J Health Syst Pharm. 2007;64:2447–61.
9. Paice JA, Penn RD, Shott S. Intraspinal morphine for chronic pain: a retrospective, multicenter study. J Pain Symptom Manag. 1996;11:71–80.
10. Winkelmüller M, Winkelmüller W. Longterm effects of continuous intrathecal opioid treatment in chronic pain of nonmalignant etiology. J Neurosurg. 1996;85:458–67.
11. Doleys DM. Preparing patients for implantable technology. In: Turk DC, Gatchel RJ, editors. Psychological approaches to pain management. New York: The Guilford Press; 2002. p. 334–48.
12. Doleys DM. Psychologic evaluation for patients undergoing neuroaugmentative procedures. Neurosurg Clin N Am. 2003;14:409–17.
13. Nelson DV, Kennington M, Novy DM, Squitieri P. Psychological selection criteria for implantable spinal cord stimulators. Pain Forum. 1996;5:93–103.
14. Celestin J, Edwards RR, Jamison RN. Pretreatment psychosocial variables as predictors of outcomes following lumbar surgery and spinal cord stimulation: a systematic review and literature synthesis. Pain Med. 2009;10:639–53.
15. Doleys DM, Olson K. Psychological assessment and intervention in implantable pain therapies (monograph). Minneapolis, MN: Medtronic Neurological; 1997. p. 1–20.
16. Centers for Disease Control and Prevention. National diabetes fact sheet, 2007. http://www.cdc.gov/chronicdisease/resources/publications/aag/diabetes.htm
17. American Diabetes Association. All about diabetes. http://www.diabetes.org/about-diabetes.jsp. Accessed 28 Jul 2009.
18. National Diabetes Information Clearinghouse (NDIC). Diabetic neuropathies: the nerve damage of diabetes. NIH Publication No. 09-3185; 2009. Accessed 28 Jul 2009.
19. Krein SL, Heisler M, Piette JD, Makki F, Kerr EA. The effect of chronic pain on diabetes patients, self-management. Diabetes Care. 2005;28:65–70.
20. Greenhalgh DG. Wound healing and diabetes mellitus. Clin Plast Surg. 2003;30:37–45.
21. Follet KA, Boortz-Marx RL, Drake JM, DuPen S, Schneider S, et al. Prevention and management of intrathecal drug delivery and spinal cord stimulation system infections. Anesthesiology. 2004;100:1582–94.
22. Van den Berghe G. How does blood glucose control with insulin save lives in intensive care? J Clin Invest. 2004;114:1187–95.

23. Ogden CL, Carrol MD, McDowell MA, Flegal KM. Obesity among adults in the United States—no statistically significant change since 2003–2004. NCHS Data Brief. 2007;1:1–6.
24. National Sleep Foundation. Obstructive sleep apnea and sleep. https://sleepfoundation.org/sleep-disorders-problems/sleep-apnea. Accessed Jul 2016.
25. Farney RJ, Walker JM, Cloward TV, Rhondeau S. Sleep-disordered breathing associated with long-term opioid therapy. Chest. 2003;123:632–9.
26. Horlocker TT, Burton AW, Connis RT, Hughes S, Nickinovich D, Palmer C, et al. Practice guidelines for the prevention, detection, and management of respiratory depression associated with neuraxial opioid administration. Anesthesiology. 2009;110:218–30.
27. Horlocker TT, Wedel DJ, Benzon H, Brown DL, Enneking FK, Heit JA, et al. Regional anesthesia in the anticoagulated patient: defining the risks (the second ASRA Consensus Confererence on Neuraxial Anesthesia and Anticoagulation). Reg Anesth Pain Med. 2003;28:172–97.
28. Chaney MA. Intrathecal and epidural anesthesia and analgesia for cardiac surgery. Anesth Analg. 2006;102:45–64.
29. Knight KH, Brand FM, Mchaourab AS, Veneziano G. Implantable intrathecal pumps for chronic pain: highlights and updates. Croat Med J. 2007;48:22–34.
30. Stearns L, Boortz-Marx R, Du Pen S, Friehs G, Gordon M, Halyard M, et al. Intrathecal drug delivery for the management of cancer pain: a multidisciplinary consensus of best clinical practices. J Support Oncol. 2005;3:399–408.
31. Deer TR, Krames E, Levy RM, Hassenbusch SJ, Prager JP. Practice choices and challenges in the current intrathecal therapy environment: an online survey. Pain Med. 2009;10:304–9.
32. Martin CT, Gao Y, Duchman KR, Pugely AJ. The impact of current smoking and smoking cessation on short-term morbidity risk after lumbar spine surgery. Spine. 20161;41:577–84.

Chapter 31
Intrathecal Drug Delivery: Medication Selection

Andrea C. Wong and Salim M. Hayek

31.1 Introduction

The appropriate selection of medications is key to the accomplishment of symptom control when using an intrathecal drug delivery system (IDDS). Medications must be preservative-free, safe for intrathecal use, and efficacious. For control of chronic pain, a number of intrathecal agents are commonly used, including opioids, the local anesthetic bupivacaine, the peptide ziconotide, and clonidine. Morphine and ziconotide are the only medications approved by the US Food and Drug Administration (FDA) for the intrathecal treatment of chronic pain. Baclofen is the only FDA-approved medication for treatment of spasticity using intrathecal drug delivery (IDD).

The selection of medications is highly dependent not only on their functional efficacy but also on their pharmacokinetics and side effect profile. Appropriate dosing can be initiated based on the type and location of pain, the patient's age and medical condition or prognosis, and the patient's opioid medication requirements prior to the initiation of intrathecal therapy.

A.C. Wong (✉)
University at Buffalo Neurosurgery, 180 Park Club Lane, Williamsville, NY 14221, USA
e-mail: awong@ubns.com

S.M. Hayek
Department of Anesthesiology and Pain Management,
University Hospitals Cleveland Medical Center, Cleveland, OH, USA
e-mail: Salim.Hayek@UHhospitals.org

S. Diwan, T.R. Deer (eds.), *Advanced Procedures for Pain Management*,
https://doi.org/10.1007/978-3-319-68841-1_31

31.2 Patient Characteristics

Many patient variables should be considered in trialing subjects with chronic pain; a standard pre-set approach may not work for all. Patient characteristics to consider include age, sex, symptomatic distribution, etiology of symptoms, type of pain, comorbidities, and prognosis.

Retrospective studies have determined that the rate of intrathecal opioid dose escalation was greater in younger patients over a period of 12–24 months' use [1, 2]. Therefore, the intrathecal opioid requirements in younger patients would be expected to rise at a faster pace than that seen in older patients. Sex also may have a role in daily opioid requirements: females were found to have a lower dose requirement at 24 months of IDD [2], though this finding was not substantiated in other studies.

Pain that is localized to one or a few adjacent dermatomes may be better targeted by IDD than generalized body pain. Intrathecal drug delivery through implanted pumps uses slow infusion rates whereby drug distribution is limited [3]. The location of the catheter tip must therefore coincide with localization of nerve fibers conducting pain to be effective in treating a patient's symptoms. Diffuse pain states will therefore not be treated well with IDD. Chronic pain may be neuropathic or a combination of nociceptive and neuropathic pain. Neuropathic pain is commonly difficult to treat and may lead to medication dose escalation in IDD patients [4].

It is important to consider patient comorbidities when determining the appropriateness of IDD and the selection of medications. In 2010, Coffey et al. [5] found that multiple comorbidities were associated with increased risk of postoperative mortality in patients with an IDDS, including concomitant use of oral opioids, muscle relaxants, hypnotics such as benzodiazepines, and other CNS depressants. Patients with a number of comorbidities are also more likely to require general anesthesia for IDD implantation, potentially contributing to respiratory compromise. Outcome analysis of patients with multiple comorbid conditions undergoing surgical neuromodulation procedures has shown a greater risk of hemodynamic instability, inadequate pain control, and delayed PACU stay [6]. This study also found that IDDS complications were the most common cause of re-operation. Appropriate patient selection is thereby paramount.

Intrathecal drug therapy may be particularly useful for patients with cancer-related pain. These patients experience improved pain scores as well as a reduction in the severity of ill-tolerated opioid-induced side effects including sleep disorders, daytime drowsiness, constipation, and nausea [7]. A randomized clinical trial by Smith et al. in 2002 [7] investigated the differences in outcomes between cancer patients who were managed with IDDS and those who were medically managed. The study found that IDDS patients had greater reduction in pain scores and toxicity, as well as improved survival. The patient's overall prognosis should be taken into account when considering targeted IDD, as patients with a shortened expected survival secondary to cancer-related pain may be limited by timing and thus unable to fully benefit from implantation of an IDDS.

Based on the above patient factors, decisions may be made as to what intrathecal agent(s) may be most appropriate. Following initiation of intrathecal drug delivery, frequent office visits are scheduled to determine the effectiveness of the medication for each patient. Initially, the pain medicine specialist may need to make several changes to the infusion rate, bolus amount, and frequency, as well as drug concentration. The changes are made depending on feedback from the patient. If there is a lack of efficacy following repeated adjustments, or if symptoms are not well tolerated, other intrathecal medication(s) may be selected and fine-tuned. To guide selection, expected effects and common possible side effects will be discussed.

31.3 Opioids

Opioids delivered intrathecally diffuse to the substantia gelatinosa, where they are able to act directly on the opioid receptors [8]. This is a significant advantage in pharmacologic availability when compared with opiates that are delivered orally or intravenously, as intrathecal administration bypasses the blood-brain barrier and the hepatic first effect. Many of the side effects that are commonly experienced through systemic delivery are lessened, and the amount of opioid required for clinical effect is also decreased. Though morphine, hydromorphone, and fentanyl have all commonly been used in IDDS, morphine is the only FDA-approved intrathecally delivered opioid.

It has been well established that the bioavailability of each opioid differs according to its lipid solubility profile. In 1971, Herz and Teschemacher demonstrated that hydrophilic intrathecal opioids, which would include morphine and hydromorphone, are able to diffuse farther into neural tissue than highly lipid-soluble drugs [9]. Herz et al. had also found in 1970 that morphine injected into the lateral ventricles of rabbits had deeper uptake into the grey matter than hydrophobic opioids [8]. Hydrophobic opioids such as fentanyl and sufentanil tend to diffuse through dura mater into epidural fat and subsequently the vasculature, so they have a larger volume of distribution [9]. Hence, hydrophilic opioids have a greater bioavailability to act on target receptors of the substantia gelatinosa. The effect of all opioids in the intrathecal compartment is terminated with redistribution into plasma and eventual hepatic metabolism and renal excretion [10].

31.3.1 Morphine, Hydromorphone, Fentanyl, Sufentanil

As previously noted, morphine is the only intrathecal opioid FDA-approved for treatment of chronic pain. Secondary to its hydrophilic nature, it remains longer in cerebrospinal fluid and is able to diffuse well into the dorsal horn. It is noted to be a first-line drug in intrathecal drug selection for the treatment of chronic nociceptive and neuropathic pain [11]. Hydromorphone is similar to morphine in lipid

Table 31.1 Recommended dosing of intrathecal opioids

Intrathecal opioid	Starting dose	Bolus	Maximum dose per day	Maximum concentration, mg/mL
Morphine	0.1–0.5 mg/day	0.1–0.5 mg	15 mg	20
Hydromorphone	0.01–0.15 mg/day	0.025–0.1 mg	10 mg	15
Fentanyl	25–75 μg/day	15–75 μg	1000 μg	10
Sufentanil	10–20 μg/day	5–20 μg	500 μg	5

solubility, but both have been implicated in catheter tip granuloma formation, which will be discussed further in the Adverse Events section [12]. Fentanyl and sufentanil are more potent and hydrophobic opioids. Therefore, they tend to diffuse through the dura and distribute in epidural fat 'sinks' [9]. The recommended initial dosing, bolus, maximum recommended dose, and maximum concentrations were reviewed by the Polyanalgesic Consensus Conference and are listed in Table 31.1 [11].

31.3.2 Adverse Effects of Opioids

There are significant possible adverse effects of intrathecal opioids, which is why it is important to closely monitor each patient on initiation and throughout maintenance of intrathecal administration. Respiratory depression is one of the greatest concerns. In a case series of nine patients who died from overdose, it was suggested that iatrogenic causes or concomitant use of other CNS depressant medications were implicated [13]. Device malfunction was not implicated in any of these patients. Secondary to their hydrophilic nature, morphine and hydromorphone tend to remain in the CSF and therefore are more likely to distribute cephalad towards the respiratory centers of the CNS [5]. Other effects that can be quite troublesome to patients include pruritus, urinary retention, gastrointestinal immotility, and peripheral edema. Peripheral edema was studied in a case series of five patients who had been treated with continuous infusions of hydromorphone or morphine [14]. The case series noted that resolution of the lower limb edema occurred within weeks or up to a few months of substituting intrathecal fentanyl for these opioid infusions.

The continued escalation of opioids to control similar pain stimuli is referred to as tolerance, and is a challenge with both systemic and intrathecally administered medication. It has been found that younger patients, especially those less than 50 years of age, are more susceptible [15]. This problem could possibly be mitigated by a low-opioid dosing strategy following an opioid weaning strategy [16, 17]. It is suggested that intrathecal drug delivery is more efficacious if patients are weaned from opioid medications prior to initiation of IDD, a concept known as 'microdosing' or low-opioid dosing. Grider et al. [16] and Hamza et al. [17] showed that when opioid dosing was initiated at a lower dose following oral opioid weaning, the patients experienced sustained pain relief with a slower rate of dose escalation and less requirement for concomitant oral opioids. This factor should be considered prior to implantation, but it may not be applicable to all patients, including those with cancer pain, who may not tolerate opioid weaning.

Withdrawal syndrome can occur with failure to refill the pump when required, iatrogenic pump programming or refill error, and catheter or pump malfunction. A case series of IDD device motor stalls showed that prevalence was higher with off-label medications, but device failure could also occur while using approved medications [18]. The length of time from implantation was found to be most correlated with motor stall. Patients should be educated to recognize withdrawal symptoms, as well as the critical error alarm of the device, so that they can seek medical assistance in an appropriate and timely manner. Patients suffering from withdrawal will experience hyperalgesia followed by 'flu-like' symptoms [19]. These symptoms, arising within 72 h of cessation of the infusion, include diarrhea, nausea, vomiting, ataxia, and/or an impairment in olfactory ability [20, 21].

Granuloma formation at the intrathecal catheter tip has been implicated with chronic use of a high concentration or dose of intrathecal opioids. Enlargement of the granuloma may eventually lead to compression of the spinal cord and neurologic injury [12]. Neurologic deficits include paralysis, loss of sensation, or bladder and/or bowel incontinence, but the earliest manifestation of an intrathecal granuloma is increased pain. Granulomas leading to neurologic deficits may require surgical resection [22]. Otherwise, granuloma resorption can be attempted by cessation of opiate drug delivery and replacement of the pump solution with preservative-free normal saline [23]. Among commonly used intrathecal opioids, infusion of morphine and hydromorphone in canine subjects has shown that these medications lead to aggregation of inflammatory cells and fibroblasts following meningeal mast cell degranulation [24]. Intrathecal infusion of fentanyl did not lead to such an inflammatory response. Figure 31.1 shows a granuloma at the fenestration of an intrathecal catheter following surgical removal [25]. Figure 31.2 illustrates MRI imaging of a granuloma along a catheter tip.

31.4 Local Anesthetics

Intrathecal bupivacaine is often used concomitantly with an opioid. In combination, the drugs may act synergistically to decrease the overall dose requirement for therapeutic pain relief, as seen in the treatment of acute pain in animal studies. This effect was shown in a retrospective study of patients with non-cancer pain, in whom the rate of dose escalation was decreased by 65% through the first year of intrathecal drug delivery [1]. However, the concomitant use of bupivacaine with opioid may not provide additional analgesic therapeutic effect [26]. The maximal daily bupivacaine dosage in that study was 8 mg/day, which was less than the average 10 mg/day in other studies [1, 27, 28]. A recent study examined the use of an admixture of bupivacaine and hydromorphone in a homogeneous cohort of patients with lumbar

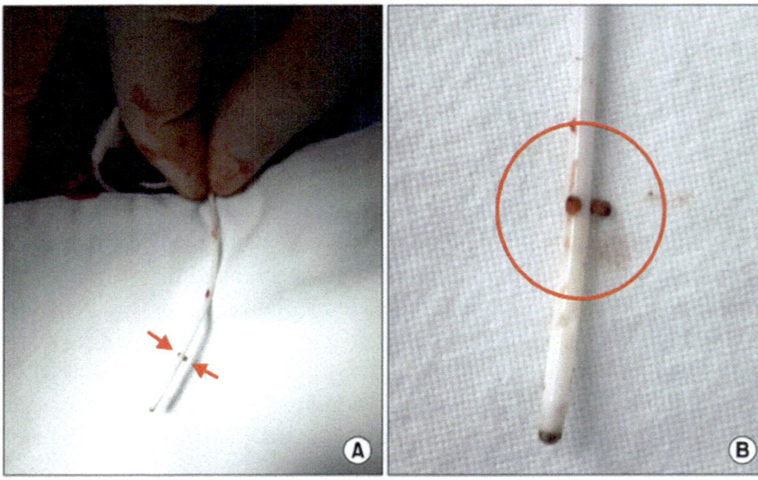

Fig. 31.1 Granuloma formation at the fenestration of an intrathecal catheter [25]. (**a**) Removal of the catheter from the patient. The side hole of the catheter was plugged. (**b**) Magnified picture of the catheter tip

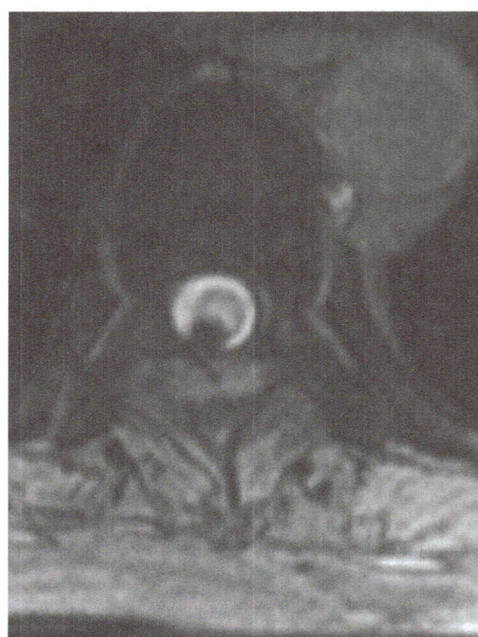

Fig. 31.2 T2-weighted MRI imaging of thoracic spine in axial view, showing granuloma formation along the catheter tip, causing compression of the spinal cord

post-laminectomy syndrome from the trial outset and followed the patients for 24 months [28]. The study showed that persistent pain relief was maintained through 2 years after implantation and was augmented by the use of a patient-activated bolus device. As discussed previously, the importance of limiting high-dose intrathecal

Table 31.2 Recommended dosing of intrathecal non-opioids

Intrathecal non-opioid	Starting dose	Bolus	Maximum dose per day	Maximum concentration
Ziconotide	0.5–1.2 μg/day (to 2.4 μg/day per product labeling)	1–5 μg	19.2 μg	100 μg/mL
Bupivacaine	0.01–4 mg/day	0.5–2.5 mg	10 mg	30 mg/mL
Clonidine	20–100 μg/day	5–20 μg	600 μg	1000 μg/mL

opioid therapy is centered on decreasing dose escalation leading to tolerance, as well as possibly limiting the advent of catheter tip granuloma formation and other opioid-related adverse events that were previously noted. It should be noted that there is not yet any strong evidence of the prevention of such events.

The mechanism of action of all local anesthetics involves the inactivation of membrane-bound voltage-gated sodium channels on neurons. Local anesthetics have been shown to have preferential effect on the nerve rootlets that attach to the spinal cord, also known as the fila radicularia [29]. The recommended initial dosing, bolus, maximum recommended dose, and maximum concentrations were discussed at the Polyanalgesic Consensus Conference [11] and are listed in Table 31.2.

31.4.1 Adverse Effects of Local Anesthetics

Uncommonly, circulating levels of local anesthetics can lead to neurotoxicity and cardiotoxicity, but intrathecal delivery of these medications results in almost insignificant circulating levels unless there is intravascular cannulation. Signs of neurotoxicity include dizziness, tinnitus, and seizures [30, 31]. Ropivacaine, a local anesthetic that has both similar chemical structure and pharmacologic properties to bupivacaine, has been shown to carry a lower risk of neurotoxicity in multiple animal studies [32–34]. There are few data from human studies demonstrating its safety and efficacy in IDD, however. Cardiotoxicity generally occurs with a plasma concentration 3.5–6.7 times higher than the concentration that causes neurotoxicity [35]. Myocardial contractility is impaired, and the conduction velocity is decreased. Patients may experience profound vasodilatation, bradycardia, arrhythmias, or even asystole [31]. Levobupivacaine has been found to have less cardiotoxic potential than bupivacaine, but its use has not been validated in IDD systems [36].

More common complaints from patients include hypotension, urinary retention, paresthesia, and motor weakness [32, 37, 38]. If these effects become intolerable for the patient, the concentration of bupivacaine can be decreased. Patients experience no drug withdrawal phenomenon if a catheter or pump failure occurs or if medication changes dictate removing bupivacaine.

31.5 Ziconotide

Ziconotide is the only other intrathecal drug approved by the FDA for treatment of chronic pain not responsive to systemic medications or any other adjunctive therapies aside from morphine. It is also considered a first-line option for the intrathecal treatment of both nociceptive and neuropathic pain [11]. Multiple randomized controlled trials have demonstrated its safety and efficacy in IDD systems [39–41].

Ziconotide was originally derived from the venom of *Conus magus*, a sea snail [42]. Its mechanism is based on the inactivation of presynaptic neuronal calcium channels [43]. This leads to a decrease in release of substance P, glutamate, and calcitonin gene-related peptide, all of which have been implicated in the transmission of the pain-signaling pathways. The drug effect is terminated following diffusion into plasma and metabolism by plasma peptidases and proteases [44]. The recommended initial dosing, bolus, maximum recommended dose, and maximum concentrations were discussed at the Polyanalgesic Consensus Conference. An interdisciplinary expert panel convened and published their recommendations, which are listed in Table 31.2 [11].

31.5.1 Adverse Effects of Ziconotide

Many studies have shown ziconotide to be safe and effective, but its use is limited by significant cerebrovestibular and neuropsychological adverse effects. Titration of this drug must be performed slowly to limit possible impairment. Possible neurologic effects include nausea, vomiting, dizziness, nystagmus, confusion, and impaired memory [45, 46]. Psychological effects can include depression and suicidal ideation; patients who have had a past medical history of comorbid psychiatric conditions are particularly susceptible [47]. A thorough psychiatric history prior to selecting this medication is required, and its use should be limited in patients with a history of depression and suicidal risk. Adverse effects are generally proportional to the dosing of the medication, patient age, and increased titration rate [39]. Discontinuation secondary to intolerance of side effects has been noted to be as high as 61% in one study [45]. In 2008, Ver Donck et al. [48] found that adverse events were experienced by 90.1% of patients during titration; they suggested that a short-term trial is sufficient to determine both effectiveness and intolerance of the medication. Ziconotide is not associated with withdrawal phenomena, granuloma formation, respiratory depression, or cardiotoxicity, as described for opioids and local anesthetics.

31.6 Clonidine

Intrathecal clonidine has also been used in the treatment of chronic pain. A retrospective study by Ackerman et al. [49] found that patients who received the medication experienced at least a 50% decrease in visual analog scale scores. The success of pain control was dependent on concomitant opioid use, which was also recommended in the Polyanalgesic Consensus Conference [11]. Recommendations for its use are also listed in Table 31.2. Clonidine is an α2-adrenergic agonist that decreases sympathetic outflow by inhibition of NF-κB and p38 in neurons, thereby inhibiting the upregulation of inflammatory cytokines [50]. In rodent studies, high doses of clonidine can lead to hypotension, bradycardia, and withdrawal symptoms [51]. Animal studies have not shown neurotoxicity, but its use is limited by effects that include night terrors, insomnia, depression, and severe dry mouth [52]. Pump failure in patients using intrathecal clonidine can lead to acute withdrawal syndrome. Withdrawal symptoms may first appear as hypertensive crisis, followed by high-output cardiac failure [53]. Other possible symptoms can include hyperthermia, diaphoresis, and tachycardia.

31.7 Polyanalgesic Consensus Conference Guidelines

A multidisciplinary expert panel convenes at the Polyanalgesic Consensus Conference every few years and publishes guidelines for intrathecal therapy based on the best available evidence. The guidelines of 2016 created algorithms for treatment approaches to neuropathic and nociceptive pain, both cancer-related and not cancer-related. Symptomatic locality was also used to delineate treatment guidelines. Table 31.3 is an algorithmic approach towards treating localized nociceptive or neuropathic pain related to cancer or another terminal condition, and Table 31.4 is an algorithmic approach towards treating this kind of diffuse pain. Table 31.5 is an algorithmic approach towards treating localized nociceptive or neuropathic pain that is not cancer-related, and Table 31.6 is an algorithmic approach towards treating diffuse pain of this type.

31.8 Baclofen for Treatment of Spasticity

Baclofen is the only FDA-approved intrathecal medication recommended for use in the treatment of spasticity. It has been used in patients with multiple sclerosis, cerebral palsy, tardive dystonia, cerebral and spinal cord injury, tetanus, stiff-person syndrome, and complex regional pain syndrome [54].

As an inhibitory neurotransmitter, baclofen functions as a selective agonist of the $GABA_B$ G-protein coupled receptor [54]. Activation of this receptor leads to

Table 31.3 Treatment of localized nociceptive or neuropathic pain related to cancer or other terminal conditions

<table>
<tr><td>Line 1A</td><td colspan="2">Ziconotide</td><td colspan="4">Morphine</td></tr>
<tr><td>Line 1B</td><td colspan="2">Fentanyl</td><td colspan="4">Morphine or fentanyl + bupivacaine</td></tr>
<tr><td>Line 2</td><td>Hydromorphone</td><td>Hydromorphone + bupivacaine</td><td colspan="2">Hydromorphone or fentanyl or morphine + clonidine</td><td colspan="2">Morphine or hydromorphone or fentanyl + ziconotide</td></tr>
<tr><td>Line 3</td><td>Hydromorphone or morphine or fentanyl + bupivacaine + clonidine</td><td>Ziconotide + bupivacaine</td><td colspan="2">Ziconotide + clonidine</td><td>Hydromorphone or morphine or fentanyl + bupivacaine + ziconotide</td><td>Sufentanil</td></tr>
<tr><td>Line 4</td><td>Sufentanil + ziconotide</td><td>Sufentanil + bupivacaine</td><td>Baclofen</td><td>Sufentanil + clonidine</td><td>Bupivacaine + clonidine + ziconotide</td><td>Bupivacaine + clonidine</td></tr>
<tr><td>Line 5</td><td colspan="6">Sufentanil + bupivacaine + ziconotide</td></tr>
<tr><td>Line 6</td><td colspan="6">Opioid[a] + bupivacaine + clonidine + adjuvants[b]</td></tr>
</table>

[a]All known intrathecal opioids

[b]Adjuvants include midazolam, ketamine, octreotide

Table 31.4 Treatment of diffuse nociceptive or neuropathic pain related to cancer or other terminal conditions

<table>
<tr><td>Line 1A</td><td colspan="4">Ziconotide</td><td colspan="2">Morphine</td></tr>
<tr><td>Line 1B</td><td colspan="4">Hydromorphone</td><td colspan="2">Morphine or hydromorphone + bupivacaine</td></tr>
<tr><td>Line 2</td><td colspan="4">Hydromorphone or morphine + clonidine</td><td colspan="2">Morphine or hydromorphone + ziconotide</td></tr>
<tr><td>Line 3</td><td>Hydromorphone or morphine or fentanyl + bupivacaine + clonidine</td><td>Ziconotide + bupivacaine</td><td colspan="2">Ziconotide + clonidine</td><td>Hydromorphone or morphine or fentanyl + bupivacaine + ziconotide</td><td>Sufentanil</td></tr>
<tr><td>Line 4</td><td>Sufentanil + ziconotide</td><td>Baclofen</td><td>Sufentanil + bupivacaine</td><td>Sufentanil + clonidine</td><td>Bupivacaine + clonidine + ziconotide</td><td>Bupivacaine + clonidine</td></tr>
<tr><td>Line 5</td><td colspan="2">Sufentanil + bupivacaine + clonidine</td><td colspan="3">Sufentanil + bupivacaine + ziconotide</td><td>Sufentanil + clonidine + ziconotide</td></tr>
<tr><td colspan="3">Line 6</td><td colspan="4">Opioid[a] + bupivacaine + clonidine + adjuvants[b]</td></tr>
</table>

[a]All known intrathecal opioids
[b]Adjuvants include midazolam, ketamine, octreotide

Table 31.5 Treatment of localized nociceptive or neuropathic pain not related to cancer

Line 1A	Ziconotide		Morphine	
Line 1B	Fentanyl		Fentanyl + bupivacaine	
Line 2	Fentanyl + clonidine	Hydromorphone or morphine + bupivacaine	Fentanyl + bupivacaine + clonidine	Bupivacaine
Line 3	Fentanyl + ziconotide + bupivacaine	Morphine or hydromorphone + clonidine	Ziconotide + clonidine or bupivacaine or both	Bupivacaine + clonidine
Line 4	Sufentanil + bupivacaine or clonidine	Baclofen	Bupivacaine + clonidine + ziconotide	
Line 5	Sufentanil + bupivacaine + clonidine		Sufentanil + ziconotide	

Table 31.6 Treatment of diffuse nociceptive or neuropathic pain not related to cancer

<table>
<tr><td>Line 1A</td><td colspan="2">Morphine</td><td colspan="2">Ziconotide (should be used as first choice in patients with >120 morphine equivalents or fast systemic dose escalation, in the absence of history of psychosis)</td></tr>
<tr><td>Line 1B</td><td colspan="2">Hydromorphone</td><td colspan="2">Morphine or hydromorphone + bupivacaine</td></tr>
<tr><td>Line 2</td><td>Hydromorphone or morphine + clonidine</td><td colspan="2">Fentanyl + bupivacaine</td><td>Ziconotide + morphine or hydromorphone</td></tr>
<tr><td>Line 3</td><td>Hydromorphone or morphine + bupivacaine + clonidine</td><td>Fentanyl + ziconotide</td><td>Sufentanil + bupivacaine or clonidine</td><td>Ziconotide + clonidine or bupivacaine or both</td></tr>
<tr><td>Line 4</td><td>Fentanyl or sufentanil + bupivacaine or clonidine</td><td colspan="2">Sufentanil + ziconotide</td><td>Baclofen</td></tr>
<tr><td>Line 5</td><td colspan="4">Opioid + ziconotide + bupivacaine or clonidine</td></tr>
</table>

Table 31.7 Modified Ashworth spasticity scale

Score	Criteria
1	No increase in tone
2	Slight increase in tone, giving a "catch" when moved in flexion and/or extension
3	More marked increase in tone but affected part(s) easily flexed
4	Considerable increase in tone; passive movement difficult
5	Affected part(s) rigid in flexion or extension

decreased cyclic AMP, leading to decreased presynaptic calcium ion conductance and hyperpolarization by means of increased postsynaptic potassium ion conductance [55]. The drug acts on $GABA_B$ receptors located in the dorsal horn, thalamic nuclei, cerebellum, interpeduncular nucleus, and cerebral cortex. Similar to other intrathecally delivered medications, its bioavailability is much greater than it is with systemic administration. Baclofen is well absorbed orally, but it cannot effectively penetrate the blood-brain barrier [55]. Administration can lead to neurologic complaints including nausea, sedation, muscle weakness, hypotonia, hypotension, ataxia, and a lowered seizure threshold [56]. Baclofen is slightly hydrophilic and therefore has a large bioavailability when used intrathecally; plasma concentrations are almost undetectable when delivered via this route [54]. In 1991, Kroin and Penn [57] demonstrated that there is a concentration gradient in intrathecal baclofen: the concentration is higher in the lumbar CSF, which may be beneficial for efficacy and the reduction of unwanted neurologic symptoms.

Patients who do not respond well to oral baclofen or who become intolerant of adverse effects are candidates for IDD. Both safety and clinical efficacy to decrease spasticity have been well established in randomized controlled studies [58, 59]. A successful trial is described as a decrease of one or two points on the Modified Ashworth Spasticity Scale, suggesting that IDDS implantation would also be successful (Table 31.7). Dosing of baclofen varies greatly and is dependent on the patient's symptoms. Generally, the daily infusion dose is initiated at once to twice the effective dose determined during the trial period [54]. The daily recommended intrathecal dosage for treatment of spasticity from cancer pain can be 10–1000 mg/day, with the maximum recommended concentration at 2 mg/mL [60]. There is presently a clinic trial pending that is testing the safety of 3 mg/mL. Overdose from the medication appears as exaggerated effect and can be treated supportively with respiratory support, in addition to intravenous physostigmine, which is an acetylcholinesterase inhibitor.

Withdrawal from baclofen can be life-threatening. Should iatrogenic error or pump failure occur, patients will present with hypertonicity, fever, pruritus, seizures, and/or hallucinations. If not emergently treated with oral or intrathecal baclofen, symptoms can lead to life-threatening conditions through rhabdomyolysis, multisystem organ failure, and disseminated intravascular coagulopathy. The use of benzodiazepine infusion has also been reported effective in treating withdrawal, if baclofen is not available [55]. If discontinuation of intrathecal baclofen is required, weaning should occur over a period of 2–4 weeks.

31.9 Conclusions

There are many factors to consider in determining appropriate medication selection for patients who have IDDS used for chronic pain. The clinician must take into account patient characteristics that include the location of symptoms, etiology, and the patient's sex and age. The side-effect profile of intrathecal medications must also be considered, with the clinician able to make changes to the infused drug, drug concentrations, and dosing as directed by the observed level of patient efficacy and in consideration of poorly tolerated adverse effects. Tables 31.1 and 31.2 list some guidelines as to appropriate concentrations, starting doses, and maximum doses.

References

1. Veizi IE, Hayek SM, Narouze S, Pope JE, Mekhail N. Combination of intrathecal opioids with bupivacaine attenuates opioid dose escalation in chronic noncancer pain patients. Pain Med. 2011;12:1481–9.
2. Dominguez E, Sahinler B, Bassam D, Day M, Lou L, Racz G, et al. Predictive value of intrathecal narcotic trials for long-term therapy with implantable drug administration systems in chronic non-cancer pain patients. Pain Pract. 2002;2:315–25.
3. Flack SH, Bernards CM. Cerebrospinal fluid and spinal cord distribution of hyperbaric bupivacaine and baclofen during slow intrathecal infusion in pigs. Anesthesiology. 2010;112:165–73.
4. Mekhail N, Mahboobi R, Farajzadeh Deroee A, Costandi S, Dalton J, et al. Factors that might impact intrathecal drug delivery (IDD) dose escalation: a longitudinal study. Pain Pract. 2014;14:301–8.
5. Coffey RJ, Owens ML, Broste SK, Dubois MY, Ferrante FM, Schultz DM, et al. Medical practice perspective: identification and mitigation of risk factors for mortality associated with intrathecal opioids for non-cancer pain. Pain Med. 2010;11:1001–9.
6. Urman RD. National perioperative outcomes for intrathecal pump, spinal cord stimulator, and peripheral nerve stimulator procedures. Pain Physician. 2015;18:547–54.
7. Smith TJ, Staats PS, Deer T, Stearns LJ, Rauck RL, Boortz-Marx RL, et al. Implantable Drug Delivery Systems Study Group. Randomized clinical trial of an implantable drug delivery system compared with comprehensive medical management for refractory cancer pain: impact on pain, drug-related toxicity, and survival. J Clin Oncol. 2002;20:4040–9.
8. Herz A, Albus K, Metys J, Schubert P, Teschemacher H. On the central sites for the antinociceptive action of morphine and fentanyl. Neuropharmacology. 1970;9:539–51.
9. Herz A, Teschemacher HJ. Activities and sites of antinociceptive action of morphine-like analgesics and kinetics of distribution following intravenous, intracerebral and intraventricular application. Adv Drug Res. 1971;6:79–119.
10. Ummenhofer WC, Arends RH, Shen DD, Bernards CM. Comparative spinal distribution and clearance kinetics of intrathecally administered morphine, fentanyl, alfentanil, and sufentanil. Anesthesiology. 2000;92:739–53.
11. Deer TR, Pope JE, Hayek S, Bux A, Buchser E, Eldabe S, et al. The polyanalgesic consensus conference (PACC): recommendations on intrathecal drug infusion systems best practices and guidelines. Neuromodulation. 2017. https://doi.org/10.1111/ner.12538.
12. North RB, Cutchis PN, Epstein JA, Long DM. Spinal cord compression complicating subarachnoid infusion of morphine: case report and laboratory experience. Neurosurgery. 1991;29:778–84.

13. Coffey RJ, Owens ML, Broste SK, Dubois MY, Ferrante FM, Schultz DM, et al. Mortality associated with implantation and management of intrathecal opioid drug infusion systems to treat noncancer pain. Anesthesiology. 2009;111:881–91.
14. Veizi E, Tornero-Bold M, Hayek SM. Resolution of intrathecal hydromorphone or morphine-induced peripheral edema by opioid rotation to fentanyl: a case series. Pain Pract. 2016;16:E94–8.
15. Hayek SM, Veizi IE, Narouze SN, Mekhail N. Age-dependent intrathecal opioid escalation in chronic noncancer pain patients. Pain Med. 2011;12:1179–89.
16. Grider JSH, Harned ME, Etscheidt MA. Patient selection and outcomes using a low-dose intrathecal opioid trialing method for chronic nonmalignant pain. Pain Physician. 2011;14:343–51.
17. Hamza M, Doleys D, Wells M, Weisbein J, Hoff J, Martin M, et al. Prospective study of 3-year follow-up of low-dose intrathecal opioids in the management of chronic nonmalignant pain. Pain Med. 2012;13:1304–13.
18. Galica R, Hayek SM, Veizi IE, Lawrence MM, Khalil AA, McEwan MT. sudden intrathecal drug delivery device motor stalls: a case series. Reg Anesth Pain Med. 2016;41:135–9.
19. Singla A, Stojanovic MP, Chen L, Mao J. A differential diagnosis of hyperalgesia, toxicity, and withdrawal from intrathecal morphine infusion. Anesth Analg. 2007;105:1816–9.
20. Compton P, Athanasos P, Elashoff D. Withdrawal hyperalgesia after acute opioid physical dependence in nonaddicted humans: a preliminary study. J Pain. 2003;4(9):511.
21. Devulder J, Bohyn P, Castille F, De Laat M, Rolly G. A case of uncommon withdrawal symptoms after a short period of spinal morphine administration. Pain. 1996;64:589–91.
22. Tomycz ND, Ortiz V, McFadden KA, Urgo L, Moossy JJ. Management of symptomatic intrathecal catheter-associated inflammatory masses. Clin Neurol Neurosurg. 2012;114:190–5.
23. Deer TR, Prager J, Levy R, Rathmell J, Buchser E, Burton A, et al. Polyanalgesic consensus conference—2012: consensus on diagnosis, detection, and treatment of catheter-tip granulomas (inflammatory masses). Neuromodulation. 2012;15:483–95.
24. Yaksh TL, Allen JW, Veesart SL, Horais KA, Malkmus SA, Scadeng M, et al. Role of meningeal mast cells in intrathecal morphine-evoked granuloma formation. Anesthesiology. 2013;118:664–78.
25. Rhee SM, Choi EJ, Lee PB, Nahm FS. Catheter obstruction of intrathecal drug administration system—a case report. Korean J Pain. 2012;25:47–51.
26. Mironer YE, Haasis JC, Chapple I, Brown C, Satterthwaite JR. Efficacy and safety of intrathecal opioids/bupivacaine mixture in chronic nonmalignant pain: a double blind, randomized, crossover, multicenter study by the National Forum of Independent Pain Clinicians (NFIPC). Neuromodulation. 2002;5:208–13.
27. Deer TR, Caraway DL, Kim CK, Dempsey CD, Stewart CD, McNeil KF. Clinical experience with intrathecal bupivacaine in combination with opioid for the treatment of chronic pain related to failed back surgery syndrome and metastatic cancer pain of the spine. Spine J. 2002;2:274–8.
28. Hayek SM, Veizi E, Hanes M. Intrathecal hydromorphone and bupivacaine combination therapy for post-laminectomy syndrome optimized with patient-activated bolus device. Pain Med. 2016;17:561–71.
29. Boswell MV, Iacono RP, Guthkelch AN. Sites of action of subarachnoid lidocaine and tetracaine: observations with evoked potential monitoring during spinal cord stimulator implantation. Reg Anesth. 1992;17:37–42.
30. Schug SA, Saunders D, Kurowski I, Paech MJ. Neuraxial drug administration: a review of treatment options for anaesthesia and analgesia. CNS Drugs. 2006;20:917–33.
31. Naguib M, Magboul MM, Samarkandi AH, Attia M. Adverse effects and drug interactions associated with local and regional anaesthesia. Drug Saf. 1998;18:221–50.
32. Zhong Z, Qulian G, Yuan Z, Wangyuan Z, Zhihua S. Repeated intrathecal administration of ropivacaine causes neurotoxicity in rats. Anaesth Intensive Care. 2009;37:929–36.

33. Malinovsky JM, Charles F, Baudrimont M, Pereon Y, Le Corre P, Pinaud M, et al. Intrathecal ropivacaine in rabbits: pharmacodynamic and neurotoxicologic study. Anesthesiology. 2002;97:429–35.
34. Yamashita A, Matsumoto M, Matsumoto S, Itoh M, Kawai K, Sakabe T. A comparison of the neurotoxic effects on the spinal cord of tetracaine, lidocaine, bupivacaine, and ropivacaine administered intrathecally in rabbits. Anesth Analg. 2003;97:512–9.
35. Liu PL, Feldman HS, Giasi R, Patterson MK, Covino BG. Comparative CNS toxicity of lidocaine, etidocaine, bupivacaine, and tetracaine in awake dogs following rapid intravenous administration. Anesth Analg. 1983;62:375–9.
36. Morrison SG, Dominguez JJ, Frascarolo P, Reiz S. A comparison of the electrocardiographic cardiotoxic effects of racemic bupivacaine, levobupivacaine, and ropivacaine in anesthetized swine. Anesth Analg. 2000;90:1308–14.
37. Sjoberg M, Nitescu P, Appelgren L, Curelaru I. Long-term intrathecal morphine and bupivacaine in patients with refractory cancer pain. Results from a morphine:bupivacaine dose regimen of 0.5:4.75 mg/ml. Anesthesiology. 1994;80:284–97.
38. Nitescu P, Dahm P, Appelgren L, Curelaru I. Continuous infusion of opioid and bupivacaine by externalized intrathecal catheters in long-term treatment of "refractory" nonmalignant pain. Clin J Pain. 1998;14:17–28.
39. Rauck RL, Wallace MS, Leong MS, Minehart M, Webster LR, Charapata SG, et al. A randomized, double-blind, placebo-controlled study of intrathecal ziconotide in adults with severe chronic pain. J Pain Symptom Manag. 2006;31:393–406.
40. Staats PS, Yearwood T, Charapata SG, Presley RW, Wallace MS, Byas-Smith M, et al. Intrathecal ziconotide in the treatment of refractory pain in patients with cancer or AIDS: a randomized controlled trial. JAMA. 2004;291:63–70.
41. Wallace MS, Charapata SG, Fisher R, Byas-Smith M, Staats PS, Mayo M, et al. Intrathecal ziconotide in the treatment of chronic nonmalignant pain: a randomized, double-blind, placebo-controlled clinical trial. Neuromodulation. 2006;9:75–86.
42. Miljanich GP. Ziconotide: neuronal calcium channel blocker for treating severe chronic pain. Curr Med Chem. 2004;11:3029–40.
43. McGivern JG. Ziconotide: a review of its pharmacology and use in the treatment of pain. Neuropsychiatr Dis Treat. 2007;3:69–85.
44. Wermeling D, Drass M, Ellis D, Mayo M, McGuire D, O'Connell D, et al. Pharmacokinetics and pharmacodynamics of intrathecal ziconotide in chronic pain patients. J Clin Pharmacol. 2003;43:624–36.
45. Wallace MS, Rauck R, Fisher R, Charapata SG, Ellis D, Dissanayake S. Intrathecal ziconotide for severe chronic pain: safety and tolerability results of an open-label, long-term trial. Anesth Analg. 2008;106:628–37.
46. Hayek SM, Hanes MC, Wang C, Veizi IE. Ziconotide combination intrathecal therapy for noncancer pain is limited secondary to delayed adverse effects: a case series with a 24-month follow-up. Neuromodulation. 2015;18:397–403.
47. Maier C, Gockel HH, Gruhn K, Krumova EK, Edel MA. Increased risk of suicide under intrathecal ziconotide treatment? A warning. Pain. 2011;152:235–7.
48. Ver Donck A, Collins R, Rauck RL, Nitescu P. An open-label, multicenter study of the safety and efficacy of intrathecal ziconotide for severe chronic pain when delivered via an external pump. Neuromodulation. 2008;11:103–11.
49. Ackerman LL, Follett KA, Rosenquist RW. Long-term outcomes during treatment of chronic pain with intrathecal clonidine or clonidine/opioid combinations. J Pain Symptom Manag. 2003;26:668–77.
50. Feng X, Zhang F, Dong R, Li W, Liu J, Zhao X, et al. Intrathecal administration of clonidine attenuates spinal neuroimmune activation in a rat model of neuropathic pain with existing hyperalgesia. Eur J Pharmacol. 2009;614:38–43.

51. Naruse T, Ishida T, Ishii R, Tagawa T, Namba K. Relationship between hypotensive effects and plasma concentrations of clonidine in spontaneously hypertensive rats: continuous treatment and sudden termination of clonidine infusion. Gen Pharmacol. 1994;25:1421–5.
52. Bevacqua BK, Fattouh M, Backonja M. Depression, night terrors, and insomnia associated with long-term intrathecal clonidine therapy. Pain Pract. 2007;7:36–8.
53. Lee HM, Ruggoo V, Graudins A. Intrathecal clonidine pump failure causing acute withdrawal syndrome with 'stress-induced' cardiomyopathy. J Med Toxicol. 2016;12:134–8.
54. Penn RD, Kroin JS. Continuous intrathecal baclofen for severe spasticity. Lancet. 1985;2(8447):125–7.
55. Hayek SM, Joseph PN, Mekhail NA. Pharmacology of intrathecally administered agents for treatment of spasticity and pain. Semin Pain Med. 2003;1(4):238–53.
56. Gracies JM, Nance P, Elovic E, McGuire J, Simpson DM. Traditional pharmacological treatments for spasticity. Part II: general and regional treatments. Muscle Nerve Suppl. 1997;6:S92–120.
57. Kroin JS, Penn RD. Cerebrospinal fluid pharmacokinetics of lumbar intrathecal baclofen. In: Lakke JP, Delhaas EM, Rutgers AW, editors. Parenteral drug therapy in spasticity and Parkinson's disease. New York, NY: Parthenon; 1991. p. 73–83.
58. Hoving MA, van Raak EP, Spincemaille GH, Palmans LJ, Becher JG, Vles JS, Dutch Study Group on Child Spasticity. Efficacy of intrathecal baclofen therapy in children with intractable spastic cerebral palsy: a randomised controlled trial. Eur J Paediatr Neurol. 2009;13:240–6.
59. Hoving MA, van Raak EP, Spincemaille GH, Palmans LJ, Sleypen FA, Vles JS, Dutch Study Group on Child Spasticity. Intrathecal baclofen in children with spastic cerebral palsy: a double-blind, randomized, placebo-controlled, dose-finding study. Dev Med Child Neurol. 2007;49:654–9.
60. Stearns L, Boortz-Marx R, Du Pen S, Friehs G, Gordon M, Halyard M, et al. Intrathecal drug delivery for the management of cancer pain: a multidisciplinary consensus of best clinical practices. J Support Oncol. 2005;3:399–408.

Chapter 32
Intrathecal Drug Delivery: Trialing

Lucas W. Campos and Jason E. Pope

Use of an implanted intrathecal drug delivery system (IDDS) in the treatment of intractable cancer and non-cancer chronic pain has been a valuable therapy over the last three decades [1]. In addition to cancer-related pain, intrathecal drug therapy (IDT) is also used in spasticity, failed back surgery syndrome, complex regional pain syndrome, and vertebral compression fractures when other conservative measures have failed [2]. There has been a paradigm shift. The recent consensus guidelines from the Polyanalgesic Consensus Conference (PACC) of 2017 review the best trial practices, such as appropriate first line agents, trial methods, and medication trial dosing, among many other practices [3]. This chapter reviews these and other concerns surrounding trials for long-term intrathecal infusion.

32.1 Introduction

With intrathecal delivery, medications are delivered directly to the spinal cord, avoiding first-pass metabolism and the blood-brain barrier [4]. This allows analgesia to occur with much smaller doses and a lower incidence of toxicity [5]. Success with IDT hinges on a thorough understanding of the pain condition, careful patient selection, and agreement between the patient and provider of what a successful outcome looks like. With advances in intrathecal (IT) pump technology and decreases in the cost of intrathecal hardware, along with a growing body of meaningful, functional outcomes, this therapeutic option has grown far beyond a salvage therapy [6]. Quality-of-life measures and overall healthcare utilization costs are decreased when IT drug delivery is compared with conventional medical management alone [7].

L.W. Campos (✉) • J.E. Pope
Summit Pain Alliance, Santa Rosa, CA, USA
e-mail: lwcamposmdphd@gmail.com; popeje@me.com

S. Diwan, T.R. Deer (eds.), *Advanced Procedures for Pain Management*,
https://doi.org/10.1007/978-3-319-68841-1_32

Trialing was introduced to offer the clinician and patient a preview of what could result with longer term infusion by an implanted pump. Unfortunately, no trialing method has proven to be superior to another in regard to predicting long-term efficacy of IT infusion [2]. Understanding this divergence may come from better data regarding pharmacokinetic and pharmacodynamic of medications in the IT space, as well as an improved understanding of the IT environment itself [8–10].

Despite a lack of evidence of its necessity, an intrathecal trial has been considered the standard of care [11]. A trial was considered reasonable because some measure of established efficacy supports the risk and cost of implanting this type of pain-control device. A trial is still required by many insurers, even as the necessity and predictive value of the trial has come under increasing scrutiny [12]. In 2012, the PACC revised their recommendations on IT trialing, stating that the need for trialing was debatable, particularly in patients with cancer pain [13]. Their reasoning was that a trial may underestimate potential side effects and the failure rate of the therapy. If medications are delivered in the same manner as intended for chronic delivery, the trial may hold more relevance.

32.2 Background and Historical Perspective

Historically, the use of bolus intrathecal drug trialing was thought to be superior to continuous or epidural trial methods. In a retrospective review, Maniker et al. reported that epidural infusion is an effective trialing method, but it overestimates the IT dosages needed for pain control [14]. Results from the epidural-trialed patients may be even more confounded due to the lack of an established dose equivalency when considering rate of infusion and volume infused. Anderson et al. showed more side effects during IT bolus trials compared to continuous infusions, but no difference in efficacy [15]. Krames [16] suggested that bolus trials were limited because of their inherent short duration, possible placebo effects, and lack of simulation of final pump implant. Mohammed et al. [43] and later Pope et al. [44] demonstrated a dual diagnostic strategy for the investigation of pump candidacy and dose, suggesting a better representative trial to permanent ratio. Later, Hamza et al. [17, 18] showed that there is no superior trialing method. There are equal levels of evidence for single shot trialing, bolus trialing, and continuous infusion [3].

32.3 Indications

A definable pain diagnosis that covers the regional area of interest, such as peripheral neuropathy, complex regional pain syndrome, severe rheumatoid or osteoarthritis, should be well established, and failure of conservative medical care should be confirmed. The on-label use of intrathecal therapy is "intractable pain of the trunk or limb." Patient candidacy hinges on the ability to place an intrathecal catheter regionally in the posterior intrathecal space that allows for coverage. Understandably, other variables exist, including previous treatment failure, age, physiochemical properties of the medication employed, and life expectancy [42]. Further, patients who receive substantial pain relief from oral opiates but develop intolerable sedation, constipation, and other adverse effects, are ideal candidates for IDDS placement. IT delivery allows many patients to achieve analgesia while avoiding the cognitive and gastrointestinal side effects. Refractory pain, not salvage pain treatment, is the appropriate position within the pain care algorithm.

32.4 Patient Selection

Judicious patient selection is perhaps the most important strategy for achieving lasting success with IT drug therapy, and this involves input from the interventionalist, mental health professionals, patients, and their caregivers. Several stepwise algorithms to identify candidates for consideration of intrathecal drug delivery have been suggested, all with a focus on evaluating and optimizing the multiple comorbidities on which chronic pain has an impact [3, 19]. First, a pain diagnosis is established. Second, a possible IDDS solution is presented to the patient, and expectations, comprehension, and support networks are assessed. It is vital for practitioners to set realistic expectations and to establish the patient's definition of a successful outcome. Third, patients are evaluated and treated for psychological comorbidities [16]. The psychological evaluation is particularly important when considering the use of ziconotide, as a history of psychosis is a contraindication [3, 20, 21]. Preexisting psychopathology is thought to predispose patients to new adverse psychiatric events after initiation of ziconotide therapy [22]. Patient dissatisfaction with IT therapy remains a significant reason for premature revision or removal of IDDS, although the majority report satisfaction with the therapy 12 months after implant [23]. Patient selection centers on evaluating how the patient will engage with his or her IDDS device.

32.5 Trial Success

If a trial is performed, it is critical to define what constitutes trial success. The trial provides information regarding improvement in function, likelihood of side effects, and appropriate starting doses of the trial medication. Each of these variables is measured and evaluated is based on a patient's expectations. The pain relief endpoint of an IT trial is generally defined, in both research protocols and clinical practice, as a 50% decrease in pain [24–26].

32.6 Function

Many implanters consider improvement of function as an important endpoint [26, 27]. Referral to a physical therapist during a trial is one approach. Expectations for function may vary based on the underlying disease and life expectancy. Functional assessment during an IT trial can be obtained by evaluating the Oswestry Disability Index (ODI) or other functional objective measures, such as moving from supine to sitting position, sitting to standing, picking up objects from the floor, and tolerance of ambulation [28].

32.7 Trialing Method

An intrathecal trial can be accomplished via a single bolus, multiple boluses, or continuous infusion technique via a catheter inserted into the intrathecal space [18]. Continuous infusion mimics the pharmacokinetics of delivery via an implanted pump, and avoids fluctuating drug levels seen with repeated intermittent bolus trials [3, 29]. Continuous catheter trials allow for dose titration targeting a particular dermatome, and direct observation of the patient throughout the trial. Continuous catheter trials have been accomplished using either epidural or IT route, although the intrathecal route is recommended [15, 30–32]. The recommended starting doses by the 2017 PACC are listed in Table 32.1.

A single-bolus IT injection allows for a quicker trial, fewer confounders of possible side effects, less infection risk, and viability in an outpatient setting compared to an indwelling catheter trial [17, 33]. Bolus trials may result in a more widespread distribution of injected substances within the IT space, which is possibly due to increased kinetic energy during the injection process [34, 35]. However, patients may need to have repeat injections. Single-bolus IT injections, titrated to effect on separate days, have been used in trialing morphine, ziconotide, and baclofen [36, 37]. The recommended starting doses by the 2017 PACC are listed in Table 32.2.

Site of service needs to be considered when trialing opioids. It is critical to maintain conservative dosing when opioid trials are performed as an outpatient. The PACC of 2017 specifically addressed trialing and the reader is directed there for in-depth discussion [3].

Table 32.1 Starting infusion trial dosage ranges for single medications intended for continuous IT trial recommended by the 2016 polyanalgesic consensus conference (PACC)

Drug	Dose
Morphine	0.1–0.5 mg/day
Hydromorphone	0.01–0.15 mg/day
Ziconotide	0.5–2.4 μg/day
Fentanyl	25–75 μg/day
Bupivacaine	0.01–4 mg/day

Table 32.2 Doses ranges for IT bolus trialing recommended by the 2016 polyanalgesic consensus conference (PACC)

Drug	Dose
Morphine	0.1–0.5 mg
Hydromorphone	0.025–0.1 mg
Ziconotide	1–5 μg
Fentanyl	15–75 μg
Bupivacaine	0.5–2.5 mg
Clonidine	5–20 μg

32.8 Combination Therapy

The 2017 Polyanalgesic Consensus Conference noted that a patient should first undergo a trial with an FDA-approved medication (Morphine, Ziconotide, and Baclofen) before attempting a trial using a combination of IT medications [3]. Despite the prevalent use of combination therapy throughout the world, there is a paucity of data on IT trialing with combinations of medications. A prospective observational pilot study was conducted using 26 patients with lumbar postlaminectomy pain, each of whom received an IT regimen consisting of morphine combined with bupivacaine, clonidine, or midazolam [30]. They found that intrathecal morphine combined with non-opioid drugs improved analgesic efficacy with few side effects. However, Medtronic issued a warning regarding increased risk of motor stall with use of unapproved drugs or admixture in the SynchroMed II pump [38], while the Prometra II pump by Flowonix does not have reduction in dosing accuracy or longevity to date.

32.9 Oral Opioids During Trialing

Reduction or elimination of oral opioids before trialing has become increasingly common. The 2017 PACC noted that systemic opioid reduction or elimination during the trial period was a strongly recommended goal [17]. However, in the absence of a personal therapy manager (PTM) for breakthrough pain, this goal may be difficult to achieve. During a Ziconotide trial, the risks of low-dose intermittent opioid rescue are small. Several small studies and case series demonstrate successful opiate tapering at or within 24 h of the initiation of the trial [15, 39]. Hamza et al. reported opioid reduction prior to trialing, with complete elimination of systemic opioids prior to implantation [17]. This study also resulted in stable analgesia over a 3-year period at relatively low IT doses. The presence of opioid-induced hyperalgesia could negatively impact the trial interpretation [13, 40]. Taken together, the evidence in favor of systemic opioid reduction is supported by multiple studies and case series [39, 41].

32.10 Conclusion

Advances in intrathecal pharmacology and intrathecal drug delivery systems have allowed for a range of medications to be trialed. IT therapy allows for reduced opiate doses, which can decrease the side effects typically associated with oral or parenteral delivery. There is no strong evidence that one trialing method is superior to another, or that a trial is even necessary. Recent expert panel consensus guidelines have provided care paths in the treatment of nociceptive, neuropathic, and mixed pain syndromes [42]. IT therapy is a rewarding offering that is vital in the community, and care needs to be taken when building a practice to serve this need.

References

1. Onofrio BM, Yaksh TL, Arnold PG. Continuous low-dose intrathecal morphine administration in the treatment of chronic pain of malignant origin. Mayo Clin Proc. 1981;56:516–20.
2. Burton AW, Deer TR, Wallace MS, Rauck RL, Grigsby E. Considerations and methodology for trialing ziconotide. Pain Physician. 2010;13:23–33.
3. Deer TR, Hayek SM, Pope JE, Lamer TJ, Hamza M, Grider JS, et al. The polyanalgesic consensus conference (PACC): recommendations for trialing of intrathecal drug delivery infusion therapy. Neuromodulation. 2017;20:133–54.
4. Yaksh TL, Rudy TA. Analgesia mediated by a direct spinal action of narcotics. Science. 1976;192:1357–8.
5. Li DF, Bahar M, Cole G, Rosen M. Neurological toxicity of the subarachnoid infusion of bupivacaine, lignocaine or 2-chloroprocaine in the rat. Br J Anaesth. 1985;57:424–9.
6. Bottros MM, Christo PJ. Current perspectives on intrathecal drug delivery. J Pain Res. 2014;7:615–26.
7. Taylor RS, Taylor RJ. The economic impact of failed back surgery syndrome. Br J Pain. 2012;6:174–81.
8. Cohen SP, Dragovich A. Intrathecal analgesia. Anesthesiol Clin. 2007;25:863–82. viii
9. Bernards CM. Understanding the physiology and pharmacology of epidural and intrathecal opioids. Best Pract Res Clin Anaesthesiol. 2002;16:489–505.
10. Przybyl JS, Follett KA, Caraway D. Intrathecal drug therapy: general considerations. Sem Pain Med. 2003;1:228–33.
11. Prager J, Deer T, Levy R, Bruel B, Buchser E, Caraway D, et al. Best practices for intrathecal drug delivery for pain. Neuromodulation. 2014;17:354–72; discussion 372.
12. Deer TR, Smith HS, Burton AW, Pope JE, Doleys DM, Levy RM, et al. Comprehensive consensus based guidelines on intrathecal drug delivery systems in the treatment of pain caused by cancer pain. Pain Physician. 2011;14:E283–312.
13. Deer TR, Prager J, Levy R, Burton A, Buchser E, Caraway D, et al. Polyanalgesic consensus conference—2012: recommendations on trialing for intrathecal (intraspinal) drug delivery: report of an interdisciplinary expert panel. Neuromodulation. 2012;15:420–35; discussion 435.
14. Maniker AH, Krieger AJ, Adler RJ, Hupert C. Epidural trial in implantation of intrathecal morphine infusion pumps. N J Med. 1991;88:797–801.
15. Anderson VC, Burchiel KJ, Cooke B. A prospective, randomized trial of intrathecal injection vs. epidural infusion in the selection of patients for continuous intrathecal opioid therapy. Neuromodulation. 2003;6:142–52.

16. Krames ES, Olson K. Clinical realities and economic considerations: patient selection in intrathecal therapy. J Pain Symptom Manag. 1997;14:S3–13.
17. Hamza M, Doleys D, Wells M, Weisbein J, Hoff J, Martin M, et al. Prospective study of 3-year follow-up of low-dose intrathecal opioids in the management of chronic nonmalignant pain. Pain Med. 2012;13:1304–13.
18. Hamza M, Doleys DM, Saleh IA, Medvedovsky A, Verdolin MH, Hamza M. A prospective, randomized, single-blinded, head-to-head long-term outcome study, comparing intrathecal (IT) boluses with continuous infusion trialing techniques prior to implantation of drug delivery systems (DDS) for the treatment of severe intractable chronic nonmalignant pain. Neuromodulation. 2015;18:636–49.
19. Ver Donck A, Vranken JH, Puylaert M, Hayek S, Mekhail N, Van Zundert J. Intrathecal drug administration in chronic pain syndromes. Pain Pract. 2014;14:461–76.
20. Maier C, Gockel H-H, Gruhn K, Krumova EK, Edel MA. Increased risk of suicide under intrathecal ziconotide treatment? A warning. Pain. 2011;152:235–7.
21. Thompson JC, Dunbar E, Laye RR. Treatment challenges and complications with ziconotide monotherapy in established pump patients. Pain Physician. 2006;9:147–52.
22. Schmidtko A, Lötsch J, Freynhagen R, Geisslinger G. Ziconotide for treatment of severe chronic pain. Lancet. 2010;375:1569–77.
23. Veizi IE, Hayek SM, Narouze S, Pope JE, Mekhail N. Combination of intrathecal opioids with bupivacaine attenuates opioid dose escalation in chronic noncancer pain patients. Pain Med. 2011;12:1481–9.
24. Smith TJ, Staats PS, Deer T, Stearns LJ, Rauck RL, Boortz-Marx RL, et al. Randomized clinical trial of an implantable drug delivery system compared with comprehensive medical management for refractory cancer pain: impact on pain, drug-related toxicity, and survival. J Clin Oncol. 2002;20:4040–9.
25. Lee J-W, Han KR, Kim S-H, Lee J-Y, Kim D-W, Kim C. Repetitive single subarachnoid injections for trial administration of the intrathecal morphine pump in patients with intractable non-cancer pain – a case report. Korean J Anesthesiol. 2011;60:138–41.
26. Knight KH, Brand FM, Mchaourab AS, Veneziano G. Implantable intrathecal pumps for chronic pain: highlights and updates. Croat Med J. 2007;48:22–34.
27. Falco FJE, Patel VB, Hayek SM, Deer TR, Geffert S, Zhu J, et al. Intrathecal infusion systems for long-term management of chronic non-cancer pain: an update of assessment of evidence. Pain Physician. 2013;16:SE185–216.
28. Grider JS, Harned ME, Etscheidt MA. Patient selection and outcomes using a low-dose intrathecal opioid trialing method for chronic nonmalignant pain. Pain Physician. 2011;14:343–51.
29. Kumar K, Kelly M, Pirlot T. Continuous intrathecal morphine treatment for chronic pain of nonmalignant etiology: long-term benefits and efficacy. Surg Neurol. 2001;55:79–86. discussion 86–8
30. Rainov NG, Heidecke V, Burkert W. Long-term intrathecal infusion of drug combinations for chronic back and leg pain. J Pain Symptom Manag. 2001;22:862–71.
31. Ruan X, Tadia R, Couch JP, Ruan J, Chiravuri S. Severe peripheral edema during an outpatient continuous epidural morphine infusion trial in a patient with failed back surgery syndrome. Pain Physician. 2008;11:363–7.
32. Wilkes D, Cook M, Solanki D. Intrathecal catheter-syringe adaptor for short-term intrathecal analgesia with an externalized pump: a case report. Pain Physician. 2010;13:151–6.
33. Dominguez E, Sahinler B, Bassam D, Day M, Lou L, Racz G, et al. Predictive value of intrathecal narcotic trials for long-term therapy with implantable drug administration systems in chronic non-cancer pain patients. Pain Pract. 2002;2:315–25.
34. Papisov MI, Belov VV, Gannon KS. Physiology of the intrathecal bolus: the leptomeningeal route for macromolecule and particle delivery to CNS. Mol Pharm. 2013;10:1522–32.
35. Rieselbach RE, Chiro GD, Freireich EJ. Subarachnoid distribution of drugs after lumbar injection. N Engl J Med. 1962;267:1273–8.

36. Pope JE, Deer TR. Intrathecal drug delivery for pain: a clinical guide and future directions. Pain Manag. 2015;5:175–83.
37. Dahm P, Nitescu P, Appelgren L, Curelaru I. Efficacy and technical complications of long-term continuous intraspinal infusions of opioid and/or bupivacaine in refractory nonmalignant pain: a comparison between the epidural and the intrathecal approach with externalized or implanted catheters and infusion pumps. Clin J Pain. 1998;14:4–16.
38. Smyth C, Ahmadzai N, Wentzell J, Pardoe A, Tse A, Nguyen T, et al. Intrathecal analgesia for chronic refractory pain: current and future prospects. Drugs. 2015;75:1957–80.
39. Shaladi A, Saltari MR, Piva B, Crestani F, Tartari S, Pinato P, et al. Continuous intrathecal morphine infusion in patients with vertebral fractures due to osteoporosis. Clin J Pain. 2007;23:511–7.
40. Deer TR. A critical time for practice change in the pain treatment continuum: we need to reconsider the role of pumps in the patient care algorithm. Pain Med. 2010;11:987–9.
41. Kim D, Saidov A, Mandhare V, Shuster A. Role of pretrial systemic opioid requirements, intrathecal trial dose, and non-psychological factors as predictors of outcome for intrathecal pump therapy: one clinician's experience with lumbar postlaminectomy pain. Neuromodulation. 2011;14:165–75; discussion 175.
42. Deer TR, Pope JE, Hayek SM, Bux A, Buchser E, Eldabe S, et al. The polyanalgesic consensus conference (PACC): recommendations on intrathecal drug infusion systems best practices and guidelines. Neuromodulation. 2017;20:96–132.
43. Mohammed SI, Eldabe S, Simpson KH Brookes M, Madzinga G, Gulve A, et al. Bolus intrathecal injection of ziconotide (Prialt) to evaluate the option of continuous administration via an implanted intrathecal drug delivery (ITDD) system: a pilot study. Neuromodulation. 2013;16(6):576–81; discussion 582.
44. Pope JE, Deer TR. Intrathecal pharmacology update: novel dosing strategy for intrathecal therapy and monotherapy ziconotide. Neuromodulation. 2015;18(5):414–20.

Chapter 33
Intrathecal Drug Delivery: Implantation

Lucas W. Campos and Jason E. Pope

33.1 Pre-op Considerations

A thorough understanding of the patient's spinal anatomy is absolutely required and begins with visual inspection of the spine. Determining the spinal level location for needle placement is imperative, along with previous back interventions and surgery. This decision can mean the difference between the ability or inability to pass the catheter through the intrathecal (IT) space at that level. Spine imaging, including plain films, CT, and MRI, of both lumbar and thoracic spine levels, shows many complex post-surgical or congenital spine deformities. Careful operative planning of reservoir placement is important to determine, along with the course of the catheter, with a clear dialogue with the patient. Catheter tunneling should be carefully marked on the skin after visual inspection of the patient's body. By convention, the pump is typically placed on the right abdomen, as it reduces presentation challenges from left-sided abdominal pain in the typical older aged patient population served by the therapy. Reasons to avoid a specific site include lack of body fat, previous surgeries, skin infection near the site, and poor quality of skin texture [1].

33.2 Antibiotics

Preoperative antibiotics are recommended within 60 minutes of incision to reduce the risk of surgical site infection. Antibiotic selection and dosing need to be determined pre-operatively as well. Cefazolin is typically given and dosed by body weight, usually 2 or 3 g IV. Clindamycin 600–900 mg IV is used if there is a true

L.W. Campos (✉) • J.E. Pope
Summit Pain Alliance, Santa Rosa, CA, USA
e-mail: lwcamposmdphd@gmail.com; popeje@me.com

S. Diwan, T.R. Deer (eds.), *Advanced Procedures for Pain Management*,
https://doi.org/10.1007/978-3-319-68841-1_33

cephalosporin allergy. Patients known to have Methicillin-resistant Staphylococcus aureus (MRSA) need Vancomycin 1 g IV given over 60 min before incision.

33.3 Positioning, Prepping, and Draping

The most common patient positioning during IDT permanent placement is lateral decubitus with flexion of the hips and cervical spine. This position facilitates pump placement in the abdominal wall. The skin is then prepped with alcohol and then chlorhexidine before draping the surgical site. The implant incision sites are mapped out using fluoroscopic images one to two vertebral bodies below the planned site of entry. Local anesthetic is then injected along all anticipated incision sites [2].

33.4 Catheter Placement

The catheter is the most common cause of system failure [3, 4]. Common catheter-related complications include kinking, dislodgment from IT space, disconnection from the pump, breaks, and occlusions. Catheter complications that need surgical correction occur in approximately 20–25% of implants [5–7]. Needle and catheter placement is essential for long-term success [8]. It is best to use a paramedian approach for catheter entry. This avoids constant stress and strain from spinous process impingement. Needle trajectory is similar to the needle trajectory for spinal cord stimulation, 15–20° of the sagittal plane and 15–20° of the skin. The needle is touched down on lamina caudal to the intralaminar entry site and, under fluoroscopic guidance, is walked off into the intrathecal space (Fig. 33.1). If

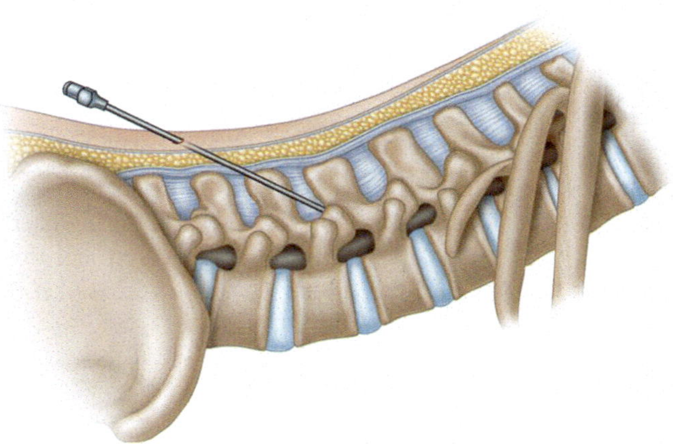

Fig. 33.1 Proper needle angle placement at 30° (*Reproduced with permission from* Deer et al. [11])

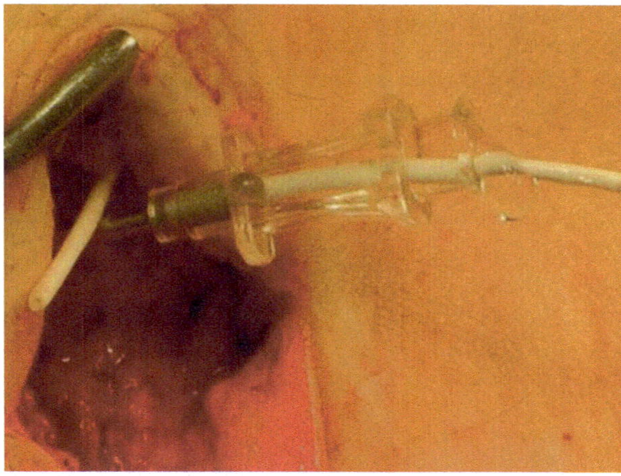

Fig. 33.2 Continuous CSF flow from the distal end of the catheter is needed to ensure the tip is still in the IT space (*Reproduced with permission from* Deer et al. [11])

identification of the epidural space or depth is of concern, it is suggested to find the epidural space first. Angles that exceed 60° will cause excessive pressure on the catheter, leading to fractures and occlusion due to subsequent kinking [9].

Once the needle is positioned in the intrathecal space, the stylet is removed and a free flow of cerebrospinal fluid should be observed. Excellent CSF flow through the catheter is essential to maintain and should be checked at various times during the procedure (Fig. 33.2) [4, 8]. This is avoided by using a low angle of entry into the IT space. The highest predictor of a positive outcome is tip placement closest to the spinal cord level matching the dermatomal level of pain site [10]. The area of tip placement for chronic pain treatment throughout the body is almost entirely in the thoracic spinal cord. To treat neck and arm pain the catheter is placed between T3–6 for back and leg pain, the catheter tip is placed from T8 to T10 [11]. It is critical that patients be conversant when the catheter is placed, and the presence of new radicular symptoms needs to be evaluated. If present, the catheter needs to be withdrawn and replaced.

Some prefer to place the catheter below the conus to reduce the complication severity of a granuloma, but this practice is no longer suggested [12–14]. A myelogram with compatible contrast confirms intrathecal placement at the target level. The physicochemical properties of the intrathecal medication and the individual CSF fluid dynamics will increase or limit cephalocaudal spread [15, 16].

33.5 Anchoring

Anchoring the catheter is a critical task. This secures the catheter in the optimal location, along with preventing dural CSF leak. Operatively, one can perform the surgical dissection of the paraspinal site, with dissection down to the lumbodorsal fascia, and then place the needle for catheter placement, or vice versa. Some surgeons suggest placement of a purse-string suture, which is placed along the fascia to anchor the catheter (Figs. 33.3 and 33.4). The goals of a purse-string suture are to secure the tissue surrounding the catheter to reduce the short-term risk of CSF leak around the catheter, and to reduce catheter migration by allowing the tissue to fibrose around the catheter [17–19]. A non-absorbable suture such as Ethibond or silk suture is placed into the fascia and spinous ligaments with at least four bites in a circular pattern around the needle [20]. The suture is then tied while the needle is still in place. This allows for a tight occlusion of the tissue without causing fracture or occlusion of the catheter [21, 22]. An anchor is sutured in place to ensure the catheter tip does not migrate (Fig. 33.5) [23]. It is critical that the placement of the catheter and the course to the intrathecal reservoir is smooth with no kinks present [15]. Total dependence on the type of anchor can lead to poor outcomes [3, 20].

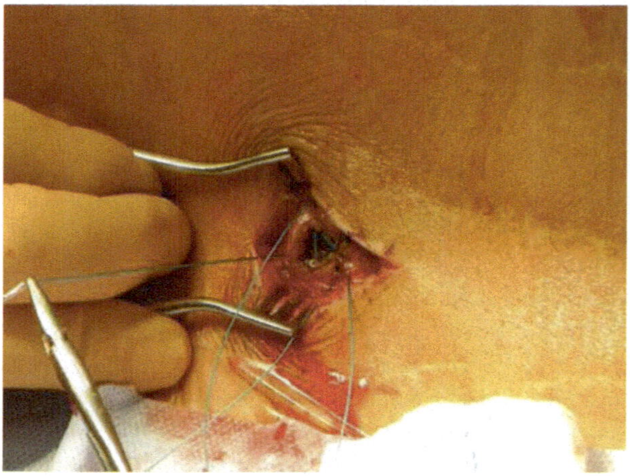

Fig. 33.3 Purse string suture placed into fascia (*Reproduced with permission from* Deer et al. [11])

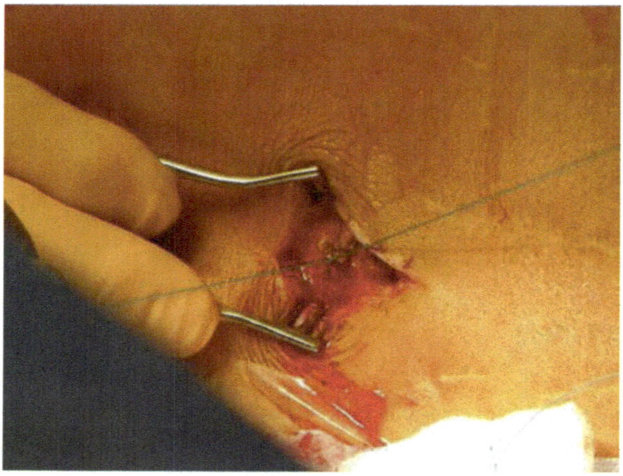

Fig. 33.4 Placement of purse string suture (*Reproduced with permission from* Deer et al. [11])

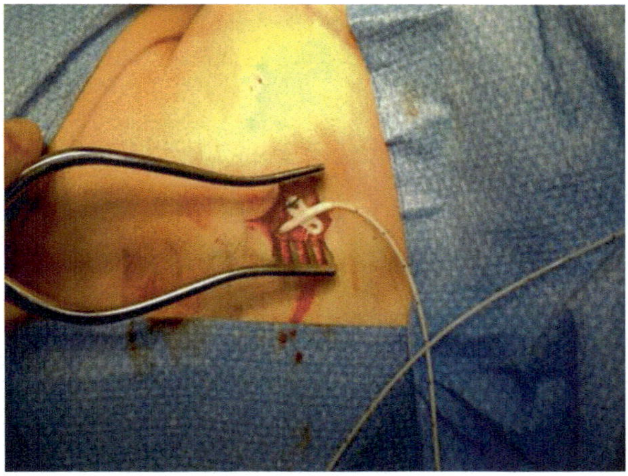

Fig. 33.5 Anchoring catheter after the tip reaches its indicated cephalocaudal level based on region of the body to be treated (*Reproduced with permission from* Deer et al. [11])

33.6 Pocket Formation

Prior to incision of the pocket site, the patient must be properly anesthetized with either local anesthesia or intravenous sedation, or a combination of these options. The pocket can be dissected out using sharp and blunt dissection with the surgeon's hand or a blunt surgical instrument (Fig. 33.6). Placement is typically in the abdomen, although some are placing pockets in the buttock or flank. The pocket should be 110–120% of the total volume of the pump [24]. If the pocket is too large, pump migration or pump flipping are more likely [25]. If the pocket is too small, the risks of increased tissue pressure causing severe pump implant site pain and dehiscence due to tissue erosion are increased [3, 25].

Careful hemostasis and tissue handling are critical for optimal surgical outcomes. Careful sharp and blunt dissection, with hemostasis, is critical to avoid complication of hematoma and seroma [26]. Pump movement can be mitigated by utilizing the suture loops (at three points) or the use of a pouch [17, 27]. The downside of a Dacron pouch is subsequent scarring, which makes future revisions difficult. As the pump is placed in the pocket, the location of the side port and pump catheter connector should be noted and the catheter placed behind the pump [28]. The patient's body habitus should be considered when placing the side port and the connector, and the position should be noted in the operative notes if it varies in individual patients.

33.7 Tunneling

Once the pocket has been created and properly sized, tunneling can begin (Fig. 33.7). Tunneling rods may cause tissue damage due to improper tunneling depth. Bending the tunneling device to the contours of the body can avoid this complication [3]. The

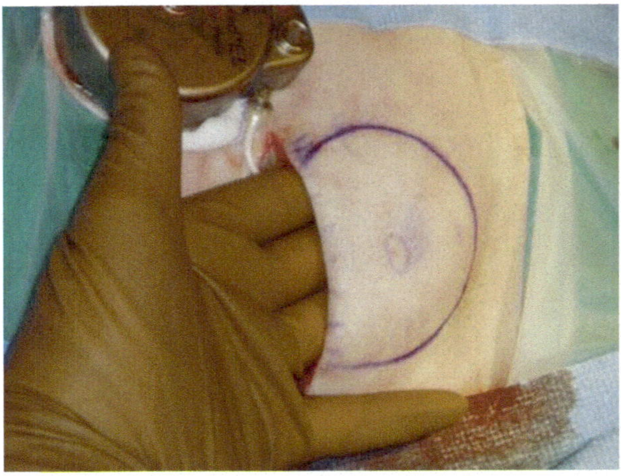

Fig. 33.6 Blunt dissection of the pocket site (*Reproduced with permission from* Deer et al. [11])

Fig. 33.7 Beginning of tunneling portion of the procedure (*Reproduced with permission from* Deer et al. [11])

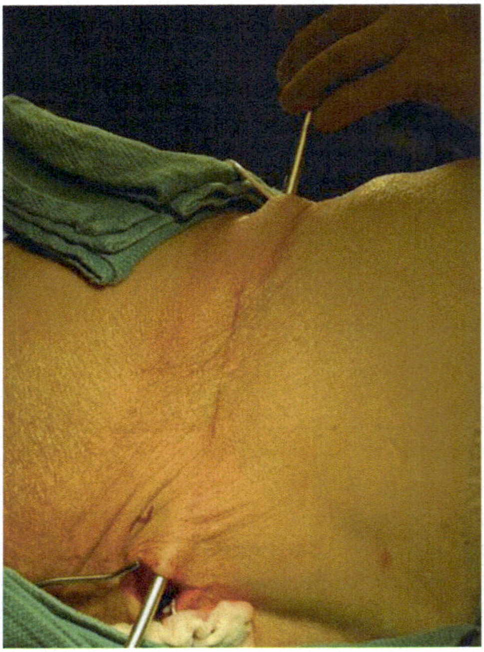

tip of the tunneling device should be constantly palpated to determine that the tunneling rod stays at the proper depth throughout (Fig. 33.8). Tunneling should remain in the subcutaneous tissue, deep enough to avoid penetrating the dermis and

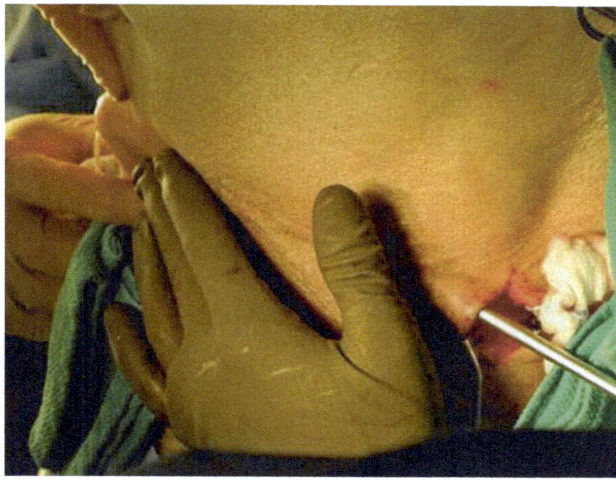

Fig. 33.8 Constant palpation of the tip of tunneling device ensures proper depth throughout this step in the procedure (*Reproduced with permission from* Deer et al. [11])

superficial enough to avoid organ penetration [29]. For obese patients, the tunneling distance required should be measured in the holding area prior to transport to the operating room. The tunneling distance should be compared to the length of the tunneling tool. If the distance is longer than the tunneling device, a two-step technique should be used [11, 30]. This technique will lead to a successful procedure and reduce the risk of improper depth of tunneling [26, 31].

33.8 Wound Closure

Langer's lines are the natural orientation of collagen fibers in the dermis (Fig. 33.9). Incisions parallel to Langer's lines heal better and produce less scarring than those that cut across these lines [32, 33]. Conversely, incisions perpendicular to Langer's lines tend to produce obvious scars and predispose the patient to scar neuromas [33].

Before closure, the pocket and tunneling tract should be irrigated vigorously with antibiotic solution and then the tissue brought together with a two- or three-layer closure. Careful attention must be paid when closing pericatheter tissues, to avoid piercing the catheter with the needle. This will lead to CSF and medication leak, causing system failure [3, 11, 34]. Skin closure can be done using absorbable monofilament subcuticular suturing or skin staples. Abdominal binder placement reduces postoperative pain and the incidence of pocket seroma or hematoma.

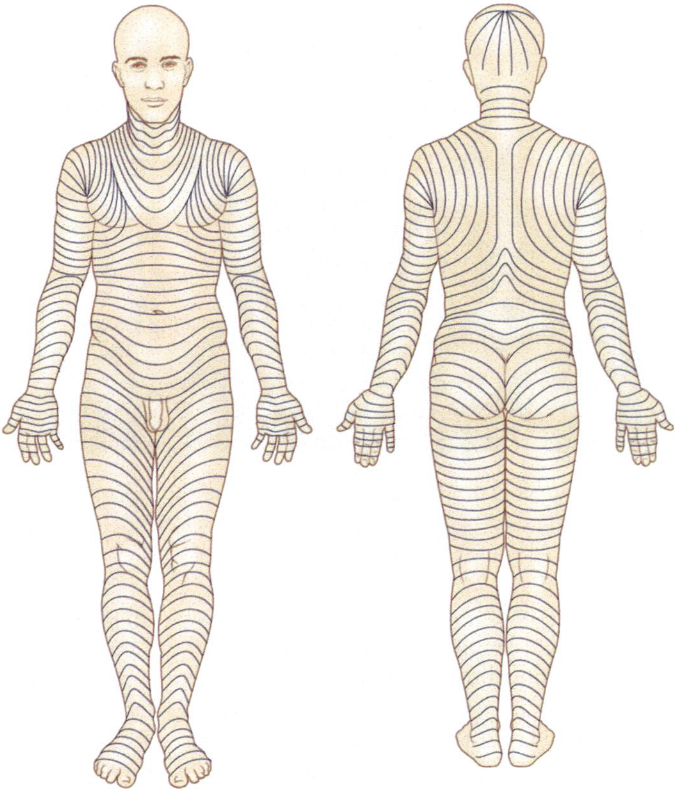

Fig. 33.9 Depicts Langer's lines (*Reproduced with permission from* Deer et al. [11])

33.9 Potential Problems During IT Implantation

The most significant risk during catheter placement is injury to the spinal cord or nerve roots [1, 3, 28]. Injuries range from nerve inflammation to spinal cord injury. Monitored sedation with direct patient communication will provide an early warning of impending nerve injury or spinal cord damage [18, 28]. Avoiding nerve or spinal cord injury also depends on proper needle alignment [3, 15]. The fluoroscopic image should be modified to correct for patient rotation, spinal kyphosis, scoliosis, or abnormal body habitus to facilitate proper needle placement and catheter entry. The contralateral oblique (CLO) view may obviate some of these concerns, particularly with buttock placement of the pump (Fig. 33.10).

Entries into the intrathecal space will cause significant CSF leakage, which can lead to hygroma formation and subsequent risk of infection [34]. Injection of a flowable hemostatic foam or placement of Gelfoam around the purse-string suture site may be helpful in tissue healing and CSF leakage [20]. Constant CSF leakage can also lead to severe spinal headache symptoms [35]. This complication may require

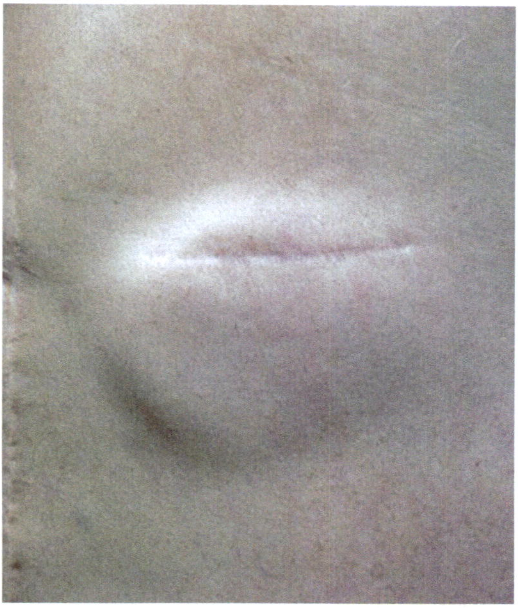

Fig. 33.10 Healed wound site over pocket site (*Reproduced with permission from* Deer et al. [11])

placement of a blood patch, neurosurgical sealing of the dural tear, and possible explantation of the entire system [36]. Ventral placement of the catheter may lead to poor pain control, as medications have limited circumferential spread [12].

Catheter damage including tearing, fracture, or accidental removal may occur during needle or stylet removal [4]. The catheter should not be completely withdrawn through the needle if the desired catheter course is not initially achieved [3].

The purse-string or anchoring suture of the catheter may lead to catheter occlusion or obstructed flow. If one chooses to perform a purse-string suture, it is important to secure it around the needle and tie the suture prior to removing the needle [19, 37]. Tying the suture after removing the needle can lead to occlusion of the catheter and system failure.

Careful attention should be given to resistance when withdrawing the needle or stylet. Pulling the needle out against significant resistance can cause catheter damage.

33.10 Conclusions

The use of ITT to treat chronic refractory pain has increased dramatically since its inception in the 1980s. IT pump placement is a complex procedure that requires significant training for precise clinical execution. Each step of this process must be carefully planned and performed. Proper anchoring and pocket location are crucial for long-term success of this treatment. Simple awareness of these issues increases the odds dramatically for a successful patient outcome. Armed with the strong surgical techniques outlined in this chapter, ITT therapy will remain an excellent treatment for spasticity, cancer pain, and non-cancer pain by ensuring the safety and efficacy of the implanted system.

References

1. Prager J, Deer T, Levy R, Bruel B, Buchser E, Caraway D, et al. Best practices for intrathecal drug delivery for pain. Neuromodulation. 2014;17:354–72.
2. Pope JE, Deer TR, Bruel BM, Falowski S. Clinical uses of intrathecal therapy and its placement in the pain care algorithm. Pain Pract. 2016. https://doi.org/10.1111/papr.12438.
3. Follett KA, Burchiel K, Deer T, Dupen S, Prager J, Turner MS, et al. Prevention of intrathecal drug delivery catheter-related complications. Neuromodulation. 2003;6:32–41.
4. Follett KA, Naumann CP. A prospective study of catheter-related complications of intrathecal drug delivery systems. J Pain Symptom Manag. 2000;19:209–15.
5. Penn RD, York MM, Paice JA. Catheter systems for intrathecal drug delivery. J Neurosurg. 1995;83:215–7.
6. Penn RD. Catheter implant systems for intrathecal drug delivery. J Neurosurg. 1996;84:713.
7. Levin AB, Sperling KB. Complications associated with infusion pumps implanted for spasticity. Stereotact Funct Neurosurg. 1995;65:147–51.
8. Naumann C, Erdine S, Koulousakis A, Van Buyten JP, Schuchard M. Drug adverse events and system complications of intrathecal opioid delivery for pain: origins, detection, manifestations, and management. Neuromodulation. 1999;2:92–107.
9. Robinson S, Robertson FC, Dasenbrock HH, O'Brien CP, Berde C, Padua H. Image-guided intrathecal baclofen pump catheter implantation: a technical note and case series. J Neurosurg Spine. 2017;26(5):621–7.
10. Cohen SP, Dragovich A. Intrathecal analgesia. Anesthesiol Clin. 2007;25:863–82. viii
11. Deer TR, Pope JE, editors. Atlas of implantable therapies for pain management. New York, NY: Springer; 2016.
12. Blount JP, Remley KB, Yue SK, Erickson DL. Intrathecal granuloma complicating chronic spinal infusion of morphine. Report of three cases. J Neurosurg. 1996;84:272–6.
13. Ver Donck A, Vranken JH, Puylaert M, Hayek S, Mekhail N, Van Zundert J. Intrathecal drug administration in chronic pain syndromes. Pain Pract. 2014;14:461–76.
14. Shields DC, Palma C, Khoo LT, Ferrante FM. Extramedullary intrathecal catheter granuloma adherent to the conus medullaris presenting as cauda equina syndrome. Anesthesiology. 2005;102:1059–61.
15. Pope JE, Deer TR. Intrathecal drug delivery for pain: a clinical guide and future directions. Pain Manag. 2015;5:175–83.
16. Deer TR, Pope JE, Hayek SM, Bux A, Buchser E, Eldabe S, et al. The polyanalgesic consensus conference (PACC): recommendations on intrathecal drug infusion systems best practices and guidelines. Neuromodulation. 2017;20:96–132.
17. Albright AL, Turner M, Pattisapu JV. Best-practice surgical techniques for intrathecal baclofen therapy. J Neurosurg. 2006;104:233–9.
18. Onofrio BM, Yaksh TL. Long-term pain relief produced by intrathecal morphine infusion in 53 patients. J Neurosurg. 1990;72:200–9.
19. Haranhalli N, Anand D, Wisoff JH, Harter DH, Weiner HL, Blate M, et al. Intrathecal baclofen therapy: complication avoidance and management. Childs Nerv Syst. 2011;27:421–7.
20. Deer TR, Verdolin MH, Pope JE. Securing and anchoring permanent intrathecal catheters. In: Deer TR, Pope JE, editors. Atlas of implantable therapies for pain Management. New York, NY: Springer; 2016. p. 263–9.

21. Awaad Y, Rizk T, Siddiqui I, Roosen N, McIntosh K, Waines GM. Complications of intrathecal baclofen pump: prevention and cure. ISRN Neurol. 2012;2012:575168.
22. Knight KH, Brand FM, Mchaourab AS, Veneziano G. Implantable intrathecal pumps for chronic pain: highlights and updates. Croat Med J. 2007;48:22–34.
23. Pope JE, Deer TR. Intrathecal pharmacology update: novel dosing strategy for intrathecal monotherapy ziconotide on efficacy and sustainability. Neuromodulation. 2015;18:414–20.
24. Deer TR, Smith HS, Burton AW, Pope JE, Doleys DM, Levy RM, et al. Comprehensive consensus based guidelines on intrathecal drug delivery systems in the treatment of pain caused by cancer pain. Pain Physician. 2011;14:E283–312.
25. Bolash R, Mekhail N. Intrathecal pain pumps: indications, patient selection, techniques, and outcomes. Neurosurg Clin N Am. 2014;25:735–42.
26. Krames E. Implantable devices for pain control: spinal cord stimulation and intrathecal therapies. Best Pract Res Clin Anaesthesiol. 2002;16:619–49.
27. Albright AL, Ferson SS. Intrathecal baclofen therapy in children. Neurosurg Focus. 2006;21:e3.
28. Vender JR, Hester S, Waller JL, Rekito A, Lee MR. Identification and management of intrathecal baclofen pump complications: a comparison of pediatric and adult patients. J Neurosurg. 2006;104:9–15.
29. Byers K, Axelrod P, Michael S, Rosen S. Infections complicating tunneled intraspinal catheter systems used to treat chronic pain. Clin Infect Dis. 1995;21:403–8.
30. Waldman SD. Atlas of interventional pain management. Philadelphia, PA: Elsevier Health Sciences; 2014.
31. Krames ES. Intraspinal opioid therapy for chronic nonmalignant pain: current practice and clinical guidelines. J Pain Symptom Manag. 1996;11:333–52.
32. Courtiss EH, Longarcre JJ, Destefano GA, Brizic L, Holmstrand K. The placement of elective skin incisions. Plast Reconstr Surg. 1963;31:31–44.
33. Kraissl CJ. The selection of appropriate lines for elective surgical incisions. Plast Reconstr Surg (1946). 1951;8:1–28.
34. Flückiger B, Knecht H, Grossmann S, Felleiter P. Device-related complications of long-term intrathecal drug therapy via implanted pumps. Spinal Cord. 2008;46:639–43.
35. Jagannathan DK, Arriaga AF, Elterman KG, Kodali BS, Robinson JN, Tsen LC, et al. Effect of neuraxial technique after inadvertent dural puncture on obstetric outcomes and anesthetic complications. Int J Obstet Anesth. 2016;25:23–9.
36. Bendel MA, Moeschler SM, Qu W, Hanley E, Neuman SA, Eldrige JS, et al. Treatment of refractory postdural puncture headache after intrathecal drug delivery system implantation with epidural blood patch procedures: a 20-year experience. Pain Res Treat. 2016;2016:2134959.
37. Belverud S, Mogilner A, Schulder M. Intrathecal pumps. Neurotherapeutics. 2008;5:114–22.

Chapter 34
Intrathecal Drug Delivery Maintenance: Refill and Programming

Brenda Beck and Salim M. Hayek

34.1 Introduction

Treatment of noncancer pain with intrathecal opioids in patients with chronic intractable pain has been an important breakthrough in the pain management field over the past four decades [1]. It has been increasingly used in patients with chronic intractable pain in whom conservative therapies have failed, or those who cannot tolerate side effects of oral opioid medications. Delivering opioids within the cerebrospinal fluid allows the administration of only a small amount of opioid to provide analgesia without the overt systemic side effects that may be experienced when the drugs are given orally or intravenously. A number of reviews have documented the safety and efficacy of intrathecal drug delivery (IDD) therapy in patients with chronic pain. IDD therapy for noncancer pain is effective, cost-neutral, and appropriate [1]. Although the overall safety of IDD systems has been documented, there have been case reports of adverse events. Most notably, respiratory depression with concomitant use of central nervous system depressant medications such as benzodiazepines has been implicated in IDD-related fatalities [1]. Potential problems also can occur during the pump refill, such as a pocket fill. Although respiratory depression is rare in patients who are opioid tolerant, missed refill dates may predispose the patient to an opioid-naïve state in which a medication refill of morphine at the same concentration and dose may result in delayed respiratory depression [2]. (Early respiratory depression has not been reported with morphine.) A number of other important matters need particular care and attention during the refill and

B. Beck (✉) • S.M. Hayek
Department of Anesthesiology and Pain Management, University Hospitals Cleveland Medical Center, Cleveland, OH, USA
e-mail: Brenda.Beck@UHHospitals.org; Salim.Hayek@UHhospitals.org

S. Diwan, T.R. Deer (eds.), *Advanced Procedures for Pain Management*,
https://doi.org/10.1007/978-3-319-68841-1_34

maintenance process, to avoid likely complications. Proper physician training and understanding of the pharmacology and dosing of intrathecal medications is imperative to limit life-threatening complications including pocket fills and respiratory depression.

34.2 Refill

A typical IDD refill kit consists of extension tubing with a clamp, filter, noncoring needles, syringes, fenestrated drape, and a refill template (Fig. 34.1) Palpation of the patient's abdomen for identification and location of the IDD system (and thus the reservoir fill port) should be relatively easy. However, difficulties with refills may arise despite the use of a commercially available template that is designed to align the edges of the IDD pump to facilitate accurate placement of the noncoring needle for refills. To facilitate the identification of the reservoir fill port, newer IDD models such as the Prometra Programmable Pump (Flowonix Medical; Mt. Olive, NJ) allow the reservoir fill port to be located via palpation secondary to it being raised (Fig. 34.2). This newer IDD pump depends on a higher-pressure system for refills than the Medtronic SynchroMed® II IDD pump (Medtronic; Minneapolis, MN).

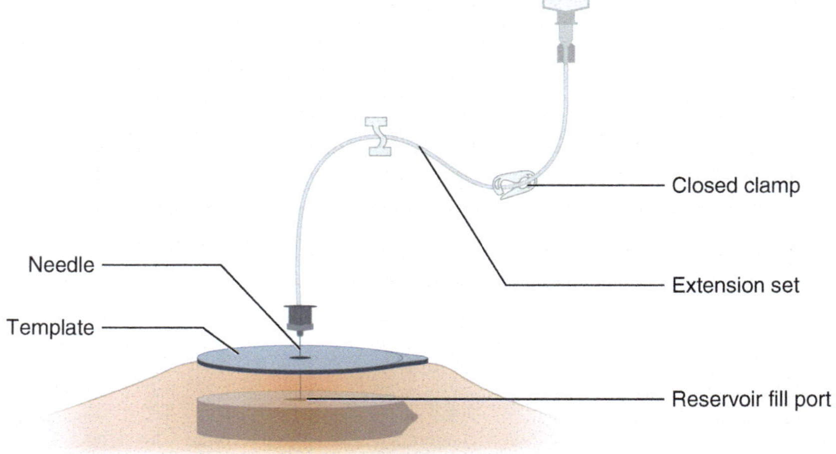

Fig. 34.1 Assembled intrathecal drug delivery (IDD) kit with template overlying the IDD system

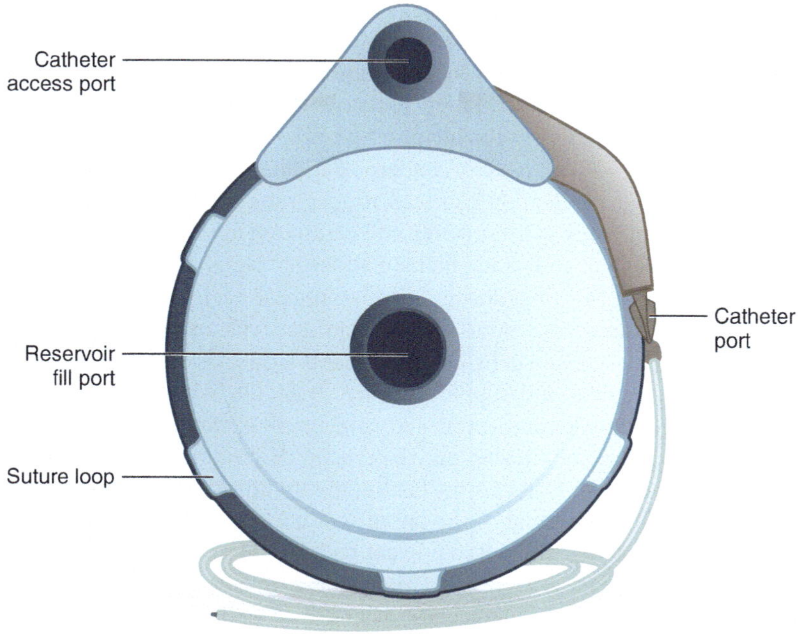

Fig. 34.2 Labeled schematic of an IDD system

Not yet approved by the Food and Drug Administration (FDA), the Arrow International Medallion Therapeutics (Valencia, CA) IDD pump uses a negative pressure system that allows for immediate withdrawal of the residual medication upon entry to the reservoir fill port by the refill needle.

Difficulties placing the needle through the septum of the reservoir fill port can be due to a number of factors:

- Obesity
- Weight gain after IDD implantation
- Pump movement within the pocket
- Presence of scar tissue at the IDD system implant site
- Deep implant
- Patient position (sitting *vs* lying down)
- Pump tilted within the pocket
- Inexperience of the practitioner

Complete aspiration of the old medication should occur prior to refilling with the new medication. It is recommended to use the manufacturer's template to identify the puncture site as a blind technique can lead to inaccurate identification of the fill port, which may result in a pocket fill from improper positioning of the needle [3]. Pocket fills can be avoided by injecting a small volume of the medication and re-aspirating that volume. Correct aspiration of the small volume injected ensures that the needle is in the reservoir fill port. A discrepancy in the amount aspirated may indicate an inappropriate needle placement that could lead to a pocket fill. Readjustment and evaluation of needle placement are critical.

Pocket fills occur when intrathecal medications are inadvertently injected into the subcutaneous tissue and/or the pump pocket. Pocket fills can lead to devastating complications that may be life-threatening and may require supportive care and intensive monitoring. Symptoms of underdosing may manifest as withdrawal. Overdosing of opioid medication can lead to respiratory depression. Local anesthetic toxicity can manifest with seizures and cardiotoxicity that can lead to death. Hypertension, confusion, and visual hallucinations are signs and symptoms related to clonidine overdose [4]. Overdosing with intrathecal baclofen (used in patients with spasticity or spinal cord injuries) can manifest with respiratory depression, hypotension, somnolence, and delirium [5]. Patients suspected of baclofen overdose require emergent medical and supportive care. Baclofen withdrawal can lead to rebound spasticity, tachycardia, fever, and seizures that requires prompt medical attention. Intensive care monitoring may be crucial. High-dose intravenous benzodiazepine therapy may be initiated for baclofen withdrawal. Prompt evaluation of the IDD device and reinstitution of the intrathecal baclofen therapy is necessary as oral baclofen may not be sufficient to prevent withdrawal [5].

Successive refills can also lead to medication overdose. A case report by Perruchoud *et al.* [4] reported medication overdose secondary to severe damage of the silicone septum of the refill reservoir port secondary to successive refills [4]. In addition, life-threatening inadvertent injection into the catheter access port (Fig. 34.2) can cause fatal drug overdose. It is crucial to properly identify and secure needle access to the IDD system reservoir fill port for patient safety (Fig. 34.3).

Some publications have suggested the use of ultrasound imaging to facilitate the identification of the reservoir fill port and proper access, especially when an IDD pump and its fill port are difficult to identify: Gofeld and McQueen [6] described a technique in which a linear ultrasound transducer was used to identify the reservoir fill port (which appears rectangular and hypoechoic under ultrasound). The transducer should be placed slightly caudal to the IDD system. With a 45-degree tilt of the

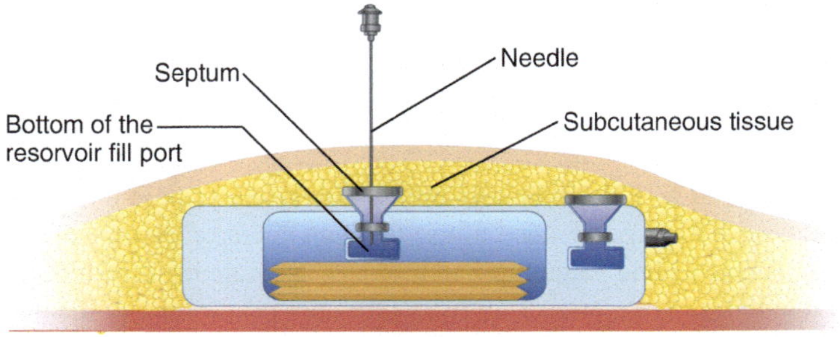

Fig. 34.3 Proper placement of 22-G noncoring needle into the septum of the reservoir fill port (Medtronic, Inc. Minneapolis, MN)

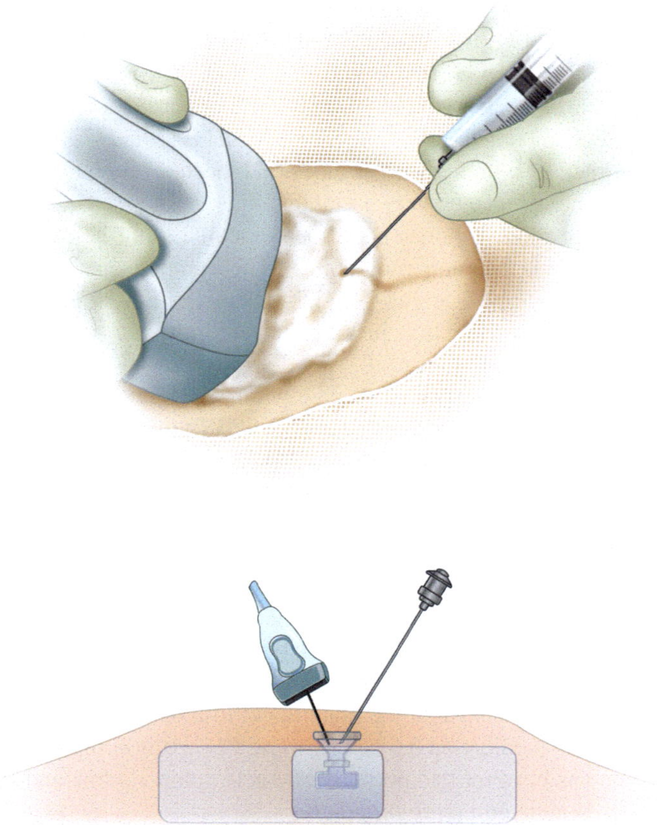

Fig. 34.4 *Top*, Position of linear ultrasound transducer and needle insertion site. *Bottom*, Schematic of the angled transducer, port, and needle entry into the reservoir fill port

transducer and the reservoir port in the middle of the screen, the needle can be entered cephalic to the transducer and can successfully enter the reservoir fill port (Fig. 34.4).

Color flow Doppler can be utilized for additional confirmation that the intrathecal medication has been injected within the reservoir fill port. A "color column" will be seen within the reservoir fill port [6]. The use of ultrasound to identify a difficult-to-access refill port may be advantageous: itscost is low, it is portable and easy to use, it offers reduced exposure to fluoroscopy, and its real-time imaging may show other structures that could be contributing to difficult needle placement, such as the formation of a postsurgical seroma [7].

Medication choice and therapy algorithm recommendations have been established by an expert panel based on the patient's pain complaint. Two medications that are currently approved by the FDA for intrathecal use are morphine (Infumorph; West-Ward Pharmaceuticals, Eatontown, NJ) and ziconotide (Prialt; Jazz Pharmaceuticals, Palo Alto, CA). Other non-FDA (*ie*, off-label) drugs used for intrathecal therapy include fentanyl, bupivacaine, hydromorphone, and clonidine. IDD therapy may be initiated with one medication or with a combination of medications. A documented concern for the use of compounded off-label medications includes pump failure secondary to corrosion and motor stall, with a failure rate of 7.0% (Medtronic SynchroMed II), compared with 2.4% when FDA-approved drugs are used [1]. It is recommended, based on chemical stability and FDA sanctions, that refills for monotherapy with intrathecal Infumorph occur every 6 months, and refills for combination therapy occur every 3 months [8].

The aspirated residual volume should be compared with the expected residual volume as indicated via the pump programmer. This comparison allows the clinician to evaluate the IDD pump's accuracy [9]. Discrepancies may be due to motor stall, catheter obstruction or malfunction, incomplete withdrawal, or an undetected pocket fill of medication at the previous refill. Any discrepancies in the aspirated residual volume compared with the expected volume within the intrathecal pump should be investigated promptly, either via a catheter dye study (pump myelogram) to rule out kink and/or malfunction, or with a thoracic MRI to rule out intrathecal granuloma formation [7]. Accuracy of medication delivery can be inferred by comparing the actual measured reservoir volume to the aspirated residual volume [9]. Accuracy of medication delivery has been reported to be as high as 97.9% for the Prometra IDD system, which uses a valve-gated dose regulation system rather than the peristaltic pump roller system of the Medtronic SynchroMed® II [10]. Nonetheless, discrepancies should alert the physician to a malfunction of either the pump (less common) or the catheter [9]. Patient complaints or manifestations of withdrawal, loss of efficacy, or overdosing may also alert the practitioner to IDD malfunction.

Once the existing medication has been removed from the pump reservoir and the new medication has been refilled properly, the new pump volume and any changes will be recorded via the pump programmer.

34.3 Programming

When programming, it is important to input all the pertinent information correctly, including the patient's name, drug information, and infusion mode. Whether the patient's medication is monotherapy or combination therapy, the opioid medication is always programmed as the primary medication. In addition, it is important to be vigilant when inputting the medication concentration and concentration units. One may also program the reservoir volume. Older IDD pumps offer 40 mL and 20 mL sizes, whereas newer models currently offer only 20 mL pumps.

As required by the individual patient, the IDD system's compatible pump programmer can adjust the medication dose in various ways: by manipulating the infusion mode, by increasing or decreasing the flow rate, or by altering the mode of administration (continuous mode, scheduled boluses, and/or step function dosing) [9].

A simple continuous delivery of medication allows for the medication to be continuously delivered at a specific programmed dose over a period of 24 h. A simple continuous delivery mode may be the only mode programmed, or it can be accompanied by a bolus dose self-administered by the patient. Bolus doses can be programmed to deliver a set amount of medication over a specific duration. A bolus may be administered to the patient throughout the 24-h period, with dose restrictions within that time frame as set by the clinician, programmed with a maximum number of activations per day, with a lockout period (a minimum time between doses).

Boluses may also be administered as a priming bolus or a bridge bolus. A priming bolus rapidly fills empty pump tubing and/or catheter tubing. It is important to program the priming bolus according to where the medication is located. For example, for a new implant or pump replacement with fluid aspirated from the catheter, the priming bolus should be programmed to include the pump tubing volume as well as the catheter volume. However, during a catheter replacement or contrast study, only the catheter volume should be included in the priming bolus. A bridge bolus is programmed when medication solutions and/or concentrations have been changed, to avoid underdosing or overdosing of the new medication. The bridge bolus delivers the medication remaining in the IDD pump tubing and catheter based on the old medication dose. Once the bridge bolus is completed, the IDD pump will return to its programmed infusion mode.

Dose titration of intrathecal medications should be done at a slow rate, to allow the patient to develop tolerance and avoid adverse effects. Safe ceiling doses of opioids have not been established, and variability to the response of opioids is patient-specific. Medication side effects of intrathecal opioids are individualized and not dose-dependent in a linear fashion [1]. Rapid dosage changes may be suitable for patients with cancer pain, but it is advised that aggressive changes of more than 20% of the total daily infused dose (to also include the bolus dose) should be avoided, to minimize the risk of overdose [1]. Patients should be monitored for respiratory depression with the start or restart of intrathecal opioid therapy, with a fully equipped staff and standard monitoring for at least 24 h [1]. A 2009 analysis by Coffey et al. of nine cases found respiratory depression to be the contributing cause of mortality within 24 h of implantation of the IDD device [11]. Vigilance with programming and accuracy in dosing intrathecal opioids is crucial to prevent life threatening complications.

34.4 Complications

IDD therapy is an important therapeutic modality for patients who experience end-of-life pain or chronic, debilitating pain. Vigilance by an adequately trained clinician familiar with the IDD system and its management is important to avoid complications that can be associated with IDD therapy. Adverse events related to IDD therapy may include respiratory depression resulting from interactions with other systemic medications (such as benzodiazepines) with inadequate monitoring; the development of a granuloma (inflammatory mass) from high doses or high concentrations of opioids; dosing errors in the medication concentration and/or pump programming error; and inadvertent pocket fills during pump refilling [12].

References

1. Prager J, Deer T, Levy R, Bruel B, Buchser E, Caraway D, et al. Best practices for intrathecal drug delivery for pain. Neuromodulation. 2014;17:354–72.
2. Ruan X, Couch JP, Liu H, Shah RV, Wang F, Chiravuri S. Respiratory failure following delayed intrathecal morphine pump refill: a valuable, but costly lesson. Pain Physician. 2010;13:337–41.
3. Maino P, Koetsier E, Perez RS. The accuracy of template-guided refill technique of intrathecal pumps controlled by fluoroscopy: an observational study. Neuromodulation. 2014;18:428–32.
4. Perruchoud C, Bovy M, Rutschmann B, Durrer A, Buchser E. Silicone septum leakage at the origin of a drug overdose in a patient implanted with an intrathecal pump. Neuromodulation. 2012;16:467–70.
5. Watve SV, Sivan M, Raza WA, Jamil FF. Management of acute overdose or withdrawal state in intrathecal baclofen therapy. Spinal Cord. 2012;50:107–11.
6. Gofeld M, McQueen CK. Ultrasound-guided intrathecal pump access and prevention of the pocket fill. Pain Med. 2011;12:607–11.
7. Shankar H. Ultrasound-guided localization of difficult-to-access refill port of the intrathecal pump reservoir. Neuromodulation. 2009;12:215–8.
8. Shields DE, Aclan J, Szatkowski A. Chemical stability of admixtures containing 25 mcg/mL ziconotide and 10 mg/mL or 20 mg/mL morphine sulfate during simulated intrathecal administration. Int J Pharm Compounding. 2008;12:552–7.
9. Wesemann K, Coffey RJ, Wallace MS, Tan Y, Broste S, Buvanendran A. Clinical accuracy and safety using the SynchroMed II intrathecal drug infusion pump. Reg Anesth Pain Med. 2014;39:341–6.
10. Rauck R, Deer T, Rosen S, Padda G, Barsa J, Dunbar E, Dwarakanath G. Long-term follow-up of a novel implantable programmable infusion pump. Neuromodulation. 2012;16:163–7.
11. Coffey RJ, Owens ML, Broste SK, Dubois MY, Ferrante FM, Schultz DM, et al. Mortality associated with implantation and management of intrathecal opioid drug infusion systems to treat noncancer pain. Anesthesiology. 2009;111:881–91.
12. Kamran S, Wright BD. Complications of intrathecal drug delivery systems. Neuromodulation. 2001;4:111–5.

Chapter 35
Intrathecal Drug Delivery Maintenance: Catheter Evaluation

Salim M. Hayek and Mahesh Mohan

35.1 Introduction

This chapter covers the troubleshooting management of an intrathecal drug delivery system (IDDS) when it loses its efficacy. The potential scenarios to consider when IDDS efficacy is lost are problems with the pump device or the catheter system, or the development of tolerance. Of the first two situations, catheter-related dysfunction is more frequent. Potential catheter-related problems include catheter tip migration, kink or occlusion, fracture of the catheter, inadvertent puncture, or loosening of connections. Long-term follow-up studies have shown 37–55% malfunction for catheter and/or pump malfunction [1]. The relative frequency of catheter-related complications include disconnection from the pump (6–10%); leak from breakage, cut, or puncture (5–16%); and catheter tip migration (3–11%) [1]. The same study reported pump malfunction in less than 14%. A more recent study of intrathecal therapy showed that 15.8% had catheter-related problems within 2 years. Of these, 5% were catheter migrations, 5% were kinks, and 5% were leaks [2]. The same study also showed 10.5% pump malfunction. In another recent series of 144 pumps, there was pump failure in 9.03% [3].

S.M. Hayek
Department of Anesthesiology and Pain Management,
University Hospitals Cleveland Medical Center, Cleveland, OH, USA
e-mail: Salim.Hayek@UHhospitals.org

M. Mohan (✉)
ORA Orthopedics, Moline, IL, USA
e-mail: mohaneras@gmail.com

S. Diwan, T.R. Deer (eds.), *Advanced Procedures for Pain Management*,
https://doi.org/10.1007/978-3-319-68841-1_35

35.2 Clinical Evaluation and Testing

Patients who are receiving chronic intrathecal drug delivery may present with the complaint of loss of efficacy. The clinician must then investigate a number of reasons that would account for decreased response. A good starting point would be clinical evaluation, including a detailed history and physical examination. It may be helpful to ask when the pump lost its efficacy, whether the loss was acute or gradual in onset, and whether patient-activated bolus dosing offers any relief. The physical examination should note any differences from previous baseline exams, especially from a neurological standpoint. If the patient is receiving bupivacaine in the intrathecal solution, testing the dermatomes around the catheter tip with a cold object may reveal differences when compared with a control region (e.g., skin of the forehead); differences suggest a functional system. This test is more definitive if it is done immediately following a patient-activated bolus when the solution contains bupivacaine.

The next step should include pump interrogation, with special attention to residual volume and use pattern. Checking whether the programmed settings and expected residual volume agree with the actual residual volume is important at every refill and may shed light on potential system malfunction (underinfusion or overinfusion). It may be appropriate to aspirate to check and confirm the residual volume in the pump even if a pump refill is not due. The presence of more fluid than expected may suggest catheter blockade or kink, or reduced output by the pump motor. Evidence of overinfusion should prompt pump replacement.

A change in the patient's neuronal motor or sensory function with or without loss of IDDS efficacy should alert the clinician to the possibility of catheter tip granuloma [4]. Indeed, loss of efficacy and increased pain is often the first sign of an intrathecal catheter tip granuloma.

As a third step, consider radiological assessment. Simple radiographs can potentially show catheter breakage, kinking, or dislodgement. Of note, some catheters such as the Ascenda (Medtronic) are not radiopaque, so a roentgenogram may yield no information.

Next, a catheter access port (CAP) study can be performed. Aspiration through the CAP is first performed. With a normally functioning catheter, one should be able to aspirate cerebrospinal fluid (CSF) without difficulty. In most cases, more than 0.4 mL should be drained to empty both the catheter and the internal pump tubing before injecting contrast, but it is always better to double-check with a pump reading. The minimal volume to discard can be found by looking at catheter data from interrogation. One should avoid injecting into the catheter port if the CSF aspiration does not empty the tubing, unless the clinician is prepared to deal with the consequences of a bolus overdose. If injection is considered in the absence of CSF aspiration, the clinician should expect overdosing from medication in the tube, should know the amount and effect of such a medication overdose, and should be prepared to manage it. The effects of an overdose may be immediate in the presence of agents such as bupivacaine (hypotension/cardiovascular collapse) or delayed in the case of an opioid (respiratory depression/apnea).

A rotor test can be done to show that the pump mechanism is working. This study is done by first taking a radiograph perpendicular to the plane of the pump and then programming 0.01 mL of priming bolus delivered over 1 min. Then the x-ray is repeated to see how much the rotors have moved. If the pump is working normally, a SynchroMed EL pump should have moved 90° and a SynchroMed II pump should have moved 120° (Medtronic; Minneapolis, MN).

35.3 Catheter Dye Study

A catheter dye study (Fig. 35.1) is done with C-arm guidance while following strict sterile precautions, as in pump refill. It is also important to use the catheter access port (CAP) kit with the proper template and needle gauge. (The ones supplied by Medtronic are purple for SynchroMed II and red for SynchroMed EL).

The process then involves identifying the CAP using fluoroscopy, aligning the edges of the pump so that the x-ray beam is perpendicular to the pump, and carefully inserting the needle through the port. It is important to aspirate and avoid injecting anything before draining the fluid in the catheter. While injecting into the CAP, it is recommended to use the bacterial filter supplied with the kit. Contrast material approved for intrathecal use (such as iohexol) can be injected for the study.

The catheter is followed with C-arm fluoroscopy from its exit from the pump, to look for any leaks and make sure that contrast is flowing to the CSF through the catheter tip. It is important to rule out contrast pooling under the pump by a

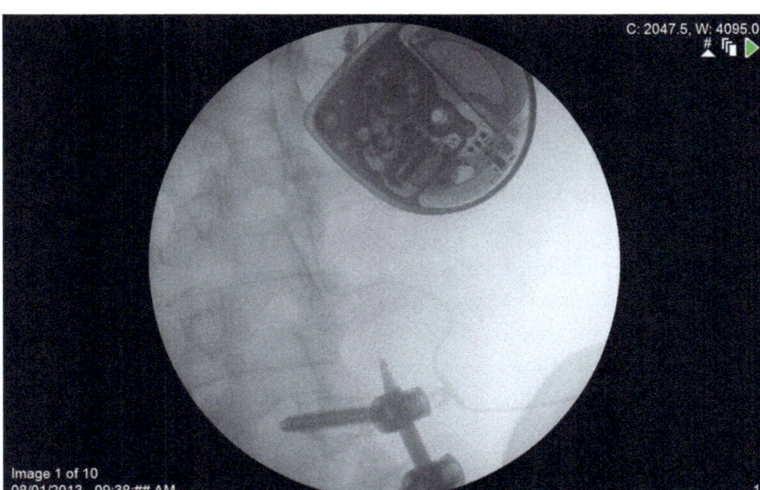

Fig. 35.1 Catheter dye study

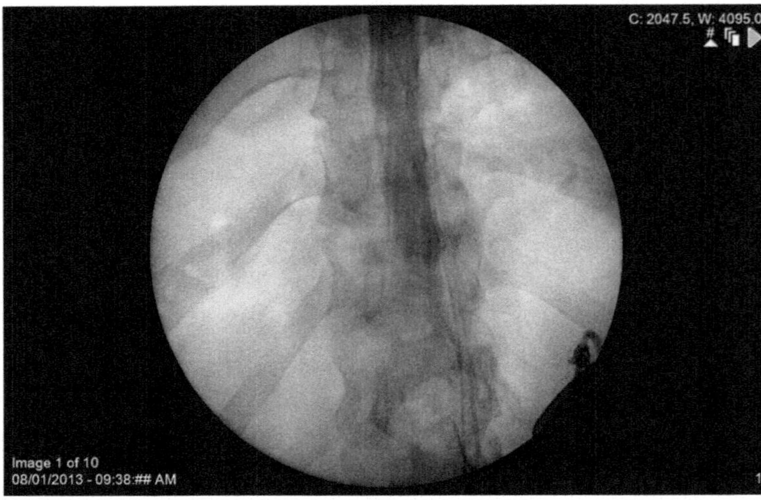

Fig. 35.2 Catheter myelogram antero-posterior view

tangential view. In addition, it is important to view contrast all along the catheter, especially at areas of connection.

Catheter contrast fluoroscopy can show a leak in macroscopic perforations and connector leaks, dislodgement of the catheter from the pump, and catheter tip dislodgement or migration. The limitation of the catheter myelogram is poor sensitivity, especially in the face of microleaks. High-definition three-dimensional (3-D) CT immediately following the catheter myelogram could be helpful if the specific site of a leak is not clear from fluoroscopy [5], which may be most likely with a small-volume leak from a microfracture within the catheter wall.

Catheter-related problems such as migration, kink, block, fracture, or dislodgement will require revision of the catheter (Figs. 35.2, 35.3, 35.4 and 35.5).

35.4 Catheter Tip Granuloma

A more dreaded complication is catheter tip granuloma; if there are features of neural compression, spine surgery consultation is needed. For catheter tip granuloma in the absence of neurologic deficits, the pump is filled with saline. After a few months, the catheter can be pulled back a few centimeters and the pump solution can be switched to non-granuloma-inducing medication such as fentanyl, bupivacaine, or ziconotide [6, 7]. There have been occasional reports of catheter tip granuloma with sufentanil [8] and one case report with fentanyl, but this is very rare and possibly more of a reflection of the use of a very high concentration. Indeed, no granuloma was seen in 18 patients with fentanyl at a dose of 50 μg/mL in solution, with an average follow-up of 24 months [9].

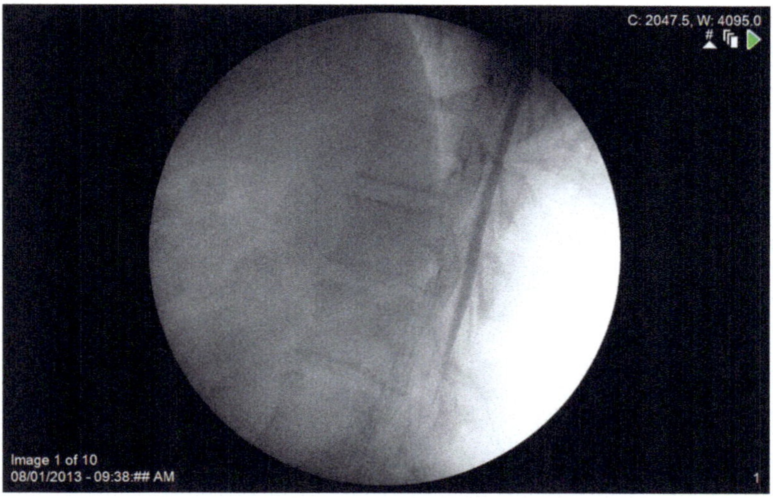

Fig. 35.3 Catheter myelogram later view

Fig. 35.4 Kink in catheter

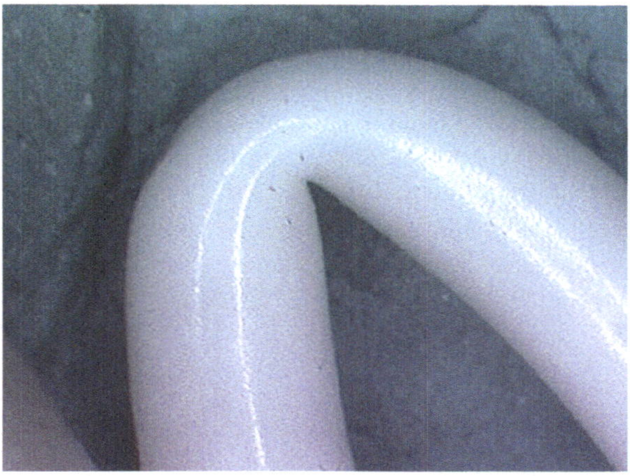

For suspected catheter tip granuloma, MRI using T1-weighted views with gadolinium contrast would be ideal to examine an enhancing lesion, using narrow slices through the tip of the catheter [7]. It is important to differentiate an enhancing catheter tip lesion from catheter tip artifact. Whenever an MRI scan is performed, a follow-up with interrogation to confirm that the pump has recovered from stall is indicated with the Medtronic pump. A different pump, the first generation from Flowonix Medical (Mt. Olive, NJ), must be emptied before the MRI. For its second generation, Prometra II, it is recommended to aspirate the pump contents until fully empty, program a demand bolus to deliver 0.03 mL concentration over 2 min (this will not displace drug, since the reservoir is empty), and then proceed with the refill process immediately after the MRI. CT scans with contrast can also be helpful if

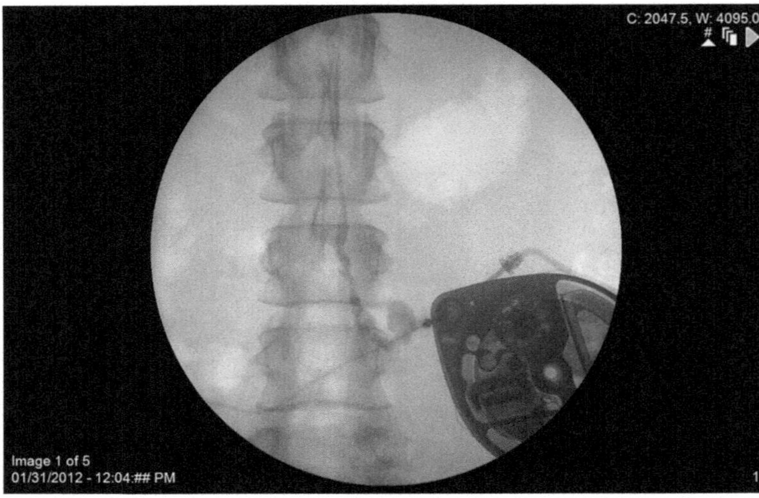

Fig. 35.5 Catheter leak

MRI is not available; the contrast could be added through the CAP procedure. Contrast should not be injected in the face of resistance or patient complaints of pain at the beginning of the slow injection process.

Acute withdrawal of baclofen is a potentially life-threatening condition. In the face of acute withdrawal of baclofen or opioids, these drugs could be supplemented orally or intrathecally through a temporary percutaneous catheter [10]. In addition to supportive care, one may consider the use of benzodiazepines for baclofen withdrawal [11].

35.5 Nuclear Medicine Scintigraphy

Nuclear medicine scintigraphic imaging is typically reserved for cases unresolved with radiological modalities. The criticism for fluoroscopic studies is that the infusion is done at a faster rate, whereas scintigraphic imaging allows for use of a drug reservoir and pumping of the radiotracer at the slow speeds used in therapeutics, together with the drug or instead of drug alone. A disadvantage of scintigraphic imaging is its relatively poor spatial resolution and the lack of anatomical landmarks in the image. Hence, using this modality to pinpoint the precise location of an occlusion, leak, or catheter position is difficult. The paucity of spatial resolution in scintigraphy can be overcome by image registration using dual-mode SPECT-CT scanners (scintigraphic and x-ray tomography registered and then displayed simultaneously) [12]. Given the slow process, scintigraphic studies are not useful in diagnosis or management when time is of the essence, as in potential withdrawal cases.

^{111}In-DTPA and ^{99m}Tc-DTPA are commonly used. For radioisotope study, ^{111}In-DTPA is typically the preferred radiopharmaceutical because of its long half-life, which allows radioactivity to be monitored for 7 days as it travels through the catheter and into the subarachnoid space. In a DTPA study, DTPA is injected into the reservoir, followed by sequential scanning. It can detect blockages, stalled motor, and large leaks. It is costly, often takes 2–3 days to perform, and has low sensitivity. It requires calculation of the flow rate and time until the isotope clears the pump tubing and catheter, to predict when the final images should be taken [13]. DTPA is injected at a dose of 0.5–0.6 mCi into the reservoir without interrupting the delivery of baclofen; if withdrawal is not a concern, the reservoir can be emptied and refilled with radiopharmaceutical solution.

35.6 Conclusions

Proper evaluation of the IDDS is an important tool in the armamentarium of the physician managing targeted intrathecal drug delivery. A thorough understanding of the system used, the effects and adverse effects of the medication(s) in the pump reservoir, and the potential advantages and limitations of interventions used to explore system malfunction is needed for appropriate investigation and troubleshooting.

References

1. Miracle AC, Fox MA, Ayyangar RN, Vyas A, Mukherji SK, Quint DJ. Imaging evaluation of intrathecal baclofen pump-catheter systems. AJNR Am J Neuroradiol. 2011;32:1158–64.
2. Hayek SM, Veizi E, Hanes M. Intrathecal hydromorphone and bupivacaine combination therapy for post-laminectomy syndrome optimized with patient-activated bolus device. Pain Med. 2015;pii:pnv021.
3. O'Connell M, Wong TZ, Forkheim KE, Jain M, Shipes SW, Fuchs HE. Comparison of Tc99m-DTPA and indium-111 DTPA studies of baclofen pump function. Clin Nucl Med. 2004;29:578–80.
4. Ellis JA, Leung R, Winfree CJ. Spinal infusion pump-catheter leak detected by high-resolution 3D computed tomography. J Neurosurg Spine. 2011;15:555–7.
5. Deer T, Krames ES, Hassenbusch S, Burton A, Caraway D, Dupen S, et al. Management of intrathecal catheter-tip inflammatory masses: an updated 2007 consensus statement from an expert panel. Neuromodulation. 2008;11:77–91.
6. Deer TR, Levy R, Prager J, Buchser E, Burton A, Caraway D, et al. Polyanalgesic consensus conference—2012: recommendations to reduce morbidity and mortality in intrathecal drug delivery in the treatment of chronic pain. Neuromodulation. 2012;15:467–82; discussion 482.
7. Gupta A, Martindale T, Christo PJ. Intrathecal catheter granuloma associated with continuous sufentanil infusion. Pain Med. 2010;11:847–52.
8. Veizi IE, Hayek SM, Hanes M, Galica R, Katta S, Yaksh T. Primary hydromorphone-related intrathecal catheter tip granulomas: is there a role for dose and concentration? Neuromodulation. 2016;19:760–9.

9. Hsieh JC, Penn RD. Intrathecal baclofen in the treatment of adult spasticity. Neurosurg Focus. 2006;21:e5.
10. Mohammed I, Hussain A. Intrathecal baclofen withdrawal syndrome—a life-threatening complication of baclofen pump: a case report. BMC Clin Pharmacol. 2004;4:6.
11. Teodorczyk J, Szmuda T, Siemiński M, Lass P, Słoniewski P. Evaluation of usefulness of scintigraphic imaging in diagnosis of intrathecal drug delivery system malfunction – a preliminary report. Pol J Radiol. 2013;78:21–7.
12. Stinchon JF, Shah NP, Ordia J, Oates E. Scintigraphic evaluation of intrathecal infusion systems: selection of patients for surgical or medical management. Clin Nucl Med. 2006;31:1–4.
13. Galica R, Hayek SM, Veizi IE, Lawrence MM, Khalil AA, McEwan MT. Sudden intrathecal drug delivery device motor stalls: a case series. Reg Anesth Pain Med. 2016;41:135–9.

Chapter 36
Intrathecal Drug Delivery: Innovation

Lucas W. Campos and Jason E. Pope

36.1 A History of Intrathecal Pain Treatment

The first documented human spinal anesthetic utilized cocaine and occurred in 1898 at the Royal Surgical Hospital of the University of Kiel [1]. The German surgeon August Bier injected cocaine into the cerebrospinal fluid (CSF) of a series of six patients who were to undergo lower extremity surgery [2]. The first patient was injected to avoid general anesthesia for his ankle operation. After administering the cocaine, Dr. Bier was able to perform the surgery with the patient awake and in no apparent distress. This success created much interest in this technique and its popularity grew [3]. Soon after, American surgeon Dr. Rudolph Matas administered the first spinal anesthetic in the United States, and showed that mixing morphine with cocaine mitigated the adverse symptoms associated with intrathecal cocaine [4, 5].

The move from single-shot anesthesia to continuous catheter use was pioneered by Dr. Grafton Love in 1935. Dr. Love was a neurosurgeon at the Mayo Clinic, and had much experience treating hydrocephalus by using continuously draining ureteral catheters placed in lateral ventricles [2]. The first clinical application of continuous spinal anesthesia was done in a series of 200 patients by a Philadelphia surgeon, Dr. William Leonard [2]. Dr. Leonard administered procaine through a syringe using a malleable, surgically placed needle. This technique was primarily used for inpatients when a general anesthetic was too great a risk. Later, Dr. Samuel Manalan, an obstetrician from Indianapolis, administered intermittent boluses of caudal anesthesia using a nylon catheter [6].

In 1944, Edward Tuohy introduced a new catheter to deliver repeated dosages of procaine during surgery. In his method, a needle and catheter directed the catheter tip to a specific location above the spinal cord [7]. The delivery of spinal

L.W. Campos (✉) • J.E. Pope
Summit Pain Alliance, Santa Rosa, CA, USA
e-mail: lwcamposmdphd@gmail.com; popeje@me.com

S. Diwan, T.R. Deer (eds.), *Advanced Procedures for Pain Management*,
https://doi.org/10.1007/978-3-319-68841-1_36

anesthetics was further advanced through permanent spinal implantation of the intrathecal catheter [8, 9]. Here, the medications were infused by accessing a subcutaneous port. In 1982, the first programmable IT pump implant was performed and by 1991 Medtronic Neurological was making this system readily available for medical use [10].

Fixed-rate devices can deliver only a specific dose of medication based on the concentration of the instilled medication. The only way to modify the dose is to empty the reservoir and instill a different medication concentration [11]. Fixed-rate pumps are less expensive than variable-rate delivery pumps, and are theorized to last a lifetime because there is no battery required [11]. These devices typically have a larger drug reservoir, so refills are less frequent [12].

36.2 Current State of the Technology

Programmable devices operated by a handheld control to communicate to the implanted device, allow delivery of variable drug doses. With the same handheld control device, these pumps are also able to deliver medication boluses. This therapy offers a means to reduce pain scores, opioid-related side effects, and oral analgesic intake. It also increases patient satisfaction and quality of life. A programmed device allows the patient to self-administer a percentage of his or her total daily intrathecal dose using their handheld remote. Safety features include a pre-programmed lockout interval and limitation of a maximum number of daily boluses [13, 14].

Programmable devices require a battery, which has a reported lifespan of 4–10 years [15]. Recently, the US Food and Drug Administration (FDA) approved two fully implantable and programmable pumps: Prometra II pump by Flowonix and the Synchromed II pump by Medtronic. The Prometra™ pump differs from the Synchromed II by its double-gated microvalve dose-regulation system. This configuration maintains accurate drug delivery despite pressure and temperature changes. A recent study demonstrated that this design functions accurately despite reservoir volume and appears to be the most accurate pump on the market to date [16]. The Medtronic Synchromed II has it is peristaltic delivery system. Both pumps are MRI conditional, as the Prometra II pump requires resetting of the flow-activated valve (FAV) after an MRI, while the Medtronic device requires interrogation.

The Medstream™ pump (Codman & Shurtleff Inc.) is approved for the IT delivery of Baclofen. This delivery system uses compressed gas as the driving force, and a ceramic drive flow valve system. Another system, awaiting FDA approval, is the Medallion™ (Alfred Mann Foundation). Like the Prometra II system, the Medallion™ offers a negative pressure reservoir that draws medications out of the syringe during pump refills, reducing the risk of a pocket-fill. There is also a pressure sensor at the tip of the catheter, which provides an alert with changes in flow [17].

36.3 Innovation

Innovation with this technology centers around device hardware, including the pump and catheter, as well as the infusion strategies employed, especially the kinetics of drug delivery. [38]. The recent PACC guidelines of 2017 highlight these advancements [39]. Thus, the demand for device companies to innovate is much reduced. Any device innovation is going to come by way of an emphasis on miniaturization, durability, dosing accuracy, and catheter design [18, 19]. The development of new pharmacological agents that utilize current pump device technology will be the likely focus of future innovation.

36.4 Resiniferatoxin

Resiniferatoxin is an ultrapotent capsaicin analog, derived from a cactus-like plant called *Euphorbia Resinifera.* This molecule targets the transient receptor vanilloid 1 (TRPV1) receptor, which transduces noxious heat stimulus applied to peripheral C-fibers. The prolonged TRPV1 ion channel activation causes a calcium influx and cell death of only those sensory neuronal cell bodies in the dorsal root ganglia which express receptor [20, 21]. Mechanistically, this makes Resiniferatoxin a promising therapeutic agent for chronic pain syndromes [22]. It is currently in a phase I study to examine its safety and analgesic effects on advanced cancer patients [23]. Brown et al. recently published a single-blind RCT in companion dogs with bone cancer pain. Intrathecal Resiniferatoxin (1.2 mg/kg) demonstrated improved analgesia and decreased lameness [24]. There was no evidence of anesthesia dolorosa, which can be seen with some other neurolytic therapies.

36.5 AYX1

Early growth response protein 1 (EGR1) is a transcription factor transiently upregulated in the spinal cord and dorsal root ganglia during acute pain. EGR1 triggers gene transcription that establishes mechanical hypersensitivity, leading to long-term movement-evoked pain. AYX1 is an investigational drug that acts by locally inhibiting EGR1 activity. It has a favorable safety profile and does not seem to alter normal neuronal function. In 2013, AYX1 was granted Fast Track designation by the FDA for the prevention of chronic pain after surgery. In 2014, a study was published that IT application of AYX1 prevented mechanical hypersensitivity in several rat models of surgically induced pain [25]. In February 2017, Adynxx initiated a phase II trial for intrathecal use of AYX1 in postoperative pain prevention [26].

36.6 Conopeptides

Cone snails produce a mixture of venomous peptides for capturing prey. Conopeptides are small peptides ranging from 10–40 amino acids in length. The conopeptides are potent and specific for mammalian targets, but exhibit a variety of pharmacologic actions, including: neurotensin-R agonism; N-methyl-D-aspartate receptor antagonism; n-acethylcholine receptor inhibition; NET inhibition; voltage-gated calcium; and sodium channel inhibition [27]. Some conopeptides are stable and exhibit long half-lives in the CSF [28, 29]. There are more than 700 cone snail species, and each may produce up to 200 conopeptides. Thus, the library of possible bioactive peptides that could have therapeutic utility is very large [30]. Several conopeptides have been identified as having analgesic potential by inhibiting peripheral nociceptors and facilitating descending pain inhibition mechanisms [31]. Some of the conopeptides identified with potential IT application include: Xen2174, a χ-conopeptide isolated from the venom of Conus Marmoreus; CGX-1160, a conopeptide-based drug that acts on the neurotensin, NTR1 receptor; and AM336, a synthetic analog of the ω-conotoxin that serves as a novel N-type, calcium channel blocker [28, 32].

36.7 Hybrid Therapy

The idea of combining IT therapy and spinal cord stimulation therapy (SCS) is garnering increased attention, and emerging literature recognizes the value of this combination. Preliminary data suggest that IT therapy can convert SCS trial non-responders into responders [33, 34]. It is theorized that the combined effect of intrathecal pharmaceutical and spinal electrical stimulation modulates GABAergic, adrenergic, serotonergic, and cholinergic spinal and supraspinal mechanisms [33, 35, 36]. Intrathecal Baclofen, the GABA-B receptor agonist that is commonly used both orally and intrathecally for the treatment of spasticity, has been evaluated prospectively [37]. Out of 48 patients who received an intrathecal baclofen bolus during SCS trial, 20 obtained a pain relief reduction of >50%. Seven of these patients were then implanted with an intrathecal baclofen pump and SCS system [37]. After an average follow-up of 6 years, these patients continued with more than 50% improvement in their previously noted pain scores. The dose of baclofen had to be gradually increased over the years, and the range of daily IT doses was 140–270 μg [37].

36.8 Conclusion

IT therapy effectively treats chronic pain and offers interventional pain physicians a high degree of flexibility such that analgesic selection and dose scheduling can be individually tailored to meet the unique needs of each patient. Innovations in pharmaceutical mechanisms of pain relief and delivery of these new medications combined with a more comprehensive understanding of the pathophysiology of pain will lead to better outcomes and improved patient quality of life. Adherence to best practices and advancement of clinical and basic science research are necessary to ensure continued progress with IT therapy.

References

1. Wulf HF. The centennial of spinal anesthesia. Anesthesiology. 1998;89:500–6.
2. Deer TR. History of intrathecal drug delivery. In: Deer TR, editor. Atlas of implantable therapies for pain management. New York, NY: Springer; 2011. p. 139–41.
3. Drasner K. Spinal anaesthesia: a century of refinement, and failure is still an option. Br J Anaesth. 2009;102:729–30.
4. Onofrio BM, Yaksh TL, Arnold PG. Continuous low-dose intrathecal morphine administration in the treatment of chronic pain of malignant origin. Mayo Clin Proc. 1981;56:516–20.
5. Matas R. Local and regional anesthesia: a retrospect and prospect. Am J Surg. 1934;25:189–96.
6. Mccormick CO, Huber CP, Spahr JF, Gillespie CF. An experience with one hundred cases of continuous caudal analgesia. Am J Obstet Gynecol. 1944;47:297–311.
7. Tuohy EB. The use of continuous spinal anesthesia: utilizing the ureteral catheter technic. JAMA. 1945;128(4):262.
8. Dahm P, Nitescu P, Appelgren L, Curelaru I. Efficacy and technical complications of long-term continuous intraspinal infusions of opioid and/or bupivacaine in refractory nonmalignant pain: a comparison between the epidural and the intrathecal approach with externalized or implanted catheters and infusion pumps. Clin J Pain. 1998;14:4–16.
9. Turner JA, Sears JM, Loeser JD. Programmable intrathecal opioid delivery systems for chronic noncancer pain: a systematic review of effectiveness and complications. Clin J Pain. 2007;23:180–95.
10. Belverud S, Mogilner A, Schulder M. Intrathecal pumps. Neurotherapeutics. 2008;5:114–22.
11. de Leon-Casasola OA. Interventional procedures for cancer pain management: when are they indicated? Cancer Invest. 2004;22:630–42.
12. Bedder MD, Burchiel K, Larson A. Cost analysis of two implantable narcotic delivery systems. J Pain Symptom Manage. 1991;6:368–73.
13. Hayek SM, Hanes MC. Intrathecal therapy for chronic pain: current trends and future needs. Curr Pain Headache Rep. 2014;18:388.
14. Bolash R, Mekhail N. Intrathecal pain pumps: indications, patient selection, techniques, and outcomes. Neurosurg Clin N Am. 2014;25:735–42.
15. Smyth C, Ahmadzai N, Wentzell J, Pardoe A, Tse A, Nguyen T, et al. Intrathecal analgesia for chronic refractory pain: current and future prospects. Drugs. 2015;75:1957–80.
16. Rauck R, Deer T, Rosen S, Padda G, Barsa J, Dunbar E, et al. Accuracy and efficacy of intrathecal administration of morphine sulfate for treatment of intractable pain using the Prometra(®) programmable pump. Neuromodulation. 2010;13:102–8.
17. Bottros MM, Christo PJ. Current perspectives on intrathecal drug delivery. J Pain Res. 2014;7:615–26.
18. De Andres J, Asensio-Samper JM, Fabregat-Cid G. Advances in intrathecal drug delivery. Curr Opin Anaesthesiol. 2013;26:594–9.
19. Lawson EF, Wallace MS. Current developments in intraspinal agents for cancer and noncancer pain. Curr Pain Headache Rep. 2010;14:8–16.
20. Karai L, Brown DC, Mannes AJ, Connelly ST, Brown J, Gandal M, et al. Deletion of vanilloid receptor 1_expressing primary afferent neurons for pain control. J Clin Invest. 2004;113:1344–52.

21. Caterina MJ, Schumacher MA, Tominaga M, Rosen TA, Levine JD, Julius D. The capsaicin receptor: a heat-activated ion channel in the pain pathway. Nature. 1997;389:816–24.
22. Holzer P. The pharmacological challenge to tame the transient receptor potential vanilloid-1 (TRPV1) nocisensor. Br J Pharmacol. 2008;155:1145–62.
23. Resiniferatoxin to treat severe pain associated with advanced cancer. ClinicalTrials.gov. https://clinicaltrials.gov/show/NCT00804154. Accessed 13 Nov 2016.
24. Brown DC, Agnello K, Iadarola MJ. Intrathecal resiniferatoxin in a dog model: efficacy in bone cancer pain. Pain. 2015;156:1018–24.
25. Mamet J, Klukinov M, Yaksh TL, Malkmus SA, Williams S, Harris S, et al. Single intrathecal administration of the transcription factor decoy AYX1 prevents acute and chronic pain after incisional, inflammatory, or neuropathic injury. Pain. 2014;155:322–33.
26. Study to evaluate safety/efficacy of a single preop dose of AYX1 injection to treat pain after knee replacement surgery. ClinicalTrials.gov. https://clinicaltrials.gov/ct2/show/NCT02807428. Accessed 13 Nov 2016.
27. Lewis RJ, Dutertre S, Vetter I, Christie MJ. Conus venom peptide pharmacology. Pharmacol Rev. 2012;64:259–98.
28. Deer T, Krames ES, Hassenbusch S, Burton A, Caraway D, Dupen S, et al. Future directions for intrathecal pain management: a review and update from the interdisciplinary polyanalgesic consensus conference 2007. Neuromodulation. 2008;11:92–7.
29. Kern SE, Allen J, Wagstaff J, Shafer SL, Yaksh T. The pharmacokinetics of the conopeptide contulakin-G (CGX-1160) after intrathecal administration: an analysis of data from studies in beagles. Anesth Analg. 2007;104:1514–20.
30. Daly NL, Craik DJ. Conopeptides as novel options for pain management. Drugs Future. 2011;36:25–32.
31. Essack M, Bajic VB, Archer JAC. Conotoxins that confer therapeutic possibilities. Mar Drugs. 2012;10:1244–65.
32. Lewis RJ. Conotoxins: molecular and therapeutic targets. Prog Mol Subcell Biol. 2009;46:45–65.
33. Lind G, Meyerson BA, Winter J, Linderoth B. Intrathecal baclofen as adjuvant therapy to enhance the effect of spinal cord stimulation in neuropathic pain: a pilot study. Eur J Pain. 2004;8:377–83.
34. Truin M, Janssen SPM, van Kleef M, Joosten EA. Successful pain relief in non-responders to spinal cord stimulation: the combined use of ketamine and spinal cord stimulation. Eur J Pain. 2011;15:1049.e1–9.
35. Slavin KV. Spinal stimulation for pain: future applications. Neurotherapeutics. 2014;11:535–42.
36. Song Z, Ultenius C, Meyerson BA, Linderoth B. Pain relief by spinal cord stimulation involves serotonergic mechanisms: an experimental study in a rat model of mononeuropathy. Pain. 2009;147:241–8.
37. Lind G, Schechtmann G, Winter J, Meyerson BA, Linderoth B. Baclofen-enhanced spinal cord stimulation and intrathecal baclofen alone for neuropathic pain: long-term outcome of a pilot study. Eur J Pain. 2008;12:132–6.
38. Pope J, McRoberts WP, Deer T, Poree L. Are bolus dosing strategies the intrathecal version of novel waveforms with spinal cord stimulation? Neuromodulation. 2015;18(8):776–7.
39. Deer TR, Pope JE, Hayek SM, Bux A, Buchser E, Eldabe S, et al. The polyanalgesic consensus conference (PACC): recommendations on intrathecal drug infusion systems best practices and guidelines. Neuromodulation. 2017;20(2):96–132.

Part III
Advanced Regenerative Medicine

Corey W. Hunter and Timothy Davis

The field of regenerative medicine has grown substantially over the past 30 years, not only in the number of providers utilizing it but in the amount of innovation we have seen during that time. Traditionally, stem cell therapy was out of reach for the common, everyday practitioner, but now it is available to whoever wishes to use it. While it has shown a great deal of promise, the lack of regulation by the U.S. Food and Drug Administration (FDA) has prevented any form of standardization in the therapy, resulting in practitioners relying on anecdotal experiences and weekend courses rather than evidence-based medicine. The purpose of this section is to give interested physicians the tools to use this therapy correctly and ethically by giving readers the ability to rely on hard evidence as presented by experts in the field. This section is truly a first of its kind—never before has there been a comprehensive, unbiased compilation of the various types of regenerative therapies currently available. As interest in this therapy continues to grow, our hope is for this *Atlas* to mark the point at which regenerative medicine starting being used in accordance with evidence rather than opinion.

Chapter 37
History of Regenerative Medicine

Houman Danesh and Lee P. Hingula

Until relatively recently, regenerative *medicine* has been a research term used to describe engineering or regrowing tissue to re-establish normal function [1]. Though research in this field and its clinical applications are novel, the central tenets are ancient. The idea that noxious stimuli applied to injured tissue can induce healing is traceable to 500 BC in Rome, where soldiers with joint dislocations were treated with hot needle therapy [2]. In the twentieth century, a practice known as prolotherapy, in which hyperosmolar substances were injected into damaged tissue, was popularized. As we have learned more about inflammation and its mediators, platelet-rich plasma (PRP) injections have been investigated as a method to regenerate tissue in a manner that is theoretically similar to prolotherapy. It is reasoned that because platelets contain inflammatory mediators and these molecules are critical to the healing process, injecting a higher than physiologic concentration of platelets could induce tissue regeneration with normal cell architecture.

The newest innovation in regenerative medicine is the use of stem cell therapy, although it is associated with considerable ethical and legal concerns. Human stem cells can broadly be categorized into embryonic, placental, and adult. Embryonic stem cells are pluripotent cells derived from human blastocysts prior to uterine implantation (Fig. 37.1) [3]. Because they require the creation of a fertilized human embryo, federal funding for their study in the United States until recently has been restricted to a finite number of existing cell lines. Fortunately, stem cells have been discovered in a variety of tissues, including in umbilical cord blood [4], amniotic

H. Danesh (✉)
Integrative Pain Management, Department of Anesthesiology, Perioperative and Pain Medicine, Mount Sinai Hospital, New York, NY, USA
e-mail: houmanmd@gmail.com

L.P. Hingula
Division of Pain Management, Department of Anesthesiology and Critical Care Medicine, Memorial Sloan-Kettering Cancer Center, New York, NY, USA
e-mail: lphingula@gmail.com

S. Diwan, T.R. Deer (eds.), *Advanced Procedures for Pain Management*,
https://doi.org/10.1007/978-3-319-68841-1_37

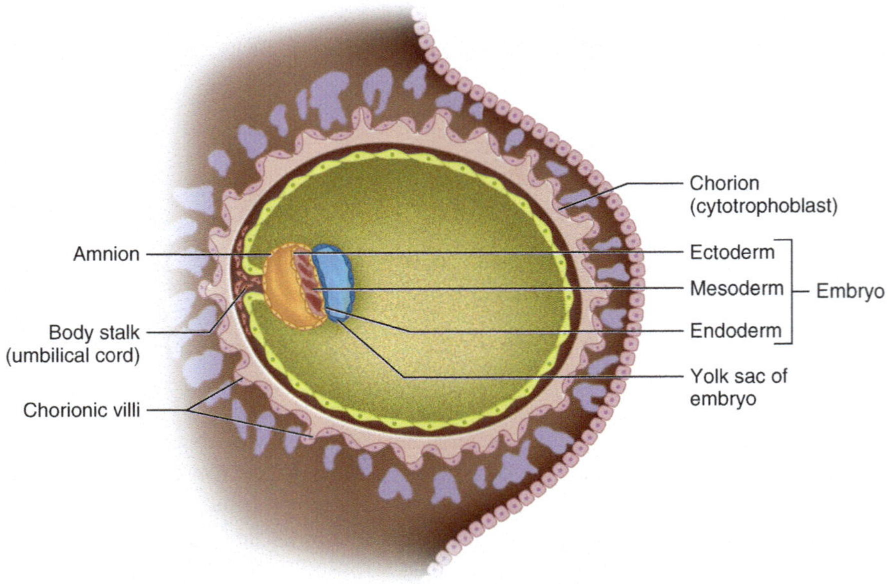

Fig. 37.1 The chorion, amnion, and embryo

fluid [5], chorionic tissue [6], and adult organs. Placenta-derived stem cells and adult stem cells lack some of the ethical concerns pertaining to embryonic stem cells, but their use has also been limited in clinical practice because of the tissue processing required to use them. The promise for novel therapies continues to grow as new technologies are developed to coax adult cells to dedifferentiate into immature precursor cells (so-called induced-pluripotent stem cells) [7]. As stem cell therapy and platelet-rich plasma are becoming increasingly popular in pain management and throughout the field of medicine, future research is likely to help guide the clinical applications of regenerative medicine.

37.1 Prolotherapy

In the 1930s, physicians developed prolotherapy, short for *proliferation therapy*, a technique of injecting irritant solutions into joints or tendons. It is reasoned that inflammation is the first step in healing, and that injecting inflammatory mediators into damaged tissue may speed convalescence. The practice expanded in the 1950s. Dr. George S. Hackett, a general surgeon in the Unites States, began using prolotherapy in an effort to repair tendons and ligaments [8]. Today the practice is less common in allopathic medicine, and in 1999 CMS (Medicare and Medicaid) reviewers decided to continue to not pay for the procedure [9]. More recent systematic reviews suggest that there may be moderate evidence for prolotherapy in the treatment of lateral epicondylitis, though the included studies have a high likelihood of bias [10, 11]. A more recent systematic review corroborates the evidence that prolotherapy for lateral epicondylitis may be beneficial [12]. Though prolotherapy may prove to be an outdated treatment modality, it has helped propel the field of regenerative medicine forward and has led to further advances, including platelet-rich plasma.

37.2 Platelet-Rich Plasma

37.2.1 Definition and Classification

Platelet-rich plasma (PRP) can be defined as plasma with a supraphysiologic concentration of platelets as well as other cell types and cell fragments of varying concentration. Most studies regarding PRP have not standardized the number of platelets, leukocytes, and red blood cells, and the addition of exogenous substances to activate the platelets. As the uses of PRP expand, so too has our understanding of the importance of its contents. The "PLRA" classification system proposed by Mautner and colleagues [13] is one of several systems that have been used, but none is currently standard of practice (Table 37.1).

37.2.2 Derivation

The mainstay of PRP preparation involves centrifuging blood into its components (Fig. 37.2). There are two common methods, the PRP method and the buffy coat method. In the PRP method, whole blood is centrifuged twice. The first centrifugation is slow and produces two layers, a red blood cell layer and another layer containing proteins, white blood cells, and platelets. This second layer is then further centrifuged to separate out the platelet fraction with varying amounts of white blood

Table 37.1 Proposed PLRA classification system for platelet-rich plasma (PRP) preparations [13]

Category	Criteria	Final score	
P	Platelet	P volume injected	M cells/microliter
L	Leukocyte content	>1% <1%	+ −
R	Red blood cell count	>1% <1%	+ −
A	Activation	Yes No	+ −

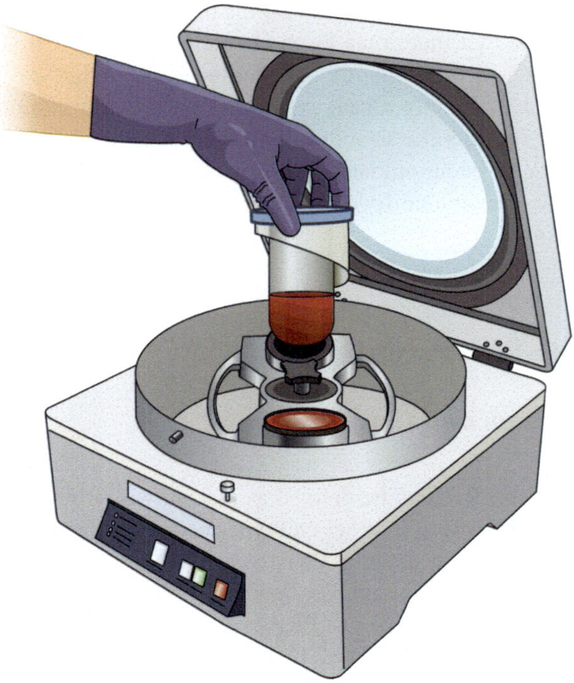

Fig. 37.2 A device used for the preparation of platelet-rich plasma (PRP)

cells and proteins, including fibrin, fibronectin, and vitronectin. The buffy coat method uses one high-speed centrifugation to separate whole blood into three fractions composed of red blood cells, plasma, and platelets/white blood cells. The platelet/white blood cell fraction can then either be centrifuged again, or leukocyte filtration can be used. Some authors recommend activating platelets with calcium or thrombin, although data to suggest which approach is optimal are insufficient [14].

37.2.3 History

High platelet concentrates were first used as a means to increase inflammation in the 1970s. In 1987, PRP was first used during open heart surgery in Italy [15]. Its use increased during the 1990s, particularly in oral and maxillofacial surgery. Plastic and orthopedic surgeons were also interested in PRP to improve flap survival and bone healing. The best evidence for PRP has been in the treatment of lateral epicondylitis, although studies examining this use often suffer from methodological flaws

[10, 11]. Increased use of PRP among amateur athletes is almost certainly due in part to its use among celebrity athletes, such as Hines Ward and Troy Polamalu, who went on to win the Super Bowl, and pro golfer Tiger Woods [16].

37.2.4 Research and Uses

PRP is most commonly used in the treatment of enthesopathies such as tennis elbow, golfers' elbow and Achilles tendonitis. There have been numerous uses throughout its history, but it has been difficult to draw conclusions across meta-analyses because each injectate's platelet concentration may differ by logs. In addition, control groups in PRP studies range from dry needling to corticosteroid injections to whole blood, or even no intervention [17]. PRP preparation kits are numerous as well. As a blood product, PRP falls under the jurisdiction of the FDA's Center for Biologics Evaluation and Research guidelines. It does not have to go through the traditional avenues of animal trials and clinical testing used for drugs. Even the devices used for PRP preparation do not have to undergo rigorous evaluation. They are given 501(k) clearance, which allows devices to be cleared for use if they are "substantially equivalent" to existing approved devices [18]. The therapeutic role of PRP is likely be more clearly defined as the number of PRP studies increase and protocols are standardized.

37.3 Stem Cells

37.3.1 Highlights of the First Stem Cell Uses

1956: Dr. E Donnall Thomas performs the first bone marrow transplant on a patient with leukemia, whose donor was his identical twin [19].

1958: French oncologist Georges Mathé performed several transplants on patients exposed to radiation poisoning [20].

1981: The first mouse stem cell line was created [21].

1995: The first nonhuman primate's stem cells could be grown in vitro [22].

1997: Dolly was the first sheep to be fully cloned (Fig. 37.3). The success of Dolly was particularly ethically important, as somatic cell nuclear transfer was the process by which the embryo was created [23]. Using this method, there is no manipulation of a previously fertilized embryo, but rather an adult cell's nuclear contents are transferred into an unfertilized egg.

1998: Thomson and Shamblott independently developed the first in vitro human embryonic stem cell lines [24, 25].

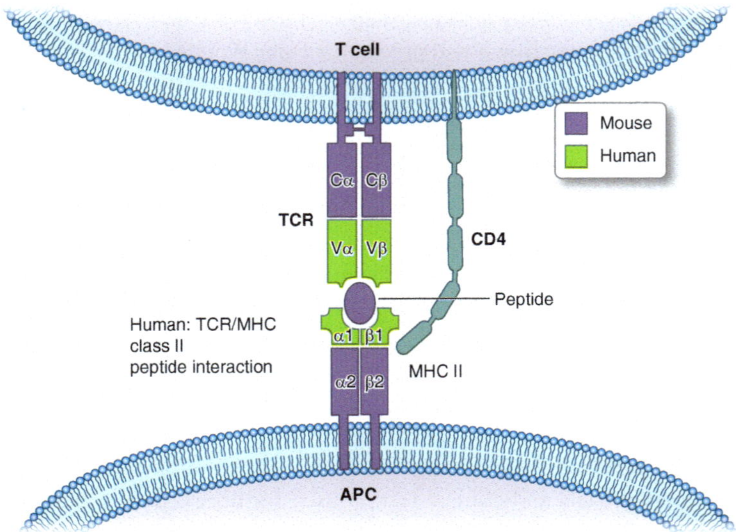

Fig. 37.3 The role of HLA proteins and the major histocompatibility complex (MHC) in antigen presentation and graft survival. *APC* antigen-presenting cell, *TCR* T-cell receptor

There was a gradual increase in the number of human stem cell lines that were produced, but government regulation in the United States had already begun to change the landscape for stem cell research.

37.3.2 Discovery of Different Types of Stem Cells

1961: Hematopoietic stem cells were described by McCulloch and Till in 1961 [26].

1978: Umbilical stem cells were discovered [4].

1992: Reynolds and Rietze found neural stem cells [27].

2001: Zuk and colleagues [28] discovered stem cells in adipose tissue.

2006: Japanese investigators inserted four functional genes (*OCT4*, *SOX2*, *KLF4*, and *MYC*) into mouse skin cells and induced a pluripotent-like state [7].

2006: Adult skin cells are used to create induced-pluripotent stem cells and grow lines of cardiomyocytes, neurons, liver cells, and hematopoietic cell lines [29].

2007: Anthony Atala's group found stem cells in amniotic fluid [30].

Although the above lines are partially fated and limited in their ability to grow into different tissue types, they have been used with some success in the field of regenerative medicine (Table 37.2). There is some evidence that adipose-derived stem cells have chondrogenic potential, and they have been used in patients with

Table 37.2 Stem cell categories

Type	Source	Differentiation potential
Amniotic	Amniotic fluid, fetal cells	Multipotent, three germ layers
Embryonic	Fertilized blastocysts	Totipotent
Bone marrow mesenchymal	Bone marrow, rare cell type	Multipotent, non-hematopoietic
Bone marrow hematopoietic	Bone marrow, abundant	Hematopoietic cell lines, perhaps others
Adipose	Lipoaspirate	Multipotent
Induced-pluripotent	Adult differentiated cells	Unknown

osteoarthritis to rebuild joint cartilage [31], although randomized controlled trials are lacking. Companies like Regenexx (Broomfield, CO) market off-the-shelf concentrated bone marrow-derived stem cells for use in peripheral joint disease. Placental tissue matrices utilizing amnion and chorion tissue preparations have been applied in many fields of medicine, including pain management. There is evidence that these tissue types are anti-inflammatory, have angiogenic potential, and exert paracrine effects that induce healing, rather than actively differentiate into native tissue [32]. It will likely be years before induced-pluripotent stem cells are regularly used for pain management.

37.3.3 Current Uses and Research of Stem Cell Therapies

There have been more setbacks than successes in the clinical application of stem cells. Shortly after the introduction of bone marrow transplantation, graft versus host disease was identified as a major source of morbidity and mortality [33]. Rejection of foreign tissue continues to stymie the success of transplantation and tissue graft survival. Modern advances in anti-rejection immunosuppressive therapy have improved the survival of graft tissue, but the risks are considerable. Placental tissue matrices have made stem cell therapies more attractive in the setting of pain management, as their use may be associated with a lower risk of complications. Amniotic tissue lacks HLA II antigens that are important in eliciting an immune response [34]. Recent research has also shown that amniotic stem cells can induce osteogenic differentiation of bone marrow–derived stem cells [35]. Adult (mesenchymal) stem cells also represent a potentially important source of chondrocytes, which are difficult to grow in vitro [36]. Bone marrow–derived stem cells express CD105 and TGF-beta, which appear to be key in their ability to differentiate into chondrocytes [37]. Unfortunately, bone marrow aspiration is associated with a high rate of pelvic fracture, which is likely to be an unacceptable risk to patients undergoing treatment for pain. Yet with the exception of the *Stro-1* gene, bone marrow-derived and adipocyte-derived stem cells appear to express the same surface markers, including CD66, CD105, CD55, CD54, CD44, and CD13 [38]. When exposed to BMP-2, adipocyte-derived stem cells can differentiate into chondrocytes that express mature cartilage markers, such as type II collagen [39]. Though these advances are promising, clinical trials for many of these therapies are years from complete. Nevertheless, certain applications are currently being used and have promising evidence.

37.3.3.1 Osteoarthritis

Although many of the studies of mesenchymal cells in the treatment of osteoarthritis are of short duration and small sample sizes, some trials have been promising. Mesenchymal stem cells (MSCs) are showing promising evidence for the treatment of osteoarthritis. These cells have both a regenerative potential and anti-inflammatory properties [40].

Three promising articles show how these cells can be used in osteoarthritis. One study showed improved quality of life outcomes and improved cartilage on MRI at 1 year [41]. it is important to note that this study included 40×10^6 million cells. Many of the studies done involve clonally expanded cells, which is not allowed in the United States. In 2009, Fennema et al. showed that bone marrow aspiration contains approximately 26×10^6 cells [42]. This is an important consideration both when reviewing the literature and when deciding to proceed with stem cells in the United States. Another study using adipose-derived stem cells showed promise in elderly patients (>65 years) with knee osteoarthritis. This study found that 88% demonstrated improved cartilage status at 2 years, and all patients were able to avoid total knee replacements during that time [43].

Another study investigated patients with unicompartmental knee osteoarthritis with varus alignment undergoing high tibial osteotomy and microfracture. The results showed improved clinical, patient-reported, and MRI-based outcomes in a group receiving a preoperative MSC injection compared with a control group that received tibial osteotomy and microfracture alone [44].

It is still too early to make a blanket recommendation on the use of the type of stem cell, concentrations, timing of use (pre-op or post-op), and the right patient population.

37.3.3.2 Tendinopathy

Tendon injuries are potentially prime candidates for stem cell therapy. The healing potential of tendons has long been an issue, as it is inferior to that of bone and other connective tissues [45]. The problem is further compounded by the fact that the repaired tendons are biomechanically inferior and show histological structure inferior to that of native tissue [46].

The standard of care has long been the use of steroids, but a Cochrane review in 2003 showed no difference at 2 weeks and 8 weeks when the supraspinatus tendon was treated with steroids or with placebo [47]. Another study showed that steroids are no more effective than NSAIDs and that they are more effective in the subacute period (<12 weeks) [48]. There is also some evidence of reduced tensile strength and mechanical properties [49].

Human treatment of tendinopathies with stem cells has scarcely been studied to date. One study took eight patients with refractory patellar tendinopathy treated with injection of autologous bone marrow MSCs and reported successful results at 2- to 5-year follow-up, with significant improvements in patient-reported outcome measures for 100% of patients. Of the eight patients, seven (87.5%) noted that they would undergo the procedure again [50].

Another study took 28 sports-related Achilles tendon ruptures in 27 patients treated with open repair and injection of bone marrow aspirate concentrate (BMAC). At a mean follow-up of 29.7 months, the authors reported no re-ruptures, with 92% of the patients returned to sport at 5.9 months, and excellent clinical outcomes [51]. It is important to note that this study is a surgical outcome and it is difficult to extrapolate to outpatient injectable settings.

37.3.4 Summary

Our understanding of the use of stem cells and their indications has expanded exponentially over the past decade. Stem cell treatment has particularly infiltrated the world of operative and nonoperative sports medicine [52]. Stem cell therapy offers a potentially effective therapy for a multitude of pathologies because of these cells' anti-inflammatory, immunoregulatory, angiogenic, and paracrine effects [53].

The ideal stem cell sources (including allogeneic or autologous), preparation, cell number, timing, and means of application continue to be evaluated, and those advantageous pathologies need to be researched further. To better answer these pertinent questions, we need to make sure we have a safe, economic, and ethically acceptable means for stem cell translational research efforts. More high-level studies with standardized protocols need to be performed. It is necessary to improve national and international collaboration in research, as well as collaboration with governing bodies, to attempt to further scientific advancement in this field of research [53, 54].

Overall, the evidence for the use of stem cells in outpatients is still in the nascent stages. Caution must be used when reviewing the literature and when using them in clinic settings.

37.3.5 History of Stem Cell Laws

1995: The Dickey-Wicker Amendment is written and signed into law by President Clinton; it prohibits the Department of Health and Human Services from using funds to create human embryos for the purpose of research, or destroying existing human embryos [56] (Fig. 42.6).

2000: The National Institutes of Health (NIH) publishes guidelines for research involving pluripotent stem cells. The guidelines require that stem cell lines used for research originate from fertility clinics, use private funds, be in excess of donors' needs, and be obtained with consent from the donor [56].

2001: George W. Bush signs an executive order prohibiting federal funding from being used for any embryonic stem cell line that originated after August 9th, 2001 [56]. This policy does not affect any research in the private sector or research conducted with state funding. Adult stem cell research is not affected by this order.

2005 and 2007: Congress passes the Stem Cell Research Enhancement Act to expand federal funding for embryonic stem cell research, but President Bush vetoes the act both times [56]. A two-thirds majority needed by the House of Representatives to override the presidential veto was not reached in either year.

2009: President Obama reversed President Bush's stance on embryonic stem cells and orders the NIH to write new guidelines regarding embryonic stem cell research. The new guidelines expanded federal funding for embryonic stem cells so that new lines of cells can be created and used for research [57].

The debate over federal funding for embryonic stem cell research has continued, and as recently as 2011 the Supreme Court refused to hear an appeal of *Sherley v Sebelius*, which challenged the legality of NIH funding for stem cell research [58]. Further legislation in the field of embryonic stem cells is almost certain, but new research on adult (mesenchymal), placental-derived, and induced-pluripotent stem cells may decrease the need for embryonic stem cells in the future. Each of the stem cells has different advantages and disadvantages (Tables 37.3 and 37.4).

Although mesenchymal stem cells have not been in the legal spotlight as much as embryonic stem cells, a number of regulations exist to govern their use. In 1997, the Tissue Reference Group (TRG) was created by the FDA to regulate cellular and tissue-based products. Since its inception, the group has published multiple updates and used the phrase "more than minimally manipulated" to distinguish those tissue types that require no FDA regulation and those that would be considered a medical device after such manipulation, thus necessitating an FDA approval process [59]. The first instance of this terminology being used to regulate stem cells was in 2006, when the TRG issued an update that umbilical cord cells enzymatically treated to increase engraftment were more than minimally manipulated [59]. Today, adipose-derived stem cells, many amniotic membrane products, and bone marrow-derived MSCs are contemporary examples of tissue that is more than minimally manipulated, as enzymatic processes or complex extraction is required to increase yield or make them suitable for reintroduction into the body. It is likely that further advances in stem cell technologies also will require tissue processing that will subject them to this regulation and require approval by the FDA.

Table 37.3 Advantages and disadvantages of stem cells [55]

Stem cell type	Source	Advantages	Disadvantages
Embryonic	Embryonic tissue	Pluripotent to all three germ layers: mesoderm, endoderm, ectoderm	Oncogenic potential; allogenic rejection; ethical and legal constraints
Induced pluripotent	Adult somatic tissue transfected with embryonic transcription factors	Pluripotent; decreased ethical concerns due to adult source; no allogenic rejection	Oncogenic potential; modest induction yield
Mesenchymal	Multiple fetal and adult tissue (umbilical cord, umbilical blood, placenta, skin, bone marrow, blood vessels, adipose, synovium, periosteum, dental pulp)	Can differentiate into tissues of interest: bone, cartilage, and tendon; immunosuppressive, allowing for allo- and xeno-transplantation	Limited differentiation capacity; modest yield from host tissue

Table 37.4 Common sources for mesenchymal stem cells with documented tissue-type differentiation and source advantages [55]

Mesenchymal stem cell source	Differentiation potential	Source	Advantages
Bone marrow	Chondrocyte, muscle, osteoblast, cardiocyte, mesangial cell, hepatocyte	Chondrocyte, muscle, osteoblast, cardiocyte, mesangial cell, hepatocyte	Highest differentiation potential
Adipose	Adipose	Chondrocyte, muscle, osteoblast, stromal cell	Easily accessible, higher colony formation compared to bone marrow derived cells
Synovium	Adipocyte, chondrocyte, muscle, osteoblast [22]	Adipocyte, chondrocyte, muscle, osteoblast [22]	Applicable for cartilage and tendon healing
Periosteum	Periosteum	Chondrocyte [22], osteoblast [23]	Applicable to fracture nonunion healing

37.4 Conclusion

Regenerative medicine as a concept has existed for hundreds of years. The idea that inflammation is necessary for healing and that inducing inflammation may be beneficial has existed since ancient Rome. Prolotherapy and PRP are the modern versions of this concept. More recently, stem cell therapies have been utilized in clinical practice for pain management and regenerative medicine. Embryonic stem cell use has been limited by legislation, but research into adult and placental stem cells circumvents many of those ethical concerns. Novel therapies utilizing these cell types have shown promise in regenerating cartilage and providing pain relief. Induced-pluripotent stem cells may be used in the future as an easy-to-harvest and abundant source of stem cells.

References

1. Horch RE, Popescu LM, Polykandriotis E. History of regenerative medicine. In: Steinhoff G, editor. Regenerative medicine: from protocol to patient. Dordrecht: Springer; 2011. p. 1–19.
2. Goswami A. Prolotherapy. J Pain Palliat Care Pharmacother. 2012;26:376–8.
3. Chen Y, Lai D. Pluripotent states of human embryonic stem cells. PLoS One. 2014;13:9–11.
4. Prindull G, Prindull B, Meulen N. Haematopoietic stem cells (CFUc) in human cord blood. Acta Paediatr Scand. 1978;67:413–6.
5. Dziadosz M, Basch RS, Young BK. Human amniotic fluid: a source of stem cells for possible therapeutic use. Am J Obstet Gynecol. 2016;214:321–7.
6. Ziadlour R, Shahhoseini M, Safari F, Sayahpour F, Eslaminejad M. Comparative analysis of neural differentiation potential in human mesenchymal stem cells derived from chorion and adult bone marrow. Cell Tissue Res. 2015;362(2):367–77.
7. Takahashi K, Yamanaka S. Induction of pluripotent stem cells from mouse embryonic and adult fibroblast cultures by defined factors. Cell. 2006;126:663–76.
8. Schwartz RG, Sagedy N. Prolotherapy: a literature review and retrospective study. J Neurol Orthop Med Surg. 1991;12:220–3.
9. Bagley GP, Bisguier E, Honemann D. Decision memo for prolotherapy for chronic low back pain (CAG-00045N). Centers for Medicare and Medicaid Services. 1999. https://www.cms.gov/medicare-coverage-database/details/nca-decision-memo. Prolotherapy+for+Chronic+Low+Back+Pain. Accessed 4 Feb 2016.
10. Judson CH, Wolf JM. Lateral epicondylitis: review of injection therapies. Orthop Clin North Am. 2013;44:615–23.
11. Krogh TP, Bartels EM, Ellingsen T, Stengaard-Pedersen K, Buchbinder R, Fredberg U, et al. Comparative effectiveness of injection therapies in lateral epicondylitis: a systematic review and network meta-analysis of randomized controlled trials. Am J Sports Med. 2013;41:1435–46.
12. Dong W, Goost H, Lin XB, Burger C, Paul C, Wang ZL, et al. Injection therapies for lateral epicondylalgia: a systematic review and Bayesian network meta-analysis. Br J Sports Med. 2016;50:900–8.
13. Mautner K, Malanga GA, Smith J, Shiple B, Ibrahim V, Sampson S, Bowen JE. A call for a standard classification system for future biologic research: the rationale for new PRP nomenclature. PM R. 2015;7(4 Suppl):S53–9.
14. Dhurat R, Sukesh MS. Principles and methods of preparation of platelet-rich plasma: a review and author's perspective. J Cutan Aesthet Surg. 2014;7:189–97.
15. Ferrari M, Zia S, Valbonesi M. A new technique for hemodilution, preparation of autologous platelet-rich plasma and intraoperative blood salvage in cardiac surgery. Int J Artif Organs. 1987;10:47–50.
16. Storrs C. Is platelet-rich plasma an effective healing therapy? Sci Am; 2009. https://www.scientificamerican.com/article/platelet-rich-plasma-therapy-dennis-cardone-sports-medicine-injury. Accessed 4 February 2016.
17. Moraes VY, Lenza M, Tamaoki MJ, Faloppa F, Belloti JC. Platelet-rich therapies for musculoskeletal soft tissue injuries. Cochrane Database Syst Rev. 2013;12:CD010071.
18. Beitzel K, Allen D, Apostolakos J, Russell RP, McCarthy MB, Gallo GJ, et al. US definitions, current use, and FDA stance on use of platelet-rich plasma in sports medicine. J Knee Surg. 2015;28:29–34.

19. Storb R. Edward Donnall Thomas (1920–2012). Nature. 2012;491(7424):334.
20. Jansen J. The first successful allogeneic bone-marrow transplant: Georges Mathé. Transfus Med Rev. 2005;19:246–8.
21. Bongso A, Richards M. History and perspective of stem cell research. Best Pract Res Clin Obstet Gynaecol. 2004;18:827–42.
22. Thomson JA, Kalishman J, Golos TG, Durning M, Harris CP, Hearn JP. Pluripotent cell lines derived from common marmoset (Callithrix jacchus) blastocysts. Biol Reprod. 1996;55:254–9.
23. McLaren A. Cloning: pathways to a pluripotent future. Science. 2000;288:1775–80.
24. Thomson JA, Itskovitz-Eldor J, Shapiro SS, Waknitz MA, Swiergiel JJ, Marshall VS, Jones JM. Embryonic stem cell lines derived from human blastocysts. Science. 1998;282:1145–7.
25. Shamblott MJ, Axelman J, Wang S, Bugg EM, Littlefield JW, Donovan PJ, et al. Derivation of pluripotent stem cells from cultured human primordial germ cells. Proc Natl Acad Sci U S A. 1998;95:13726–31.
26. Sharkis SJ. Canadian stem cell scientists take the prize. Cell. 2005;122:817–9.
27. Rietze RL, Reynolds BA. Neural stem cell isolation and characterization. Methods Enzymol. 2006;419:3–23.
28. Zuk PA, Zhu M, Ashjian P, De Ugarte DA, Huang JI, Mizuno H, et al. Human adipose tissue is a source of multipotent stem cells. Mol Biol Cell. 2002;13:4279–95.
29. Robinton DA, Daley GQ. The promise of induced pluripotent stem cells in research and therapy. Nature. 2012;481:295–305.
30. Olson JL, Atala A, Yoo JJ. Tissue engineering: current strategies and future directions. Chonnam Med J. 2011;47(1):13.
31. Perdisa F, Gostyńska N, Roffi A, Filardo G, Marcacci M, Kon E. Adipose-derived mesenchymal stem cells for the treatment of articular cartilage: a systematic review on preclinical and clinical evidence. Stem Cells Int. 2015;2015:597652.
32. Silini AR, Cargnoni A, Magatti M, Pianta S, Parolini O. The long path of human placenta, and its derivatives, in regenerative medicine. Front Bioeng Biotechnol. 2015;3:162.
33. Porada CD, Atala AJ, Almeida-Porada G. The hematopoietic system in the context of regenerative medicine. Methods. 2016;99:44–61.
34. Kubo M, Sonoda Y, Muramatsu R, Usui M. Immunogenicity of human amniotic membrane in experimental xenotransplantation. Invest Ophthalmol Vis Sci. 2001;42:1539–46.
35. Wang Y, Jiang F, Liang Y, Shen M, Chen N. Human amnion-derived mesenchymal stem cells promote osteogenic differentiation in human bone marrow mesenchymal stem cells by influencing the ERK1/2 signaling pathway. Stem Cells Int. 2016;2016:4851081.
36. Raghunath J, Salacinski HJ, Sales KM, Butler PE, Seifalian AM. Advancing cartilage tissue engineering: the application of stem cell technology. Curr Opin Biotechnol. 2005;16:503–9.
37. Majumdar MK, Thiede MA, Haynesworth SE, Bruder SP, Gerson SL. Human marrow-derived mesenchymal stem cells (MSCs) express hematopoietic cytokines and support long-term hematopoiesis when differentiated toward stromal and osteogenic lineages. J Hematother Stem Cell Res. 2000;9:841–8.
38. Gronthos S, Franklin DM, Leddy HA, Robey PG, Storms RW, Gimble JM. Surface protein characterization of human adipose tissue-derived stromal cells. J Cell Physiol. 2001;189:54–63.
39. Ullah I, Subbarao RB, Rho GJ. Human mesenchymal stem cells – current trends and future prospective. Biosci Rep. 2015;35:e00191.
40. Pers YM, Ruiz M, Noël D, Jorgensen C. Mesenchymal stem cells for the management of inflammation in osteoarthritis: state of the art and perspectives. Osteoarthr Cartil. 2015;23:2027–35.
41. Vega A, Martín-Ferrero MA, Del Canto F, Alberca M, García V, Munar A, et al. Treatment of knee osteoarthritis with allogeneic bone marrow mesenchymal stem cells: a randomized controlled trial. Transplantation. 2015;99:1681–90.
42. Fennema EM, Renard AJ, Leusink A, van Blitterswijk CA, de Boer J. The effect of bone marrow aspiration strategy on the yield and quality of human mesenchymal stem cells. Acta Orthop. 2009;80:618–21.

43. Koh YG, Choi YJ, Kwon SK, Kim YS, Yeo JE. Clinical results and second-look arthroscopic findings after treatment with adipose-derived stem cells for knee osteoarthritis. Knee Surg Sports Traumatol Arthrosc. 2015;23:1308–16.
44. Wong KL, Lee KB, Tai BC, Law P, Lee EH, Hui JH. Injectable cultured bone marrow-derived mesenchymal stem cells in varus knees with cartilage defects undergoing high tibial osteotomy: a prospective, randomized controlled clinical trial with 2 years' follow-up. Arthroscopy. 2013;29:2020–8.
45. Thomopoulos S, Parks WC, Rifkin DB, Derwin KA. Mechanisms of tendon injury and repair. J Orthop Res. 2015;33:832–9.
46. Müller SA, Todorov A, Heisterbach PE, Martin I, Majewski M. Tendon healing: an overview of physiology, biology, and pathology of tendon healing and systematic review of state of the art in tendon bioengineering. Knee Surg Sports Traumatol Arthrosc. 2015;23:2097–105.
47. Buchbinder R, Green S, Youd JM. Corticosteroid injections for shoulder pain. Cochrane Database of Syst Rev. 2003;1:CD004016.
48. Gaujoux-Viala C, Dougados M, Gossec L. Efficacy and safety of steroid injections for shoulder and elbow tendonitis: a meta-analysis of randomised controlled trials. Ann Rheum Dis. 2009;68:1843–9.
49. Dean BJ, Lostis E, Oakley T, Rombach I, Morrey ME, Carr AJ. The risks and benefits of glucocorticoid treatment for tendinopathy: a systematic review of the effects of local glucocorticoid on tendon. Semin Arthritis Rheum. 2014;43:570–6.
50. Pascual-Garrido C, Rolón A, Makino A. Treatment of chronic patellar tendinopathy with autologous bone marrow stem cells: a 5-year followup. Stem Cells Int. 2012;2012:953510.
51. Kopka M, Bradley JP. The use of biologic agents in athletes with knee injuries. J Knee Surg. 2016;29:379–386. Erratum. https://doi.org/10.1055/s-0037-1599135.
52. Stein BE, Stroh DA, Schon LC. Outcomes of acute achilles tendon rupture repair with bone marrow aspirate concentrate augmentation. Int Orthop. 2015;39(5):901.
53. Valencia Mora M, Ruiz Ibán MA, Díaz Heredia J, Barco Laakso R, Cuéllar R, García Arranz M. Stem cell therapy in the management of shoulder rotator cuff disorders. World J Stem Cells. 2015;7:691–9.
54. Zlotnicki JP, Geeslin AG, Murray IR, Petrigliano FA, LaPrade RF, Mann BJ, Musahl V. Biologic treatments for sports injuries II think tank-current concepts, future research, and barriers to advancement, part 3: articular cartilage. Orthop J Sports Med. 2016;4:2325967116642433.
55. Saltzman BM, Kuhns BD, Weber AE, Yanke A, Nho SJ. Stem cells in orthopedics: a comprehensive guide for the general orthopedist. Am J Orthop (Belle Mead NJ). 2016;45:280–326.
56. Robertson JA. Embryo stem cell research: ten years of controversy. J Law Med Ethics. 2010;38:191–203.
57. Obama B. Executive order 13505 — removing barriers to responsible scientific research involving human stem cells. 9 Mar 2009. Fed Regist Vol. 74, No. 46. https://www.gpo.gov/fdsys/pkg/FR-2009-03-11/pdf/E9-5441.pdf. Accessed 2 Feb 2016.
58. Baynes T. U.S. high court won't review federal embryonic stem cell funds. Reuters 7 2013. http://www.reuters.com/article/us-usa-court-stemcell-idUSBRE9060IQ20130107. Accessed 2 Feb 2016.
59. Tissue Reference Group. U S Food and Drug Administration 19 Jun 2015. https://www.fda.gov/BiologicsBloodVaccines/TissueTissueProducts/RegulationofTissues/ucm152857.htm. Accessed 2 Feb 2016.

Chapter 38
Platelet-Rich Plasma

Corey W. Hunter, Timothy Davis, and Priyal Fadadu

38.1 Introduction

Platelet-rich plasma (PRP) is most concisely defined as a volume of plasma that contains a concentrate of platelets above that of baseline blood levels [1]. PRP, while considered experimental to most third-party payers, has been used for over 30 years as an aid in recovery following certain surgical, orthopedic, and dental procedures, with thousands of research articles having been published over that time on the safety and efficacy of its application. It is an autologous blood product that can be injected into virtually any damaged area of the body to deliver platelet-derived growth factors (PDGF) to promote healing [2]. Given the autologous nature of PRP, potential side effects or complications are theoretically reduced; moreover, as it is one's own blood simply being re-administered, many view PRP as a holistic treatment methodology.

To understand the conceptual benefit of PRP, we will briefly review the phases of healing. In an acute injury, platelets aggregate to form a plug at the site of injury, followed by a fibrin clot. After the platelets aggregate, they are then activated and

C.W. Hunter (✉)
Ainsworth Institute of Pain Management, New York, NY, USA

Department of Physical Medicine and Rehabilitation, Mount Sinai Hospital, New York, NY, USA
e-mail: corey.hunter@me.com

T. Davis
Orthopedic Pain Specialists, Santa Monica, CA, USA
e-mail: ttdavis23@gmail.com

P. Fadadu
Orthopedic Pain Specialists, Fremont, CA, USA
e-mail: fadadu.priyal@mayo.edu

S. Diwan, T.R. Deer (eds.), *Advanced Procedures for Pain Management*,
https://doi.org/10.1007/978-3-319-68841-1_38

induce inflammatory responses from monocytes, neutrophils, and lymphocytes [3]. Degranulation of alpha granules then release seven fundamental growth factors to initiate the healing process [1]. This stage is triggered by the clotting process of blood and typically occurs within 10–15 min after injection, with more than 95% of factors secreted within the first hour [4]. The proliferative phase then begins, stimulating fibroblasts to create new connective tissue (collagen), which replaces the fibrin clot. Endothelial cells promote angiogenesis, which is required to supply nutrients to the healing region. Remodeling and scar maturation is the final stage of healing [1, 2].

Interrupted wound healing occurs when there is inadequate blood supply to an injured area. This is one of the theories of chronic musculoskeletal injury. Tendons, ligaments, and joints have poor blood supply in comparison to bone, skin, and other tissues. This fact dictates their ability to heal in a timely manner and makes them prone to re-injury. PRP has been proposed as a means to "kickstart" a stalled healing mechanism in chronically inflamed tissues that have substandard blood supply. The concept is to recreate the cascade that occurs after an acute injury by artificially transplanting a platelet-rich volume to an injured area with circulatory deficiency [2].

The popularity of PRP has been steadily growing, particularly among boutique and contemporary medical practices, with some of the most novel applications at the time of this publication dwelling commonly within the cosmetic and elective realms (e.g., facelifts, hair regrowth, and improving one's libido); however, these modalities lack evidence and typically rely mostly on anecdotal data. As it pertains to pain management and conventional medicine, the use of PRP for ligament, tendon, and musculoskeletal pathologies has achieved a great deal of acceptance. Numerous studies have shown PRP to be effective in the treatment and management of tendonopathy and ligamentous injuries, with the most persuasive data to date being on lateral epicondylitis (tennis elbow) [5]. Another popular application for PRP is osteoarthritis (OA)—particularly knee OA [6–9].

The thinking behind PRP is that since platelets are the body's natural mechanism for healing, concentrating and directing these healing agents into a particular area of injury could effectively focus and even accelerate the restoration process. Inherent to a concentration of platelets are seven fundamental protein growth factors that have been proven to be actively secreted by platelets to initiate the healing process [1]. PRP works via the activation and subsequent degranulation of the alpha granules in the platelets—these contain the synthesized and prepackaged growth factors.

Despite the lack of coverage by insurance companies, PRP has become a burgeoning industry with newer customized kits and more advanced equipment for obtaining PRP becoming readily available. Conventionally, PRP was created through manual laboratory preparation—standard blood collection, transferring to conical vials, centrifuging to separate the blood, and extracting the platelet-rich portion. Commercially available systems are now widely accessible with the promise of greater ease while offering more theoretical precision, higher platelet yields, and better consistency [10].

Table 38.1 PRP Indications based on supporting scientific evidence [11]

Evidence	Definition[a]	Indications
Level I	Evidence obtained from at least one properly designed randomized controlled trial	• Lateral epicondylitis (tennis elbow) [12–14] • Hip pain secondary to OA and labral tears • Knee pain secondary to OA and soft tissue injuries • Maxillofacial surgery • Shoulder pain, including acromioclavicular joint and rotator cuff injuries [15]
Level II-1	Evidence obtained from well-designed controlled trials without randomization	• Patellar tendonosis (Jumper's knee) [16] • ACL and MCL repairs (animal studies) [17]
Level II-2	Evidence obtained from well-designed cohort or case-control analytic studies, preferably from more than one center or research group	• Achilles tendonitis [18] • Plantar fasciitis [19] • Medial epicondylitis (Golfer's elbow) [15]
Level II-3	Evidence obtained from multiple time series designs with or without the intervention	• Degenerative disc disease [20]

38.2 Indications

PRP is an autologous concentrate of platelets and growth factors within a relatively small volume of blood plasma designed to promote healing and regeneration. This treatment modality is effective for use in soft tissue and musculoskeletal injuries such as tendonitis and ligament tears. PRP is particularly effective in treating injured areas of the body where blood supply is scant or diminished, making it difficult for the body to deliver endogenous platelets and growth factors to heal itself. Injections of PRP to these areas can essentially circumvent a decrease in vascular access and force healing. Evidence to support several of indications such Lateral Epicondylitis, OA of the knees or hips, Maxillofacial surgery, and shoulder pain is prevalent, but further research is being done to strengthen the support of PRP use for the indications listed in Table 38.1, as well as for new indications.

38.3 Microanatomy and Biochemistry

The therapeutic effect of PRP is thought to be facilitated through the release of a variety of growth factors [21]:

- Platelet-derived growth factor AB (PDGF-AB)
- Transforming growth factor β1 (TGF β1)
- Fibroblast growth factor (FGF)

- Vascular endothelial growth factor (VEGF)
- Connective tissue growth factor (CTGF)
- Epithelial growth factor (EGF)
- Insulin-like growth factor 1&2 (ILGF)
- Keratinocyte growth factor (KGF)

In addition to these growth factors, PRP contains the chemokine Interleukin 8 (IL-8), which is believed to promote angiogenesis and improve blood flow.

These factors are located within the platelets themselves and are released upon activation, or in the case of PRP injection into the injured body part, to facilitate a focused and highly localized healing process.

PRP also contains the three proteins in blood known to act as cell adhesion molecules for osteoconduction, and which also serve as a matrix for bone, connective tissue, and epithelial migration:

- Fibrin
- Fibronectin
- Vitronectin

One aspect of PRP preparation touches on a topic of some debate—whether to include the "buffy coat" in the injectate. The buffy coat is a layer of white blood cells visible within a sample of fractionate blood after centrifuging. The buffy coat is also dense with platelets. Proponents of the inclusion of the buffy coat claim that by including it, there is a decreased likelihood of infection due to the presence of the white blood cells creating an inflammatory process to draw further attention from the body and increase the healing process. Opponents of the buffy coat claim the buffy coat increases pain and discomfort after the procedure as well as creating a detrimental inflammatory process that can cause damage rather than healing.

38.4 Basic Concerns and Contraindications

PRP is a minimally invasive procedure with a low risk profile. While there is a good deal of evidence to support its use in a variety of procedures, third-party payers consider it to be "experimental." The most important thing to address before considering PRP or Regenerative Injection Therapy is that many painful conditions can be adequately treated through established treatment methods—some involve surgery while others are more conservative.

Some basic concerns about PRP are the following:

- Immunocompromised patients are potentially at high risk for infection.
- Patients may have thrombocytopenia or bleeding disorders.
- Patients with an active cancer, history of cancer, or suspicion of cancer should consult with their oncologist prior and obtain clearance.

Contraindications for PRP include:

- Infection, systemic or localized
- Coagulopathy
- Distorted or complicated anatomy
- Patients on long-term and/or constant Non-Steroidal Anti-Inflammatory Drugs (NSAIDs) therapy
- Patient refusal

38.5 Preoperative Considerations

- Provide a proper explanation of all potential complications and get the patient's informed consent.
- Anti-coagulation is less of a concern in PRP than for a neuraxial procedure; however, excessive bleeding can occur due to the injection process, thus increasing the likelihood of a hemarthrosis.
- Physically examine the area for evidence of infection, skin ulceration or necrosis, and extent of disease.
- The patient should take no NSAIDs for one week prior to the procedure (e.g., Aspirin, Ibuprofen, Naproxen, etc.).
- The patient should take no steroids of any kind for 10 days prior to the procedure (e.g., prednisone, Medrol dose packs, cortisone, cortisone injections, etc.).
- The patient should be free of systemic infections for a minimum of one week (e.g., common cold, sore throat, cough, etc.). Any antibiotics should be completed prior to the procedure.
- If using radiographic guidance, evaluate the patient for any contrast allergies prior to the procedure.
- Consider the amount of blood to draw. Depending on the size of the area in need of treatment (e.g., elbow vs. hip) or the number of joints (e.g., unilateral vs. bilateral), more or less blood may need to be drawn to derive a large enough portion of PRP. Many vendors provide kits in 30 and 60 mL denominations to suit this consideration.

38.6 Radiographic Guidance

PRP injections can be easily performed "blind"; however, due to the limited amount of injectate available after the extraction of PRP from fractionated whole blood and the need to deliver as much as possible in the necessary area, radiographic guidance is recommended.

- Fluoroscopy—when injecting into joints such as the knee, shoulder, or hip, one can perform an arthrogram under fluoroscopy to confirm needle placement

within the joint capsule prior to injecting the PRP, thus optimizing the likelihood of delivering the maximum amount to the desired location.
- Ultrasound—the literature suggests ultrasound guidance can offer improved accuracy for injection as compared to fluoroscopy [22]. When injecting into tendons, ligaments, and other soft tissue, one can directly visualize in real time the target area, position of the needle tip, and spread of the injectate, thus making ultrasound a must for these types of PRP injections.

38.7 Equipment

Currently there are two general methods for obtaining PRP:

1. Conventional: This method is akin to traditional laboratory methods for blood collection and preparation as the materials and equipment are all obtained individually (e.g., conical vials, vacutainer, needles, etc.), and then the blood is prepared from scratch according to one of several accepted protocols (e.g., Anitua [23], Landesberg [24], etc.).
2. Device or Prepackaged Kits: There are an abundance of vendors and medical device companies that currently offer upscale kits with specially designed collection receptacles and modified centrifuges with preset timers customized for collection and harvesting PRP from whole blood; these are designed for convenience as well as with the claim of higher platelet counts than conventional harvesting methods and their competitors.

Equipment needed for conventional PRP harvesting—to collect 30 mL of blood and produce 4–6 mL of PRP—is as follows:

- Centrifuge
- 20 mL conical vial (2)
- 18-gauge blunt tip needle (2)
- 20 mL syringe
- 10 mL syringe
- Venous blood collection tubes (3) (*contents of vial varies depending on protocol)*
  - Landsberg [24]: 5 mL vials with 0.5 mL of 0.129 mol/L sodium citrate (Becton Dickinson, Franklin Lackes, NJ)
  - Landsberg [25]: 10 mL vials 1.0 mL of ACD Solution B (Becton Dickinson, Franklin Lackes, NJ)
  - Ethylenediaminetetraacetic acid (EDTA) has been found to yield higher concentrations of platelets when used as the anticoagulant contained with the blood collection vials; however, EDTA may damage the platelets, so it should therefore be avoided [24].

- 21-G butterfly blood collection set (smaller gauge needles may cause premature activation of the platelet [26])
- Tourniquet

*ACE Surgical Supply Company offers a "PRP Collection Kit," in which all the materials to collect and prepare PRP conventionally come prepackaged.

38.8 Technique

Both single- and double-centrifuge techniques have been reported in the literature. While excellent results have been reported with PRP obtained from a single-spin technique (enhancement and acceleration of bone regeneration and more rapid and predictable soft-tissue healing in future sites for implants), platelet concentrations were not reported in those studies [27]. Other authors have reported platelet concentrations as high as 356% with single-spin techniques [28]. Marx et al. [29], however, have stated that a double-spin is necessary to obtain a truly optimal concentration of platelets.

We advocate using the double-spin method described by Landesberg [24]. This protocol has shown consistently reproducible platelet concentrations and growth factors.

38.8.1 Landesberg Protocol [24, 25]

Using sterile technique, obtain venous access with the butterfly needle and withdraw 30 mL of blood into the blood collection vials

- Tubes are then placed in the centrifuge and spun at 200 × *g* for 15 min.
- Using the 20 mL syringe with the 18-G blunt tip needle attached, the plasma and buffy coat are then drawn from the vials and transferred to the conical vial.
- The conical vial with the plasma and the buffy coat is then placed back into the centrifuge.
- The second conical vial is filled with water to match the volume with plasma and the buffy coat to serve as a counterweight.
- The centrifuge is then run a second time at 200 × *g* for 10 min.
- The conical vial with sample is removed from the centrifuge.
- Using the 10 mL syringe with the second blunt-tip needle attached, the upper half of the plasma is drawn up—this is the Platelet Poor Plasma (PPP).
- The PPP is discarded.
- The remaining volume in the conical vial is PRP and should yield 4–6 mL.

38.8.2 Commercially Available Kits

- Several kits are available to choose from, depending on desired platelet, white blood cell, and growth factor concentration (see Authors' Note, Sect. 38.12).
- Each vendor will provide a specific set of instructions exclusive to their particular product.
- In many cases, the vendor will also provide a centrifuge with preset times for spinning the blood sample.

38.9 Post-procedure Considerations

- No NSAIDs and/or Steroids for one month after the procedure.
- The positive effects of the injection may occur within the first week when treating tendons, ligaments, soft-tissue injuries, and bursitis. Joints and other osteoarthritic conditions may take as long as 6 weeks to respond.
- Normal activity with no extra exercise for the first 48 h.
- After 10–12 days, start light exercise without stressful activity for 6 weeks. Returning to stressful activity before 6 weeks will result in incomplete healing of the treated tissue.
- Depending on the severity of the injury or pathology, added treatments may be necessary. To date, there are no published studies that have established a paradigm for the number of treatments or amount of PRP needed to treat different conditions.

38.10 Potential Complications and Pitfalls

As with any medical or surgical procedure, there is always a risk of potential complication—even with the use of autologous-derived blood as the injectate.

- Irritation at the injection site.
- Localized soreness or discomfort from the injection itself.
- Increased pain or inflammation in the area where the PRP was deposited, due to inflammation from the PRP, and lasting up to 10 days post-procedure. In many cases this can be due to the body intentionally creating some inflammation in and around the area where the PRP was injected. This inflammation is the body's response to the introduction of PRP into an injured area and attempting to offer additional assistance by luring growth factors and inflammatory markers.
- Infection—this can occur due to the nature of a simple injection if aseptic technique is not strictly adhered to or from contamination of the blood during the transfer process.

- Graft rejection—this is a theoretical possibility in the event multiple samples from several patients are obtained and prepared simultaneously and PRP from one patient is accidently injected into another. One should either carefully label each sample and perform "time-out" procedures before commencing with the injection, or prepare samples one at a time to avoid this possibility.

38.11 Clinical Pearls

- There is a wide variety of indications for which PRP can used to either induce or accelerate healing. It is most effective in cases of lateral epicondylitis, OA of the knees or hips, maxillofacial surgery, and shoulder pain.
- Despite a lack of coverage by third-party payers for being considered "experimental," there is good evidence to support the use of PRP, including a number of blinded, randomized controlled trials.
- A larger-bore needle is recommended during the blood draw, as a narrow needle can shear the platelets and cause premature activation.
- EDTA should be avoided in the blood collection phase.
- When preparing PRP from scratch (without the use of a commercially purchased kit), a double-spin is recommended.
- Buffy coat should not be included with PRP for injection, as it can cause unwanted increases in inflammation.
- NSAIDs should be avoided for 7 days prior to PRP treatment, and steroids should be avoided for 10 days prior. Both should be avoided for 1 month following treatment.
- Multiple treatments may be necessary.

38.12 Authors' Note

As of the date of this publication, there are over 30 blood concentration kits for regenerative medicine. The authors realize the complexity providers are met with when various vendors present unstandardized data. Therefore, in an attempt to standardize the data presented throughout the literature, we have created a chart with normalized values to provide a like-for-like comparison (Table 38.2). We would like to draw your attention to the first three numerical columns in Table 38.2: PRP Platelet Concentration, Platelet Factor Increase from Whole Blood, and White Blood Cell Concentration. PRP systems primarily aim to concentrate platelets among other blood factors, and the systems in Table 38.2 show a wide range of values, which are also presented as a "Platelet Factor Increase from Whole Blood" value for ease of comparison. It is currently debated whether white blood cells are advantageous or detrimental in PRP due to the creation of an inflammatory response, so we expect the white blood cell concentration to vary between systems depending

Table 38.2 Comparison of published protocols and commercially available kits

System	Reference	Platelet-rich plasma				Preparation			Platelet-derived growth factors		
		Platelet × 10^3/μL	Platelet factor increase from whole Blood	White blood cells × 10^3/μL	PRP vol (mL)	Blood vol (mL)	Force	Centrifuge, time (min)	PDGF-AB (ng/mL)	TGF-B1 (ng/mL)	VEGF (ng/mL)
Whole blood	**[30]**	**273.8**		**6.4**							
ACE Surgical	[1]	493 ± 245	1.8	–	7.8 ± 0.6	–	–	–	35 ± 17.2	43.0 ± 17.9	–
Anitua Protocol	[1]	433 ± 129	1.9	–	9.5 ± 4.1	–	–	–	35 ± 11.3	52.0 ± 7.6	–
Arteriocyte MagellanPRP™	[30]	780.2 ± 24.7	2.8 ± 0.8	11.0 ±8.2	6.0	26	1200 × *g*	17	34.4 ±10.7	0.2 ± 0.1	1.2 ± 0.8
	[31]	1520	9.05	0.0014	3.0	60	610 × *g*; 1240 × *g*	4; 6	74.8	1719[a]	0.05[a]
Arthrex ACP®	[32]	261	1.7	2.80	4.0	9.0	–	–	27.65	15.98	0.1
Arthrex Angel®	[33]	774.2 ± 324.0	4.8 ± 0.7	–	6.9	70	–	17	–	–	–
Biomet 3i PCCS®	[1]	939 ± 284	3.24	–	7.0 ± 1.5		–	–	103 ± 27	144 ± 31	–
	[34]	1095.2[b]	4.0[c]	–	8.5 ± 3.5	50	–	10	103 ± 27	–	–
Biomet GPS®II	[35]	477	1.89[d]	7.94	6.01	50	180 × *g*	15	–	–	–
Biomet GPS®II (Biomet® Biologics Drucker centrifuge)	[36]	2136[e]	6.2 to 9.4	312.88	6.2	52	3200 rpm	15	–	–	–
Biomet GPS®III	[30]	566.2 ± 292.6	2.07 ± 1.1	34.4 ± 13.6	6.0	55	1100 × *g*	15	18.7 ±12.8	0.10 ± 0.08	2.4 ± 1.1
Biomet GPS®III (Biomet® Biologics Drucker centrifuge)	[36]	2135.6[e]	7.3 to 8.3	275.4	6.6	52	3200 rpm	15	–	–	–

Biotechnology Institue PRGF®-Endoret®	[34]	201.75[b]	0.737[c]	–	9.5 ± 4.1	20	–	–	47 ± 21	–	–
Clinaseal Sealed Technology Centrifuge	[1]	401 ± 267	1.64	–	7.6 ± 1.5	–	–	–	46 ± 15.3	55 ± 19	–
Curasan® AG	[1]	344 ± 192	1.39	–	7.6 ± 1.5	–	–	–	39 ± 11.4	39 ± 16	–
	[34]	178.3[b]	0.65[c]	–	7.6 ± 1.6	15	–	–	35 ± 17	–	–
	[35]	693.8	2.75[d]	320	1.0	8.5	1000 × *g*; 2300 × *g*	10; 15	–	–	–
DePuy PEAK®	[37]	1242.4	6.9	32[f]	3.3	27	–	3	–	–	–
Emcyte GenesisCS	[38]	1643 ± 421	9.13	20 ± 7.4	–	52	2400 rpm	12	–	–	–
	[32]	1355	9.7	49.7	5.0	55	–	–	198.22	38.54	0.442
Emcyte Pure PRP™	[32]	1128 ± 319	6.7 ± 0.3	0.0149	6.6 ± 0.2	48	2500 × *g*; 2500 × *g*	1.5; 4	–	–	–
	[33]	1067.6 ± 253	6.9 ± 0.7	–	7.4	75	3800 rpm; 3800 rpm	1.5[g]; 5	–	–	–
Fibrinet® PRFM	[34]	323.6[b]	1.18[c]	–	4.4 ± 0.2	8.0	–	–	105 ± 30	–	–
Friadent-Schütze Protocol	[39]	1440.5 ± 501.7	5.2[i]	21.69 ± 16.43	0.8	7.5	24,000 rpm; 3600 rpm	10; 15	251.6 ±115.4	196.8 ± 109.6	–
Glofinn GLO PRP	[31]	891	5.28	0.0101[h]	0.6	8.5	1800 × *g*; 1800 × *g*	3; 6	67.3	1370[a]	0.039[a]
Harvest® Smart PReP	[39]	1228 ± 312	4.43[i]	19.26 ± 8.08	7.0	52 (female); 48 (male)	–	12	208 ± 85.2	77.2 ± 54.8	–
	[1]	1086 ± 227	4.04	–	7.4 ± 0.5	–	–	–	133 ± 29.2	170 ± 42	–
	[34]	917.3[b]	3.35[c]	–	10.0	50	–	–	133 ± 29	–	–

(continued)

Table 38.2 (continued)

System	Reference	Platelet-rich plasma				Preparation			Platelet-derived growth factors		
		Platelet × 10^3/µL	Platelet factor increase from whole Blood	White blood cells × 10^3/µL	PRP vol (mL)	Blood vol (mL)	Force	Centrifuge, time (min)	PDGF-AB (ng/mL)	TGF-B1 (ng/mL)	VEGF (ng/mL)
Japan Paramedic Co., JP200	[31]	871	5.16	0.026	1.0	20	1000 × *g*; 800 × *g*	6; 8	93.5	1563[a]	0.041[a]
Korea Melsmon Co., Thrombo Kit	[31]	700[h]	4.14	0.0149	1.0	8.5	1720 × *g*	8	39[h]	910[a]	0.030[a]
KYOCERA®	[31]	1312	7.77	0.014[h]	2.0	20	600 × *g*; 2000 × *g*	7; 5	76.2	1508.2[a]	0.043[a]
Landesberg Protocol (Mistral 3000i centrifuge)	[1, 24]	336 ± 141	1.5	–	10.6 ± 2.4	–	200 × *g*; 200 × *g*	10; 10	26 ± 13.7	50 ± 11	–
Landesberg Protocol	[34]	465[b]	1.7[c]	–	10.6 ± 2.4	60	–	–	33 ± 7	–	–
Liège University Hospital Protocol (Jouan BR4i centrifuge)	[35]	447.8	1.78[d]	0.210	2.08	8.0	180 × *g*	10	–	–	–
MTF Cascade® PRP	[30]	443.8 ± 24.7	1.62 ± 0.1	1.1 ± 0.2	7.5	18	1100 × *g*	6	9.7 ± 3.6	0.10 ± 0.08	0.3 ± 0.3
	[40]	136 ± 61	0.7	–	4.1 ± 0.5	9.0	1100 × *g*; 1450 × *g*	6; 15	5.31 ± 3.17	–	–
MyCells®	[31]	840[h]	4.97	0.005[h]	1.0	10	2054 × *g*	7	72.2	1350[a]	0.038[a]

		Platelet-rich plasma				Preparation			Platelet-derived growth factors		
System	Reference	Platelet × 10^3/µL	Platelet factor increase from whole Blood	White blood cells × 10^3/µL	PRP vol (mL)	Blood vol (mL)	Force	Centrifuge, time (min)	PDGF-AB (ng/mL)	TGF-B1 (ng/mL)	VEGF (ng/mL)
Plateltex®	[34]	346.1[b]	1.264[c]	–	5.0 ± 0.4	8.0	180 × *g*	10	60 ± 20	0.755	0.36
	[35]	864.6	3.43[d]	5.76	0.34	6.0	180 × *g*; 1000 × *g*	10; 10	–	–	–
Regenlab RegenKit®	[34]	492.3[b]	1.8[c]	–	5.0 ± 0.5	10	–	–	140 ± 14	–	–
	[35]	390.6	1.55[d]	0.020	3.07	6.0	300 × *g*	5	–	–	–
Selphyl®	[31]	88	0.52	0.0003	2.0	8.0	525 × *g*	15	12.2	384[a]	0.029[a]
Vivostat®	[34]	1117[b]	4.08[c]	–	5.0	120	–	–	130 ± 29	–	–

[a]Value approximated from chart in Kushida [31]. However, there is a conversion discrepancy between the units provided in the chart and the text, so the values and units from the chart were used for consistency

[b]Value approximated from the % platelet recovery value in the paper using the average WB platelet concentration and % platelet capture efficacy = (volumePRP × [platelet-PRP])/(volumeWB × [plateletWB]) from Castillo [30]

[c]Factor increase calculated using the average WB platelet concentration from Castillo [30]

[d]Factor increase (PRP platelet concentration/Whole Blood platelet concentration) calculated using average Whole Blood (WB) platelet concentration given in paper (2.52×10^5 platelet/µL)

[e]PRP platelet concentration was not given in paper. Value approximated using the average Factor Increase Value and average WB platelet concentration from Castillo [30]

[f]Value approximated from the average WB White Blood Cell concentration from Castillo [30]

[g]Value discrepancy in text (1.5 min) and Table (2.5 min)

[h]Value approximated from chart in paper (exact value not given in paper)

[i]Factor increase calculated using the average WB platelet concentration given in paper (2.7681×10^5 platelet/µL)

on the indication the PRP is formulated for. In addition, it is interesting to note how even the same system can concentrate platelets, white blood cells, and growth factors in varying amounts depending on the centrifuge used, protocol followed, and patient's blood composition.

References

1. Marx RE. Platelet-rich plasma: evidence to support its use. J Oral Maxillofac Surg. 2004;62:489–96.
2. Foster TE, Puskas BL, Mandelbaum BR, Gerhardt MB, Rodeo SA. Platelet-rich plasma: from basic science to clinical applications. Am J Sports Med. 2009;37:2259–72.
3. Golebiewska EM, Poole AW. Platelet secretion: from haemostasis to wound healing and beyond. Blood Rev. 2015;29:153–62.
4. Kevy SV, Jacobson MS. Preparation of growth factors enriched autologous platelet gel. Proceedings of the 27th annual meeting of service biomaterials, Apr 2001.
5. Pourcho AM, Smith J, Wisniewski SJ, Sellon JL. Intraarticular platelet-rich plasma injection in the treatment of knee osteoarthritis: review and recommendations. Am J Phys Med Rehabil. 2014;93:S108–21.
6. Al-Ajlouni J, Awidi A, Samara O, Al-Najar M, Tarwanah E, Saleh M, et al. Safety and efficacy of autologous intra-articular platelet lysates in early and intermediate knee osteoarthritis in humans: a prospective open-label study. Clin J Sport Med. 2015;25(6):524–8.
7. Patel S, Dhillon MS, Aggarwal S, Marwaha N, Jain A. Treatment with platelet-rich plasma is more effective than placebo for knee osteoarthritis: a prospective, double-blind, randomized trial. Am J Sports Med. 2013;41:356–64.
8. Kon E, Mandelbaum B, Buda R, Filardo G, Delcogliano M, Timoncini A, et al. Platelet-rich plasma versus hyaluronic acid viscosupplementation as treatments for cartilage pathology: from early degeneration to osteoarthritis. Arthroscopy. 2011;27:1490–501.
9. Sun Y, Feng Y, Zhang CQ, Chen SB, Cheng XG. The regenerative effect of platelet-rich plasma on healing in large osteochondral defects. Int Orthop. 2010;34:589–97.
10. Kevy SV, Jacobson MS. Comparison of methods for point of care preparation of autologous platelet gel. J Extra Corpor Technol. 2004;36:28–35.
11. US Preventive Services Task Force. Guide to clinical preventive services: report of the U.S. preventive services task force. Baltimore, MD: Williams and Wilkins; 1989.
12. Tetschke E, Rudolf M, Lohmann CH, Stärke C. Autologous proliferative therapies in recalcitrant lateral epicondylitis. Am J Phys Rehabil. 2015;94:696–706.
13. Thanasas C, Papadimitriou G, Charalambidis C, Paraskevopoulos I, Papanikolaou A. Platelet-rich plasma versus autologous whole blood for the treatment of chronic lateral elbow epicondylitis: a randomized controlled clinical trial. Am J Sports Med. 2011;39:2130–4.
14. Gosens T, Peerbooms JC, van Laar W, den Oudsten BL. Ongoing positive effect of platelet-rich plasma versus corticosteroid injection in lateral epicondylitis: a double-blind randomized controlled trial with 2-year follow-up. Am J Sports Med. 2011;39:1200–8.
15. Nguyen RT, Borg-Stein J, McInnis K. Applications of platelet-rich plasma in musculoskeletal and sports medicine: an evidence-based approach. PM R. 2011;3:226–50.
16. Filardo G, Kon E, Della Villa S, Vincentelli F, Fornasari PM, Marcacci MM. Use of platelet-rich plasma for the treatment of refractory jumper's knee. Int Orthop. 2010;34:909–15.
17. Middleton KK, Barro V, Muller B, Terada S, Fu FH. Evaluation of the effects of platelet-rich plasma (PRP) therapy involved in the healing of sports-related soft tissue injuries. Iowa Orthop J. 2012;32:150–63.
18. Diehl JW. Platelet-rich plasma therapy in chronic Achilles tendonopathy. Tech Foot Ankle Surg. 2011;10:2–6.

19. Tinsley BA, Ferreira JV, Dukas AG, Mazzocca AD. Platelet-rich plasma nonoperative injection therapy—a review of indications and evidence. Oper Tech Sports Med. 2012;20:192–200.
20. Kepler CK, Anderson DG, Tannoury C, Ponnapan RK. Intervertebral disc degeneration and emerging biologic treatments. J Am Acad Orthop Surg. 2011;19:534–53.
21. Civinini R, Nistri L, Martini C, Redl B, Ristori G, Innocenti M. Growth factors in the treatment of early osteoarthritis. Clin Cases Miner Bone Metab. 2013;10:26–9.
22. Narouze S. Atlas of ultrasound-guided procedures in interventional pain management. 1st ed. New York, NY: Springer; 2011.
23. Anitua E. The use of plasma rich growth factors (PRGF) in oral surgery. Pract Proced Aesthet Dent. 2001;13:487–93.
24. Landesberg R, Roy M, Glickman RS. Quantification of growth factor levels using a simplified method of platelet rich plasma gel preparation. J Oral Maxillofac Surg. 2000;58:297–300.
25. Landesberg R, Burke A, Pinksy D, Katz R, Vo J, Eisig SB, et al. Activation of platelet-rich plasma using thrombin agonist receptor peptide. J Oral Maxillofac Surg. 2005;63:529–35.
26. Lippi G, Salvagno GL, Montagnana M, Poli G, Guidi GC. Influence of the needle bore size on platelet count and routine coagulation testing. Blood Coagul Fibrinolysis. 2006;17:557–61.
27. Anitua E. Plasma rich in growth factors: preliminary results of use in the preparation of sites for implants. Int J Oral Maxillofac Implants. 1999;14:529–35.
28. Eby EW. Platelet-rich plasma: Harvesting with a single-spin centrifuge. J Oral Implantol. 2002;28:297–301.
29. Marx RE, Carlson ER, Eichstaedt RM, Schimmele SR, Strauss JE, Georgeff KR. Platelet-rich plasma: Growth factor enhancement for bone grafts. Oral Surg Oral Med Oral Pathol Oral Radiol Endod. 1998;85:638–46.
30. Castillo TN, Pouliot MA, Kim HJ, Dragoo JL. Comparison of growth factor and platelet concentration from commercial platelet-rich plasma separation systems. Am J Sports Med. 2011;39(2):266–71.
31. Kushida S, Kakudo N, Morimoto N, Hara T, Ogawa T, Mitsui T, et al. Platelet and growth factor concentrations in activated platelet-rich plasma: a comparison of seven commercial separation systems. J Artif Organs. 2014;17:186–92.
32. Mandle RJ. Analysis of EmCyte Corporation concentrating systems: an independent review of pre-clinical performance data. 2nd ed. Cambridge, MA: BioSciences Research Associates, Inc.; 2013.
33. Mandle RJ. Research study comparison of angel whole blood separation system and EmCyte PurePRP®. Cambridge, MA: BioSciences Research Associates, Inc.; 2014.
34. Mazzucco L, Balbo V, Cattana E, Borzini P. Platelet-rich plasma and platelet gel preparation using Plateltex®. Vox Sang. 2008;94:202–8.
35. Kaux JF, Le Goff C, Seidel L, Péters P, Gothot A, Albert A, et al. Comparative study of five techniques of preparation of platelet-rich plasma. Pathol Biol (Paris). 2011;59(3):157–60.
36. Kaux JF, Le Goff C, Renouf J, Peters P, Lutteri L, Gothot A, et al. Comparison of the platelet concentrations obtained in platelet-rich plasma (PRP) between the GPS™ II and GPS™ III systems. Pathol Bio (Paris). 2011;59(5):275–7.
37. Mandle RJ. Analysis of PEAK™ platelet rich plasma system: a pre-clinical evaluation of device performance. Cambridge, MA: BioSciences Research Associates, Inc.; 2014.
38. Kevy SV, Jacobson MS, Mandle RJ. Analysis of GenesisCS component concentrating system: preparation of concentrated platelet product. Cambridge, MA: BioSciences Research Associates, Inc.; 2006.
39. Weibrich G, Kleis WK, Buch R, Hitzler WE, Hafner G. The harvest smart PRepPTM system versus the Friadent-Schutze platelet-rich plasma kit. Clinc Oral Implants Res. 2003;14:233–9.
40. Arthrex Research and Development. Plasma-based autologous blood systems: Arthrex ACP®, MTF Cascade®, and Orthovita® CellPaker®/Vitagel™. Naples, FL, Arthrex, Inc.; 2016.

Chapter 39
Alpha-2-Macroglobulin: Protease Inhibitor Treatment (PRP Variant)

Gaetano J. Scuderi and Lewis Hanna

Alpha-2-macroglobulin (A2M) is a major plasma glycoprotein best known for its ability to inhibit a broad spectrum of metalloproteases and inflammatory cytokines by a unique "bait-and-trap" method. As a result, A2M has emerged as a unique potential treatment for cartilage-based pathology and inflammatory arthritides. This chapter describes the unique method by which A2M not only can inhibit the associated inflammatory cascade but also can disrupt the catabolic process of cartilage degeneration. Additionally, recent work has shown that recombinant A2M may be able to enhance cartilage regeneration. Autologous concentrated A2M from plasma is currently used successfully by some providers to treat various painful arthritides, including mild to moderate osteoarthritis, post-traumatic osteoarthritis, enthesopathies, and spinal discogenic back pain. The discovery of A2M as the body's own healing mechanism, with anti-inflammatory and disease-modifying potential, offers great promise.

39.1 Potential Indications

A2M can be concentrated from an autologous source and injected into diseased tissue to enhance healing, prevent further degradation, and protect normal tissue. Though most research has been related to cartilage degeneration, some work has

G.J. Scuderi (✉)
Department of Orthopedic Surgery, Jupiter Medical Center, Jupiter, FL, USA
e-mail: scuderimd@aol.com

L. Hanna
Cytonics Corporation, Jupiter, FL, USA
e-mail: lewis.hanna@cytonics.com

S. Diwan, T.R. Deer (eds.), *Advanced Procedures for Pain Management*,
https://doi.org/10.1007/978-3-319-68841-1_39

been done on tendon and ligament pathology [1, 2]. Potential treatments can be categorized as follows:

- Tendonitis (lateral epicondylitis, rotator cuff tendinopathy)
- Ligament Injury (anterior and posterior cruciate ligaments [ACL, PCL])
- Fasciitis (plantar, palmar)
- Osteoarthritis (OA), in any diarthrodial joint
- Cartilage injury (labral tears of the shoulder or hip, meniscal tear)
- Degenerative disc disease [3]

In short, any pathology that is protease-mediated may benefit from A2M therapy. Additionally, in the future it may be applied perioperatively or postoperatively to protect normal cartilage, for example, from excess protease activity.

39.2 Microanatomy and Biochemistry

The etiology of OA is complex. It is still not fully understood, but a growing body of evidence suggests that a cycle of cartilage catabolism follows changes in the normal physiology of chondrocytes, leading to upregulation of metalloproteases that break down cartilage [4–6]. OA is mediated by numerous biomechanical and biochemical processes involved in its pathophysiology.

Four groups are known to contribute to cartilage catabolism:

- Cytokines, such as interleukin-6 (IL-6), TNFα, and IL-1
- Metalloproteases, such as matrix metalloproteinase (MMP) 1, 2, 3, 7, 12, or 13
- A disintegrin and metalloprotease with thrombospondin motifs (ADAMTS-4, ADAMTS-5, etc.)
- Cartilage breakdown products, such as fibronectin-aggrecan complex (FAC), nitric oxide, advanced glycation end products (AGEs), and C-telopeptide fragments of collagen type II (CTX-II)

Inflammation in OA is mediated primarily by TNFα, IL-1β, and IL-6 [7]. Along with their roles in mediating inflammation, TNFα and IL-1β downregulate the production of extracellular matrix proteins in chondrocytes [8–10] and induce the upregulation of matrix metalloproteases (MMPs), including those that degrade collagen, such as MMP-1, MMP-3, and MMP-13.

ADAMTS-4 is also upregulated by IL-1β, though ADAMTS-5 operates by a different mechanism [11–13]. Importantly, transgenic mouse models with a modified *ADAMTS-5* gene have attenuated OA pathology, suggesting that inhibitors of ADAMTS-5 should be included in any therapy that targets proteases.

The degradative products of cartilage catabolism can also stimulate production of inflammatory mediators. Fragments of fibronectin and collagen stimulate the production of inflammatory cytokines, chemokines, and MMPs [6, 14, 15]. Consequently, the fragments of extracellular matrix proteins and other degradative products in OA contribute to the inflammatory response that stimulates further protease production. Moreover, proteases that cleave aggrecan to release the G3 domain (MMP-2, -7, -9 and -13) are responsible for the formation of the fibronectin-aggrecan complex (FAC) [16].

Fibronectin (an extracellular matrix protein) and its fragments can stimulate cytokine production and activation of MMPs [15, 16]. Aggrecan (a proteoglycan component of articular cartilage) undergoes extensive degeneration during aging and triggers signaling cascades, which augment joint and cartilage damage [17]. This cartilage degradation product, the fibronectin-aggrecan complex (FAC), has been shown to be associated with joint pathology, and it also predicts response to lumbar epidural steroid injection in patients with radiculopathy in lumbar vertebral disc herniation [18, 19].

Identification of FAC associated with painful cartilage conditions leads to the theory that if we can devise a therapeutic agent that prevents the formation of the G3 domain of aggrecan, this agent will reduce the fibronectin-aggrecan G3 complex, resulting in an efficacious treatment for painful cartilage pathophysiology. Because the production of the G3 domain of aggrecan is catalyzed by different known classes of proteases, a common inhibitor of all of these proteases may represent an ideal therapeutic agent, again suggesting the potential and proposed mechanism of efficacy of A2M as a multipurpose protease inhibitor and anti-inflammatory mediator.

Not surprisingly, inhibitors of metalloproteinases have received increasing attention as possible targets for therapeutic intervention in preventing or treating degenerative cartilage pathology [14, 20–22]. Similar to inhibitors of inflammatory cytokines, inhibitors of metalloproteases would need to have broad specificity to be effective at preventing OA pathology. Therapeutic targets based on inhibiting one mediator have failed clinically [23] secondary to the complex crosstalk in the pathogenesis of OA. A2M is a unique molecule, which can stop degradation of cartilage from all four groups of known protease activity (Fig. 39.1). It is a therapy that will reduce cartilage degradation and may delay or reduce the necessity of joint replacement [24].

The therapeutic effect of A2M is thought to be facilitated through its unique bait and trap mechanism:

- After transcription of A2M, it assumes a tetrameric shape of two dimers linked by disulfide bonds. In the center of each dimer is a bait region, which entraps proteases (Fig. 39.2).
- It inhibits breakdown due to numerous cytokines involved in musculoskeletal inflammation, such as TNFα and IL-1β (Fig. 39.3).
- A2M can also inhibit the enzymatic activity leading to the formation of the FAC via MMPs that degrade cartilage (Fig. 39.4).
- A2M also inhibits the protease activity of ADAMTS-4 and -5 (Fig. 39.5).

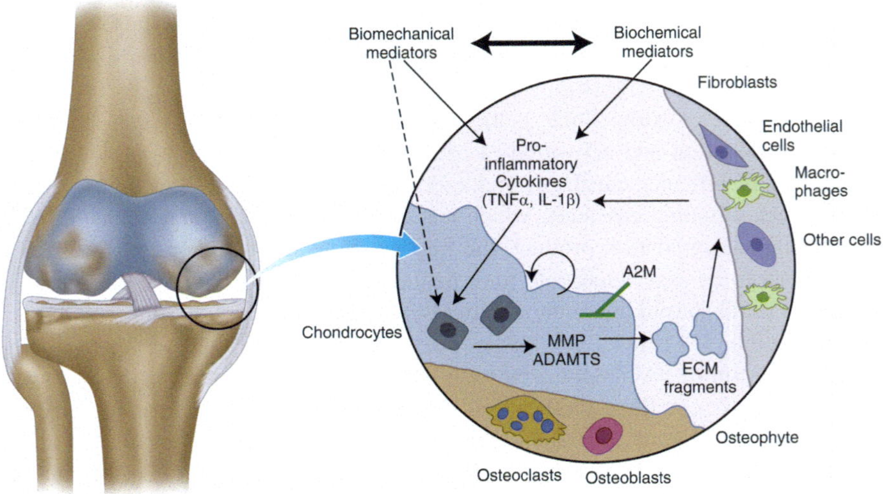

Fig. 39.1 Schematic of the inflammatory cascade that occurs in osteoarthritis (OA): Cartilage breakdown from cytokines, matrix metalloproteinases (MMPs), and ADAMTSs leads to extracellular matrix (ECM) breakdown products such as fibronectin-aggrecan complex (FAC), which then stimulate the release of inflammatory cytokines, leading to a vicious cycle of further cartilage breakdown (positive feedback loop. These can all be inhibited by alpha-2-macroglobulin (A2M)

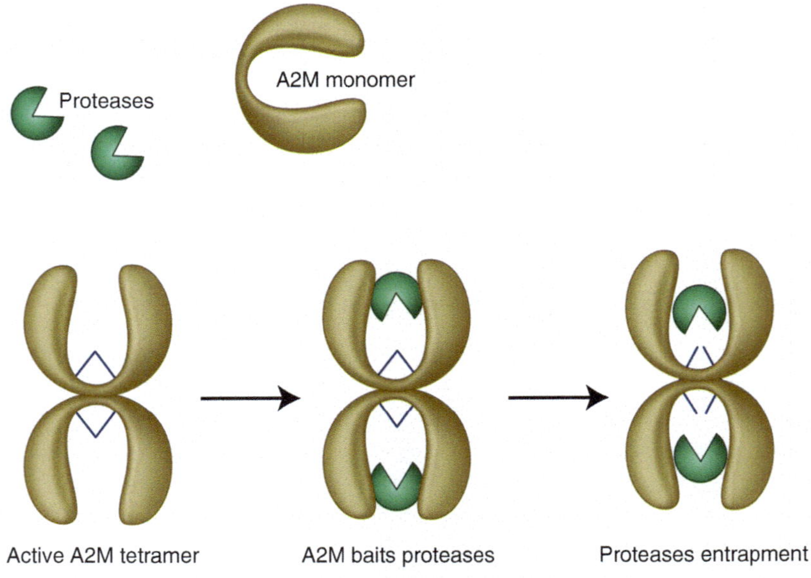

Fig. 39.2 A2M assumes a tetrameric shape and traps proteases. Each dimer traps a single protease. The second trapped protease causes conformational change to allow excretion

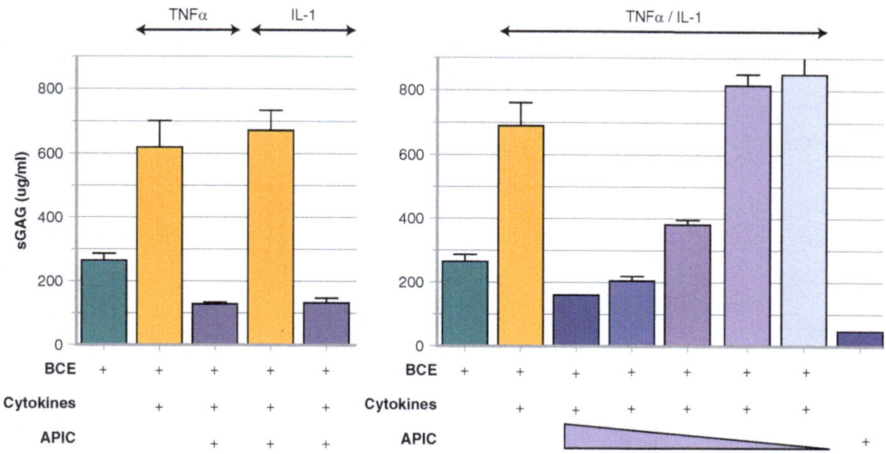

Fig. 39.3 Treatment of bovine cartilage explants (*green column*) with pro-inflammatory cytokines TNFα and IL-1β (*orange column*) induces chondrocytes within the cartilage to produce or activate proteases resulting in increased production of sulfated glycosaminoglycan (sGAG), a cartilage breakdown product. Treatment with purified human A2M (*purple column*) potently inhibited cartilage catabolism, with a pharmacologic effect with increasing concentration

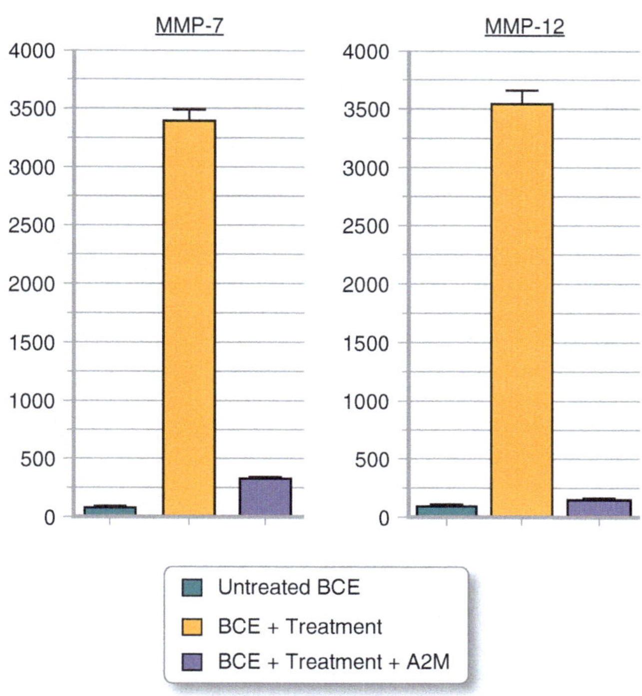

Fig. 39.4 A2M can inhibit the degradation of cartilage from MMP-7 and MMP-12. In turn, G3 formation is prevented, so FAC cannot form

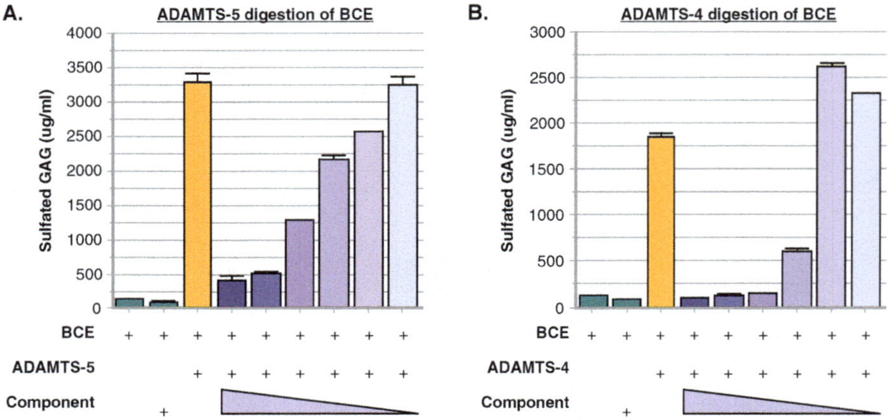

Fig. 39.5 A2M can inhibit the degradation of cartilage from ADAMTS-4 and -5. This also prevents G3 formation, so FAC cannot form

39.3 Basic Concerns and Contraindications

A2M injection is considered a minimally invasive procedure with a low risk profile, similar to other autologous procedures such as platelet-rich plasma (PRP). Although there is a good deal of evidence to support its use in a variety of procedures, third party payers consider it to be "experimental."

There is no known disease state of excess A2M in humans. Additionally, the A2M injected locally comes from the plasma, so there is no "amplification" of A2M. The patient gets back only the amount of A2M removed, which is why A2M procedures require a higher volume of blood draw than traditional PRP.

Contraindications for A2M include active infection or coagulopathy. I would not recommend A2M injection in the following patient populations:

- Immunocompromised patients
- Patients with a bleeding disorder
- Patients with cancer

39.4 Preoperative Considerations

Before beginning the treatment, patients should receive an explanation of alternative treatments and potential complications. Informed consent should be obtained.

Standard intravenous access precautions should be used, along with standard precautions typically in place for joint injections.

39.5 Equipment

Currently there is only one method for obtaining an autologous A2M concentration. It involves using a specialized filter (Fig. 39.6). A hemoconcentrator, though it does concentrate A2M, removes only water, so it concentrates all the molecules in the blood and plasma. One cannot achieve high concentrations of A2M by this method, as other molecules take additional space. Most importantly, the hemoconcentrator also concentrates pro-inflammatory cytokines, which will be deleterious to the tissue and will result in a greater likelihood of a "post-injection flare." A specialized filter that dilutes unnecessary molecules results in a safer injectate with no post-injection pain, and a therapy that more closely targets the pathology.

Equipment for conventional A2M harvesting (for 114 mL collection of blood to produce 8–10 mL of injectate):

- Centrifuge
- Three 50 mL conical vials
- Peristaltic pump system
- One 50 mL syringe

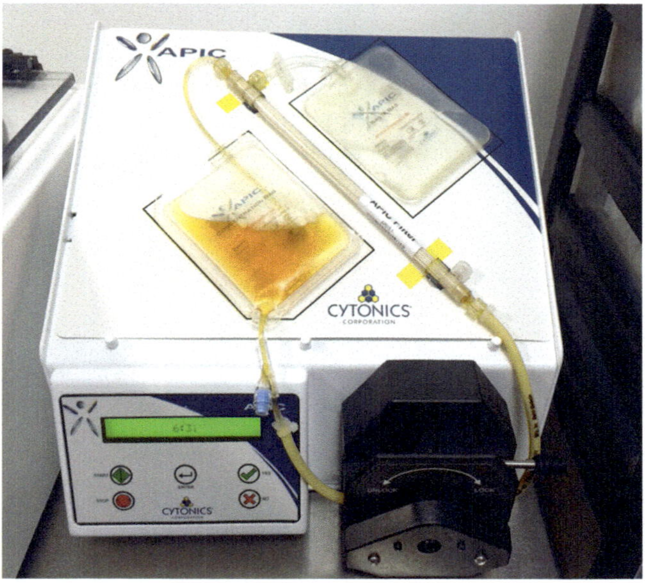

Fig. 39.6 System that concentrates A2M from a sample of blood using a peristaltic pump

39.6 Post-procedure Considerations

- It is not necessary to recommend stopping NSAIDs or steroids.
- A sensation of fullness is common, but there is little to no pain for 24–48 h.
- The positive effects of the injection often occur within the first week.
- Normal activity is allowed.

39.7 Potential Complications and Pitfalls

As with any medical or surgical procedure, there is always a risk of potential complications, even with the use of autologous-derived blood as the injectate. Localized soreness or discomfort from the injection itself may occur. As with any injection, infection is possible if aseptic technique is not strictly adhered to or if the blood becomes contaminated during the transfer process.

39.8 Clinical Pearls

- A2M can be used to either induce or accelerate healing for a wide variety of indications. It seems most effective in cases of plantar fasciitis, lateral epicondylitis or OA of the knees or hips.
- Despite a lack of coverage by third party payers for being considered "experimental," there is early evidence to support A2M's use.
- Because of the viscosity of the injectate, a larger-bore needle (generally 22 G) is recommended for the injections. A small needle requires a longer time to inject.
- The half-life is quite long, so successful treatment can result in months of pain relief. Treatment twice yearly should be considered for patients with chronic disease.

References

1. Bedi A, Kovacevic D, Hettrich C, Gulotta LV, Ehteshami JR, Warren RF, Rodeo SA. The effect of matrix metalloproteinase inhibition on tendon-to-bone healing in a rotator cuff repair model. J Shoulder Elb Surg. 2010;19:384–91.
2. Demirag B, Sarisozen B, Ozer O, Kaplan T, Ozturk C. Enhancement of tendon-bone healing of anterior cruciate ligament grafts by blockage of matrix metalloproteinases. J Bone Joint Surg Am. 2005;87:2401–10.
3. Scuderi GJ, Cuellar JM, Montesano PX. Intradiscal injection of autologous alpha-2-macroglobulin (A2M) concentrate alleviates back pain in FAC-positive patients. ISASS 2016, Abstract 202. http://www.isass.org/m/h/03_2029.html.
4. Cawston TE, McLaughlin P, Hazleman BL. Paired serum and synovial fluid values of alpha 2-macroglobulin and TIMP in rheumatoid arthritis. Br J Rheumatol. 1987;26:354–8.

5. Ades EW, Hinson A, Chapuis-Cellier C, Arnaud P. Modulation of the immune response by plasma protease inhibitors. I. Alpha 2-macroglobulin and alpha 1-antitrypsin inhibit natural killing and antibody-dependent cell-mediated cytotoxicity. Scand J Immunol. 1982;15:109–13.
6. Fichter M, Körner U, Schömburg J, Jennings L, Cole AA, Mollenhauer J. Collagen degradation products modulate matrix metalloproteinase expression in cultured articular chondrocytes. J Orthop Res. 2006;24:63–70.
7. Lefebvre V, Peeters-Joris C, Vaes G. Modulation by interleukin 1 and tumor necrosis factor alpha of production of collagenase, tissue inhibitor of metalloproteinases and collagen types in differentiated and dedifferentiated articular chondrocytes. Biochim Biophys Acta. 1990;1052:366–78.
8. Saklatvala J. Tumour necrosis factor alpha stimulates resorption and inhibits synthesis of proteoglycan in cartilage. Nature. 1986;322:547–9.
9. Goldring MB, Fukuo K, Birkhead JR, Dudek E, Sandell LJ. Transcriptional suppression by interleukin-1 and interferon-gamma of type II collagen gene expression in human chondrocytes. J Cell Biochem. 1994;54:85–99.
10. Stöve J, Huch K, Günther KP, Scharf HP. Interleukin-1beta induces different gene expression of stromelysin, aggrecan and tumor-necrosis-factor-stimulated gene 6 in human osteoarthritic chondrocytes in vitro. Pathobiology. 2000;68:144–9.
11. Glasson SS, Askew R, Sheppard B, Carito B, Blanchet T, Ma HL, et al. Deletion of active ADAMTS5 prevents cartilage degradation in a murine model of osteoarthritis. Nature. 2005;434:644–8. Erratum in: Nature 2007;446:102
12. Rogerson FM, Chung YM, Deutscher ME, Last K, Fosang AJ. Cytokine-induced increases in ADAMTS-4 messenger RNA expression do not lead to increased aggrecanase activity in ADAMTS-5-deficient mice. Arthritis Rheum. 2010;62:3365–73.
13. Tortorella MD, Malfait AM, Deccico C, Arner E. The role of ADAM-TS4 (aggrecanase-1) and ADAM-TS5 (aggrecanase-2) in a model of cartilage degradation. Osteoarthritis Cartilage. 2001;9:539–52. Erratum in: Osteoarthritis Cartilage 2002;10:82
14. Miller RE, Lu Y, Tortorella MD, Malfait AM. Genetically engineered mouse models reveal the importance of proteases as osteoarthritis drug targets. Curr Rheumatol Rep. 2013;15:350.
15. Homandberg GA, Wen C, Hui F. Cartilage damaging activities of fibronectin fragments derived from cartilage and synovial fluid. Osteoarthr Cartil. 1998;6:231–44.
16. Scuderi GJ, Woolf N, Dent K, Golish SR, Cuellar JM, Cuellar VG, et al. Identification of a complex between fibronectin and aggrecan G3 domain in synovial fluid of patients with painful meniscal pathology. Clin Biochem. 2010;43:808–14.
17. Scuderi GJ, Golish SR, Cook FF, Cuellar JM, Bowser RP, Hanna LS. Identification of a novel fibronectin-aggrecan complex in the synovial fluid of knees with painful meniscal injury. J Bone Joint Surg Am. 2011;93:336–40.
18. Scuderi GJ, Cuellar JM, Cuellar VG, Yeomans DC, Carragee EJ, Angst MS. Epidural interferon gamma-immunoreactivity: a biomarker for lumbar nerve root irritation. Spine (Phila Pa 1976). 2009;34:2311–7.
19. Golish SR, Hanna LS, Bowser RP, Montesano PX, Carragee EJ, Scuderi GJ. Outcome of lumbar epidural steroid injection is predicted by assay of a complex of fibronectin and aggrecan from epidural lavage. Spine (Phila Pa 1976). 2011;36:1464–9.
20. Meszaros E, Malemud CJ. Prospects for treating osteoarthritis: enzyme-protein interactions regulating matrix metalloproteinase activity. Ther Adv Chronic Dis. 2012;3:219–29.
21. Rothenberg ML, Nelson AR, Hande KR. New drugs on the horizon: matrix metalloproteinase inhibitors. Stem Cells. 1999;17:237–40.
22. Amar S, Fields GB. Potential clinical implications of recent matrix metalloproteinase inhibitor design strategies. Expert Rev Proteomics. 2015;12:445–7.
23. Jotanovic Z, Mihelic R, Sestan B, Dembic Z. Role of interleukin-1 inhibitors in osteoarthritis: an evidence-based review. Drugs Aging. 2012;29:343–58.
24. Wang S, Wei X, Zhou J, Zhang J, Li K, Chen Q, et al. Identification of α2-macroglobulin as a master inhibitor of cartilage-degrading factors that attenuates the progression of posttraumatic osteoarthritis. Arthritis Rheumatol. 2014;66:1843–53.

Chapter 40
Bone Marrow Derived Stem Cells and Their Application in Pain Medicine

Christopher J. Centeno, Matthew W. Hyzy, and Christopher J. Williams

Bone marrow is increasingly being used to treat musculoskeletal disorders. There is promising early clinical data on the treatment of knee, hip, and shoulder osteoarthritis, as well as intervertebral disc disease [1–10]. The most common type of therapy uses bone marrow concentrate (BMC), which is comprised of the isolation of the buffy coat found within centrifuged bone marrow aspirate [11]. It is considered that the active components within bone marrow are mesenchymal stem cells, but other cells are also present.

Treatment with BMC is allowing for a shift in orthopedic care from surgeries to remove or modify tissue to precise, image-guided injections to help the healing of injured or degenerated tissues. The advantages to this approach are obvious: the ability to reduce the morbidity associated with more invasive surgical procedures, as well as the ability to prompt tissue healing. Finally, the implications for pain management clinicians are also game-changing, as their interventional skill set fits well with these new approaches to orthopedic problems.

40.1 Indications

As of 3 April 2016, a total of 8428 patients had been treated for orthopedic conditions with any type of bone marrow stem cell therapy and had their results (outcomes or adverse events) published and listed in the U.S. Library of Medicine. Table 40.1 lists the disease areas with the most published outcome information for bone marrow concentrate (BMC).

C.J. Centeno • M.W. Hyzy • C.J. Williams (✉)
The Centeno-Schultz Clinic, Broomfield, CO, USA
e-mail: Centenooffice@centenoschultz.com; MHyzy@centenoschultz.com; CWilliams@centenoschultz.com

S. Diwan, T.R. Deer (eds.), *Advanced Procedures for Pain Management*,
https://doi.org/10.1007/978-3-319-68841-1_40

Table 40.1 Summary of evidence for common orthopedic conditions treated with bone marrow concentrate

Pathology	Total treated, *n*	References
Osteonecrosis	342	[12]
Knee osteoarthritis	1018	[4, 13]
Shoulder rotator cuff	200	[1, 6]
Hip osteoarthritis	201	[17, 18]
Degenerative disc disease	47	[7–9, 19, 20]
Ankle disorders	92	[18, 21]
Epicondylitis	30	[22]

40.1.1 Osteonecrosis

The largest published study is Hernigou et al. ($n = 342$) [12]. Hips of Association Research Circulation Osseous (ARCO) grade 1 or 2 showed approximately an 80% long-term likelihood of not requiring arthroplasty. With more severe grades (ARCO grades 3 and 4), there was declining success.

40.1.2 Knee Osteoarthritis

Table 40.2 summarizes the major studies, including both BMC and culture-expanded mesenchymal stem cells (MSCs) for the treatment of knee osteoarthritis (OA):

- Published data demonstrate good clinical results. The Vangsness study [13] revealed an increase in meniscus size in one in four patients, and the Vega study [14] showed improvement in cartilage signal on follow-up MRI.
- We have published a large case series demonstrating promising pain and functional outcomes; the addition of a fat graft did not improve outcomes over injecting BMC alone [15].

40.1.3 Shoulder Rotator Cuff

Two published studies support the use of BMC for shoulder OA and rotator cuff tears (Table 40.3):

- Hernigou et al. [6] published a comparison trial of surgical shoulder rotator cuff repair with or without the use of injected BMC. The BMC group had approximately one half the re-tear rate of the surgery-only group.
- The authors have completed a case series of 102 patients with shoulder OA and rotator cuff tears who demonstrated significant reductions in pain and increases in validated functional metrics [1].

Table 40.2 Summary of published research using BMC or culture-expanded bone marrow MSCs for knee osteoarthritis

Study	Study type	Intervention	Patients, *n*	Stem cells used	Functional improvement	Notes
Vangsness et al. [13]	DB RCT	Partial menisctomy with MSC injection	55	Allo cultured bone marrow MSCs	Yes	1 in 4 patients with increased meniscus volume
Centeno et al. [15]	Prospective case series	Image-guided injection	840	BMC	Yes	2/3 of patients were TKA candidates
Kim et al. [16]	Prospective case series	Injection	49	Autologous cultured bone marrow MSCs	Yes	Full-thickness chondral lesions <6 cm/2 responded best
Vega et al. [14]	RCT	Injection of MSCs vs HA	30	Allo cultured bone marrow MSCs	Yes	Improved cartilage signal on MRI T2 mapping

BMC bone marrow concentrate, *DB* double blind, *HA* hyaluronic acid, *MSCs* mesenchymal stem cells, *RCT* randomized, controlled trial, *TKA* total knee arthroplasty

Table 40.3 Summary of published research using BMC for shoulder osteoarthritis and rotator cuff tear

Study	Study type	Intervention	Patients, *n*	Stem cells used	Functional improvement	Notes
Centeno et al. [1]	Prospective case series	Image-guided injection	105	BMC	Yes	Patients failed conservative management
Hernigou et al. [6]	Prospective case controlled	Arthroscopic rotator cuff repair with MSCs *vs* repair only group	45	BMC	Yes	100% healing of tendon on MRI *vs* 67% in control group at 6 months; intact tendon in 87% *vs* 44% at 10 years

BMC bone marrow concentrate, *MSCs* mesenchymal stem cells

Table 40.4 Summary of published research using BMC for hip osteoarthritis

Study	Study type	Intervention	Patients, *n*	Stem cells used	Functional improvement	Notes
Centeno et al. [17]	Prospective case series	Image-guided injection	196	BMC	Yes	Majority of patients were THA candidates
Emadedin et al. [18]	Prospective case series	Unknown	5	Culture-expanded bone marrow MSCs	Yes	Severity unknown

BMC bone marrow concentrate, *MSCs* mesenchymal stem cells, *THA* total hip arthroplasty

40.1.4 Hip Osteoarthritis

The response rates are generally lower in severe disease. Table 40.4 summarizes published research using BMC for hip OA:

- The author's case series of 196 patients treated through injection of BMC demonstrated that patients over age 55 (i.e. likely those with more severe disease) showed poorer outcomes [17].
- Emadedin et al. published a smaller case series of five patients treated with culture-expanded bone marrow MSCs [18].

40.1.5 Lumbar Intervertebral Disc (Degenerative Disc Disease)

Table 40.5 summarizes the published clinical data on BMC for degenerative disc disease (DDD):

- Pettine et al. published 1- and 2-year results, in which patients with the highest MSC dose (as demonstrated by Colony Forming Units) reported the best outcomes [8, 9].
- Other published studies have used isolated and culture-expanded MSCs, autologous nucleus pulposus cells, allogeneic culture-expanded cord blood MSCs, and autologous cord blood MSCs [7, 19, 20].

Table 40.5 Summary of published research using BMC, culture-expanded MSCs, and other cell types to treat degenerative disk disease

Study	Study type	Intervention	Patients, *n*	Stem cells used	Functional improvement	Notes
Mochida et al. [19]	Prospective case series	Surgical implant	9	Autologous nucleus pulposus cells	No—minimal MRI changes	Safety study
Pettine et al. [8, 9]	Prospective case series	Injection into IVD	26	BMC	Yes	Possible slight changes in MRI, but within error of DDD grading scale
Pang et al. [20]	Prospective case series	Surgical implantation	2	Autologous cord blood MSCs	Yes	No imaging
Orozco et al. [7]	Prospective case series	Injection into IVD	10	Autologous culture-expanded bone marrow MSCs	Yes	No improvement in disc height, some increase in T2 signal

BMC bone marrow concentrate, *DDD* degenerative disc disease, *IVD* intervertebral disc, *MSCs* mesenchymal stem cells

40.1.6 Ankle Disorders

- A study published in 2015 that used cultured MSCs for the treatment of osteoarthritis of the ankle showed a significant reduction in pain, improved function, and a decrease in subchondral edema on MRI 6 months after the procedure, in a subset of the patients [18].
- Hernigou et al. [21] published a study on the treatment of ankle non-union in diabetic patients. One arm of the study received the standard treatment with an iliac crest bone graft; the other arm was treated with autologous BMC. Those treated with BMC had a success rate of 82% *versus* 62% in those treated with the bone graft.

40.1.7 Epicondylitis

A case series of 30 patients treated with a single injection of BMC for lateral epicondylitis showed a significant reduction in symptoms at short and medium follow-up intervals [22].

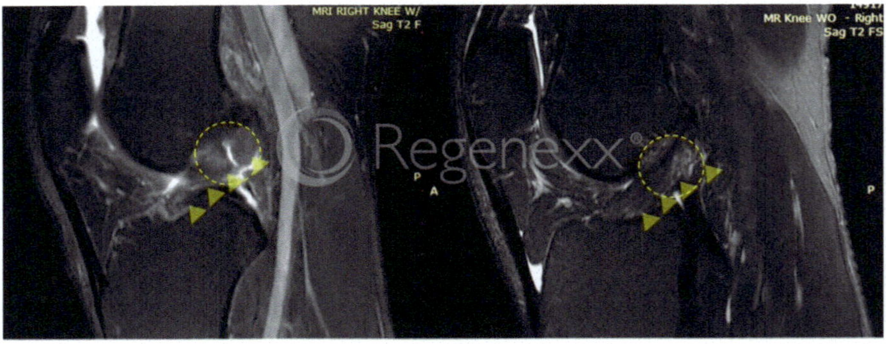

Fig. 40.1 Exemplar MRIs showing improved complete anterior cruciate ligament (ACL) tear signal on sagittal T2 MRI before and 3 months after precise ACL bone marrow concentrate (BMC) injection with fluoroscopic guidance and contrast confirmation. The left image is the pre-procedure knee ACL tear. It shows a white tear (inside the *yellow dashed circle*) diagonally through the dark-appearing ACL. The right image shows the follow-up MRI at 3 months after the injection of the patient's own BMC. No tear is seen inside the *yellow dashed circle*. The *yellow triangles* in both images delineate the course of the ACL

40.1.8 Anterior Cruciate Ligament (ACL) Tears

A small case series published by Centeno et al. [23] demonstrated healing on pre- and post-procedure MRI after treatment with BMC for partial and complete ACL tears (Fig. 40.1).

40.2 Microanatomy and Biochemistry

What is a stem cell? At its most basic, it is a cell that has the following three properties:

- Undifferentiated
- Capable of differentiating into many cell types
- Can divide through mitosis to give rise to new stem cells

The fact that bone marrow contains stem cells was first discovered in the 1960s [24]. Since then, a number of stem cell types that are potentially important to pain management physicians have been discovered:

- *Mesenchymal stem cells (MSCs)*: Multipotent, adult stem cells that show clinical potential as therapeutic agents in regenerative medicine [1–5].
  - Also known as *marrow stromal cells*, these cells are also derived from other mesodermal tissues. MSCs were later assayed and renamed "colony forming fibroblasts" in the 1970s [7].
  - Experiments through the 1980s and 1990s demonstrated that local environmental clues differentiated MSCs into different cell types. For example, cul-

turing these cells with ascorbic acid, inorganic phosphate, or dexamethasone could differentiate cells to osteoblasts, whereas exposure to TGFβ caused cells to differentiate into chondrocytes [1].
  - More recent research has revealed that MSCs are actually a heterogeneous population of similar cells rather than one distinct cell type [8].
  - International groups have attempted to provide a definition of MSC that consists of adherence to plastic, MSC-specific cell surface markers, and multilineage mesodermal tissue differentiation [9].

- *Hematopoietic stem cells (HSCs)*: These cells give rise to the nucleated cells of the blood but also are secondarily involved in muscle repair [25].
  - In the body, HSCs are routinely recruited from the bone marrow when local muscle satellite cells are unable to complete muscle repair.
- *Endothelial progenitor cells (EPCs)*: These cells are recruited from the bone marrow to facilitate vascular homeostasis and neovasculogenesis [26].
  - Because many chronically injured musculoskeletal tissues have poor blood supply, this cell type may be useful for reestablishing vascularity.
- *Pericytes*: These cells are also recruited from the bone marrow for neovasculogenesis, as these cells reside around blood vessels [27].
  - Some believe that pericytes can differentiate into MSCs when injury is detected [28].
- *Osteochondral reticular cells*: These recently discovered cells are concentrated in the metaphysis of long bones, but not in the perisinusoidal space.
  - These cells can differentiate into osteoblasts, chondrocytes, and reticular marrow stromal cells [29].
- *Multilineage-differentiating stress-enduring (MUSE) cells*: These cells can differentiate into all three embryonic layers (endoderm, mesoderm, and ectoderm).
  - These cells act as a reserve cell source; they are difficult to kill and are activated by physical stress. They are also involved in regenerative homeostasis and tissue repair.

40.2.1 Bone Marrow Concentrate Versus Adipose?

Several sources have suggested that adipose contains a higher stem cell count than bone marrow [30, 31]. This misconception seems to be the result of a difference in nucleated cell content between the two tissues:

- Bone marrow has as many or more stem cells per unit volume as adipose tissue.
- Adipose tissue is less cellular and has a much lower nucleated cell content per volume than bone marrow. For example, bone marrow has approximately 100 times more total cells than adipose tissue [32].

- Adipose tissue has a much higher percentage of stem cells, as compared with nucleated cells; 1–5% are MSCs, *versus* 0.01–0.5% in bone marrow.
- Adipose tissue contains significantly fewer HSCs (4×10^{-6}% *versus* 1–2%).

40.3 Basic Concerns and Contraindications

BMC safety in orthopedic diseases has been well established via two large studies:

- Hernigou et al. [33]: 1873 patients monitored for 12.5 years for the occurrence of neoplasm (not all adverse events).
- Centeno et al. [34]: 2372 patients treated at multiple sites, followed for up to 9 years for all adverse events, showing an excellent safety profile. 1835 patients received BMC; the remainder received cultured expanded MSCs.

Common contraindications include anemia, uncontrolled bleeding disorders, and active neoplasm or a history of neoplasm. The paper by Hernigou et al. [33] showed that cancer patients treated with BMC injections for orthopedic conditions did not show any increase in new neoplasm rates. Hence, though injecting MSCs directly into a tumor is ill-advised because of a risk that the cells may differentiate into tumor cells or promote cell proliferation, an existing neoplasm may be a relative contraindication.

40.4 Preoperative Considerations

- Explanation of potential complications and alternative treatments.
- Hematocrit and overall patient health as appropriate for a surgical procedure.
- Anticoagulation and bleeding disorders that may prevent or complicate the clotting process after penetration of the periosteum.
- Physical examination of the area of potential harvest for infection, skin ulceration, or necrosis.
- Heparin produces fewer clots in bone marrow aspirate (BMA) than ACD (acid-citrate-dextrose). It is essential to ensure that the patient has no history of heparin-induced thrombocytopenia. If this is suspected, ACD should be used in place of heparin.

Research on maximizing the MSC yield from BMC has yielded several key points:

- The posterior superior iliac spine contains double the nucleated cells of other bone aspiration sites, like the tibia [35].
- Drawing a large volume (>20 mL) from a single bone site reduces MSC yield; drawing small volumes (5–15 mL) from many sites increases that yield [35].

- MSCs reside in the subcortical areas, and pericytes reside around blood vessels. Hence, drawing from more sites maximizes subcortical MSC yield and allows access to pericytes. Travelling through the bone marrow space sacrifices subcortical MSCs, however.
- Even small concentrations of bupivacaine or lidocaine are toxic to MSCs, so BMA should not be allowed to come in direct contact with either anesthetic. *The only safe drug to use is ropivacaine (0.25% or less)* [36, 37].

40.5 Radiographic Guidance

The hallmark of interventional orthopedics is the use of imaging guidance to precisely place cells into the damaged or diseased tissue. Both ultrasound and fluoroscopic guidance are commonly used. Each has its benefits and its drawbacks.

40.5.1 Ultrasound

- *Benefit:* Superior in imaging superficial soft tissue
- *Drawback:* Unable to image deeper structures obscured by bony tunnels or bone
- *Example*: Suggested for injecting the shoulder rotator cuff, but less than ideal for injecting the knee ACL, because the origin is buried in the trochlear groove.

40.5.2 Fluoroscopy

- *Benefit*: Superior for imaging bone and deeper structures with the aid of contrast
- *Drawback*: Unable to image soft tissues; produces radiation exposure, and cost is higher
- *Example:* Suggested for injecting stem cells into an osteonecrotic lesion of the hip, but would be less appropriate to inject a rotator cuff tear

Attempting bone marrow aspiration without either ultrasound or fluoroscopic guidance is below the standard of care, because the thick areas of the pelvis that have appropriate depth to cannulate are very close to very thin areas that cannot be cannulated (Fig. 40.2).

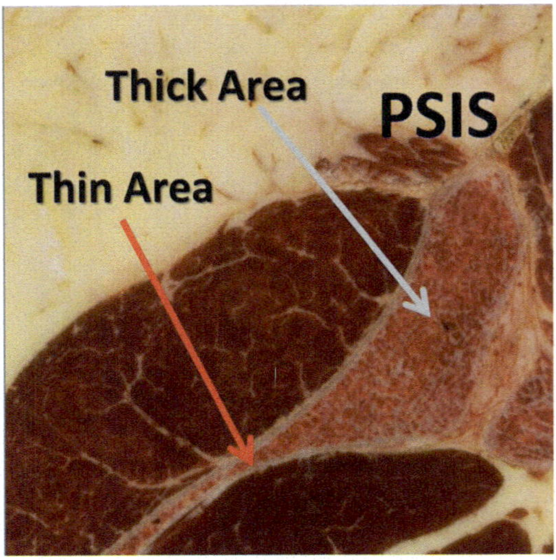

Fig. 40.2 A slice through the bony pelvis showing two marrow draw angles. The first goes through the "thin area" or the area identified as more radiolucent on plain radiographs. This is a thin area of the pelvis, where the likelihood of passing through the marrow space is very high. The "thick area" is a more opaque area on radiographs. This area has a large marrow space with less risk of passing through the marrow-rich area and much higher likelihood of aspirating whole marrow. *PSIS* posterior superior iliac spine

40.6 Equipment

- 10–15 mL of 1% lidocaine or 0.25% ropivacaine
- 5000 IU vial of heparin
- 20,000 IU and 10,000 IU vials of heparin
- Preservative-free normal saline
- 30 G needle (for anesthetizing skin)
- 25 G 3.5-in. spinal needle (for anesthetizing periosteum and underlying tissue)
- Sterile 11-G disposable trocars (one for each side of access)
- 5-mL syringe
- 30-mL syringes
  – At least one study has suggested that using multiple 5- or 10-mL syringes may increase MSC yield [38]. We have been unable to replicate these results, which may be an artifact of the larger 50-mL syringes used as comparison.

Most physicians using BMC utilize a commercially available 510 K approved bedside centrifuge, which uses a disposable kit, such as those systems listed here:

- Accelerate: Autologous Platelet Concentrating System
- Accellerated Biologics: BC 60 and BC 120 Pure
- Arthrex Angel

- Celling ART BMC
- EmCyte 544E
- EmCyte PureBMC
- GenesisCS Component Concentrating System
- Harvest Technologies SmartPReP 2
- ISTO CellPoint

Some physicians also use manual processing and a biologic safety cabinet. The advantages of a bedside centrifuge using a kit are ease of use, lower start-up costs, and a requirement for very little training. The disadvantage is that frequently a standard volume is inputted and a standard volume is delivered in this one-size-fits-all approach.

40.7 Technique

40.7.1 Harvesting BMC

Bone marrow can be obtained easily via an aspirate procedure. This is a safe procedure; one large registry in the UK, which included bone marrow aspiration and trephine biopsy, showed 15 serious adverse events in 20,323 procedures [39].

The suggested target for harvesting BMC is the pelvic crest. The steps for bone marrow aspiration are as follows:

- The patient is placed prone on a procedure table.
- After sterile prep, 10–15 mL of either 1% lidocaine (which must not come into contact with the BMA) or 0.25% ropivacaine are injected.
  - It is critical for the numbing to occur under guidance, with careful attention paid to the exact areas that are injected; straying out of the anesthetized area will cause significant pain. It is also critical that the skin, soft tissues, and periosteum are injected. In my experience with more than 1000 bone marrow aspiration procedures, the single biggest cause of pain is inadequate numbing of the soft tissues.
- Sufficient time must be allowed to pass for the area to be adequately anesthetized.
- Prep the draw syringes by adding 1000 units of heparin per milliliter drawn (or follow the instructions of the point-of-care automated centrifuge). Thus 30-mL syringes would have 30,000 units of heparin per syringe.
- Prep one additional 5-mL syringe with 5000 units of heparin in normal saline.
- If using ultrasound, the entry must be at a shallow angle to the probe (Fig. 40.3). If using fluoroscopy, the entry point is at a steeper angle (Fig. 40.4). The draw sites are around the posterior superior iliac spine (PSIS), as shown in Fig. 40.5. These target the thick areas of the bone marrow and avoid the thin areas.

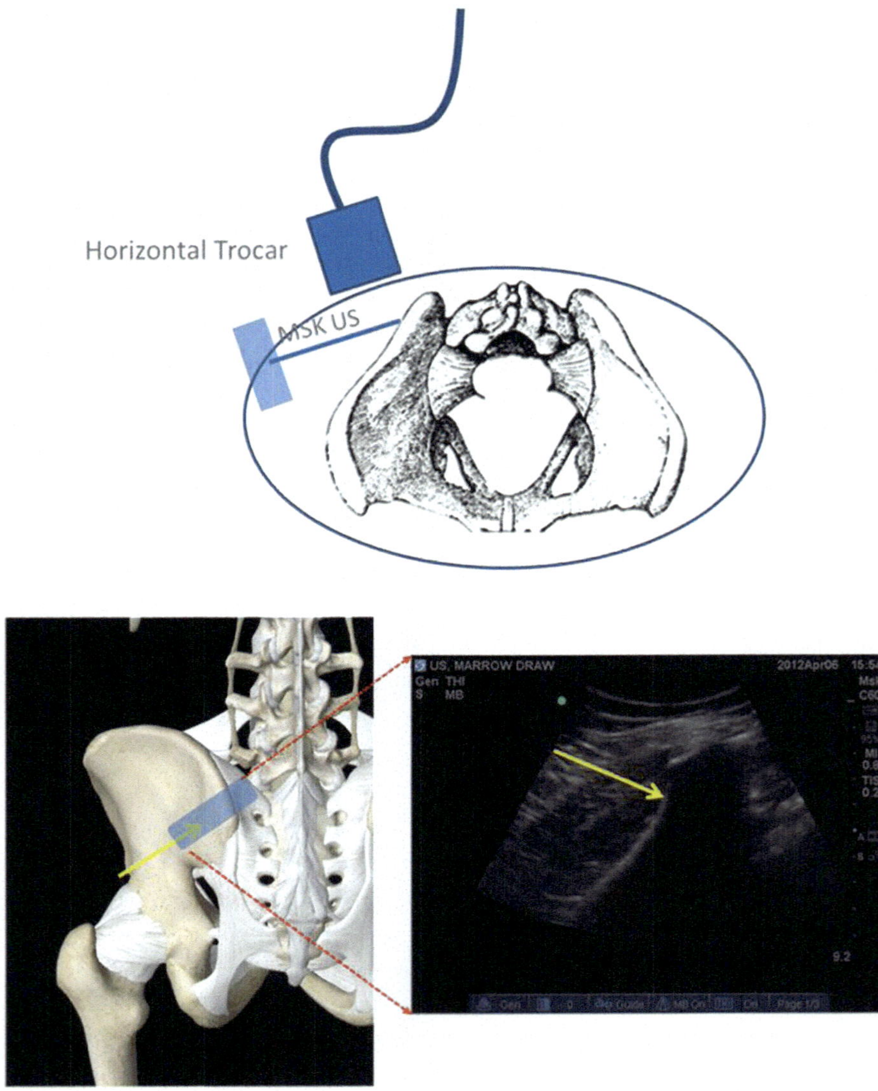

Fig. 40.3 The ideal ultrasound linear probe and trocar placement for identification of the posterior superior iliac spine (PSIS) during a bone marrow aspiration procedure. *MSK US* musculoskeletal ultrasound

- The trocar is placed against the bone cortex, and forward pressure is used while the device is turned back and forth, using the angled tip to bore a hole in the bone. The trocar is advanced 5–10 mm until it is seated in the cortex. Note that many trocars have 1-cm markers on the shaft, making it easy to gauge the depth.

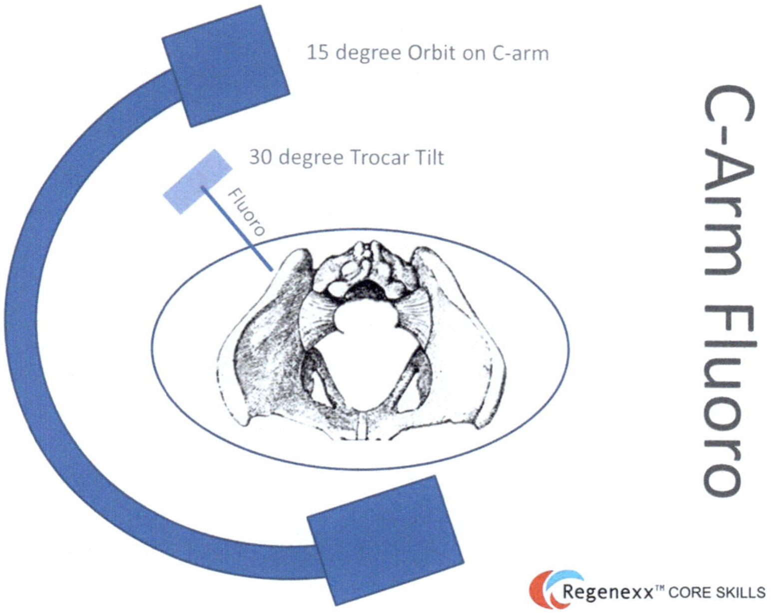

Fig. 40.4 The ideal fluoroscopic C-arm and trocar placement for identification of the PSIS during a bone marrow aspiration procedure

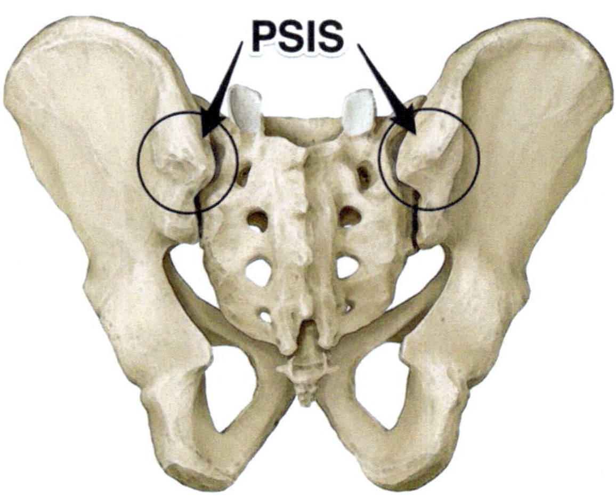

Fig. 40.5 Depiction of the PSIS located on the posterior pelvis. This is the ideal area for three or four draw sites from each PSIS

- To ensure that the trocar is properly seated in the bone, the trocar should be wiggled gently back and forth; if solid, no further advancement is required. If it can still be moved, then the trocar is advanced until it is solidly in the bone.
- Remove the stylet from the trocar and make sure the trocar is still firmly implanted in the cortex by performing a second wiggle test. If it is not firmly implanted, advance the trocar until firm, not exceeding approximately 1 cm in depth.

- Because clotting of the marrow sample traps unrecoverable MSCs in the clot, avoiding this event is important. Hence, before aspiration, the 5-mL syringe with the 5000 units of heparin is placed on the trocar and approximately 500–750 units of heparin is injected into the marrow space immediately on entry into the cortex. This is performed for each bone site entered.
- Attach the draw syringe to the trocar. Pull back on the plunger to patient tolerance. The BMA will not naturally mix with the heparin, so the first few milliliters of BMA must be mixed with the heparin using gentle agitation of the syringe.
- Once mixed, draw no more than 5–15 mL per site. Once complete, move the trocar tip to a new cortex site, using the same skin site (i.e., not removing the trocar from the skin).
- Draw volumes are dependent on patient weight and the size of the area to be treated.
  - For women less than 105 pounds, draw no more than 50 mL.
  - For women between 105 and 120 pounds, the most appropriate draw volume is 60 mL.
  - For heavier patients of either sex between 120 and 180 pounds, up to 90 mL can be drawn.
  - For men over 180 pounds, 120 mL can be drawn.

40.7.2 Processing BMC

There are many commercial systems to process BMA. Some physicians also process via manual means in a biologic safety cabinet. The goal of BMA concentration is to isolate the buffy coat, which is the smaller, grey, middle section in a centrifuged BMA sample. Automated bedside systems all concentrate the buffy coat and have developed many proprietary ways to perform this simple task. To date, little third-party research is available comparing the MSC outputs of various concentration devices.

40.7.3 Dosing BMC for Use

The dose of BMC can be quantified as follows:

- *Colony Forming Unit (CFU) assay*: BMC is placed in monolayer culture and incubated until colonies of plastic-adherent MSCs form. These are then counted as a rough metric of MSC content [40].
  - This technique is helpful for research, but is little help to the clinician at the bedside.
- *Flow cytometry*: The cells in BMC are stained via fluorescent antibodies to specific cell surface markers and run through a flow cytometer, which uses laser light

to identify collections of markers. MSCs have a known marker panel, commonly considered to be CD34−, CD14−, CD105+, CD44+, CD90+, CD73+ [41].

  - This technique can be used clinically, but the expertise required to run and analyze the results and the cost of this technology make it unlikely to be used for most clinical settings.

- *Total Nucleated Cell Count (TNC)*: The number of nucleated cells in the BMC is counted using either a manual hemocytometer or a commercial automated counting system [42].

  - TNC can be used at the bedside for clinical settings. Note that it is not a direct MSC count, but an indirect measure of a proxy for that count.

The research on dosing of BMC and clinical outcome has consistently shown that higher CFU counts or TNC counts are associated with better clinical outcome [9].

40.8 Postoperative Considerations

Our extensive experience in culturing MSCs using an autologous platelet lysate procedure has taught us that certain medications can cause cell culture failure and hence reduce MSC function. These medications should be stopped for two to three serum half-lives before a BMC procedure and at least 2–4 weeks after the procedure, where feasible:

- Nonsteroidal anti-inflammatory drugs (NSAIDs) [43]
- Corticosteroids [44]
- ACE inhibitors [45]
- Statins [46]

40.9 Potential Complications and Pitfalls

- Marcaine, bupivacaine, and lidocaine are toxic to MSCs at low concentrations. Injecting these anesthetics with BMC will significantly reduce cell viability. Ropivacaine at concentrations of 0.125–0.25% is safe to use with MSCs [36, 37].
- Incomplete anesthesia of the periosteum can lead to intense pain and even neuralgia.

  - Many clinicians numb only the skin and then the deep tissues. It is critical also to numb the mid-field soft tissues between these two areas.
  - The clinician MUST provide adequate time for the local anesthetic to take effect, typically 3–5 min. Numbing these tissues first on one side and then the other, and then drawing medications, usually provides that set time.

- When using fluoroscopy, there is an innate sense of two-dimensional anatomy, so simply remembering anatomic landmarks will help define that area.
- When using ultrasound, the cross-sectional nature of the imaging technology provides less information about the location of anesthetic. We suggest using a sterile surgical marker on the skin to better define the numbed area.
- Many physicians have been taught to pull high volumes (60 mL or more) from a single site during bone marrow aspiration. Doing so will dramatically reduce yield, as discussed above.
- Most are unaware that clots can form in the BMA and will reduce MSC yield. These clots can form when not using heparin in the BMA or not pre-heparinizing the draw sites. We suggest using heparin because it is a much more effective anticoagulant than ACD. It must be used in the BMA draw syringe (see above) and must be mixed as soon as the BMA hits the syringe, as it will not naturally mix through diffusion. In addition, the immediate injection of heparin directly into the bone site being cannulated, before the BMA is drawn, will help prevent clots in slow bone marrow aspirations due to dehydration.

40.10 Clinical Pearls

- Adipose tissue does not necessarily yield higher counts of MSCs.
- Anesthetics take time to work. The patient can be made more comfortable simply by injecting local anesthetic first, then drawing up heparin and preparing the trocar, then placing the trocar into the skin. These extra few minutes of prep time allow for a better block. Avoid using lidocaine or bupivacaine, which can be toxic to the MSCs; instead use ropivacaine or prevent the anesthetic from coming into contact with the graft.
- Using multiple collection syringes for several smaller aspirations rather than one larger one will allow for higher yields.
- Heparin is preferred over ACD because it prevents clotting, which may potentially decrease cell counts.

References

1. Centeno CJ, Al-Sayegh H, Bashir J, Goodyear S, Freeman MD. A prospective multi-site registry study of a specific protocol of autologous bone marrow concentrate for the treatment of shoulder rotator cuff tears and osteoarthritis. J Pain Res. 2015;8:269–76.
2. Daltro GC, Fortuna V, de Souza ES, Salles MM, Carreira AC, Meyer R, et al. Efficacy of autologous stem cell-based therapy for osteonecrosis of the femoral head in sickle cell disease: a five-year follow-up study. Stem Cell Res Ther. 2015;6:110.
3. Gobbi A, Scotti C, Karnatzikos G, Mudhigere A, Castro M, Peretti GM. One-step surgery with multipotent stem cells and Hyaluronan-based scaffold for the treatment of full-thickness chondral defects of the knee in patients older than 45 years. Knee Surg Sports Traumatol Arthrosc. 2016;25(8):2494–501.

4. Gobbi A, Whyte GP. One-stage cartilage repair using a hyaluronic acid-based scaffold with activated bone marrow-derived mesenchymal stem cells compared with microfracture: five-year follow-up. Am J Sports Med. 2016;44:2846–54.
5. Havlas V, Kotaška J, Koníček P, Trč T, Konrádová Š, Kočí Z, Syková E. Use of cultured human autologous bone marrow stem cells in repair of a rotator cuff tear: preliminary results of a safety study. Acta Chir Orthop Traumatol Cechoslov. 2015;82:229–34.
6. Hernigou P, Flouzat Lachaniette CH, Delambre J, Zilber S, Duffiet P, Chevallier N, Rouard H. Biologic augmentation of rotator cuff repair with mesenchymal stem cells during arthroscopy improves healing and prevents further tears: a case-controlled study. Int Orthop. 2014;38:1811–8.
7. Orozco L, Soler R, Morera C, Alberca M, Sánchez A, García-Sancho J. Intervertebral disc repair by autologous mesenchymal bone marrow cells: a pilot study. Transplantation. 2011;92:822–8.
8. Pettine K, Suzuki R, Sand T, Murphy M. Treatment of discogenic back pain with autologous bone marrow concentrate injection with minimum two year follow-up. Int Orthop. 2016;40:135–40.
9. Pettine KA, Murphy MB, Suzuki RK, Sand TT. Percutaneous injection of autologous bone marrow concentrate cells significantly reduces lumbar discogenic pain through 12 months. Stem Cells. 2015;33:146–56.
10. Zhao D, Liu B, Wang B, Yang L, Xie H, Huang S, et al. Autologous bone marrow mesenchymal stem cells associated with tantalum rod implantation and vascularized iliac grafting for the treatment of end-stage osteonecrosis of the femoral head. Biomed Res Int. 2015;2015:240506.
11. Sampson S, Botto-van Bemden A, Aufiero D. Autologous bone marrow concentrate: review and application of a novel intra-articular orthobiologic for cartilage disease. Phys Sportsmed. 2013;41:7–18.
12. Hernigou P, Poignard A, Zilber S, Rouard H. Cell therapy of hip osteonecrosis with autologous bone marrow grafting. Indian J Orthop. 2009;43:40–5.
13. Vangsness CT Jr, Farr J II, Boyd J, Dellaero DT, Mills CR, LeRoux-Williams M. Adult human mesenchymal stem cells delivered via intra-articular injection to the knee following partial medial meniscectomy: a randomized, double-blind, controlled study. J Bone Joint Surg Am. 2014;96:90–8.
14. Vega A, Martín-Ferrero MA, Del Canto F, Alberca M, García V, Munar A, et al. Treatment of knee osteoarthritis with allogeneic bone marrow mesenchymal stem cells: a randomized controlled trial. Transplantation. 2015;99:1681–90.
15. Centeno C, Pitts J, Al-Sayegh H, Freeman M. Efficacy of autologous bone marrow concentrate for knee osteoarthritis with and without adipose graft. Biomed Res Int 2014;2014:370621.
16. Kim YS, Choi YJ, Koh YG. Mesenchymal stem cell implantation in knee osteoarthritis: an assessment of the factors influencing clinical outcomes. Am J Sports Med. 2015;43:2293–301.
17. Centeno CJ, Pitts JA, Al-Sayegh H, Freeman MD. Efficacy and safety of bone marrow concentrate for osteoarthritis of the hip; treatment registry results for 196 patients. J Stem Cell Res Ther. 2014;4:242.
18. Emadedin M, Ghorbani Liastani M, Fazeli R, Mohseni F, Moghadasali R, et al. Long-term follow-up of intra-articular injection of autologous mesenchymal stem cells in patients with knee, ankle, or hip osteoarthritis. Arch Iran Med. 2015;18:336–44.
19. Mochida J, Sakai D, Nakamura Y, Watanabe T, Yamamoto Y, Kato S. Intervertebral disc repair with activated nucleus pulposus cell transplantation: a three-year, prospective clinical study of its safety. Eur Cell Mater. 2015;29:202–12; discussion 212.
20. Pang X, Yang H, Peng B. Human umbilical cord mesenchymal stem cell transplantation for the treatment of chronic discogenic low back pain. Pain Physician. 2014;17:E525–30.
21. Hernigou P, Guissou I, Homma Y, Poignard A, Chevallier N, Rouard H, Flouzat Lachaniette CH. Percutaneous injection of bone marrow mesenchymal stem cells for ankle non-unions decreases complications in patients with diabetes. Int Orthop. 2015;39:1639–43.
22. Singh A, Gangwar DS, Singh S. Bone marrow injection: a novel treatment for tennis elbow. J Nat Sci Biol Med. 2014;5:389–91.

23. Centeno CJ, Pitts J, Al-Sayegh H, Freeman MD. Anterior cruciate ligament tears treated with percutaneous injection of autologous bone marrow nucleated cells: a case series. J Pain Res. 2015;8:437–47.
24. Friedenstein AJ, Chailakhjan RK, Lalykina KS. The development of fibroblast colonies in monolayer cultures of guinea-pig bone marrow and spleen cells. Cell Tissue Kinet. 1970;3:393–403.
25. Strömberg A, Jansson M, Fischer H, Rullman E, Hägglund H, Gustafsson T. Bone marrow derived cells in adult skeletal muscle tissue in humans. Skelet Muscle. 2013;3:12.
26. Szmitko PE, Wang CH, Weisel RD, Jeffries GA, Anderson TJ, Verma S. Biomarkers of vascular disease linking inflammation to endothelial activation: part II. Circulation. 2003;108:2041–8.
27. Bergmann CE, Hoefer IE, Meder B, Roth H, van Royen N, Breit SM, et al. Arteriogenesis depends on circulating monocytes and macrophage accumulation and is severely depressed in op/op mice. J Leukoc Biol. 2006;80:59–65.
28. Crisan M, Yap S, Casteilla L, Chen CW, Corselli M, Park TS, et al. A perivascular origin for mesenchymal stem cells in multiple human organs. Cell Stem Cell. 2008;3:301–13.
29. Worthley DL, Churchill M, Compton JT, Tailor Y, Rao M, Si Y, et al. Gremlin 1 identifies a skeletal stem cell with bone, cartilage, and reticular stromal potential. Cell. 2015;160:269–84.
30. Mafi R, Hindocha S, Mafi P, Griffin M, Khan WS. Sources of adult mesenchymal stem cells applicable for musculoskeletal applications - a systematic review of the literature. Open Orthop J. 2011;5(Suppl 2):242–8.
31. Zuk PA, Zhu M, Mizuno H, Huang J, Futrell JW, Katz AJ, et al. Multilineage cells from human adipose tissue: implications for cell-based therapies. Tissue Eng. 2001;7:211–28.
32. Sakaguchi Y, Sekiya I, Yagishita K, Muneta T. Comparison of human stem cells derived from various mesenchymal tissues: superiority of synovium as a cell source. Arthritis Rheum. 2005;52:2521–9.
33. Hernigou P, Homma Y, Flouzat-Lachaniette CH, Poignard A, Chevallier N, Rouard H. Cancer risk is not increased in patients treated for orthopaedic diseases with autologous bone marrow cell concentrate. J Bone Joint Surg Am. 2013;95:2215–21.
34. Centeno CJ, Al-Sayegh H, Freeman MD, Smith J, Murrell WD, Bubnov R. A multi-center analysis of adverse events among two thousand, three hundred and seventy two adult patients undergoing adult autologous stem cell therapy for orthopaedic conditions. Int Orthop. 2016;40:1755–65.
35. Marx RE, Tursun R. A qualitative and quantitative analysis of autologous human multipotent adult stem cells derived from three anatomic areas by marrow aspiration: tibia, anterior ilium, and posterior ilium. Int J Oral Maxillofac Implants. 2013;28:e290–4.
36. Breu A, Eckl S, Zink W, Kujat R, Angele P. Cytotoxicity of local anesthetics on human mesenchymal stem cells in vitro. Arthroscopy. 2013;29:1676–84.
37. Dregalla RC, Lyons NF, Reischling PD, Centeno CJ. Amide-type local anesthetics and human mesenchymal stem cells: clinical implications for stem cell therapy. Stem Cells Transl Med. 2014;3:365–74.
38. Hernigou P, Homma Y, Flouzat Lachaniette CH, Poignard A, Allain J, Chevallier N, Rouard H. Benefits of small volume and small syringe for bone marrow aspirations of mesenchymal stem cells. Int Orthop. 2013;37:2279–87.
39. Bain BJ. Morbidity associated with bone marrow aspiration and trephine biopsy – a review of UK data for 2004. Haematologica. 2006;91:1293–4.
40. Franken NA, Rodermond HM, Stap J, Haveman J, van Bree C. Clonogenic assay ofcells in vitro. Nat Protoc. 2006;1:2315–9.
41. Boxall SA, Jones E. Markers for characterization of bone marrow multipotential stromal cells. Stem Cells Int. 2012;2012:975871.
42. Peters AE, Watts AE. Biopsy needle advancement during bone marrow aspiration increases mesenchymal stem cell concentration. Front Vet Sci. 2016;3:23.
43. Chang JK, Li CJ, Wu SC, Yeh CH, Chen CH, Fu YC, et al. Effects of anti-inflammatory drugs on proliferation, cytotoxicity and osteogenesis in bone marrow mesenchymal stem cells. Biochem Pharmacol. 2007;74:1371–82.

44. Wyles CC, Houdek MT, Wyles SP, Wagner ER, Behfar A, Sierra RJ. Differential cytotoxicity of corticosteroids on human mesenchymal stem cells. Clin Orthop Relat Res. 2015;473:1155–64.
45. Durik M, Sevá Pessôa B, Roks AJ. The renin-angiotensin system, bone marrow and progenitor cells. Clin Sci (Lond). 2012;123:205–23.
46. Izadpanah R, Schächtele DJ, Pfnür AB, Lin D, Slakey DP, Kadowitz PJ, Alt EU. The impact of statins on biological characteristics of stem cells provides a novel explanation for their pleiotropic beneficial and adverse clinical effects. Am J Physiol Cell Physiol. 2015;309:C522–31.

Chapter 41
Adipose-Derived Stromal Stem Cells

Lora L. Brown

41.1 Introduction

Autologous adipose-derived stem cells are a novel therapy for patients suffering from traumatic, degenerative, or inflammatory disease processes. Clinical data have identified adipose tissue as an alternative source of mesenchymal stem cells (MSCs). Stromal vascular tissue derived from adipose tissue contains a subset of tissue that is different from that found in blood cells. Adipose stromal tissue contains a subset of multipotent progenitor cells with adipogenic, chondrogenic, and osteogenic differentiation potential [1].

Adipose tissue is abundant, easily accessible, and easily obtainable via lipoaspiration with little patient discomfort. Additionally, a large body of in vitro research shows that adipose-derived stem cells—referred to as the stromal vascular fraction (SVF)—parallel the mononuclear cell fraction obtained from bone marrow–derived stem cells [2] (Table 41.1). In fact, 1 mL of adipose tissue contains 300 to 500 times more MSCs than 1 mL of bone marrow aspirate [3]. The cell populations present in the SVF include hematopoietic-lineage cells (stem and progenitor cells, granulocytes, monocytes, lymphocytes), endothelial cells, pericytes, and stromal cells. Collectively, these cell populations possess many advantageous characteristics, including immunomodulatory, anti-inflammatory, anti-apoptotic, angiogenic, and mitogenic properties. They also resist scar cascade initiation. These cells accomplish regenerative capabilities via complex secretion and signaling of growth factors and cytokines. These paracrine effects, as well as direct cell-to-cell interaction, exert great effects on local tissue repair by activating endogenous progenitor cells previously dormant in the affected tissue [1, 4–7]. Consequently there is a decrease in inflammation and pain, as well as regeneration of tissue in the damaged areas.

L. Brown (✉)
TruWell, PLLC, St. Petersburg, FL, USA
e-mail: LLBMD@me.com

S. Diwan, T.R. Deer (eds.), *Advanced Procedures for Pain Management*,
https://doi.org/10.1007/978-3-319-68841-1_41

Table 41.1 Comparison of bone marrow-derived and adipose-derived stem cells

Bone marrow aspirate concentration (BMAC)	Adipose-derived stem cells (SVF)
Easy to obtain	Moderate difficulty to obtain
Bone marrow aspiration	Tumescent liposuction
Centrifuge and remainder of materials come in commercially-available kits	Flow hood, incubator, tissue culture hood, plus equipment that is typically purchased a la carte
Takes less than an hour to harvest cells, process, and inject to target region	Can take an hour just to harvest cells
Lower nucleated cell concentrations	Higher nucleated cell concentrations
Progenitor and stem cell concentrations unpredictable and typically lower	Progenitor and stem cell concentrations predictable and much higher

Although limited, human studies involving MSCs for the treatment of osteoarthritis are promising. Mesenchymal stem cells derived from bone marrow aspirate and percutaneously injected into subjects with MRI-proven degenerative joint disease of the knee showed statistically significant cartilage and meniscus growth on MRI, as well as increased range of motion and decreased modified Visual Analog Scale (VAS) pain scores at 21 weeks after the injection [8]. Emadedin et al. treated six female subjects with osteoarthritis of the knee who were candidates for knee replacements with bone marrow-derived MSCs and found improvements in pain, functional status, and walking distance 6 months post-injection. MRI images at baseline and 6 months post-injection demonstrated an increase in cartilage thickness, extension of repair tissue over the subchondral bone, and a considerable decrease in the size of edematous subchondral patches [9]. In a similar study, autologous MSCs derived from adipose tissue were administered to 18 patients with osteoarthritis of the knee. The results showed that intra-articular injection of 1.0×10^8 adipose-derived (AD) MSCs into the osteoarthritic knee improved function and pain of the knee joint without causing adverse events, and it reduced cartilage defects by regeneration of hyaline-like articular cartilage [10].

Another area of interest in regenerative medicine is the treatment of degenerative disc disease. Researchers have demonstrated that intervertebral discs contain an endogenous stem cell population of skeletal progenitor cells displaying osteogenic, adipogenic, and chondrogenic characteristics, which are the same characteristics shared by MSCs derived from both bone marrow and adipose tissue. MSC implantation has been shown to stimulate nucleus pulposus cell proliferation and MSC chondrogenic differentiation, as well as increased production of cytokines, particularly transforming growth factor-beta [11, 12].

Animal studies for the treatment of disc degeneration have demonstrated that MSCs injected into the nucleus pulposus not only survive but proliferate in canine, porcine, and rabbit models. The results of these studies also showed that the transplanted stem cells influenced the production of extracellular matrix proteins, including aggrecan, proteoglycans, and type I and type II collagen. Most importantly, these injections resulted in preservation of both water content and height in the damaged disc [13–16].

Human studies utilizing stem cells for the treatment of degenerative disc disease are promising. Orozco et al. conducted a pilot study utilizing autologous culture-expanded bone marrow mesenchymal cells for intervertebral disc repair [17]. Ten subjects were followed for 1 year to evaluate back pain, disability, and quality of life. MRI measurements of disc height and fluid content were also performed. Results confirmed feasibility and safety. Patients exhibited rapid improvement of pain and disability at 85% of maximum in 3 months. MRI scans showed that although disc height was not recovered, water content was significantly elevated at 12 months.

Pettine et al. [18] investigated the use of autologous bone marrow concentrate for the treatment of discogenic pain. Twenty-six subjects received percutaneous injections in one or two intervertebral discs and were evaluated using MRI, the Oswestry Disability Index (ODI), and VAS. Results showed a substantial reduction in pain of 69.5% on the ODI and 70.6% on the VAS. Eight of 20 patients improved by one modified Pfirrmann grade at 1 year. Furthermore, recent basic research and preclinical studies have revealed that the use of adipose-derived MSCs in regenerative medicine is not limited to mesodermal tissue, but extends to ectodermal and endodermal tissues and organs as well [19].

Although there is little data to support the wide array of disease processes treated with stem cell therapy, the evidence is growing exponentially. Physicians around the world utilize adipose-derived MSCs to treat some of the most troubling maladies. Today these therapies are limited to "last resort treatments" for those who can afford them, but some day, regenerative therapies will be at the forefront of advanced medical therapies.

41.2 Indications

In the field of musculoskeletal medicine, adipose stem cell therapy has been used in the treatment of muscle, tendon, and ligament injuries as well as joint arthritis, with anecdotal success of 70%. Painful degenerative disc disease, facet arthritis, and sacroiliac joint pain are also reasonable applications for this therapy.

Although there are no clear treatment protocols defined for the use of adipose stem cell therapy, the current standard of care preserves this treatment for those patients who have failed conventional treatment options or who are not candidates for conventional treatment options.

41.2.1 Musculoskeletal Conditions Treated with Adipose-Derived MSCs

- Joint osteoarthritis and rheumatoid arthritis
- Tendon, ligament, or meniscal incomplete tears
- Shoulder or hip labral tears

- Rotator cuff disease
- Degenerative disc disease
- Facet and sacroiliac joint disease

An evolving body of evidence suggests adipose-derived stem cells also are therapeutic for systemic autoimmune and inflammatory diseases. Although these diseases may fall outside the scope of this book, it important to understand the breadth of potential therapeutic applications of this treatment.

41.2.2 Chronic Conditions Treated with Adipose-Derived MSCs

- Osteoarthritis
- Rheumatoid arthritis
- COPD
- Heart failure
- Multiple sclerosis
- Alzheimer's disease
- Parkinson's disease
- ALS
- Ulcerative colitis
- Heart failure
- Poorly healing wounds
- Spinal cord injury
- Post-stroke
- Diabetic neuropathy
- Erectile dysfunction

41.3 Microanatomy and Biochemistry

The mesenchymal stem cells (MSCs) in adult adipose tissue are powerful progenitor cells that have the amazing capacity to differentiate into specific cell types that generate mesenchymal tissue including bone, cartilage, tendon and ligament, muscle, fat dermis, and other connective tissues. These cell types include osteoblasts, chondrocytes, myoblasts, and fibroblasts, the very lineages that evolve to many of the musculoskeletal tissues targeted in regenerative medicine [1, 5–7, 19].

The characterization of adipose-derived MSCs has been described in the literature [20, 21]. The stromal vascular fraction (SVF) is composed of the following:

- Hematopoietic stem cells, 2%
- Pre/Endothelial cells, 7%

- Pericytes/smooth muscle cells, 2%
- Fibroblasts, 47%
- Other (macrophages, various blood cells), 33%
- Adipose-derived stem cells, 2–5%

Adipose-derived MSCs have trophic, immunomodulatory, and antimicrobial functions. Included in the trophic functions are angiogenic, mitogenic, anti-apoptotic, and anti-scar properties [1, 6, 7, 19, 21, 22].

Some of the cytokines found in the adipose-derived SVF include high levels of expression of several growth factors:

- Hepatocyte growth factor (HGF)
  - Major role in embryonic organ development; in adult, organ regeneration and wound healing
- Vascular endothelial growth factor (VEGF)
  - Stimulates growth of new blood vessels
- Placental growth factor (PGF)
  - Angiogenesis and vasculogenesis
- Transforming growth factor beta (TGFβ)
  - Controls proliferation, cellular differentiation, and other functions

Also found are moderate levels of expression of other factors:

- Fibroblast growth factor (FGF-2)
  - Involved in wound healing and angiogenesis
- Angiopoietin (Ang-1 and Ang-2)
  - Promotes angiogenesis and formation of blood vessels

MSCs demonstrate the ability to release bioactive molecules that are immunoregulatory. They secrete a wide array of paracrine factors that create a regenerative milieu that possesses trophic regenerative properties. Consequently, it is felt that the beneficial impact of adipose-derived MSCs on various tissues and organs may be due to soluble factors produced by the cells, rather than to their tissue differentiation capabilities. Moreover, it has also been shown that the soluble factors secreted by adipose-derived MSCs can be modulated by exposure to different agents, giving promise to the field of tissue engineering [1, 6, 7, 19, 21, 22].

Adipose-derived MSCs have an inherent ability to locate damaged tissue. Their response to molecular signaling within the body has been demonstrated in studies using radionucleotide-tagged cells [21].

41.4 Basic Concerns and Contraindications

The clinical application of cell-based therapies is somewhat controversial. Considered experimental, the therapy is not FDA-approved as of 2017. These facts must be disclosed to all prospective patients. Potential patients should also be informed that their treatment prevents them from participation in future clinical research studies.

In 2014, the FDA released two draft guidance documents [23, 24] regarding the use of human cell and tissue products used during the same surgical procedure from adipose tissue, and requested comments from the public. They brought into question the concept of "homologous use" and suggested that enzymatic digestion of adipose tissue was considered more than minimal manipulation. Adipose-derived stem cells thus would be considered and regulated as a drug, device, and/or biologic product, but these documents do not establish legally enforceable responsibilities. Instead, they describe the FDA's current thinking and should be viewed only as recommendations unless they cite specific regulatory or statutory requirements. The FDA's position on autologous adipose-derived stem cell therapy is currently evolving.

Cell-based therapies are minimally invasive, relatively safe approaches to complex diseases, though the lack of conclusive evidence creates some question as to their safety and efficacy. It is estimated, however, that hundreds of thousands of autologous stem cell treatments are done per year worldwide, with a paucity of reported complications [25].

Angiogenesis and mitosis are effective outcomes of cell-based therapies, so there is a theoretical risk of tumorigenesis or increased growth of preexisting cancers. This result has not been seen clinically. Hernigou et al. [26] reported no increased cancer risk in 1873 patients who were observed for an average of 12.5 years after treatment with autologous cell-based therapy using bone marrow–derived stromal progenitor cells. Nevertheless, many physicians consider preexisting solid tumor disease a contraindication to stem cell therapy.

Contraindications for the use of autologous stem cell therapy in musculoskeletal medicine include complete ligament or tendon tears and loose body formations in the articular space. In these cases, surgical therapy is warranted.

The use of stem cell therapy within the spine is nascent. Proper indications and contraindications will be developed as the therapy gains wider utilization, but it is clear that some findings within the spine would constitute a contraindication. These include spinal instability, disc extrusion, Pfirrmann Grade V disc disease, critical spinal stenosis, and spinal infection.

Other conditions considered to be contraindications to autologous adipose stem cell therapy are preexisting local or systemic infection, severe cardiovascular disease, and blood dyscrasias.

41.5 Preoperative Considerations

Age, general health, nutritional status, and the availability of adipose tissue should be considered when evaluating a patient for autologous stem cell therapy. In patients with advanced age or nutritional or medical compromise, autologous therapy may not be the best option and an allogeneic approach can be considered. Emaciated patients or high-performance athletes may not have an adequate volume of adipose tissue. In those cases, alternative treatments should be considered.

The health of each patient should be assessed preoperatively. Patients should be encouraged to stop smoking 4–6 weeks before treatment. Heavy alcohol consumption should be avoided. Nutrition should be optimized with clean, whole foods and nutritional supplementation.

NSAIDs should be avoided at least 2 weeks before and 4 weeks after autologous stem cell therapy. Steroid injections should be avoided for 4 weeks before and after treatment.

The patient's medical condition will determine the amount of adipose to be aspirated. Most systems utilize approximately 60 cc of adipose tissue to recover a therapeutic dose of SVF, which should contain 50–100 million stem cells. An adequate adipose harvest site must be selected. The abdomen is commonly used, but in some instances one must resort to the flank or "love handles", the hips, or thighs. Careful examination of the area should include notation of any prior operative procedures that may have produced scar tissue within or near the lipoaspiration area. Topographical, superficial skin markings performed preoperatively with the patient standing may provide a useful guide during the procedure. Although this is not a cosmetic procedure, one should attempt to provide a symmetric and appealing outcome.

A proper procedure consent should be completed and signed by the patient on the day of the procedure, prior to any sedative medication, including the following points:

- Consent for tumescent anesthesia
- Consent for lipoaspiration
- Consent for reintroduction of the final product, whether that be a joint injection; a muscle, tendon, or ligament injection; or an intravascular or intrathecal injection
- Disclosure that the procedure is experimental
- Disclosure that the procedure is not FDA-approved
- Acknowledgement that a successful outcome is not guaranteed
- Disclosure that the treatment may eliminate the patient's candidacy for future clinical research studies

Assess whether the patient would like to "bank" or cryopreserve some cells. Several FDA-listed tissue banks will cryopreserve a patient's adipose-derived MSCs for a fee. Theoretically, the tissue that is stored will always be more youthful and beneficial than tissue available in the future. Most tissue banks require 60–100 mL of adipose to be shipped overnight. The adipose tissue is processed, and the cells are expanded and cryopreserved until future need. Currently, expanded cell products are considered highly processed and consequently are subject to the Public Health Safety Act, Section 351. For such tissue to be used in the United States, it would need to be licensed by the FDA as a biological drug [23].

Preoperative IV antibiotics may be considered, as well as an anxiolytic.

41.6 Equipment

Figures 41.1 and 41.2 show some the equipment needed for lipoaspiration:

- 14 g/25 cm garden spray infiltration cannula
- 3 mm/25 cm Mercedes cannula
- 60 mL syringe snap lock
- Syringe caddy
- 2 quart stainless steel bowl
- 60 mL Luer lock syringes × 4
- 60 mL Toomey syringe × 2
- #11 blade scalpel

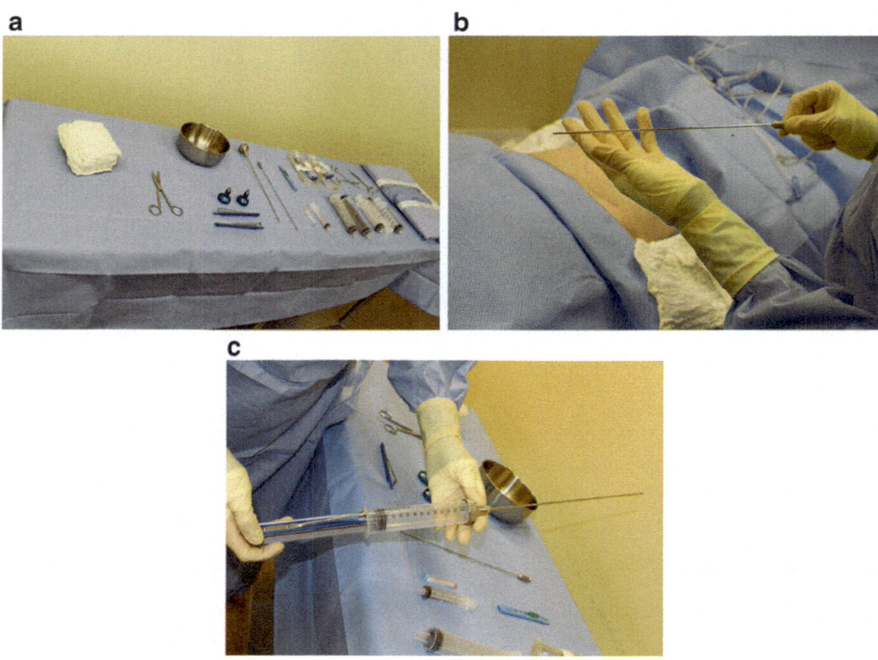

Fig. 41.1 (**a**) Back table set up for lipoaspiration procedure. (**b**) Irrigation cannula. (**c**) Lipoaspiration cannula with snap lock

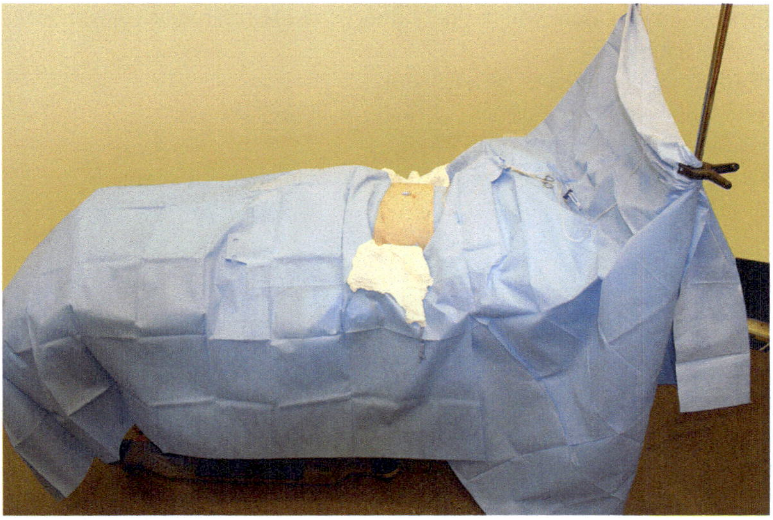

Fig. 41.2 Patient positioning and draping

- 10 mL syringe
- 18-G 1-in. needle
- 25-G 1.5-in. needle
- Sterile back cover drape
- Sterile half drape
- Sterile prep kit (povidone iodine or Hibiclens® (Mölnlycke Health Care, Norcross, GA)
- Sterile surgical marking pen

Also to be used are several medications and some items of laboratory and tissue culture equipment:

- 0.9% sodium chloride IV solution (1000 mL)
- 8.4% sodium bicarbonate, 1 mEq/mL (50-mL vial)
- Lidocaine HCl 2% (50-mL vial)
- Epinephrine 1:1000 (30-mL vial)
- HEPA-filtered Class 100 laminar flow biological cabinet
- Centrifuge
- Dry block incubator or incubator shaker
- Disposable manual stem cell isolation kit

41.7 Technique of Lipoaspiration

Rodbell and James pioneered the initial techniques used to isolate cells from adipose tissue in the 1960s. The procedure has evolved to become a safe, minimally invasive procedure [27–29]. Today the isolation procedure includes the following steps:

- Tumescent liposuction, which finely minces tissue fragments (dependent on the size of the cannula)
- Washing to remove hematopoietic cells
- Enzyme digestion
- Centrifugation to separate the SVF
- Isolating SVF with washing cells, centrifugation, and cell strainer
- Cells (SVF) prepared in final solution

41.7.1 Preparation of Tumescent Anesthetic Fluid

Tumescent technique uses the standard anesthetic solution used for liposuction procedures. Tumescent fluid premixed on the day of the procedure is infiltrated into the subcutaneous tissue in order to anesthetize the procedure site locally. The amount of tumescent fluid used is calculated based upon the amount of adipose being harvested; it is limited by the maximum lidocaine dose based upon the patient's weight (4.5 mg/kg; 7 mg/kg when combined with epinephrine). The safe dosage for tumescent lidocaine was shown to be 35 mg/kg by Klein in 1990. This has become standard of care for liposuction procedures [30].

- For harvesting small amounts of adipose tissue (60–120 mL), a 0.1% tumescent solution may be utilized. Into a 1000-mL bag of 0.9% sodium chloride, introduce the following using sterile technique:
  - 50 mL lidocaine 2%
  - 1 mL epinephrine 1:1000
  - 10 mL sodium bicarbonate 8.4%
- For harvesting large amounts of adipose tissue (>120 mL), a 0.05% tumescent solution can be utilized. Into a 1000-mL bag of 0.9% sodium chloride, introduce the following using sterile technique:
  - 25 mL lidocaine 2%
  - 1 mL epinephrine 1:1000
  - 8 mL sodium bicarbonate 8.4%

The tumescent solution should be mixed on the same day as the procedure, and the epinephrine should be added immediately prior to use. The bag should be clearly identified and dated.

41.7.2 Infiltration of Tumescent Anesthetic Fluid

The patient is taken to the procedure suite and positioned supine for abdominal adipose harvesting or lateral decubitus for flank or hip adipose harvesting. Appropriate monitoring is placed. Sterile prep and drape is performed over the lipoaspiration site

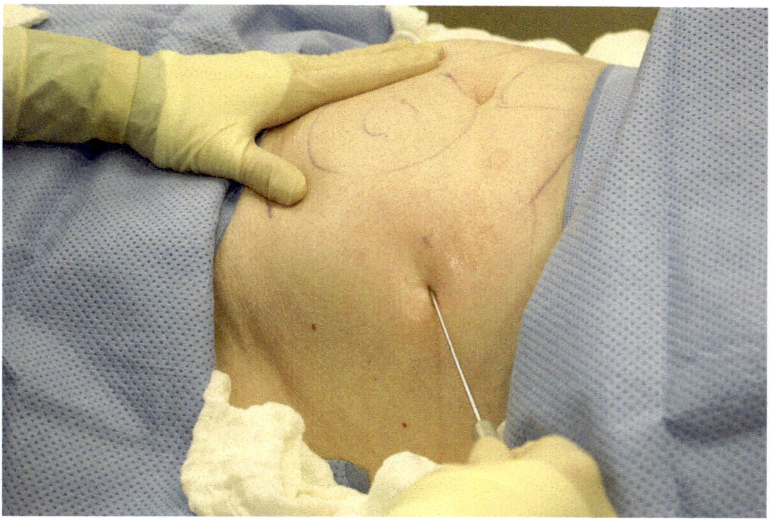

Fig. 41.3 Infiltration of tumescent fluid

(Fig. 41.2). The port placement should be considered. If the abdomen is the harvest site, the port sites should be asymmetrically placed bilaterally at the anterior axillary line, at the level of the anterior iliac spine. Place a local anesthetic skin wheal at these sites. Using a #11 blade scalpel, make a 3-mm skin incision. The tumescent fluid is then infiltrated subcutaneously using the 14 G garden spray infiltrating cannula throughout the area of lipoaspiration. The tumescent fluid IV bag maybe hung on an IV pole with pressure bag–assisted gravitational flow. As an alternative, the tumescent fluid may be delivered manually with a 60 mL syringe.

Tumescent fluid infiltration should be delivered slowly and evenly throughout the tissue. The irrigational cannula must remain parallel with the abdominal wall to avoid any unintentional transabdominal or peritoneal injury. Adequate infiltration is appreciated when the skin appears firm with turgor. There may be blanching, demarcating vasoconstriction associated with the epinephrine (Fig. 41.3).

41.7.3 Collection of Lipoaspirate

Once the tumescent fluid has been infiltrated, lipoaspiration is conducted with a 3 mm/25 cm Mercedes cannula attached to a 60-mL Toomey syringe, with approximately 18 in. of Hg pressure. This is obtained by pulling back the syringe plunger after the cannula has been placed subcutaneously. Using a “snap lock” or “Johnnie snap” will support the plunger in this position while you work (Fig. 41.4).

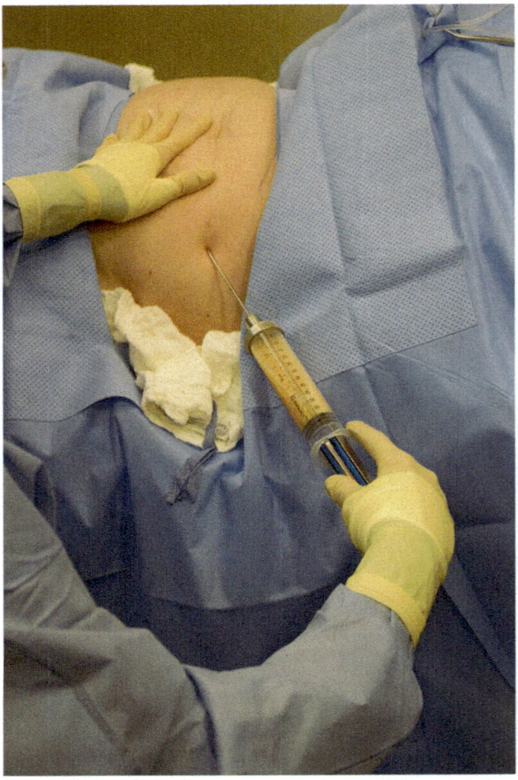

Fig. 41.4 Collection of lipoaspirate

The cannula is manipulated in a fanlike manner throughout the targeted tissue as the lipoaspirate is collected. The nondominant hand should be used as a guide to feel the tip of the cannula, ensuring that the cannula tip is not too superficial and does not extend beyond the intended treatment area (Fig. 41.4). Using this technique, deeper areas are aspirated first, followed by more shallow areas. Take care not to repeatedly course a specific area, as doing so may cause dimpling of the skin.

Continue to suction the aspirate until the syringe is full. Then place it upright in a syringe rack to allow the fat to rise above the supernatant fluid. Drain any supernatant fluid into a sterile stainless steel bowl and continue until the desired volume of fat has been harvested (Fig. 41.5).

Once collected, the harvested fat should be transferred to the processing area in a closed system. If using a syringe, cap the syringe for transport (Fig. 41.6).

41.7.4 Post-procedure Care

- Gently express any excess tumescent fluid through the port sites.
- Close the port sites with steri-strips.

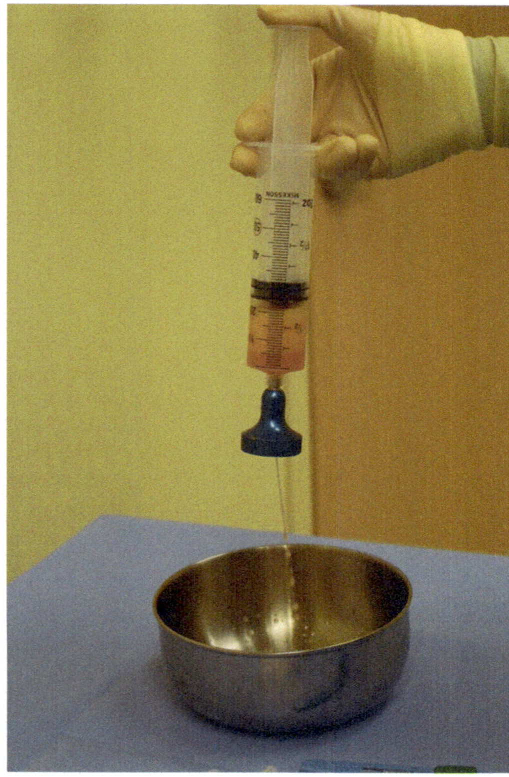

Fig. 41.5 Separation of fat from supernatant fluid

- Apply absorbent dressings over the port sites.
- Apply a compression garment. This can be a compression body suit for patients with thigh or hip lipoaspiration sites. A simple abdominal binder will suffice for most patients. The patient should be instructed to wear the compression device continuously for the first 72 hours, and then daily for the next 3–4 days. Compression aids in hemostasis, improving post-procedure bruising and discomfort, and helps with post-procedure aesthetics.
- Transfer the patient to recovery and monitor vital signs.

41.8 Adipose Processing

There are two generally accepted means for isolation of the SVF from adipose tissue: mechanical and enzymatic. Both methods are equally safe, but there are differences to be noted when choosing between them. Mechanical isolation is less costly and quicker to perform, but the end product will contain a higher concentration of blood mononuclear cells and fewer progenitor cells. When contemplating using

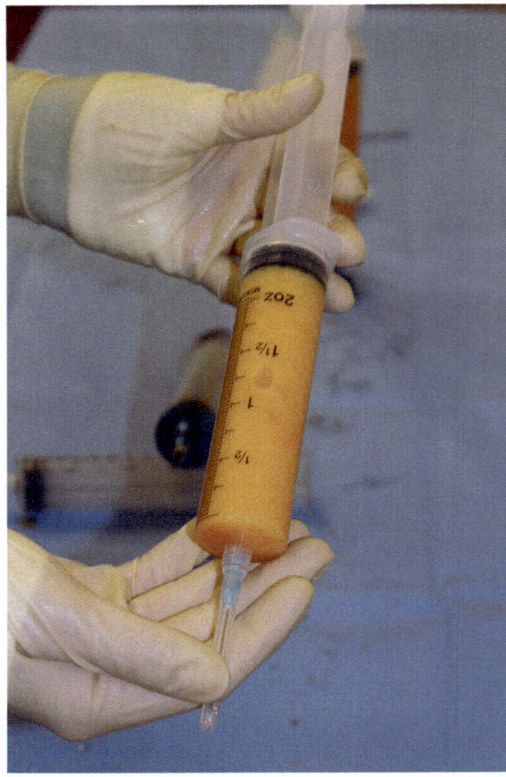

Fig. 41.6 Transport of the harvested adipose

smaller quantities of adipose tissue for SVF extraction, the mechanical method would be preferred. Enzymatic isolation, on the other hand, has been shown in studies to demonstrate a significantly greater efficiency in the separation process through a consistent and predictable digestion of the extracellular matrix (Table 41.2). For this reason, the authors advocate the enzymatic isolation method, as outlined here:

- Harvested adipose tissue should be processed in a clean setting. All specimens should be clearly marked with patient identifiers. We recommend that all tissue handling outside of the sterile procedure suite occur under a Class 100 HEPA-filtered laminar flow biological cabinet using aseptic technique.
- Several companies offer proprietary formulas including protocol steps and unique digestive enzymes, which are packaged in disposable kits. The basic steps universally utilized to isolate adipose stem cells involve a cell wash and collagenase digestion, followed by centrifugal separation and filtration to isolate the single-cell SVF from the primary adipocytes.
- The SVF is then resuspended in a carrier solution for final treatment. The carrier solutions include autologous platelet-rich plasma and preservative-free normal saline. Autologous platelet-rich plasma is the author's preferred carrier solution for musculoskeletal, intrathecal, or intravascular therapeutic applications. The total resuspension volume may range from 2 to 10 cc depending on the site of treatment.

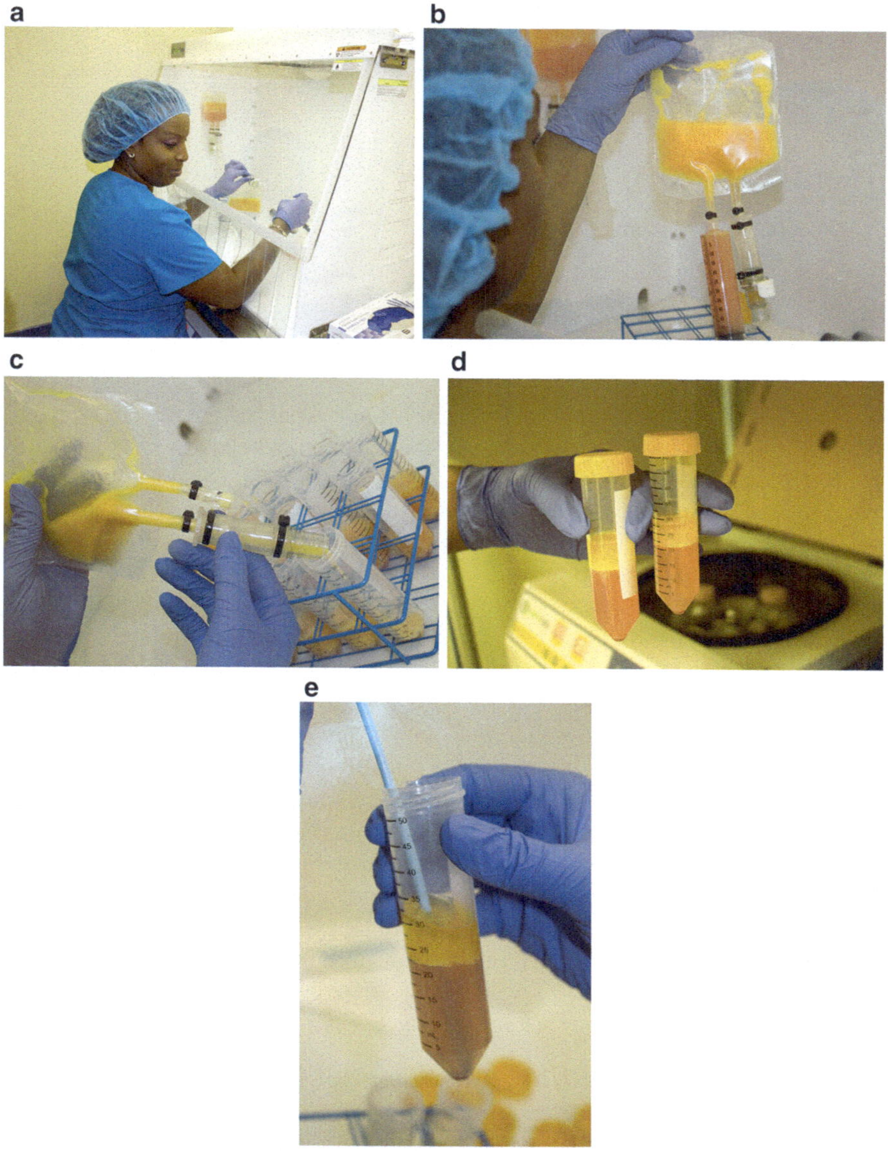

Fig. 41.7 (**a**) Processing of harvested adipose tissue under a laminar flow hood. (**b**) Processing of harvested adipose tissue: washing the adipose. (**c**) Processing of harvested adipose tissue: separating adipose into 50 mL conicals for centrifugation. (**d**) Processing of harvested adipose tissue: after centrifugation the adipose has separated into the SVF at bottom and adipose at top. (**e**) Processing of harvested adipose tissue: collecting the SVF pellet from the bottom of the conical

Table 41.2 Comparison of mechanical *vs* enzymatic isolation methods for extracting the SVF from harvested adipose tissue

	Mechanical isolation	Enzymatic isolation
Time to perform	15–30 min	2–3 h
Cost	No added cost	\$2–\$5 per gram
Cell count (nucleated cells per cc of lipoaspirate)	1.0×10^4–2.4×10^5	1.0×10^5–1.3×10^6
Progenitor cell concentrations	Lower	Higher

41.9 Reintroduction of the Adipose Stem Cell Product

For musculoskeletal applications, the patient is transferred back to the clean procedure suite and positioned appropriately for the injection, with appropriate monitoring. The injection (whether intra-articular or soft tissue) should be done with direct visualization utilizing fluoroscopy or ultrasound. Note that contrast material is cytotoxic and should not be used. Additionally, many local anesthetics are cytotoxic. One percent Lidocaine is well tolerated.

For systemic applications, the resuspended stem cell solution will be injected into a peripheral vein through an IV catheter or needle. The injection should be done as an IV push slowly over 5–10 min. The patient's pulse, oxygen saturation, and blood pressure should be monitored before, during, and after the injection.

For intradiscal, facet joint, or sacroiliac joint injections, the patient is taken to the clean procedure suite and positioned prone with monitors applied. Fluoroscopy or ultrasound guidance should be used to confirm accurate needle placement.

For intrathecal applications, the patient is taken to the clean procedure suite and positioned in a prone position with monitors applied. Sterile prep is carried out and the patient is draped for a lumbar fluoroscopically guided intrathecal injection. Do not use contrast, as it has been demonstrated to be cytotoxic. Confirmation of the intrathecal location is demonstrated by CSF flow through the hub of the needle.

41.10 Post-procedure Care and Potential Complications

- No NSAIDS/steroids for 4 weeks after treatment.
- The anti-inflammatory properties of the treatment may result in positive effects within the first couple of weeks in some cases, but the true therapeutic results may take 4–6 months to be realized.
- Normal light activity is recommended for the initial week after the procedure. Return to light exercise is recommended 6 weeks after treatment.
- Many in the field believe that repeat treatments may be needed for many patients with severe local or systemic disease processes, though there is no research to support this idea. Autologous stem cell therapy may not offer a cure, but it certainly may offer a nonpharmacological treatment alternative.

- Although autologous adipose stem cell therapy is considered a safe same-day procedure, there are potential complications:
  - Infection due to poor sterile technique or contamination of the tissue product is possible. Fortunately, MSCs have demonstrated an antibiotic propensity.
  - Harvest site pain, soreness, or bruising may occur but is usually mild and can be treated with supportive therapy such as ice, acetaminophen, or analgesics. If symptoms persist, have the patient come in for a clinical evaluation.
  - Injection site pain, soreness, or bruising also is usually mild and responsive to supportive care. If persistent, have the patient come in for a clinical evaluation.
  - Skin dimpling or other cosmetic disfigurement is possible. It is always important to practice good technique during lipoaspiration. Avoid excessive aspiration in any given area.
  - Because you are using the patient's own tissue in this therapy, there is no risk of rejection, but if you are processing tissue samples from multiple patients on the same day, there is a risk of injecting the wrong sample into a patient. Always clearly label all specimens through the entire isolation process.

41.11 Clinical Pearls

- Standard universal precautions should be followed by all personnel with potential exposure to any patient tissue.
- There have been case reports of transient hypertension and tachycardia and/or symptoms of lightheadedness, flushing, or headache upon systemic intravascular injections. Always monitor your patient and have oxygen and supportive medications available.
- Although it is highly unlikely that you will ever need it, have a crash cart and airway resuscitative equipment available. Many of your patients may have multiple comorbidities.
- Contrast, antibiotics, and many local anesthetics have been shown to be cytotoxic to mesenchymal stem cells. Use only 1–2% lidocaine, which has been shown not to be cytotoxic.
- Inject the final product with needles and catheters of 22-G or larger bore. This bore size does not disrupt the cell structure.
- Proprietary cell isolation techniques can provide safe, legal methods to consistently harvest approximately 50–100 million cells per 60–100 mL of adipose tissue, with reproducibility and validated analysis.
- Cell yield can be affected by several factors:
  - Surgical technique
  - Location of fat
  - Enzymatic digestion: Enzymatic digestion times and concentrations strongly modify the yield and viability of cells.

- Consider in advance the volume of injectate you will need for each area treated when performing your final resuspension. A small joint such as a finger or facet joint will only accommodate 1–2 mL of fluid, whereas a large joint such as a knee may require 6–8 mL.
- I frequently recommend an intravascular dose as well as an intraarticular dose in patients with osteoarthritis. Mesenchymal stem cells have demonstrated a unique homing ability. When introduced intravascularly, they make their way to the damaged tissue via cell signaling mechanisms.
- There is a theoretical benefit for the use of intravascular stem cell treatments for autoimmune and inflammatory diseases, as well as for prevention and longevity.
- Do not advertise or make therapeutic claims with regard to this therapy. The FDA is hypervigilant regarding such public statements.

References

1. Murphy M, Moncivias K, Caplan AI. Mesenchymal stem cells: environmentally responsive for regenerative medicine. Exp Mol Med. 2013;45:e54.
2. Han J, Koh YJ, Moon HR, Ryoo HG, Cho CH, Kim I, et al. Adipose tissue is an extramedullary reservoir for functional hematopoietic stem and progenitor cells. Blood. 2004;115(5):957–64.
3. Bourin P, Bunnell BA, Casteilla L, Dominici M, Katz AJ, March KL, et al. Stromal cells from the adipose tissue-derived stromal vascular fraction and culture expanded adipose tissue-derived stromal/stem cells: a joint statement of the International Federation for Adipose Therapeutics and Science (IFATS) and the International Society for Cellular Therapy (ISCT). Cytotherapy. 2013;15:641–8.
4. Traktuev DO, Merfeld-Clauss S, Li J, Kolonin M, Arap W, Pasgualini R, et al. A population of CD-34 positive adipose stromal cells share pericyte and mesenchymal surface markers, reside in a periendothelial location, and stabilize endothelial networks. Circ Res. 2008;102(1):77–85.
5. Gimble JM, Katz AJ, Bunnell BA. Adipose derived stem cells for regenerative medicine. Circ Res. 2007;100:1249–60.
6. Caplan AI. Mesenchymal stem cells. J Orthop Res. 1991;9:641–50.
7. Al C, Dennis JE. Mesenchymal stem cells as trophic mediators. J Cell Biochem. 2006;98:1076–84.
8. Centeno CJ, Busse D, Kisiday J, Keohan C, Freeman M, Karli D. Increased knee cartilage volume in degenerative joint disease using percutaneously implanted, autologous mesenchymal stem cells. Pain Physician. 2008;11(3):343–53.
9. Emadedin M, Aghdami N, Taghiyar L, Fazeli R, Moghadasali R, Jahangir S, et al. Intra-articular injection of autologous mesenchymal stem cells in six patients with knee osteoarthritis. Arch Iran Med. 2012;15(7):422–8.
10. Jo CH, Lee YG, Shin WH, Kim H, Chai JW, Jeong EC, et al. Intra-articular injection of mesenchymal stem cells for the treatment of osteoarthritis of the knee: a proof-of-concept clinical trial. Stem Cells. 2014;32(5):1254–66.
11. Longo UG, Papapietro N, Petrillo S, Franceschetti E, Maffulli N, Denaro V. Mesenchymal stem cell for prevention and management of intervertebral disc degeneration. Stem Cell Int. 2012;2012:921053.
12. Sivakamansundari V, Lufkin T. Stemming the degeneration: IVD stem cells and regenerative therapy for degenerative disc disease. Adv Stem Cells. 2013;2013:pii: 724547.
13. Hohaus C, Ganey TM, Minkus Y, Meisel HJ. Cell transplantation in lumbar spine disc degeneration disease. Eur Spine J. 2008;17(suppl 4):492.
14. Hiyama A, Mochida J, Iwashina T, Omi H, Watanabe T, Serigano K, et al. Transplantation of mesenchymal stem cells in a canine disc degeneration model. J Orthop Res. 2008;26:589–600.

15. Henriksson HB, Svanvik T, Jonsson M, Hagman M, Horn M, Lindahl A, Brisby H. Transplantation of human mesenchymal stem cells into intervertebral discs in a xenogeneic porcine model. Spine. 2009;34:141–8.
16. Sakai D, Mochida J, Iwashina T, Watanabe T, Nakai T, Ando K, et al. Differentiation of mesenchymal stem cells transplanted to a rabbit degenerative disc model: potential and limitations for stem cell therapy in disc regeneration. Spine. 2005;30:2379–87.
17. Orozco L, Soler R, Morera C, Alberca M, Sánchez A, García-Sancho J. Intervertebral disc repair by autologous mesenchymal bone marrow cells: 2 pilot study. Transplantation. 2011;92(7):822–8.
18. Pettine KA, Murphy MB, Suzuki RK, Sand TT. Percutaneous injection of autologous bone marrow concentrate cells significantly reduces lumbar discogenic pain through 12 months. Stem Cells. 2015;33(1):146–56.
19. Mizuno H, Tobita M, Uysal AC. Concise review: adipose derived stem cells as a novel tool for future regenerative medicine. Stem Cells. 2012;30(5):804–10.
20. Folgiero V, Migliano E, Tedesco M, Iacovelli S, Bon G, Torre ML, et al. Purification and characterization of adipose derived stem cells from patients with lipoaspirate transplantation. Cell Transplant. 2010;19(10):1225–35.
21. Bailey AM, Kapur S, Katz AJ. Characterization of adipose derived stem cells: an update. Curr Stem Cell Res Ther. 2010;5(2):95–102.
22. Caplan AI, Correa D. The MSC: an injury drugstore. Cell Stem Cell. 2012;9:11–5.
23. FDA draft guidance (Dec 2014): minimal manipulation of human cells, tissues and cellular and tissue-based products. http://www.fda.gov/downloads/BiologicsBloodVaccines/GuidanceComplianceRegulatoryInformartion/G/CellularandGeneTherapy/UCM427746.pdf
24. FDA draft guidance for industry (Oct 2014): same surgical procedure exemption under 21 CFR 1271.15(b): questions and answers regarding the scope of the exception. http://www.fda.gov/BiologicsBloodVaccines/GuidanceComplianceRegulatoryInformation/Guidances/Tissue/ucm419911.htm
25. Halme DG, Kessler DA. FDA regulation of stem cell based therapies. N Engl J Med. 2006;355:1730–5.
26. Hernigou P, Homma Y, Flouzat-Lachaniette CH, Poignard A, Chevailler N, Rouard H. Cancer risk is not increased in patients treated for orthopedic diseases with autologous bone marrow cell concentrate. J Bone Joint Surg Am. 2013;95:2215–21.
27. Fournier PF. Reduction syringe lipo contouring. Dermatol Clin. 1990;8:539–51.
28. Hunsted JP. Tumescent and syringe liposculture: a logical partnership. Aesthet Plast Surg. 1995;19:321–3.
29. Housman TS, Lawrence N, Mellen BG, George MN, Filippo JS, Cerveny KA, et al. The safety of liposuction: results of national survey. Dermatol Surg. 2002;28(11):971–8.
30. Klein J. Tumescent technique chronicles. Dermatol Surg. 1995;21:449–57.

Suggested Reading

Caplan AI, Correa D. The MSC: an injury drugstore. Cell Stem Cell. 2012;9:11–5.
Caplan A, Dennis JE. Mesenchymal stem cells as trophic mediators. J Cell Biochem. 2006;98:1076–84.
Longo UG, Papapietro N, Petrillo S, Franceschetti E, Maffulli N, Denaro V. Mesenchymal stem cell for prevention and management of intervertebral disc degeneration. Stem Cell Int. 2012;2012:921053.
Sivakamansundari V, Lufkin T. Stemming the degeneration: IVD stem cells and regenerative therapy for degenerative disc disease. Adv Stem Cells. 2013;2013:pii: 724547.

Chapter 42
Intradiscal Biologic Treatments: Allogeneic Stem Cells

Daniel L. Kline and Michael J. DePalma

Low back pain has been estimated to affect 15–20% of adults in any given year, and 80% over the course of their lifetime [1]. Furthermore, it has been estimated that at some point, 28% of adults will experience disabling low back pain [2]. A 2011 study found that the intervertebral disc accounted for 42% of the cases of chronic low back pain [3]. Prior studies support this finding and have estimated a similar rate of 39% for internal disc disruption (IDD) [4]. These statistics are especially troubling because of the lack of a reliable means of treating discogenic low back pain.

In IDD, internal disc structures are deranged, resulting in pain. Innervated annular fissures are the hallmark feature [5]. Annular injury initiates an inflammatory response that ultimately results in the local development of granulation tissue flanked by blood vessels and nociceptors [6–9]. It is thought that the increase in sensory fibers, combined with the presence of inflammatory mediators, creates a state of hyperalgesia that can be painful with even physiologic loading of the disc [10, 11].

Disc degeneration associated with this condition is complicated and entails reduced nutrition and removal of metabolic byproducts, altered biophysical milieu, cell loss, changes in matrix turnover, and altered biomechanics [12]. Yet the degree of disc degeneration itself does not correlate with disc-related chronic low back pain (LBP) symptoms [5].

D.L. Kline
Valley Health Interventional Spine, Winchester, VA, USA
e-mail: dkline1@gmail.com

M.J. DePalma (✉)
Virginia iSpine Physicians, PC, Richmond, VA, USA
e-mail: michaeldepalma8@gmail.com

S. Diwan, T.R. Deer (eds.), *Advanced Procedures for Pain Management*, https://doi.org/10.1007/978-3-319-68841-1_42

42.1 Indications

The primary indications for the intradiscal use of biologic technologies in the spine is chronic, discogenic LBP, along with grade III or IV annular tears associated with mild degeneration. It is important to note, however, that this indication has not yet been approved by the US Food and Drug Administration (FDA).

Imaging criteria based on changes from normal disc morphology combined with clinical findings have been developed to guide appropriate patient selection as part of FDA-regulated clinical research studies. Discography assists in identifying appropriate candidates and determining which disc is the source of symptoms. Intranuclear injection of contrast material allows the clinician to examine the structural integrity of the annulus by both direct fluoroscopic visualization of epidural extension of contrast and by tactile feel for the absence of an endpoint upon injecting the disc.

42.2 Diagnosing Discogenic Low Back Pain

Detecting a symptomatic disc is challenging. Advanced imaging has not been able to reliably discriminate painful from nonpainful discs. It has been shown that as few as 36% of asymptomatic individuals possess no bulging, degenerated, or herniated intervertebral discs [13]. Currently, there are two accepted methods for examining a suspected, symptomatic intervertebral disc: MRI and provocation discography.

42.2.1 MRI

- MRI is not dynamic; the image shows a moment in time with no relation to movement, position, or activity.
- Sensitivity of MRI in identifying internal disc disruption is less than 60%, with a 24% false-positive rate and a 38% false-negative rate [14].
- Some diagnostic value has been demonstrated in the limited circumstances where MRI demonstrates high-intensity zone lesions and moderate to severe Modic type I or II endplate changes, with a positive predictive value of 64–87% and specificity of 67–97% [15]. The low sensitivity of these findings, however, reflects the fact that not all patients with discogenic LBP exhibit these morphologic features [16, 17].
- The presence of a high-intensity zone (HIZ) or type I or II Modic endplate changes in the setting of LBP represents a small increase in the likelihood of that disc being painful upon stimulation [16, 17]. Figures 42.1 and 42.2 demonstrate type II Modic endplate changes in MRI.

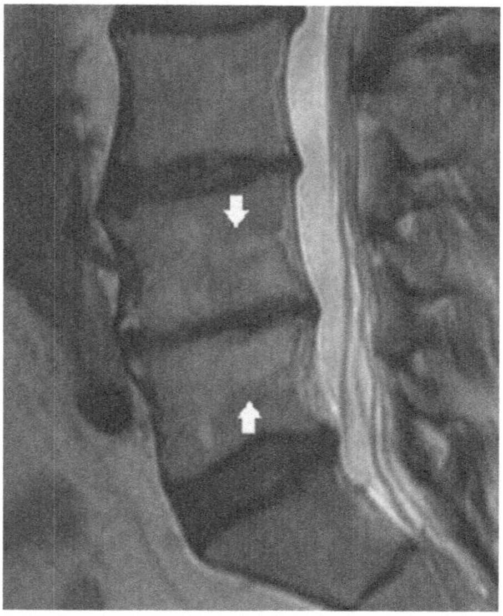

Fig. 42.1 Type II Modic endplate changes (*white arrows*) on T2-weighted MRI

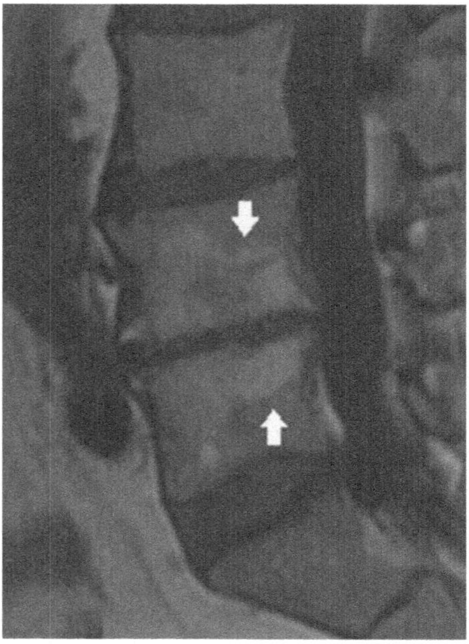

Fig. 42.2 Type II Modic endplate changes (*white arrows*) on T1-weighted MRI

42.2.2 Provocation Discography

Discography is a reliable method for diagnosing painful discs if it is performed with adherence to stringent operational criteria [18].

- Dynamic discography, in addition to visualizing a particular intervertebral disc, allows one to assess any painful attributes it may hold.
- Provocation lumbar discography (PLD) aims at reproducing identical or similar LBP upon low-pressure (<50 psi) stimulation of the disc that contains outer annular disruption. In Fig. 42.3, a post-discography CT scan demonstrates the presence of a grade IV annular tear (due to >30° circumferential tear), which was detected during disc stimulation (Fig. 42.4).

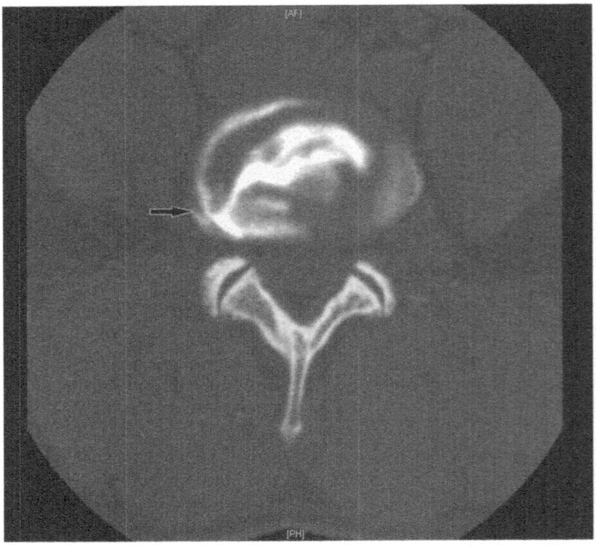

Fig. 42.3 A post-discography CT scan demonstrates the presence of a grade IV annular tear (due to >30° circumferential tear), which was detected during disc stimulation

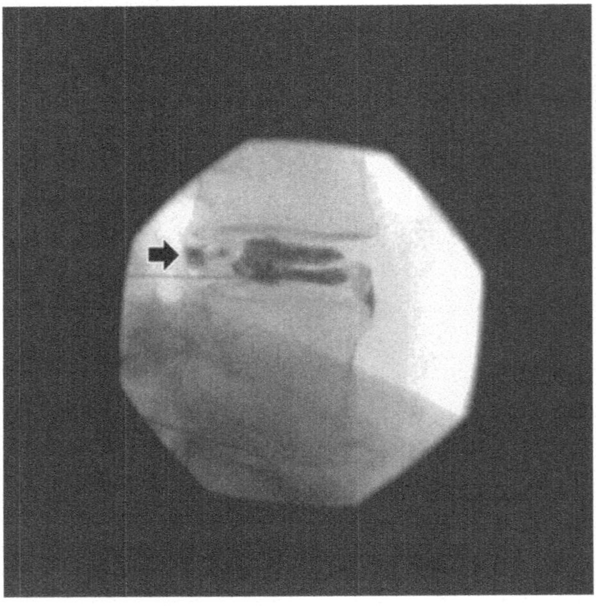

Fig. 42.4 Lateral fluoroscopic image taken post-discogram, demonstrating annular tear (*black arrow*)

- Pain severity greater than 6 out of 10 is required for diagnosis, and stimulation of adjacent discs must not reproduce the pain.

The false-positive rates of PLD have stirred controversy, as studies have had small sample sizes and wide confidence intervals and have lacked control discs or manometric monitoring. When performed with strict adherence to standards, PLD has a false-positive rate of 6% and specificity of 94% [18]. Figure 42.5 shows a lateral image taken during fluoroscopically guided PLD, and Fig. 42.6 shows an anteroposterior (AP) image.

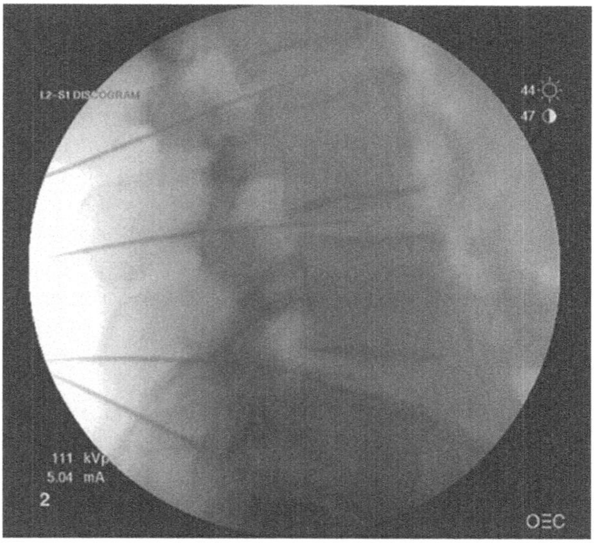

Fig. 42.5 A lateral image taken during fluoroscopically guided PLD

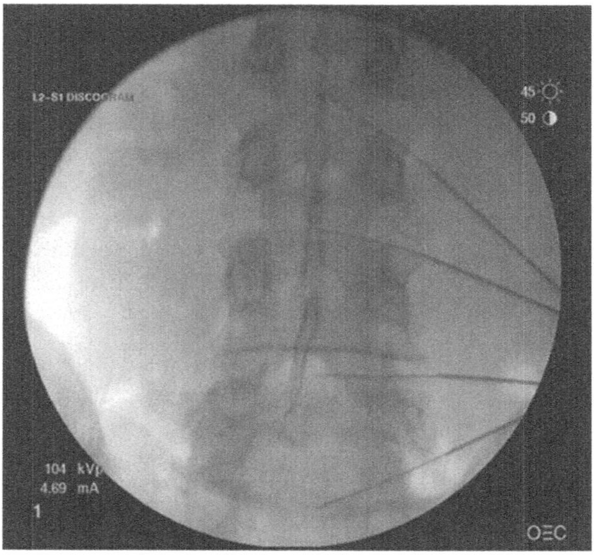

Fig. 42.6 Anteroposterior (AP) fluoroscopic image demonstrating proper intradiscal needle placement

- Published studies have not found a greater incidence of disc degeneration in patients who had undergone PLD. A 1.3% occurrence of new morphologic intradiscal abnormality discovered upon repeat discography has been reported in discs having undergone a prior PLD [19].
- Histologic findings have revealed that laceration of lamellae fibers does not occur, given that the long axis of the needle remains perpendicular to the lamellar fibers [19]. A follow-up MRI study found accelerated disc degeneration, Modic changes, and disc herniation in 66% of patients who underwent PLD [20]. However, when disc degeneration and each herniation subgroup was compared with control values, confidence intervals overlapped, revealing a lack of statistical significance for these findings, and 30% of cases were lost to follow-up [20]. Therefore, available data do not conclusively show that PLD or disc puncture is undeniably injurious to the disc.
- PLD has been found to be predictive of fusion outcomes, suggesting that it has therapeutic utility [21], which is an important feature of a useful diagnostic test. Patients with discogenic LBP undergoing fusion based on PLD findings were found to be five times more likely to return to at least 25% of their daily activities, 3.4 times more likely to return to at least 50% of their daily activities, and 3.3 times more likely to have less back pain than patients who had a positive PLD but who did not undergo surgery. Anesthetization of the painful annular fissures identified during PLD results in reduction of LBP during functional maneuvers (DePalma, unpublished, 2008).

Hence it is rational (but still unproven) that PLD may have positive therapeutic utility if positive PLD can be shown to be associated with acceptable outcomes after treatment.

42.3 Microanatomy and Biochemistry

Efforts are ongoing to establish an ideal treatment for discogenic low back pain, with perhaps the most attractive strategies focusing on the regenerative potential of biologic agents. The possibility of regenerating the underlying painful disc while avoiding alteration of structural dynamics of the lumbosacral spine is appealing. The current belief is that, in general, biologics are appropriate for mildly to moderately degenerated discs, in which there may be a higher likelihood of sufficient supporting elements. One can conceptualize these strategies in three broad categories:

- *Growth factors*: metabolic agents stimulating productivity of native cells
- *Tissue scaffolds*: substances that allow propagation of native cells in a "three-dimensional meshwork"
- *Cellular supplementation*: the introduction of productive cells to synthesize extracellular matrix

42.3.1 Growth Factors

- *Osteogenic protein-1 (OP-1)* was initially studied in vivo in the discs of rabbits. The data revealed increased disc height, as well as increased proteoglycan and annular content in the treated discs [22]. This study suggests increased anabolic activity following intradiscal injection of OP-1 into the affected disc.
- *Growth differentiation factor-5 (GDF5).* A 2010 study evaluated the effects of in vivo gene therapy using an adenoviral vector carrying the *GDF5* gene in degenerated mouse discs. At 6 and 8 weeks, T2-weighted signals were detected in the treatment group but not in the control group. At 2 weeks, the percent disc height index in the treatment group increased significantly, compared with the control group. Additionally, the discs injected with Ad-GDF5 demonstrated no decrease in glycosaminoglycan and DNA levels throughout the 8-week treatment period, whereas the control group demonstrated diminished levels at 2 and 4 weeks respectively [23].

42.3.2 Tissue Scaffolding

The use of intradiscal fibrin sealant in the treatment of IDD has also been studied because of several compelling findings. Downregulation of inflammatory cytokines and upregulation of anabolic growth factors were noted in both animal and in vitro studies. Additionally, maintenance of nuclear volume was observed in a porcine model in the setting of surgical denucleation [24, 25]. Intradiscal injection of fibrin may seal annular nociceptors from inflammatory nociceptive compounds in the nucleus [7, 26, 27]. Fibrin, acting as a degradable tissue scaffold, may also promote cellular repair of annular fissures [28].

42.3.3 Cellular Supplementation

Cell-based biologic therapies (perhaps most notably using stem cells) offer another approach to regenerate painful discs by synthesizing extracellular matrix. The cells used can be either autologous or allogeneic.

In autologous therapies, the host and recipient are the same. These techniques have demonstrated promise [29–31], but they require ex vivo expansion [32], which is expensive and is not currently FDA-approved.

In allogeneic therapies, the cells are harvested from same species, but the host and recipient are different individuals. The ex vivo expansion process is more cost-effective. Cells can be harvested from fat, umbilical cord, or bone marrow.

Mesenchymal cells are self-renewing, undifferentiated, pluripotent cells with the capacity to differentiate into osteoblasts, chondroblasts, and adipocytes [32–36]. An intervertebral disc–like phenotype has been achieved with mesenchymal cells after induction with TGF-β, dexamethasone, and ascorbate, allowing for creation of a universal donor line [37].

Allogeneic bone marrow stromal cells have been the most extensively studied, demonstrating survival and replication at 8–48 weeks after transplantation in animal studies [38–40]. Restored disc height and proteoglycan content were observed 6 months after a single injection into ovine nucleus pulposus [41]. Case studies have also been encouraging, with two reporting restored disc height and improved symptomatology after injection with allogeneic mesenchymal stem cells (MSCs) from bone marrow [42]. Hence, human application has been investigated.

Mesenchymal precursor cells (MPCs) found in human bone marrow are the precursors to MSCs, which are in turn the precursors to osteoblasts, chondroblasts, and adipocytes [34]. Use of an antibody to select for cells displaying Stro-3 in human bone marrow has provided the means by which to select multipotent MPCs [43]. These precursor cells can proliferate and differentiate into a number of different cell types [44]. MPCs have also demonstrated the ability to secrete multiple factors in response to injury and inflammation, including growth factors, enzymes, and proteoglycans [45].

Data from an FDA-regulated phase II randomized, controlled safety and effectiveness study to further investigate MPCs have been released [46, 47]. Safety results revealed that patients tolerated the treatment well, with no significant difference in adverse events between the treatment and control groups [45]. Preliminary effectiveness data from this study has shown that at 12 months after injection, 69% (95% CI: 53, 86) of patients treated with MPCs experienced >50% reduction in LBP, versus 33% (95% CI: 19, 48) of control patients. In the treatment group, 52% reported minimal residual LBP and minimal functional disability at 12 months, versus 18% in the control (saline) group [47]. The confidence intervals between the MPC and control groups do not overlap. Therefore, there appears to be a treatment effect due to the MPCs. Furthermore, radiographic improvement in disc translational motion suggests increased stability of the disc annulus [48]. Predicated on these findings, a large phase III follow-up study is currently underway.

Chondrocytic cells located in the disc nucleus are responsible for production of the proteoglycans aggrecan and versican. These hydrophilic molecules utilize negatively charged side changes, chondroitin sulfate, and keratin sulfate to attract and hold water [49]. Disc degeneration compromises the ability to produce these molecules, leading to desiccation and disc height loss and contributing to annular tears. Juvenile allogeneic chondrocytes have been studied in an effort to address the above-stated issues present in the cell, as well as for their increased productive capacity relative to adult cells [50].

A prospective study evaluating the effectiveness and safety of allogeneic juvenile chondrocytes has shown promise [49]. At 6 months, 10 of 13 patients undergoing repeat imaging revealed improvements on MRI, such as improvement in disc height. Mean pain and disability scores improved significantly. No serious adverse events were observed [49]. Based on the preliminary findings in this pilot study, a larger phase II trial is under way.

42.4 Basic Concerns and Contraindications

All intradiscal treatments (regenerative or otherwise) carry potentially devastating (yet avoidable) complications such as discitis or even rupture. These are rare, but cost/benefit considerations should be made prior to treatment, and precautions should be taken to mitigate negative outcomes. Most importantly, all available options for the treatment of discogenic pain should be thoroughly explained to allow the patient to make an informed decision, as third-party payers consider the use of stem cells to be experimental.

42.4.1 Procedure-Based Concerns

Several conditions should raise concern:

- Immunocompromise or any increased risk for infection in the patient
- INR above accepted standards for neuraxial procedures
- Thrombocytopenia
- Anatomical variations or deformities limiting percutaneous access to the suspected intervertebral disc

42.4.2 Histology-Based Concerns

Other concerns are related to conditions in the disc:

- The chemical microenvironment present in the affected disc presents a challenge, specifically regarding the survivability of injected cells, and has been shown to have a strong influence on stem cell activity [51].
  - Acidic pH in the disc may be deleterious, especially when lower than 6.8 [52].
  - Hypoxia may inhibit both viability and proliferation of MSCs [53].
  - Combination of pH, osmolarity, and glucose: Low glucose enhances matrix and cell proliferation, but high osmolarity and low pH have the opposite effect [54].
- Lack of intradiscal nutrients may not sufficiently support cellular activity; this condition naturally occurs over time, in part because the permeability of the endplate and matrix to diffusion decreases in association with degeneration and aging [55].
- Avascular disc: Endplate blood vessels supply nutrients to discs by way of diffusion; extracellular matrix breakdown is increased in the presence of decreased endplate blood supply [56, 57].

- Similarly, newly introduced cells may not have adequate signaling from appropriate growth factors to proliferate and produce appropriate extracellular matrix.

- Growth factors can stimulate bone resorption and lead to osteolysis at the endplate.

42.4.3 Contraindications

A number of conditions should be considered contraindications for intradiscal biologic treatments:

- LBP due to joint, facet, and/or sacroiliac
- Moderate to severe disc degeneration, as cells may not be able to survive and function within discs that are more severely degenerated. Cell supplementation technologies are being investigated in discs with mild degeneration
- Grade V annular tears, with full-thickness radial tears and associated leakage of contrast; these tears would permit extradiscal escape of injected cells into the epidural space
  - More concerning than the lack of therapeutic benefit would be potential consequences of the injected material's ability to produce tissue within the epidural space
- Infection (systemic and/or local)
- Allergy to any component of the injectate
- Pregnancy
- Anatomy, pathologic or not, that would prevent successful completion of the procedure
- High risk for bleeding
- Malignancy
- Inability to obtain consent

42.5 Preoperative Considerations

As with any procedure focused on treating disc-mediated LBP, appropriate identification of the problematic disc is essential.

- PLD performed using appropriate criteria plays an important role in targeting the correct disc and reliably excluding grade V annular fissures.
- Proper imaging is utilized to evaluate and verify less than 50% loss of disc height and exclude listhesis greater than grade 1 at the targeted level.

- Standard preoperative protocol for intradiscal injection, including intravenous antibiotics, must be followed.

42.6 Radiographic Guidance

Fluoroscopic guidance using a C- arm is now the standard used at most institutions when gaining access to the disc [58]. The posterolateral approach is appropriate to gain access to the disc space and safely avoid the intraforaminal nerve root. Ultrasound has not been shown to be superior to fluoroscopic guidance in gaining disc access.

42.7 Equipment

- C-arm
- Radiolucent x-ray table
- Monitoring equipment
- Sterile gloves
- Surgical gown, caps, masks
- Surgical field drapes
- Antiseptic for skin preparation
- Extension tubing
- Appropriate volume syringes
- Appropriate length and gauge needles
- Assistant(s)
- Anesthetic, antibiotics, cell solution

42.8 Technique

Per the International Spine Intervention Society guidelines, lumbar disc access involves three stages:

1. Target acquisition
2. Trajectory
3. Insertion, using either a single needle or a two-needle technique. *The two-needle technique, in which a smaller-gauge needle is inserted through a larger-gauge needle that pierces the skin, is encouraged as a precaution against infection.*

   Following are the steps in the posterolateral approach:

- Patient placed in prone position.

- AP view of the lumbar spine is centered on the target disc, with a "squared" view with regard to the vertebral endplates.
- The C-arm is obliqued to the trajectory view, preferably opposite the side of the patient's pain.
- Lateral views may be used to confirm safe needle advancement.
- The needle or needles are placed percutaneously and advanced into the disc under intermittent fluoroscopic guidance, using the standard "discogram" approach, accessing the disc within the safe zone as described by Kambin's triangle.
- Radiographic contrast dye is **not** to be used to confirm intranuclear placement, as contrast media may interfere with cell function.
- Once the needle tip is suspected to be within the proper position within the nucleus, the cell suspension is injected.
- Careful attention should be paid to ensure that the needle is "clean" so as not to track cells out of the annulus. An extremely small amount (0.5 cc) of preservative-free normal saline can be used to flush the needle in a very limited sense.

42.9 Post-procedure Considerations

Though pre-procedure antibiotics are often standard protocol and post-procedure monitoring for infection is important, discitis is rare. A systemic review of ten studies did not find sufficient evidence to support the routine use of prophylactic antibiotics in patients undergoing PLD, which carries with it the inherent risks associated with disc access. The steps critical in reducing the risk of infection are proper skin preparation and employing a two-needle approach, so the needle that pierces the annulus does not first pass through the skin [59].

Limiting activity for 1 or 2 days is simply a general post-procedure precaution. No data are currently available to suggest what restrictions, if any, or other post-procedure precautions would affect intradiscal stem cell treatment with respect to the graft viability or disc regeneration.

42.10 Potential Complications and Pitfalls

Potential complications include those associated with lumbar disc injection as well as those of the cells and related materials:

- Discitis is the most common complication associated with disc access for any purpose, but the incidence is minimal (<0.01% per disc) [59].
- Cell/graft contamination is a possibility, but this is controlled through rigorous screening methods prior to use.

- Immunogenic or inflammatory responses may occur secondary to exposure to either the cells or associated manufacturing material. These risks are not fully known, but to date they appear to be remote or minimal, based on animal data.
- Cellular lysis could occur, leading to the release of irritating cellular contents that may cause a transient post-procedure flare of LBP.

42.11 Clinical Pearls

- Any targeted and specific treatment, no matter how efficacious, will fail without proper identification of pain generators.
- PLD is a reliable method for diagnosing painful discs, if it is performed adhering to stringent operational criteria [18].
- Advanced imaging has not been able to reliably distinguish painful from non-painful discs, as 64% of asymptomatic individuals possess bulging, degenerated, or herniated intervertebral discs [13].
- PLD continues to play an important role in the diagnosis and treatment of LBP, but its prediction of which disc(s) will favorably respond to cellular supplementation is yet to be established.

References

1. Rubin DI. Epidemiology and risk factors for spine pain. Neurol Clin. 2007;25:353–71.
2. Manchikanti L. Epidemiology of low back pain. Pain Physician. 2000;3:167–92.
3. DePalma MJ, Ketchum JM, Saullo T. What is the source of chronic low back pain and does age play a role? Pain Med. 2011;12:224–33.
4. Schwarzer AC, Aprill CN, Derby R, Fortin J, Kine G, Bogduk N. The prevalence and clinical features of internal disc disruption in patients with chronic low back pain. Spine. 1995;20:1878–83.
5. Moneta G, Videman T, Kaivanto K, Aprill C, Spivey M, Vanharanta H, et al. reported pain during lumbar discography as a function of annular ruptures and disc degeneration: a re-analysis of 833 discograms. Spine. 1994;19:1968–74.
6. Coppes MH, Marani E, Thomeer RT, Groen GJ. Innervation of "painful" lumbar discs. Spine. 1997;22:2342–9.
7. Freemont AJ, Watkins A, Le Maitre C, Baird P, Jeziorska M, Knight MT, et al. Nerve growth factor expression and innervation of the painful intervertebral disc. J Pathol. 2002;197:286–92.
8. Peng B, Wu W, Hou S, Li P, Zhang C, Yang Y. The pathogenesis of discogenic low back pain. J Bone Joint Surg Br. 2005;87:62–7.
9. Peng B, Hao J, Hou S, Wu W, Jiang D, Fu X, Yang Y. Possible pathogenesis of painful intervertebral disc degeneration. Spine. 2006;31:560–6.
10. Burke JG, Watson RW, McCormack DR, Dowling FE, Walsh MG, Fitzpatrick JM. Intervertebral discs which cause low back pain secrete high levels of proinflammatory mediators. J Bone Joint Surg Br. 2002;84:196–201.
11. Cunha JM, Cunha FQ, Poole S, Ferreira SH. Cytokine-mediated inflammatory hyperalgesia limited by interleukin-1 receptor antagonist. Br J Pharmacol. 2000;130:1418–24.
12. DePalma M. NASS spineLine. Mar–April 2012:19–26.

13. Jensen MC, Brant-Zawadzki MN, Obuchowski N, Modic MT, Malkasian D, Ross JS. Magnetic resonance imaging of the lumbar spine in people without back pain. N Engl J Med. 1994;331:69–73.
14. Zhou Y, Abdi S. Diagnosis and minimally invasive treatment of lumbar discogenic pain—a review of the literature. Clin J Pain. 2006;22:468–81.
15. Thompson KJ, Dagher AP, Eckel TS, Clark M, Reinig JW. Modic changes on MR images as studied with provocation diskography: clinical relevance—a retrospective study of 2457 disks. Radiology. 2009;250:849–55.
16. Ito M, Incorvaia KM, Shiwei FY, Fredrickson BE, Yuan HA, Rosenbaum AE. Predictive signs of discogenic lumbar pain on magnetic resonance imaging with discography correlation. Spine. 1998;23:1252–8.
17. Braithwaite I, White J, Saifuddin A, Renton P, Taylor BA. Vertebral end-plate (modic) changes on lumbar spine MRI: correlation with pain reproduction at lumbar discography. Eur Spine J. 1998;7:363–8.
18. Wolfer LR, Derby R, Lee JE, Lee SH. Systematic review of lumbar provocation discography in asymptomatic subjects with a meta-analysis of false-positive rates. Pain Physician. 2007;11:513–38.
19. Johnson RG. Does discography injure normal discs? An analysis of repeat discograms. Spine. 1989;14:424–6.
20. Carragee EJ, Don AS, Hurwitz EL, Cuellar JM, Carrino J, Herzog R. 2009 ISSLS prize winner: does discography cause accelerated progression of degeneration changes in the lumbar disc: a ten-year matched cohort study. Spine. 2009;34:2338–45.
21. Derby R, Howard MW, Grant JM, Lettice JJ, Van Peteghem PK, Ryan DP. The ability of pressure-controlled discography to predict surgical and nonsurgical outcomes. Spine. 1999;24:364–71.
22. Miyamoto K, Masuda K, Kim JG, Inoue N, Akeda K, Andersson GB, An HS. Intradiscal injections of osteogenic protein-1 restore the viscoelastic properties of degenerated intervertebral discs. Spine J. 2006;6:692–703.
23. Liang H, Ma SY, Feng G, Shen FH, Li XJ. Therapeutic effects of adenovirus-mediated growth and differentiation factor-5 in a mice disc degeneration model induced by annulus needle puncture. Spine J. 2010;10:32–41.
24. Buser Z, Kuelling F, Liu J, Liebenberg E, Thorne KJ, Coughlin D, Lotz JC. Biological and biomechanical effects of fibrin injection into porcine intervertebral discs. Spine. 2011;36:E1201–9.
25. Buser Z, Liu J, Thorne KJ, Coughlin D, Lotz JC. Inflammatory response of intervertebral disc cells is reduced by fibrin sealant scaffold in vitro. J Tissue Eng Regen Med. 2014;8:77–84.
26. Aoki Y, Ohtori S, Takahashi K, Ino H, Takahashi Y, Chiba T, Moriya H. Innervation of the lumbar intervertebral disc by nerve growth factor-dependent neurons related to inflammatory pain. Spine. 2004;29:1077–81.
27. Brown MF, Hukkanen MV, McCarthy ID, Redfern DR, Batten JJ, Crock HV, et al. Sensory and sympathetic innervation of the vertebral endplate in patients with degenerative disc disease. J Bone Joint Surg Br. 1997;79:147–53.
28. Yin W, Pauza K, Olan WJ, Doerzbacher JF, Thorne KJ. Intradiscal injection of fibrin sealant for the treatment of symptomatic lumbar internal disc disruption: results of a prospective multicenter pilot study with 24-month follow-up. Pain Med. 2014;15:16–31.
29. Ganey TM, Meisel H. A potential role for cell-based therapeutics in the treatment of intervertebral disc herniation. Eur Spine J. 2002;11:S206–14.
30. Meisel HJ, Ganey T, Hutton WC, Libera J, Minkus Y, Alasevic O. Clinical experience in cell-based therapeutics: intervention and outcome. Eur Spine J. 2006;15:397–405.
31. Meisel HJ, Siodla V, Ganey T, Minkus Y, Hutton WC, Alasevic OJ. Clinical experience in cell-based therapeutics: disc chondrocyte transplantation: a treatment for degenerated or damaged intervertebral disc. Biomol Eng. 2007;24:5–21.
32. Friedenstein AJ, Gorskaja JF, Kulagina NN. Fibroblast precursors in normal and irradiated mouse hematopoietic organs. Exp Hematol. 1976;4:267–74.

33. Pittenger MF, Mackay AM, Beck SC, Jaiswal RK, Douglas R, Mosca JD, et al. Multilineage potential of adult human mesenchymal stem cells. Science. 1999;284:143–7.
34. Deans RJ, Moseley AB. Mesenchymal stem cells: biology and potential clinical uses. Exp Hematol. 2000;28:875–84.
35. Baksh D, Song L, Tuan RS. Adult mesenchymal stem cells: characterization, differentiation, and application in cell and gene therapy. J Cell Mol Med. 2004;8:301–16.
36. Lin Z, Willers C, Xu J, Zheng MH. The chondrocyte: biology and clinical application. Tissue Eng. 2006;12:1971–84.
37. Steck E, Bertram H, Abel R, Chen B, Winter A, Richter W. Induction of intervertebral disc-like cells from adult mesenchymal stem cells. Stem Cells. 2005;23:403–11.
38. Sakai D, Mochida J, Iwashina T, Watanabe T, Nakai T, Ando K, Hotta T. Differentiation of mesenchymal stem cells transplanted to a rabbit degenerative disc model: potential and limitations for stem cell therapy in disc regeneration. Spine. 2005;30:2379–87.
39. Sakai D, Mochida J, Iwashina T, Hiyama A, Omi H, Imai M, et al. Regenerative effects of transplanting mesenchymal stem cells embedded in atelocollagen to the degenerated intervertebral disc. Biomaterials. 2006;27:335–45.
40. Sheikh H, Zakharian K, De La Torre RP, Facek C, Vasquez A, Chaudhry GR, et al. In vivo intervertebral disc regeneration using stem cell-derived chondroprogenitors: laboratory investigation. J Neurosurg Spine. 2009;10:265–72.
41. Ghosh P. STRO-3 immunoselected allogeneic mesenchymal precursor cells injected into degenerate intervertebral discs reconstitute the proteoglycans of the nucleus pulposus—an experimental study in sheep. Orthopaedic Research Society Annual Scientific Meeting. Long Beach, CA, USA, 2011 Jan
42. Yoshikawa T, Ueda Y, Miyazaki K, Koizumi M, Takakura Y. Disc regeneration therapy using marrow mesenchymal cell transplantation: a report of two case studies. Spine. 2010;35:E475–80.
43. Gronthos S, Fitter S, Diamond P, Simmons PJ, Itescu S, Zannettino AC. A novel monoclonal antibody (STRO-3) identifies an isoform of tissue nonspecific alkaline phosphatase expressed by multipotent bone marrow stromal stem cells. Stem Cells Dev. 2007;16:953–64.
44. Gronthos S, Zannettino AC, Hay SJ, Shi S, Graves SE, Kortesidis A, Simmons PJ. Molecular and cellular characterisation of highly purified stromal stem cells derived from human bone marrow. J Cell Sci. 2003;116:1827–35.
45. Bae HW, Amirdelfan K, Coric D, McJunkin TL, Pettine KA, Hong HJ, et al. A phase II study demonstrating efficacy and safety of mesenchymal precursor cells in low back pain due to disc degeneration. Spine J. 2014;14:S31–2.
46. Safety and preliminary efficacy study of mesenchymal precursor cells (MPCs) in subjects with lumbar back pain. https://clinicaltrials.gov/ct2/show/study/NCT01290367. Accessed 3 May 2016.
47. DePalma M. International spine intervention society, annual scientific meeting. Jul 2014, Orlando, FL.
48. Inoue N, Orías AA. Biomechanics of intervertebral disk degeneration. Orthop Clin North Am. 2011;42:487–99.
49. Coric D, Pettine K, Sumich A, Boltes MO. Prospective study of disc repair with allogeneic chondrocytes. Presented at the 2012 Joint Spine Section Meeting: Clinical article. J Neurosurg Spine. 2013;18:85–95.
50. Adkisson HD, Milliman C, Zhang X, Mauch K, Maziarz RT, Streeter PR. Immune evasion by neocartilage-derived chondrocytes: Implications for biologic repair of joint articular cartilage. Stem Cell Res. 2010;4:57–68.
51. Moore KA, Lemischka IR. Stem cells and their niches. Science. 2006;311:1880–5.
52. Li H, Liang C, Tao Y, Zhou X, Li F, Chen G, Chen QX. Acidic pH conditions mimicking degenerative intervertebral discs impair the survival and biological behavior of human adipose-derived mesenchymal stem cells. Exp Biol Med. 2012;237:845–52.

53. Li H, Tao Y, Liang C, Han B, Li F, Chen G, Chen Q. Influence of hypoxia in the intervertebral disc on the biological behaviors of rat adipose- and nucleus pulposus-derived mesenchymal stem cells. Cells Tissues Organs. 2013;198:266–77.
54. Wuertz K, Godburn K, Neidlinger-Wilke C, Urban J, Iatridis JC. Behavior of mesenchymal stem cells in the chemical microenvironment of the intervertebral disc. Spine. 2008;33:1843.
55. Brown MD, Tsaltas TT. Studies on the permeability of the intervertebral disc during skeletal maturation. Spine. 1976;1(4):240.
56. Boos N, Weissbach S, Rohrbach H, Weiler C, Spratt KF, Nerlich AG. Classification of age-related changes in lumbar intervertebral discs: 2002 Volvo Award in basic science. Spine. 2002;27:2631–44.
57. Holm S, Maroudas A, Urban JP, Selstam G, Nachemson A. Nutrition of the intervertebral disc: solute transport and metabolism. Connect Tissue Res. 1981;8:101–19.
58. Walker J III, El Abd O, Isaac Z, Muzin S. Discography in practice: a clinical and historical review. Curr Rev Musculoskelet Med. 2008;1:69–83.
59. Willems PC, Jacobs W, Duinkerke ES, De Kleuver M. Lumbar discography: should we use prophylactic antibiotics? A study of 435 consecutive discograms and a systematic review of the literature. J Spinal Disord Tech. 2004;17:243–7.

Chapter 43
Intradiscal Biologic Treatments: Intra-annular Fibrin Disc Sealant

Kevin Pauza

Intra-annular fibrin bio-adhesive glue represents a potential treatment for patients suffering with chronic lumbar, thoracic, or cervical spine disc symptoms. Fibrin, composed of purified prothrombin and fibrinogen, and reconstituted with aprotinin and calcium, is an FDA-approved drug and biologic for several treatment indications in the human body [1–5]. In contrast to all other surgical and nonsurgical treatments of the spine at this time, including regenerative medicine techniques, this treatment possesses the unique intent to both: (1) identify each disc possessing abnormal morphology in the region of symptomatology, and (2) to treat each disc identified with annular tears in the region of symptomatology.

Fibrin glue is introduced percutaneously into the annulus fibrosus of the disc by injecting human-derived, nonautologous, prothrombin, fibrinogen, and aprotinin into annular tears, where a catalytic reaction immediately forms a three-dimensional conductive scaffold matrix sealant. Investigation confirms fibrin occupies rents, tears, and voids, sealing annulus fibrosus tears [6] and serves as a chemotactic agent, transforming the fibrin matrix into new disc tissue [7–9]. By preventing nucleus pulposus leakage through torn annulus fibrosus, fibrin has the potential to also serve as an synergistic adjunct in helping other intradiscal biologic treatments stay within discs. Other biologics include mesenchymal precursor cells (MPCs) and platelet-rich plasma (PRP), which might otherwise leak through porous annular tears. Aprotinin causes fibrin to remain intact within the annulus fibrosus for a more prolonged duration, subsequently to be replaced with collagen and other tissue regenerating the disc. A prospective, placebo-controlled, live animal investigation demonstrated the time sequence for fibrin converting to new disc tissue with improved biomechanical and biochemical characteristics. Aprotinin prolongs the duration of fibrin until it is replaced by collagen and other disc tissue [7].

K. Pauza (✉)
Texas Spine and Joint Hospital, Tyler, TX, USA
e-mail: kevinpauza@gmail.com

S. Diwan, T.R. Deer (eds.), *Advanced Procedures for Pain Management*,
https://doi.org/10.1007/978-3-319-68841-1_43

Fresh human cadaver discs injected with fibrin confirmed that a delivery device causes fibrin sealant to flow through fissures and voids of the lamella of the annulus fibrosus, evacuating chemical inflammatory constituents. Here, it rapidly solidifies into a small-pore, fibrin matrix with a high surface area [6]. Statistically superior pain relief treating with intra-annular fibrin (based on diagnostic annulograms) was confirmed superior to intra-nuclear fibrin or placebo injection (both based on diagnostic provocation discography and non-provocation annulogram) [10].

Intradiscal biologics, including MPCs and PRP, demonstrate potential value to treat internal disc disruption (IDD) and degenerative disc disease (DDD). Although results are highly encouraging, well-performed investigations demonstrate that relief is neither predictable nor definite, however [11–14].

Efficacy of other intradiscal biologics may be hindered, in part, by diagnostic or therapeutic concerns associated with their treatment. Sequential disc harvesting after treating discs of live human subjects who underwent intra-annular fibrin injection has not been undertaken, owing to strictness of the IRB. In vivo investigations of other intradiscal biologics evaluating live animal discs demonstrated that the majority of MPCs introduced intradiscally leaked from targeted discs [15]. Discs injected with radiolabeled MPCs were subsequently found void of those MPCs, and those radiolabeled MPCs were incorporated into osteophyte formations adjacent to those discs [16, 17]. Fibrin bio-adhesive annular injection minimizes leakage of torn, porous annulus fibrosus by immediately sealing tears and occupying voids within the annulus fibrosus [10], potentially minimizing extravasation of nucleus pulposus and leakage of inflammatory constituents from degenerated discs.

Likewise, fibrin may act as an adjunct to other intradiscal biologics by making discs more impervious to leakage of therapeutic intradiscal biologics. An in vivo, human trial demonstrated that fibrin immediately sealed discs, as affirmed by increased resistance to internal pressure when compared with control discs [18].

Most spine pathology, whether symptomatic or not, originates from abnormal intervertebral disc morphology. More specifically, abnormal disc morphology, reflected as internal disc disruption, disc degeneration, and disc herniation, bears two commonalities: (1) it results from tears of the lamella of the annulus fibrosus, and (2) it has the potential to influence adjacent osseous structures (including zygapophyseal joints) and nonosseous structures (including nociceptors).

In one investigation of subjects who underwent intra-annular fibrin injections, it was hypothesized that in those who experienced immediate relief, their relief may have been due to sealing off annular fissures from hyperalgesic inflammatory constituents from within the region where the nucleus pulposus leaks through the annulus fibrosis [8]. Additionally, it is hypothesized that the three-dimensional fibrin matrix structure supports the natural soft tissue healing process of the disc [7–9]. A benefit of intradiscal fibrin over surgical fusion and disc arthrodesis is that fibrin does not cause detrimental mechanical forces on adjacent segments, known to accelerate adjacent segment degeneration [19]. Likewise, fibrin does not weaken a disc's annulus fibrosus, and therefore fibrin does not accelerate disc degeneration, as does surgical discectomy occasionally employed in an attempt to treat herniated and bulged discs [20].

Published preclinical and clinical evidence has demonstrated that fibrin sealant, its components, and its degradation products all enhance normal wound healing by reducing inflammation and stimulating cellular migration, proliferation, and extracellular matrix formation [7, 8]. A randomized, double-blind, placebo-controlled investigation comparing treatment using intradiscal, nonautologous fibrin with placebo intradiscal normal saline in an animal model objectively demonstrated statistically significant improvements in all parameters evaluated, including morphological and histological growth, proteoglycan composition, cytokine content, and mechanical properties (utilizing pressure and volume testing) [7].

43.1 Indications

Treatment with intra-annular fibrin may be appropriate for patients with several conditions:

- Chronic lumbar or cervical axial or extremity symptoms recalcitrant to relief with other conservative treatments.
- Intervertebral disc abnormal annular morphology, ranging from small annular tears (with or without high-intensity zones) to profound disc disruption, as demonstrated by advanced imaging, including CT or MRI.
- Symptoms or clinical findings consistent with extremity radiculopathy or radiculitis neither preclude nor indicate intra-annular fibrin treatment. For this reason, axial pain may be greater or less than extremity pain, and isolated axial symptoms are not a prerequisite for treatment.

Precise disc levels indicated for treatment are determined through fluoroscopically guided intraprocedural annulograms (Fig. 43.1), not by MRI or CT scans alone, recognizing that advanced imaging studies do not correlate with symptomatology [21, 22].

43.2 Microanatomy and Biochemistry

Clinical and experimental evidence has confirmed that early degenerative changes in the structure of the intervertebral disc can be associated with chronic low back pain. A number of common features are associated with this early disc degeneration [23]:

- Nuclear dehydration
- Proteoglycan depletion
- Endplate calcification
- Diminished cellularity
- Annular disorganization and disruption

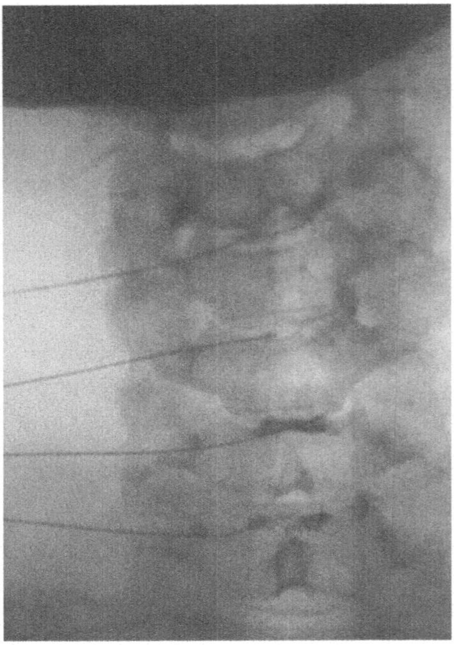

Fig. 43.1 Cervical annulogram (AP view) demonstrating multilevel cervical intervertebral disc annulus fibrosus tears

43.2.1 Progression of Discogenic Pain from Degeneration

- Tears and voids within the annulus fibrosus are known harbingers of inflammatory constituents within the intervertebral disc [21, 22], stimulating nociceptors within those tears [24].
- These stimulated annular nociceptors instigate a patient's axial symptoms and referred somatic symptoms.
- These chemical constituents also stimulate adjacent structures, including descending spinal nerves, dura, and meninges.
- Symptoms were historically attributed to the pressure of a "pinched nerve" but investigations confirm that symptom etiology is attributed to the chemical stimulation of nociceptors with or without nerve root compression, instead of compression alone [24].

Therefore, sealing annulus fibrosus tears serves to minimize extravasation of nucleus pulposus through annular tears of intervertebral discs with or without herniations, thus treating symptoms referred to as "leaky disc syndrome" or internal disc disruption (IDD) [25].

Several studies have recently confirmed that discogenic back pain is directly related to the extent and nature of nociceptive innervation in the intervertebral disc [21, 22, 24, 26, 27]. These sensory nerve endings are located within the annulus fibrosus, and disc pain is proportionally related to the extent and nature of the nociceptive innervation of the annulus fibrosus of the intervertebral disc [21]. Back pain is attributed to the interaction of these nerves with inflammatory mediators concentrated within the damaged annulus fibrosus of the disc. Persistent, long-term pain is attributed to chronic inflammation and impaired healing of annular disruptions.

Immunohistochemical techniques demonstrated that the outer third of the annulus fibrosus is vascularized and highly innervated in healthy human and animal intervertebral discs [24, 28–32]. In degenerated intervertebral discs demonstrating positive provocation discography, both blood vessels and nerves are observed to penetrate more deeply into the disc [21, 33]. These nociceptors are concentrated within annulus fibrosus tears, referred to as IDD. The nociceptors allow nociceptive pain transmission because of their proven association and reactivity with substance P, calcitonin gene-related peptide (CGRP), and vasoactive intestinal peptide (VIP) [28, 33–35].

43.3 Basic Concerns and Contraindications

Patients should have no signs or symptoms of several contraindications:

- Cauda equina syndrome
- Myelopathy
- Significant vertebral canal stenosis causing impingement on the spinal cord or thecal sac at the segmental level of disc treatment; mild to moderate vertebral canal or intervertebral stenosis is acceptable
- Infection at the planned procedure site, or active blood-borne systemic infection
- Known or suspected hypersensitivity or allergy to drugs or components of the fibrin sealant, including aprotinin (a constituent incorporated into the fibrin)

Several other conditions are relative contraindications:

- Active malignancy or tumor
- Presence of intervertebral disc extrusion or sequestration
- Lumbar intervertebral foramen stenosis at the affected level(s), resulting in moderate or significant spinal nerve root compression or impingement
- Congenital or acquired coagulopathy or thrombocytopenia
- Current use of anticoagulant, antineoplastic, antiplatelet, or thrombocytopenia-inducing medications
- Significant systemic disease, including unstable angina or autoimmune disease

Dynamic instability demonstrated on cervical or lumbar flexion and extension radiographs does not necessarily preclude treatment, but it merits understanding and discussion. This instability may result from decreased intervertebral disc height, resulting in subsequent ligamentous laxity, particularly of the anterior and posterior longitudinal ligaments, intraspinous and supraspinous ligaments, and the ligamentum flavum. The introduction of intradiscal fibrin may serve to increase disc height, thus decreasing ligamentous laxity.

43.4 Preoperative Considerations

- Mild to moderate vertebral canal or intervertebral stenosis does not necessarily preclude one from candidacy.
- Consideration of contained herniation versus non-contained herniation may dictate both the volume and location of fibrin introduced; a non-contained disc herniation potentially mandates a lesser volume of fibrin, or it may disqualify the patient from treatment.
- Results of pretreatment diagnostic medial branch blocks, sacroiliac joint blocks, and ventral ramus blocks add to the diagnostic algorithm, but these diagnostic results do not necessarily preclude or affirm the indication for intra-annular fibrin treatment.

43.5 Radiographic Guidance

43.5.1 Annulogram

- Because the intent of intra-annular fibrin treatment is to address annular tears, its pre-emptive test is a diagnostic annulogram, recognizing the correlation (or lack thereof) between disc morphology, pathology, and the patient's symptoms, each morphologically abnormal disc within the region is treated with fibrin.
- The value of the annulogram lies in its unique ability to assess dynamic contrast flow patterns through the annulus, and to assess the competency of the lamella throughout the entire depth of the annulus fibrosus, not just its inner margins.
- In comparison, provocation discography lacks the ability to routinely assess the competency of the outer margins of the annulus fibrosus [18] because discography introduces radiopaque contrast to the disc's central nucleus pulposus only, therefore potentially precluding contrast flow through the disc's outer annular region.
- Additionally, one investigation suggests that provocation discography itself may cause iatrogenic accelerated disc degeneration. Intra-annular fibrin treatment mitigates that concern by utilizing fibrin sealant subsequent to the diagnostic annulogram injection, to seal not only the tears within the annulus fibrosus but also the annulogram's needle hole.

43.5.2 Discography

- Provocation discography is not mandated for this procedure because intraprocedural annulograms allow evaluation of the competency of the peripheral annulus fibrosus, particularly in those discs possessing peripheral annular tears, which

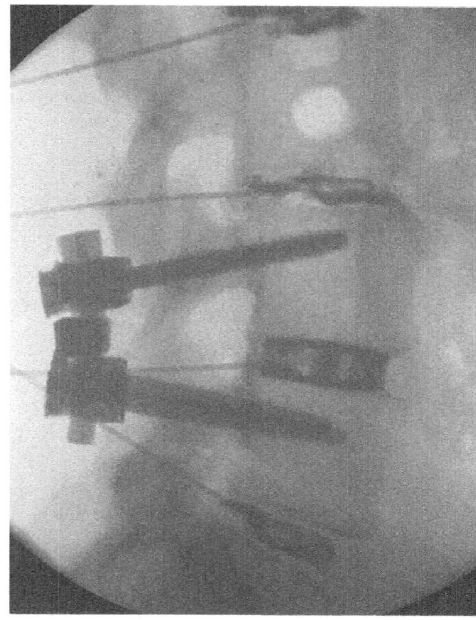

Fig. 43.2 Lumbar annulogram (lateral view) demonstrating multilevel intervertebral disc annulus fibrosus tears in a patient who experienced worsening symptoms following surgical fusion

may be noncontiguous with the nucleus pulposus. Based on annulograms performed on subjects with chronic low back pain (Fig. 43.2), 2.5% of those subjects demonstrate one or two abnormal disc levels; 92.4% of subjects demonstrate three or four abnormal disc levels; and the remaining 4.0% of subjects demonstrate five or more morphologically abnormal lumbar disc levels [18].
- Outer annular tears may remain unidentified through conventional discography techniques, which inject radiopaque contrast into the nucleus pulposus.

43.6 Equipment

- C-arm
- Radiolucent x-ray table
- Monitoring equipment
- Surgical gown, caps, masks, field drapes, and sterile gloves
- Antiseptic for skin preparation
- Extension tubing
- Appropriate volume syringes
- Spinal needles of appropriate gauge and length for standard intradiscal injection treatment
- Anesthetic, antibiotics
- Fibrin sealant

43.7 Technique

Note the technique was awarded patents and is protected because it meets all three criteria of a Congressional Act. More specifically, patent protection was granted, because this procedure meets the three criteria listed by Congress. Those criteria include: (1) causes tissue transformation; (2) made of a specific ratio of constituents; and (3) requires a device to introduce the material into the body. When performed correctly, intra-annular fibrin treatment possesses the unique intent to address all tears of all discs within the region of symptoms. This technique first employs diagnostic nonprovocative annulograms to assess the integrity of the annulus fibrosus of all proximal discs, and then subsequently treats all morphologically abnormal discs with nonautologous fibrin sealant.

This treatment differs from other biologic treatments meant to treat IDD, in that it intentionally targets the surfaces of tears within the annulus fibrosus, in an effort to mechanically adhere to lamellae surfaces, occupy voids, and form a barrier between the inner nucleus pulposus and the outer annulus fibrosus, thus minimizing the potential for leakage from the nucleus pulposus through tears in the annulus fibrosus.

- After obtaining informed consent, intravenous antibiotics for prophylaxis against discitis (e.g., cefazolin, clindamycin, or ciprofloxacin) are administered before the patient is placed prone on the procedure table.
- Mild conscious sedation is obtained using a short-acting sedative or analgesic such as midazolam or fentanyl, which is administered to the patient while monitoring his or her cardiopulmonary status.
- Using fluoroscopy, an ipsilateral oblique image is obtained of the targeted intervertebral disc so that the x-ray beam passes oblique to the prone horizontal spine axis.
- After penetrating the spine, the needle trajectory is parallel to the ring apophysis and subchondral bone of the fibrocartilage endplate of the disc.
- With maximum radiographic "crispness" of the target disc, a curved-tip, 18-gauge Tuohy needle is directed towards the posterior annulus fibrosus of the intervertebral disc.
- The needle trajectory continues passing along the lateral surface of the superior articular process of that segmental level, allowing the needle to remain medial to the ipsilateral descending spinal nerves, until purchase is made into the posterior lateral annulus fibrosus.
- This technique differs from targeting of the nucleus pulposus, as is done in discography [36] and other disc access procedures.
- In this technique, the needle tip is instead directed medially and posteriorly into the most posterior aspect of the annulus fibrosus. AP and lateral images are obtained while the needle's distal tip advances into the center, posterior aspect of the annulus fibrosus.
- Next, up to 0.5 mL of nonionic, noniodine, water-soluble radio-opaque contrast medium is diluted with 10 mg of antibiotic (e.g., cephazolin or clindamycin) per mL of contrast [36].

- The radiopaque contrast is introduced during dynamic fluoroscopy, allowing visualization of its flow pattern through the annulus fibrosus.
- Close scrutiny often reveals contrast flow into the vertebral canal and epidural space through a noncompetent annulus fibrosus.
- The needle remains in place, and if abnormal morphology is identified, the adjacent disc is tested in a similar manner.
- Each adjacent disc segmental level is sequentially tested until all discs are tested, or until a morphologically normal disc without annular tears is identified.
- The needle remains in place in all discs, including normal-appearing discs.
- Following this diagnostic portion, highly concentrated, nonautologous prothrombin, fibrinogen, aprotinin, and calcium are concurrently introduced to the surfaces of the tears of the annulus fibrosus using a multichambered device.
- The iatrogenic needle hole is also sealed in a similar manner while withdrawing the needle. Therefore, upon completion, each disc's tear is glued and sealed, returning it to its normal morphologic radiographic appearance.
- Fibrin volumes used depend upon the extent of the annular tears; volumes typically range from 1.5 to 6.0 mL per disc in the lumbar discs, and 0.2–0.5 mL in the cervical discs.
- The elicitation of symptoms during annulograms does not matter, because each annular tear will be sealed and returned to normal morphological appearance, regardless of symptoms produced while the annulus is tested.
- After sterile dressings are placed, patients are returned to the recovery room and can be discharged after 30–60 min.

43.8 Post-procedure Considerations

- Patients are instructed to notify the physician or report to the Emergency Department if they experience fever above 38 °C.
- New onset of motor weakness or bowel or bladder incontinence should be reported. Many patients experience transient increased axial or extremity symptoms.
- Patients are advised to maintain proper lifting techniques and body mechanics, including avoiding axial flexion and rotation, to avoid mechanical compressive and shear forces. This recommendation is not limited to the postoperative period.

43.9 Potential Complications and Pitfalls

Potential complications include those associated with provocation discography:

- There is a possibility of anaphylactic reaction to introduced medications or contrast medium, but there have been no reported cases of anaphylactic reaction to the components of the human-derived constituents of fibrin (including prothrombin, fibrinogen, and aprotinin). The possibility exists, however.

- There have been no incidences of transmission of blood-borne pathogens (probably because of the current refined processing techniques), but that possibility also exists.
- Because any disc pressurization technique may elicit an intraoperative vagal reflex, consider intravenous administration of glycopyrrolate (Robinul), repeated at intervals of 2–3 min, if medically appropriate.

43.10 Clinical Pearls

- Intradiscal fibrin treatment has the potential to reach and seal all tears within an affected disc when applied correctly.
- This procedure relies on annulograms rather than provocative discography.
- Because the fibrin sealant can also be used to heal the hole from the presence of the needle itself within the disc, this procedure carries the potential advantage of being able to prevent increased risk of disc degeneration inherent to intradiscal needle entry.
- Fibrin sealant is readily available for purchase and does not require the harvesting-type procedures that are commonly the case with most regenerative medicine.

References

1. United States FDA approval letter; Raplixa fibrin. 30 Apr 2015.
2. United States FDA approval letter; Evarrest fibrin. 7 Apr 2015.
3. United States FDA approval letter; TachoSil fibrin, 5 Apr 2010.
4. United States FDA approval letter; TISSEEL fibrin. December 31, 2014.
5. United States FDA approval letter for ArterX surgical sealant, 1 Mar 2013.
6. Pauza K, Thorne K. The penetration and sealing characteristics of fibrin sealant injected into cadaver IVDs. Spinal restoration FDA device performance validation report 20070927, 14 Feb 2008.
7. Buser Z, Kuelling F, Liu J, Liebenberg E, Thorne KJ, Coughlin D, Lotz JC. Biological and biomechanical effects of fibrin injection into porcine intervertebral discs. Spine (Phila Pa 1976). 2011;36:E1201–9.
8. Buser Z, Liu J, Thorne KJ, Coughlin D, Lotz JC. Inflammatory response of intervertebral disc cells is reduced by fibrin sealant scaffold in vitro. J Tissue Eng Regen Med. 2014;8:77–84.
9. Buser Z, Kuelling F, Jane L, Liebenberg E, Tang J, Thome K, et al. Fibrin injection stimulates early disc healing in the porcine model (NASS Abstract 199). Spine J. 2009;105S:9.
10. Pauza K, Wright C. Abstract. 2015. Prospective Investigation Comparing Intra-annular fibrin with intra-nuclear fibrin, and intra-nuclear placebo. American association of orthopaedic medicine annual meeting.
11. Zeckser J, Wolff M, Tucker J, Goodwin J. Multipotent mesenchymal stem cell treatment for discogenic low back pain and disc degeneration. Stem Cells Int. 2016;2016:3908389.
12. Tuakli-Wosornu YA, Terry A, Boachie-Adjei K, Harrison JR, Gribbin CK, LaSalle EE, et al. Lumbar intradiskal platelet-rich plasma (PRP) injections: a prospective, double-blind, randomized controlled study. PM R. 2016;8:1–10.

13. Wang SZ, Rui YF, Tan Q, Wang C. Enhancing intervertebral disc repair and regeneration through biology: platelet-rich plasma as an alternative strategy. Arthritis Res Ther. 2013;15:220.
14. Bae HW, Amirdelfan K, Coric D, McJunkin TL, Pettine KA, Hong HJ, et al. A phase II study demonstrating efficacy and safety of mesenchymal precursor cells in low back pain due to disc degeneration [Abstract 62]. Spine J. 2014;14:S31–2.
15. Bron JL, Helder MN, Meisel HJ, Van Royen BJ, Smit TH. Repair, regenerative and supportive therapies of the annulus fibrosus: achievements and challenges. Eur Spine J. 2009;18:301–13.
16. Crevensten G, Walsh AJ, Ananthakrishnan D, Page P, Wahba GM, Lotz JC, Berven S. Intervertebral disc cell therapy for regeneration: mesenchymal stem cell implantation in rat intervertebral discs. Ann Biomed Eng. 2004;32:430–4.
17. Vadalà G, Sowa G, Hubert M, Gilbertson LG, Denaro V, Kang JD. Mesenchymal stem cells injection in degenerated intervertebral disc: cell leakage may induce osteophyte formation. J Tissue Eng Regen Med. 2012;6:348–55.
18. Pauza K, Wright C, Fairbourn A. Treatment of annular disc tears and "leaky disc syndrome" with fibrin sealant. Tech Reg Anesth Pain Manag. 2016;19:45–9.
19. Throckmorton TW, Hilibrand AS, Mencio GA, Hodge A, Spengler DM. The impact of adjacent level disc degeneration on health status outcomes following lumbar fusion. Spine (Phila Pa 1976). 2003;28:2546–50.
20. Adams MA, Freeman BJ, Morrison HP, Nelson IW, Dolan P. Mechanical initiation of intervertebral disc degeneration. Spine (Phila Pa 1976). 2000;25:1625–36.
21. Wiesel SW, Tsourmas N, Feffer HL, Citrin CM, Patronas NA. study of computer-assisted tomography. I. The incidence of positive CAT scans in an asymptomatic group of patients. Spine (Phila Pa 1976). 1984;9:549–51.
22. Jensen M, Obuchowski F. Magnetic resonance imaging of the lumbar spine in people without back pain. N Engl J Med. 1994;331:69–73.
23. Pandit A. In vivo wound healing response to a modified degradable fibrin scaffold. J Appl Biomater. 1998;12:222–36.
24. Freemont AJ, Peacock TE, Goupille P, Hoyland JA, O'Brien J, Jayson MI. Nerve ingrowth into diseased intervertebral disc in chronic back pain. Lancet. 1997;350:178–81.
25. Melrose J, Ghosh P, Taylor TK, Hall A, Osti OL, Vernon-Roberts B, Fraser RD. A longitudinal study of the matrix changes induced in the intervertebral disc by surgical damage to the annulus fibrosus. J Orthop Res. 1992;10:665–76.
26. Vernon-Roberts B. Age-related and degenerative pathology of intervertebral discs and apophyseal joints. In: Jayson M, editor. Lumbar spine and back pain. 4th ed. Edinburgh: Churchill Livingstone; 1992. p. 24–37.
27. Singh K, Masuda K, An H. Animal models for human disc degeneration. Spine J. 2005;5:267S–79S.
28. Weinstein J, Claverie W, Gibson S. The pain of discography. Spine (Phila Pa 1976). 1988;13:1344–8.
29. Gronblad M, Weinstein J, Santavirta S. Immunohistochemical observations on spinal tissue innervation: a review of hypothetical mechanisms of back pain. Acta Orthop Scand. 1991;62:614–22.
30. Coppes MH, Marani E, Thomeer RT, Oudega M, Groen GJ. Innervation of annulus fibrosis in low back pain. Lancet. 1990;336:189–90.
31. McCarthy PW, Carruthers B, Martin D, Petts P. Immunohistochemical demonstration of sensory nerve fibers and endings in lumbar intervertebral discs of the rat. Spine (Phila Pa 1976). 1991;16:653–5.
32. Bogduk N, Tynan W, Wilson AS. The nerve supply to the human lumbar intervertebral discs. J Anat. 1981;132:39–56.
33. Jackson H, Winkelmann R, Bickel W. Nerve endings in the human lumbar spine column and related structures. J Bone Joint Surg Am. 1966;48:1272–81.
34. Malinsky I. The ontogenetic development of nerve terminals in the intervertebral discs of man. Acta Anat. 1959;38:96–113.

35. Ahmed M, Bjurholm A, Kreicbergs A, Schultzberg M, Neuropeptide Y. tyrosine hydroxylase and vasoactive intestinal polypeptide-immunoreactive nerve fibers in the vertebral bodies, discs, dura mater, and spinal ligaments of the rat lumbar spine. Spine (Phila Pa 1976). 1993;18:268–73.
36. Palmgren T, Grönblad M, Virri J, Seitsalo S, Ruuskanen M, Karaharju E. Immunohistochemical demonstration of sensory and autonomic nerve terminals in herniated lumbar disc tissue. Spine (Phila Pa 1976). 1996;21:1301–6.

Chapter 44
Amniotic Tissue

Tory L. McJunkin, Edward L. Swing, and Paul J. Lynch

44.1 Introduction

The potential for allografts of human amniotic tissues, specifically amniotic membrane (AM) and amniotic fluid (AF), to aid in tissue growth and healing has been recognized and applied for over 100 years [1, 2]. Over this time, research has extensively documented the content and properties of amniotic tissues as well as their mechanisms of action as a regenerative treatment [3]. Though it remains an experimental treatment, clinical data in humans also provide some support for applications of amniotic tissues as a therapeutic treatment. Amniotic fluid contains an array of cell types and proteins that changes over the course of gestation. A number of these components are thought to play important roles in therapeutic applications of amniotic tissues (Table 44.1).

Amniotic tissues have several properties that make them well suited to use as an allograft treatment. Human amniotic epithelial cells do not produce acute rejection when implanted in another patient [4]. Amniotic tissues have also demonstrated the potential to improve allograft tolerance [5]. Both amniotic and chorionic tissues contain mesenchymal stem cells (MSCs), with amniotic MSCs in particular acting as an immunosuppressant and improving outcomes in an animal model of graft-versus-host disease [6].

Amniotic tissues are also well suited to implantation because of their antimicrobial properties. Amnion has demonstrated antibacterial properties in in vitro studies [7]. When exposed to human interleukin (IL)-1β, amniotic epithelial cells produce elevated levels of several types of natural antimicrobial proteins: human beta defensins (HBD1, HBD2) and secretory leukocyte protease inhibitor (SLPI) [8].

T.L. McJunkin (✉) • E.L. Swing • P.J. Lynch
Arizona Pain Specialists, Scottsdale, AZ, USA
e-mail: Dr.McJunkin@ArizonaPain.com; torymcj@gmail.com; TedS@arizonapain.com; lynchmd@gmail.com

S. Diwan, T.R. Deer (eds.), *Advanced Procedures for Pain Management*,
https://doi.org/10.1007/978-3-319-68841-1_44

Table 44.1 Growth factors and cellular components of amniotic fluid and their functions in growth and regeneration of tissues

	Functions
Growth factor	
Angiogenin	Stimulates the formation of new blood vessels (angiogenesis). During wound healing, causes cell migration, invasion, and proliferation
Angiopoietin (ANG-1)	Stimulates angiogenesis. Regulates microvascular permeability as well as blood vessel adhesion, maturation, migration, and survival
Fibroblast growth factor 6 (FGF-6)	A mitogenic, proliferative growth factor that is also important for tissue repair and morphogenesis
Follistatin-like protein 3 (FLRG)	Assists TGF-β mediated signaling, regulating developmental factors Activin A and BMP2
Granulocyte colony stimulating factor (GCSF)	Stimulates formation of blood components (hematopoiesis) and nerves (neurogenesis)
Insulin-like growth factor #2 (IGF-2)	A regulatory and mitogenic fetal growth factor
Insulin-like growth factor binding proteins 2/3/4/6 (IGFBP-2/3/4/6)	Regulates cell proliferation
Monocyte chemoattractant protein #1 (MCP-1)	Recruits mesenchymal stem cells from the host
Matrix metalloproteinase 1/7/9/10 (MMP-1/7/9/10)	Remodels extracellular matrix during wound healing
Stromal cell derived factor #1 (SDF-1α)	Mesenchymal and endothelial cell chemotactic factor
Tissue inhibitor of metalloproteinases 1/2 (TIMP-1/2)	Remodels extracellular matrix during wound healing
Epidermal growth factor (EGF)	Stimulates cellular growth, proliferation, and differentiation
Basic fibroblast growth factor (bFGF)	A mitogenic, proliferative growth factor that is also important for tissue repair and morphogenesis
Endocrine gland-derived vascular endothelial growth factor (EG-VEGF)	Stimulates cellular proliferation and angiogenesis
Hepatocyte growth factor (HGF)	A morphogenic factor in wound healing and the development of organs
Platelet-derived growth factor (PDGF-AA)	Regulates angiogenesis and mitogenesis
Transforming growth factor α (TGF-α)	A mitogenic growth factor that promotes cellular proliferation during wound healing
Transforming growth factor β (TGF-β)	A signaling factor in cell proliferation that regulates inflammation and fibrosis
Cellular components	
Mesenchymal stem cells	Differentiate into tissues such as skin, cartilage, cardiac tissue, nerves, muscle, and bone
Epithelial cells	Pluripotent cells that can differentiate into cells of any of the three germ layers: endoderm, mesoderm, and ectoderm

The effective regrowth of injured tissues is aided by a supporting matrix of cells, known as a scaffold, on which new cells and tissues can grow [9]. Amniotic membrane has long been used as such a scaffold. Though tissue injury can lead to fibrosis and chronic inflammation, amniotic membrane reduces fibrosis by down-regulating transforming growth factor (TGF)β and suppressing pro-inflammatory cytokines (IL-1α and IL-1β).

44.2 Potential Indications

Amniotic fluid contains pluripotent cells and growth factors that facilitate healing and regeneration. Though injections of amniotic fluid are an experimental treatment, early research has examined has examined the potential for these injections to treat a variety of conditions, including injuries to connective tissues and degenerative conditions of joints and other tissues (Figs. 44.1, 44.2, and 44.3).

In addition to its function in stimulating the growth of new tissues, amniotic fluid can alleviate pain by serving as a tissue void filler in joint spaces lacking cartilage because of conditions such as osteoarthritis. It also may be used for other possible indications:

- Assistance with wound healing
- Knee arthritis

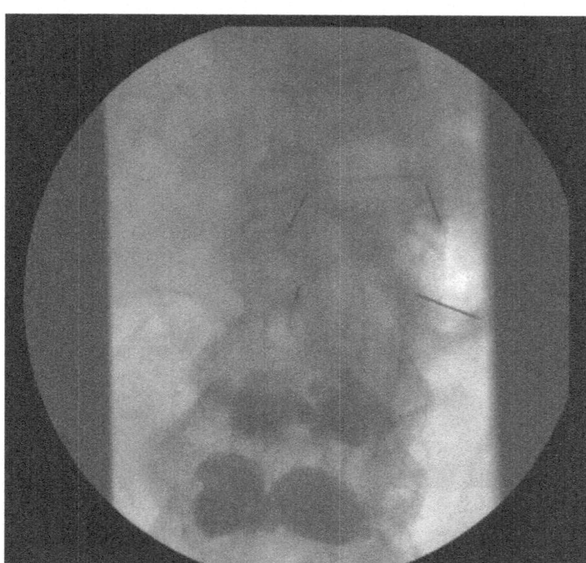

Fig. 44.1 Bilateral L1/2 and L2/3 intra-articular amniotic fluid injections in an 82-year-old man with chronic low back pain due to facet degeneration. Patient has A history of vertebral augmentation for vertebral fractures

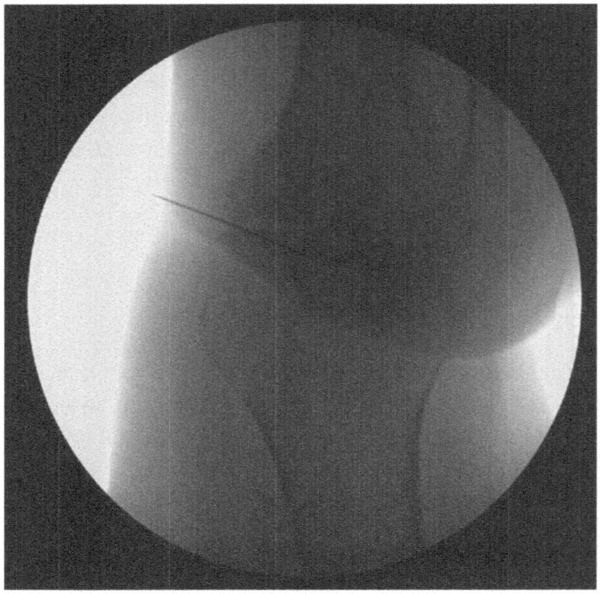

Fig. 44.2 Right knee injection of amniotic fluid in a 68-year-old woman with moderate pain due to osteoarthritis of the knee

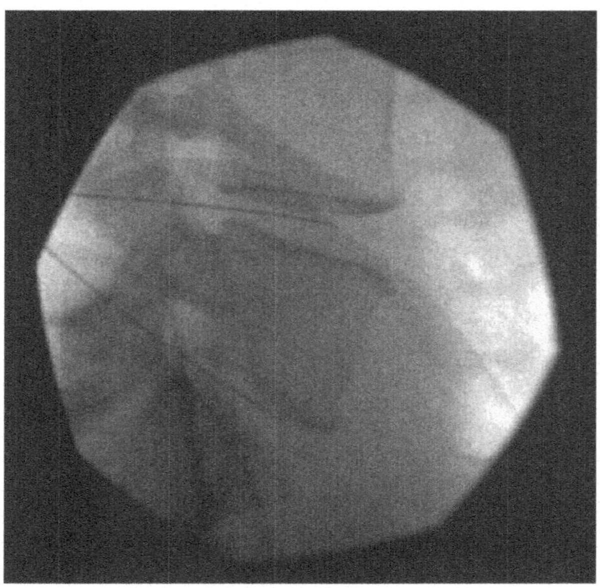

Fig. 44.3 Intradiscal injection of amniotic fluid at L4/5 and L5/S1 in a 52-year-old man with chronic low back pain due to degenerative disc disease

- Foot and ankle joint arthritis
- Achilles tendinosis/tendinopathy
- Anterior cruciate ligament (ACL) injury
- Bone fracture repair
- Spinal cord injury
- Nerve entrapment
- Neuropathy

44.3 Microanatomy and Biochemistry

Clinical evidence for the efficacy of amniotic tissue–based treatments for chronic pain conditions is generally limited to in vitro studies, in vivo animal models, case studies, and non-randomized studies. Along with randomized studies of other similar treatments (such as bone marrow-derived stem cells), these studies demonstrate some promise for amniotic tissue in treating certain types of chronic pain.

There is some clinical evidence that amniotic tissues can aid in the healing of skin wounds. An in vitro study found that amniotic fluid aided in the re-epithelialization of wounded human skin [10]. This re-epithelialization was diminished when hyaluronic acid, naturally found in amniotic fluid, was degraded. Some small, non-randomized studies in humans have found that treatment with amniotic fluid and amniotic membrane can substantially enhance healing of leg ulcers [11, 12]. In one case study, a patient treated with amniotic fluid and amniotic membrane achieved successful wound closure and limb salvage in a case of a chronically draining knee secondary to total knee arthroplasty [13].

Evidence also suggests that amniotic tissues can aid in the healing of tendons and ligaments. Amniotic membrane-derived cells were able to develop into tendon-like structures of cells in an in vitro ovine model [14]. Amniotic tissue-derived injections were effective in enhancing Achilles tendon repair in in vivo ovine and rat studies [15, 16], and another in vivo study found such injections to be effective in reducing recovery time in equine tendon and ligament injuries [17].

Some studies also suggest that amniotic tissues can aid in bone fracture repair. Human amniotic fluid was effective in enhancing the repair of bone defects in a rabbit model [18], and amniotic membrane similarly improved the repair of bone defects in a rat model [19].

Amniotic tissues have also demonstrated efficacy in treating spinal cord injury and other nerve injuries. Amniotic fluid significantly improved cell regeneration and motor recovery in a mouse model of spinal cord injury [20]. Another study found that amniotic tissues supported regrowth in a monkey model of spinal cord injury [21], and amniotic membrane-derived stem cells improved recovery in both mouse and rat models of peripheral nerve injury [22, 23].

Amniotic tissues also hold promise for treating degenerative joint conditions, such as osteoarthritis. One study found that human amniotic membrane added to human cartilage in in vitro human osteoarthritis samples caused the growth of new collagen [24]. An interim analysis of a clinical registry study in 170 patients with knee osteoarthritis found that amniotic fluid reduced pain and stiffness in the treated knee [25].

44.4 Basic Concerns and Contraindications

Treatments with amniotic tissues, such as amniotic fluid injections, generally present low risk to the patient. However, these treatments are still considered experimental and consideration should be given to various standard treatment options, particularly low-risk conservative treatments, before pursuing treatments based on amniotic tissue.

There are additional considerations involving the selection of appropriate patients and delivery of these therapies. Contraindications to the use of amniotic tissue-based treatments are similar to the contraindications to any localized injection or treatment:

- Systemic infection
- Site infection
- Coagulopathy

It is important to note that no allergic reactions have yet been reported.

44.5 Preoperative Considerations

It is imperative to understand the disease state and correctly diagnose the source of the problem. Typically, more conservative treatments will have been tried, such as physical therapy, chiropractic care, stretching, massage, and possibly other injections.

It is also important to understand the area that one is treating with an injection and the volume required for a particular area. For example, a knee might require a higher volume (2–4 mL) than a temporomandibular joint (0.5–1 mL). For any injection, standard sterile precautions should be taken. Typically, larger-gauge needles are used (22 gauge or larger), and the amniotic tissue is "peppered" or "needled" into the target area as it is deposited, to promote micro-tissue damage, increased circulation, and ultimately healing.

44.6 Radiographic Guidance

For precise placement, many physicians will use ultrasound or fluoroscopy to visualize the target area. Choosing between ultrasound and fluoroscopy usually depends on the physician's imaging expertise, the patient's pathology, and what structure is being addressed.

44.6.1 *Ultrasound*

Ultrasound is extremely helpful to diagnose pathology and to precisely place injectate into a desired target. It is the imaging modality of choice when placing medications into a ligament, tendon, bursa, or muscular area, and it is also the optimal imaging choice for placing medication into joints, including knees, hips, shoulders, wrists, ankles, and smaller joints.

44.6.2 *Fluoroscopy*

Fluoroscopy may be use to place medication into deeper structures, and also into many of the above-mentioned joints and other structures.

44.7 Clinical Pearls

- Amniotic tissues, including amniotic membrane and amniotic fluid, contain cellular components such as stem cells, as well as numerous growth factors that give amniotic tissue allografts the potential to stimulate healing and regeneration.
- Amniotic tissues have several other unique and potentially beneficial properties, including low immunogenicity, ease of harvesting, antimicrobial properties, and anti-inflammatory properties.
- Amniotic allografts are increasingly being used in medical practices for their potential benefits in treating various degenerative conditions.
- To date, the evidence for the efficacy of amniotic tissue-based treatments is limited to in vitro studies, animal models, case studies, and other non-randomized clinical studies. The available evidence is consistent with relatively low risk and beneficial responses in at least some cases.
- Because of the lack of randomized, double-blinded, placebo-controlled clinical trials, amniotic tissue-based treatments should be considered experimental. In addition to appropriate consideration of any contraindications, standard of care treatments, particularly low-risk conservative therapies, should be utilized before pursuing treatment with amniotic tissue therapies.

References

1. Davis JW. Skin transplantation with a review of 550 cases at the Johns Hopkins Hospital. Johns Hopkins Med J. 1910;15:307.
2. Shimberg M. The use of amniotic-fluid concentrate in orthopedic conditions. J Bone Joint Surg Am. 1938;20:167–77.

3. Rennie K, Gruslin A, Hengstschläger M, Pei D, Cai J, Nikaido T, Bani-Yaghoub M. Applications of amniotic membrane and fluid in stem cell biology and regenerative medicine. Stem Cells Int. 2012;2012:2–13.
4. Akle CA, Adinolfi M, Welsh KI, Leibowitz S, McColl I. Immunogenicity of human amniotic epithelial cells after transplantation into volunteers. Lancet. 1981;318:1003–5.
5. Anam K, Lazdun Y, Davis PM, Banas RA, Elster EA, Davis TA. Amnion-derived multipotent progenitor cells support allograft tolerance induction. Am J Transplant. 2013;13:1416–28.
6. Yamahara K, Harada K, Ohshima M, Ishikane S, Ohnishi S, Tsuda H, et al. Comparison of angiogenic, cytoprotective, and immunosuppressive properties of human amnion- and chorion-derived mesenchymal stem cells. PLoS One. 2014;9:e88319.
7. Kjaergaard N, Hein M, Hyttel L, Helmig RB, Schonheyder HC, Uldbjerg N, Madsen H. Antibacterial properties of human amnion and chorion in vitro. Eur J Obstet Gynaecol Reprod Biol. 2001;94:224–9.
8. Stock SJ, Kelly RW, Riley SC, Calder AA. Natural antimicrobial production by the amnion. Am J Obstet Gynecol. 2007;196:255.e1–6.
9. Niknejad H, Peirovi H, Jorjani M, Ahmadiani A, Ghanavi J, Seifalian AM. Properties of the amniotic membrane for potential use in tissue engineering. Eur Cell Mater. 2008;15:88–99.
10. Nyman E, Huss F, Nyman T, Junker J, Kratz G. Hyaluronic acid, an important factor in the wound healing properties of amniotic fluid: in vitro studies of re-epithelialisation in human skin wounds. J Plast Surg Hand Surg. 2013;47:89–92.
11. Faulk WP, Stevens PJ, Burgos H, Matthews R, Bennett JP, His BL. Human amnion as an adjunct in wound healing. Lancet. 1980;315:1156–63.
12. Mermet I, Pottier N, Sainthillier JM, Malugani C, Cairey-Remonnay S, Maddens S, et al. Use of amniotic membrane transplantation in the treatment of venous leg ulcers. Wound Repair Regen. 2007;15:459–64.
13. Swartz G, Kozak I. Wound closure and limb salvage following total knee arthroplasty using amniotic fluid and amniotic membrane. Poster presented at desert foot annual meeting, Phoenix, AZ, 19 Nov 2014.
14. Barboni B, Curini V, Russo V, Mauro A, Di Giacinto O, Marchisio M, et al. Indirect co-culture with tendons or tenocytes can program amniotic epithelial cells towards stepwise tenogenic differentiation. PLoS One. 2012;7:e30974.
15. Barboni B, Russo V, Curini V, Mauro A, Martelli A, Muttini A, et al. Achilles tendon regeneration can be improved by amniotic epithelial cell allotransplantation. Cell Transplant. 2012;21:2377–95.
16. Philip J, Hackl F, Canseco JA, Kamel RA, Kiwanuka E, Diaz-Siso JR, et al. Amnion-derived multipotent progenitor cells improve Achilles tendon repair in rats. ePlasty. 2013;13:e31.
17. Lange-Consiglio A, Tassan S, Corradetti B, Meucci A, Perego R, Bizzaro D, Cremonesi F. Investigating the efficacy of amnion-derived compared with bone marrow-derived mesenchymal stromal cells in equine tendon and ligament injuries. Cytotherapy. 2013;15:1011–20.
18. Karacal N, Kosucu P, Cobanglu U, Kutlu N. Effect of human amniotic fluid on bone healing. J Surg Res. 2005;129:283–7.
19. Starecki M, Schwartz JA, Grande DA. Evaluation of amniotic-derived membrane biomaterial as an adjunct for repair of critical sized bone defects. Adv Orth Surg. 2014;2014:1–5.
20. Bottai D, Scesa G, Cigognini D, Adami R, Nicora E, Abrignani S, et al. Third trimester NG2-positive amniotic fluid cells are effective in improving repair in spinal cord injury. Exp Neurol. 2014;254:121–33.
21. Sankar V, Muthusamy R. Role of human amniotic epithelial cell transplantation in spinal cord injury repair research. Neuroscience. 2003;118:11–7.
22. Li YN, Guo L, Ahn HS, Kim MH, Kim SW. Amniotic mesenchymal stem cells display neurovascular tropism and aid in the recovery of injury peripheral nerves. J Cell Mol Med. 2014;18:1028–34.
23. Mligiliche N, Endo K, Okamoto K, Fujimoto E, Ide C. J Biomed Mater Res. 2002;63:591–600.

24. Díaz-Prado S, Rendal-Vázquez ME, Muiños-López E, Hermida-Gómez T, Rodríguez-Cabarcos M, Fuentes-Boquete I, et al. Potential use of the human amniotic membrane as a scaffold in human articular cartilage repair. Cell Tissue Bank. 2010;11:183–95.
25. Demesmin D, Beall D, Nalamachu S, Witherby J, Rana N. Amniotic fluid as a homologue to synovial fluid: Interim analysis of prospective, multi-center outcome observational cohort registry of amniotic fluid treatment for osteoarthritis of the knee. Poster presented at the 2015 American academy of pain medicine annual meeting. http://www.painmed.org/2015posters/abstract-lb004.

Chapter 45
Platelet-Rich Plasma (PRP): Procedural Techniques for Musculoskeletal Injuries

Eric T. Lee and David Kloth

Platelet-rich plasma (PRP) and regenerative medicine has many potential applications, and advancements in its acceptance has increased its use. In terms of pain management, it appears that its greatest benefit may be to aid in healing of soft tissue injury. Many musculoskeletal structures, such as tendons, ligaments, entheses, and muscle belly, can be treated with PRP. Given the multitude of potential sites of treatment, it is important to understand the proper technique and possible complications when using such a therapy.

45.1 Introduction

Platelet-rich plasma (PRP) is a form of regenerative therapy commonly used to treat painful joints and soft tissue injuries (i.e., ligaments, tendons, cartilage, and muscles). PRP promotes natural healing using the patient's own cells and growth factors to repair damaged tissue. Appropriate targets include most types of musculoskeletal injuries, both acute and chronic, such as ligament or tendon tears, which would not or have not responded well to conservative therapies [1, 2, 3]. The number of treatments needed to achieve a therapeutic effect has yet to be established and tends to vary depending on the type and extent of injury. Most PRP injections have the potential to be "one-time treatments," but two to three treatments typically maximize the benefit of the PRP [4].

E.T. Lee
Musculoskeletal Care and Regenerative Medicine, Summit Pain Alliance, Santa Rosa, CA, USA
e-mail: eric.lee@summitpainalliance.com

D. Kloth (✉)
Connecticut Pain Care, Danbury, CT, USA
e-mail: dkmd@ctpaincare.com

S. Diwan, T.R. Deer (eds.), *Advanced Procedures for Pain Management*,
https://doi.org/10.1007/978-3-319-68841-1_45

There are a wide variety of commercially available products for PRP harvesting and preparation. Each platform has subtle differences that may yield higher or lower cell counts, increased or decreased buffy coat (white blood cells), or a change in the number of red blood cells (RBCs) ending up in the final product. Which platform is chosen may depend on the physician's preferences and the condition being treated. This chapter does not cover that decision; the source and preparation of the final PRP product used is left to the discretion of the treating physician. The procedural descriptions below assume that PRP harvesting has already taken place.

This chapter describes several techniques for the treatment of musculoskeletal injuries with PRP, including where to inject and the technique that we advocate for accomplishing it. For all procedures described here, the advantages of using ultrasound are readily apparent; it allows for visualization of the needle relative to target areas, thus maximizing accuracy and the total volume of the injectate delivered to the damaged areas. Therefore, familiarity with ultrasound and performing injections under ultrasound guidance is recommended for all physicians planning to use PRP for musculoskeletal injuries.

45.1.1 *Activation*

Activation means adding a substance, typically calcium chloride, to the PRP (usually pharmacologically) to stimulate the release of growth factors such as platelet-derived growth factors (PDGF)-AB and insulin-like growth factor (IGF-1) from the platelets [5]. This would increase the recruitment of other cells such as osteoblasts, stem cells, and epidermal cells [6]. As these cells become activated, a fibrin membrane forms, increasing cell growth and activation and leading toward healing of tissue [7]. There is some evidence, however, that both unactivated and activated platelets are more beneficial to tissue repair [8]. It has been suggested that the biological substrates already found in tissue at an injured site would be more effective [9]. We leave it to the discretion of the practicing physician as to whether or not activation is beneficial in the use of PRP.

Photo activation for PRP has been advocated for reduction in post-procedure immune response and pain and may be used at the physician's discretion.

45.2 Indications

There are many potential targets for PRP therapy. For the purposes of this chapter, we have selected the most common areas that may benefit from treatment:

- Lateral epicondylitis
- Medial epicondylitis
- Rotator cuff pathology

- Medial collateral ligament
- Lateral collateral ligament
- Shoulder labrum tear
- Hip labrum tear

Technique for treating each of these is discussed below.

45.3 Basic Concerns and Contraindications

See Sect. 38.5.2.

45.4 Preoperative Considerations

See Sect. 38.6.

45.4.1 Equipment Needed

- 18 G 1.5-in. needle
- 27 G 1.5-in. needle
- 3.5-in. spinal needle, 20 G/22 G/25 G (for shoulder and hip labrum, rotator cuff tendons)
- 1.5-in. needle, 20 G/22 G/25 G (for lateral and medial epicondyles, medial and lateral collateral ligaments)
- 3- or 5-mL syringe for local anesthetic
- 10-mL syringe for collecting PRP from the concentrating receptacle (if not included in the kit)
- 1% or 2% lidocaine (Some believe that the use of local anesthetic, such as lidocaine, may be detrimental, but we have used it without negative outcomes (while admitting that bupivacaine may be cytotoxic). While acknowledging this fact, the following procedures will mention the use of lidocaine.)
- Sterile fenestrated drape or utility drapes
- Chlorhexidine gluconate 2% or povidone-iodine
- PRP harvesting/processing kit
- Surgical marker
- Ultrasound
- Sterile sheath for ultrasound probe

45.5 Technique

45.5.1 Lateral Epicondyle

Lateral epicondyle injuries (also known as tennis elbow) can be small, acute tears or chronic, repetitive injuries. Lateral epicondylitis is characterized by tenderness of the lateral epicondyle at the confluence of the extensor tendons of the forearm (extensor carpi radials brevis, extensor digitorum, extensor digit minimi, and extensor carpi ulnaris)—more specifically, where the extensor tendons attach to the lateral epicondyle of the humerus. It is important when considering PRP for ligamentous and tendon injuries to understand that partial tears or even full-thickness tears without retraction may respond well, but a complete transection with retraction is unlikely to benefit from PRP.

PRP injections for lateral epicondylitis have been extensively studied; perhaps the most robust literature support exists for PRP injections of these conditions [10–14]. Following is the technique:

- Patient is seated with arm in front, lying on the procedure table.
- Elbow is flexed at 45°, with wrist in neutral position (Fig. 45.1).
- Lateral epicondyle is palpated to area of maximal tenderness, and the ultrasound probe is placed in either the long or short axis to allow for visualization of the common extensor tendon and lateral epicondyle on the humerus.

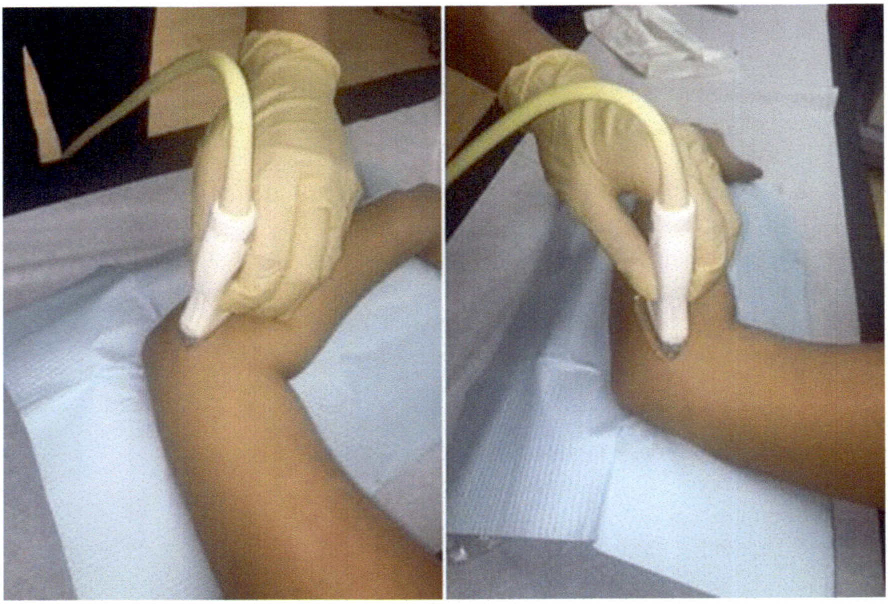

Fig. 45.1 Correct positioning of the upper extremity and placement of an ultrasound probe for the administration of platelet-rich plasma (PRP) into the lateral epicondyle

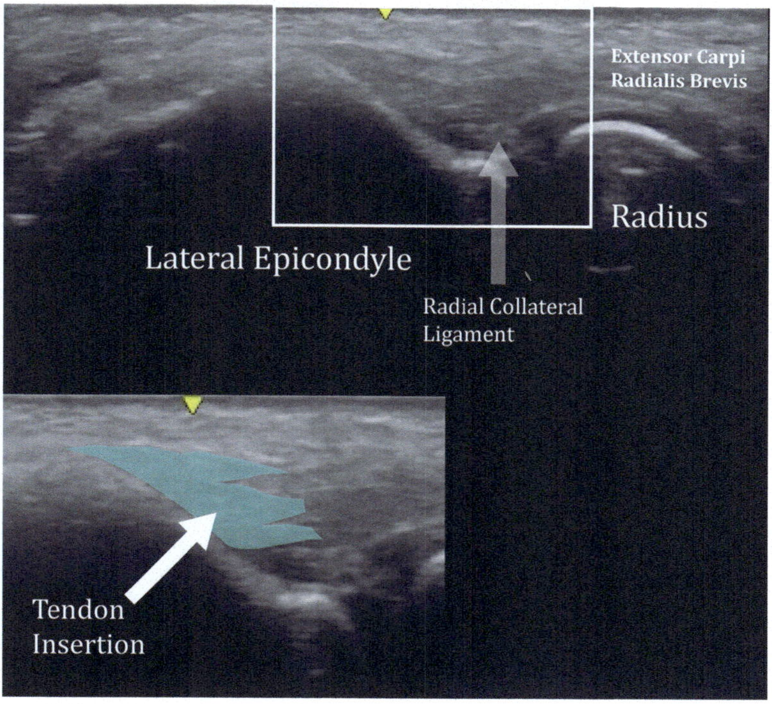

Fig. 45.2 Ultrasound image of the lateral epicondyle

- An appropriate needle entry point is marked using a surgical marker about 1 cm proximal to the area of maximum tenderness; this will allow for visualization of the needle in-plane along the ultrasound probe as it advances towards the target site.
- The skin is prepared in typical, sterile fashion.
- 3–5 mL of lidocaine is drawn up into a 3- or 5-mL syringe using an 18 G needle.
- A 27 G needle is used to anesthetize the superficial skin and underlying soft tissue.
- A sterile sheath is placed over the ultrasound probe, which is reapplied to the skin.
- A 20 or 22 G 1.5-in. needle is attached to the PRP syringe.
- The needle is advanced using "in-plane technique" toward the distal third of the lateral epicondyle (see Fig. 45.2)
- Once the needle touches periosteum, it is withdrawn 1–2 mm, and 0.5 mL of PRP is injected under visualization.
- Once the injectate is determined to be in the correct location, approximately 2.5–3 mL of PRP is injected in a fenestrating-fan technique to fully surround the damaged area with PRP.
- The needle is then withdrawn and a sterile bandage is applied.

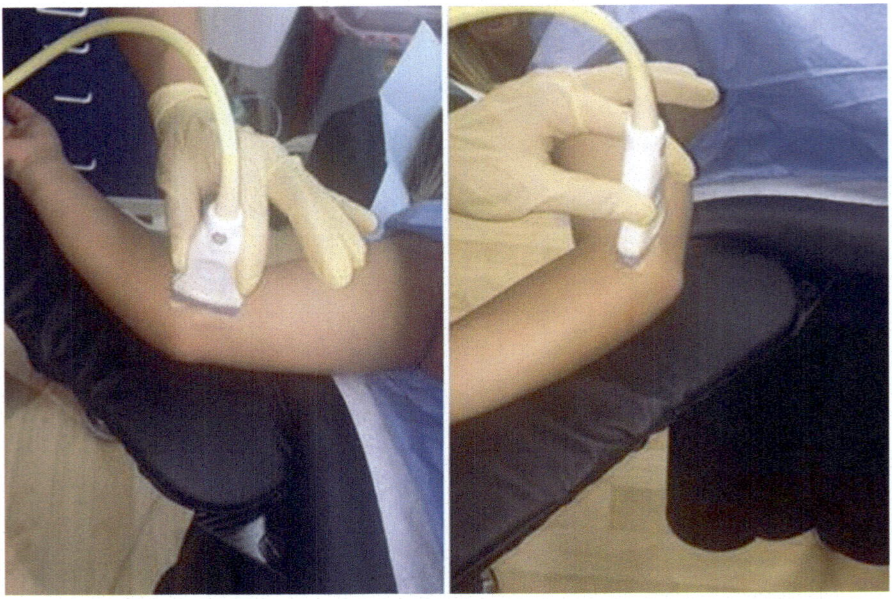

Fig. 45.3 Correct positioning of the upper extremity and placement of an ultrasound probe for the administration of PRP into the medial epicondyle

45.5.2 Medial Epicondyle

Medial epicondyle injuries (also known as golfer's elbow) can be small, acute tears or chronic, repetitive injuries. Medical epicondylitis is characterized by tenderness of the medial epicondyle, at the confluence of the flexor tendons from the forearm flexors (the pronator teres, palmaris longus, flexor carpi ulnaris, and flexor carpi radialis). The point of maximal tenderness is the insertion site of the tendons (flexors) into the medial epicondyle. Much like lateral epicondylitis, there is a wealth of data in the literature to support the use of PRP for treating medial epicondylitis [10–14]. Following is the technique:

- Patient is lying supine, with the shoulder abducted to 90°.
- Externally rotate the arm at the elbow (Fig. 45.3).
- Palpate the medial epicondyle and place the ultrasound probe in either long or short axis to allow for visualization of the interface between the pronator teres and the flexor carpi radialis origins and the medial epicondyle on the humerus.
- An appropriate needle entry point is marked using a surgical marker about 1 cm proximal to the area of maximum tenderness, to allow for visualization of the needle in-plane along the ultrasound probe as it advances towards target site.
- The skin is prepared in typical sterile fashion.
- 3–5 mL of lidocaine is drawn up into a 3- or 5-mL syringe using an 18 G needle.

- A 27 G needle is used to anesthetize the superficial skin and underlying soft tissue.
- A sterile sheath is placed over the ultrasound probe, which is reapplied to the skin.
- A 25 or 27 G 1.5-in. needle is attached to the PRP syringe.
- The needle is advanced using "in-plane technique" toward the distal portion of the medial epicondyle.
- Once the needle touches periosteum, it is withdrawn 1–2 mm and redirected slightly distal and medial; 0.5 mL of PRP is injected under direct visualization.
- Once the injectate is determined to be in the correct location, approximately 2.5–3 mL of PRP is administered in a fenestrating-fan technique to fully surround the damaged area with the PRP.
- The needle is then withdrawn and a sterile bandage is applied.

45.5.3 Rotator Cuff Tendons

The rotator cuff comprises four muscles: the supraspinatus, infraspinatus, teres minor, and subscapularis, which form a musculotendinous cuff at the glenohumeral joint. These tendons attach to the head of the humerus at the greater and lesser tuberosity, and these tendinous attachments to the humerus are often the site of tears. Overuse combined with limited blood flow makes this often-injured structure difficult to heal [15]. This also results in tendinosis and tearing; if left untreated, small tears may progress to larger tears. Athletic and trauma-induced tears often require extensive rehab. In many cases, despite appropriate measures, rotator cuff injuries will never fully heal. PRP may help to heal certain types of rotator cuff injuries, but full-thickness tears with retraction typically will not respond to PRP injection.

Anatomically, the muscles of the rotator cuff originate at the medial aspect of the scapula and insert into the humerus. The subscapularis lies on the anterior part of the scapula, while the infraspinatus and teres minor lie on the posterior aspect. The supraspinatus lies above the scapular spine on the cephalad portion of the scapula.

The ideal approach depends on where the tear being treated is located. A thorough physical exam will often diagnose the location of the injury, but it should be confirmed with ultrasound or MRI. These studies should be used to precisely identify the location of the damage along the rotator cuff tendons (attachment site, the body of the tendon, etc.). Tears are most frequently found in the distal fourth of the tendons and are in a transverse direction [16].

If the tear is at the supraspinatus or subscapularis, then an anterior rotator cuff interval approach may be best. This is a triangular space, bordered by the coracoid process, the anterior supraspinatus, and the superior portion of the subscapularis tendon.

45.5.3.1 Anterior Rotator Cuff Interval Approach

- Patient is seated with the arm placed in slight external rotation.
- The ultrasound probe is placed in a transverse plane on the anterior portion of the shoulder just superior to the greater and lesser tuberosity of the humerus.
- One may visualize the biceps tendon between the supraspinatus and subscapularis tendons.
- An appropriate needle entry point is marked using a surgical marker.
- The area is prepared in typical sterile fashion.
- Using a 25 or 27 G needle, the superficial skin and underlying soft tissue are anesthetized with 1 mL of 1–2% lidocaine.
- The ultrasound probe is reapplied with a sterile sheath.
- Place a 20 G 3.5-in. needle with approximately a 30° bend of the distal 5-mm tip, with attached PRP syringe, directed using in-plane technique toward the space just lateral to the coracoid process at the humeral head.
- The needle is advanced into the rotator cuff interval next to the supraspinatus tendon between it and the biceps tendon. (This area is inferior to the coracoid process and is also the target for the subscapularis,)
- 0.5 mL of PRP is injected under visualization.
- Once the injectate is determined to be in the correct location, the approximately 2.5–3 mL remaining in the syringe are administered in a fenestrating-fan technique to fully surround the damaged area with PRP.
- The needle is then withdrawn and a sterile bandage is applied.

45.5.3.2 Posterior Shoulder Approach

- Patient is seated with the arm hanging by the patient's side.
- Position the arm, internally rotated, resting the wrist upon the patient's ipsilateral thigh for patient comfort and to increase posterior joint space (Fig. 45.4).
- An appropriate needle entry point is marked using a surgical marker.
- Then the area is prepared in typical sterile fashion.
- Using a 27 or 25 G needle, the superficial skin and underlying soft tissue are anesthetized with 1 mL of 1–2% lidocaine.
- The ultrasound probe is reapplied with a sterile sheath.
- Place a 20 or 22 G 3.5-in. needle with approximately a 30-degree bend of the distal 5-mm tip, directed using in-plane technique toward the space just medial to the glenohumeral joint.
- Once the needle touches periosteum, it is withdrawn 2 mm and redirected slightly distal and medial.
- 0.5 mL of PRP is injected under visualization.
- Once the injectate is determined to be in the correct location, approximately 4 mL remaining in the syringe are administered in a fenestrating-fan technique to fully surround the damaged area with the PRP.
- The needle is then withdrawn and a sterile bandage is applied.

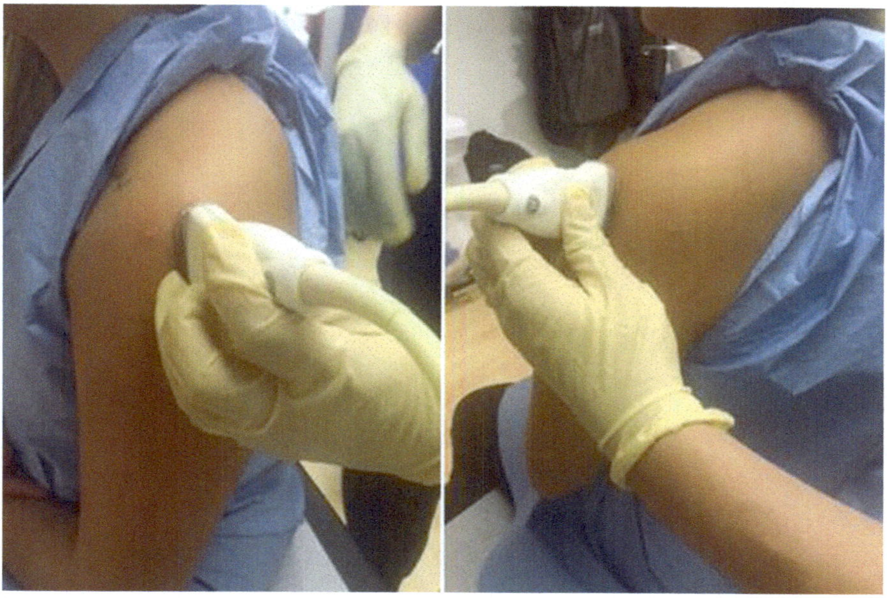

Fig. 45.4 Correct positioning of the upper extremity and placement of the ultrasound probe for the administration of PRP into the rotator cuff

45.5.4 Medial Collateral Ligament

The medial collateral ligament (MCL) provides stabilization for the knee against valgus and varus stress. The MCL is composed of two parts, the superficial and the deep. The superficial MCL attaches on the posterior aspect of medial femoral condyle and inserts distally at the metaphyseal region of the tibia, up to 4–5 cm distal to the joint, lying beneath the pes anserine; this location is important to consider when treating the distal MCL, to avoid causing unnecessary damage to the bursa. The deep MCL attaches at inserts directly into the edge of the tibia plateau and meniscus, so that MCL tears are frequently associated with medial meniscus tears.

Tears of this ligament are often treated conservatively unless trauma to the knee joint involves multiple ligaments, significantly reducing the stability of the knee [17]. Physical examination will typically reveal tenderness at the attachment points to the femoral, fibular, or tibial condyles and will help the clinician to diagnose the condition and the location of injury. Recent data show that the administration of PRP to medial and lateral collateral ligament tears improves healing and outcomes [18–20].

- Patient is lying in the lateral decubitus position with the affected limb down.
- The treatment leg should be in extension at the knee, with slight hip flexion to allow the limb receiving treatment to be anterior to the nontreated limb (Fig. 45.5).

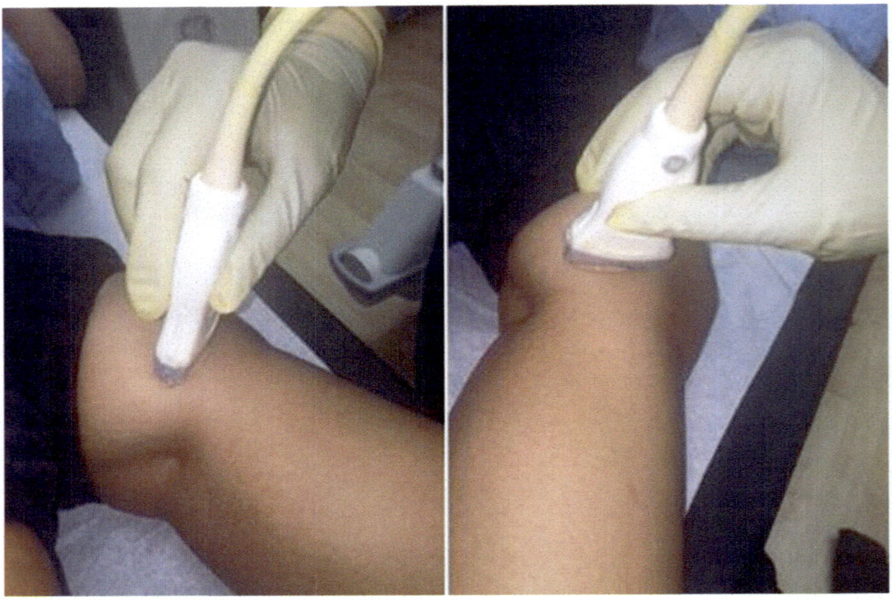

Fig. 45.5 Correct positioning of the lower extremity and placement of the ultrasound probe for the administration of PRP into the medial collateral ligament

- Starting at the superior attachment site of the MCL at the femoral condyle and moving inferiorly toward its insertion on the medial condyle of the tibia, the area of maximal tenderness is palpated.
- Surface skin marked over this area.
- Using a 27 G needle, the superficial skin and underlying soft tissue are anesthetized with 1 mL of 1–2% lidocaine.
- The ultrasound probe, in a sterile sheath, is applied to allow for visualization of the MCL.
- Keeping the probe in the short axis, the 22 or 25 G 1.5-in. needle is then introduced in plane toward the tear.
- When the distal tip of the needle is adjacent to the tear in the ligament tissue, 0.5 mL of PRP is administered.
- Once the injectate is confirmed to be spreading in the correct location, approximately 2.5–3 mL remaining in the syringe are administered in a fenestrating-fan technique to fully surround the damaged area with the PRP.
- The needle is then withdrawn and a sterile bandage is applied.

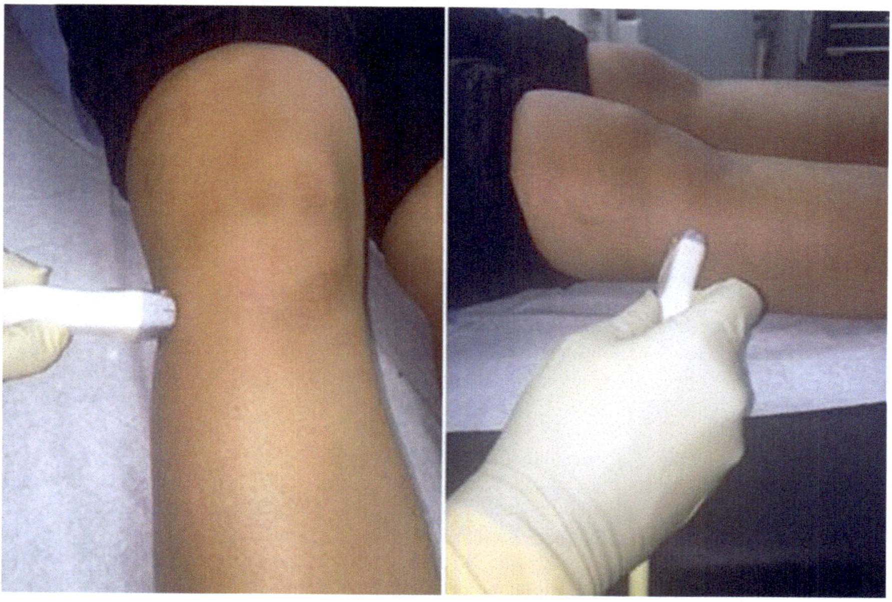

Fig. 45.6 Correct positioning of the lower extremity and placement of the ultrasound probe for the administration of PRP into the lateral collateral ligament

45.5.5 Lateral Collateral Ligaments

The lateral collateral ligament (LCL) provides stabilization for the knee against valgus and varus stress. These injuries are often treated conservatively unless trauma to the knee joint involves multiple ligaments, significantly reducing the stability of the knee [21].

The LCL attaches at the lateral femoral condyle to the lateral aspect of the fibular head. Physical examination will typically reveal tenderness at the attachment points to the femoral, fibular, or tibial condyles and will help the clinician to diagnose the condition and the location of the injury. Recent data show that administration of PRP to LCL tears improves healing and outcomes [18–20].

- Patient is lying in the supine position.
- The treatment leg should be in extension at the knee (Fig. 45.6).
- Starting at the superior attachment site of the LCL at the femoral condyle and moving inferiorly toward its insertion on the lateral condyle of the tibia, the area of maximal tenderness is palpated.
- Surface skin marked over this area.
- Using a 27 G needle, the superficial skin and underlying soft tissue are anesthetized with 1 mL of 1–2% lidocaine.
- The ultrasound probe, in a sterile sheath, is applied to allow for visualization of the LCL.

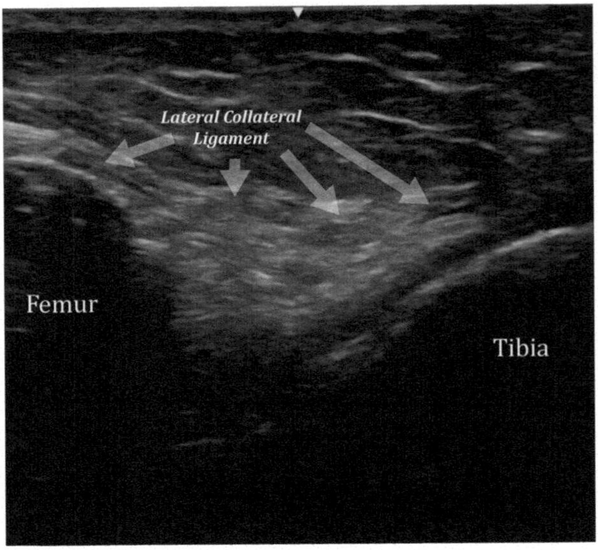

Fig. 45.7 Ultrasound image of the lateral collateral ligament

- Keeping the probe in the short axis, the 22 or 25 G 1.5-in. needle is then introduced about 1 cm proximal to the area marked, in plane toward the tear (Fig. 45.7)
- Once the distal tip of the needle is adjacent to the tear in the ligament tissue, 0.5 mL of PRP is administered.
- Once the injectate is confirmed to be spreading in the correct location, the approximately 2.5–3 mL remaining in the syringe are administered in a fenestrating-fan technique to fully surround the damaged area with the PRP.
- The needle is then withdrawn and a sterile bandage is applied.

45.5.6 Labrum: Shoulder

Labrum is a term describing the tough, fibrocartilaginous tissue structures that help encapsulate the shoulder and the hip. Given the fact that these structures are poorly vascularized, regenerative medicine provides a therapeutic option to improve the chances that these tears will heal [22–24].

Because the labrum circumscribes the shoulder, diagnosing the location of the tear with imaging may be helpful in deciding the best approach to inject the PRP to maximize delivery. If the tear is posterior, a glenohumeral posterior approach may be best. Intra-articular joint injections can be achieved in several ways; the goal when deciding which approach to use is to attempt to gain the maximum spread.

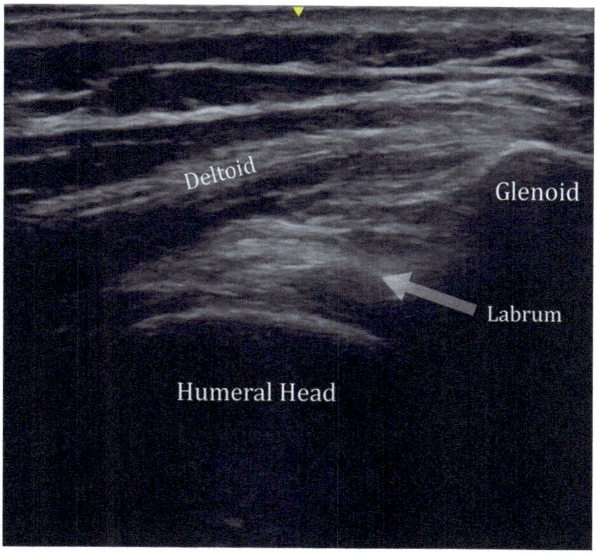

Fig. 45.8 Ultrasound image of the glenoid fossa and labrum

- Patient is in a seated position.
- To visualize the posterior labrum, adduction of the humerus will help increase the posterior joint space (see Fig. 45.4).
- The ultrasound transducer is placed parallel and just inferior to the scapular spine.
- The labrum will be seen as a hyperechoic, triangular structure between the semi-circular humeral head and the glenoid fossa (Fig. 45.8). Using lower frequency may be helpful in visualizing deeper structures in large, obese or athletic shoulders.
- Once the labrum is visualized, it is recommended to slightly rotate the shoulder to observe the humerus rotating.
- Once visualization is confirmed, the skin surface should be marked.
- Using a 27 G 1-in. needle, the superficial skin and underlying soft tissue are anesthetized with 1 mL of 1–2% lidocaine.
- Next, a 3.5-in. 20 or 22 G needle should be placed about 1 cm lateral to the lateral edge of the transducer, along the long axis. Sometimes it is helpful to bend the distal end of the needle 30° approximately 5 mm from the tip.
- Initially, the needle should be directed towards the humeral head unless the distal tip of the needle is well visualized, to avoid traversing the labrum.
- Once the humeral head is contacted, the needle should be redirected anterior towards the glenoid labrum.
- As resistance is felt, 0.5 mL of PRP is administered. Once the needle location is confirmed, approximately 2.5–3 mL remaining in the syringe is administered in a fenestrating-fan technique, to fully surround the damaged area with the PRP.
- The needle is then withdrawn and a sterile bandage is applied.

45.5.7 Labrum: Hip

Acetabular labral tears in the hip are a common injury. Anatomically, the acetabular labrum attaches to the acetabular rim, and inferiorly it is bordered by the acetabular ligament at the acetabular notch [25].

For the hip, we recommend carrying out the procedure under fluoroscopy, also using ultrasound for initial guidance. With the patient lying supine, an anterior lateral approach is recommended. Begin with palpation of the femoral neurovascular bundle, and then use the ultrasound probe to visualize and mark the skin surface overlying unwanted structures.

- Patient is positioned supine.
- Using anteroposterior fluoroscopic imaging, the hip joint should be visualized.
- The ipsilateral femoral artery and neurovascular bundle should again be palpated and an intended needle entry point should be identified and marked approximately 2–3 cm lateral to it, in line with the femoral neck.
- The skin is then draped and prepared in a typical sterile fashion.
- Thereafter, using an anterior-lateral approach, a 22 G 3.5- or 5-in. spinal needle should be advanced with intermittent fluoroscopic control toward the anterior aspect of the proximal femoral neck.
- The needle should be aspirated and found to be negative for heme.
- Thereafter, 1–2 mL of contrast may be injected under intermittent and live fluoroscopic imaging, demonstrating a positive arthrogram within the joint and hip capsule, with no intravascular uptake (Fig. 45.9).

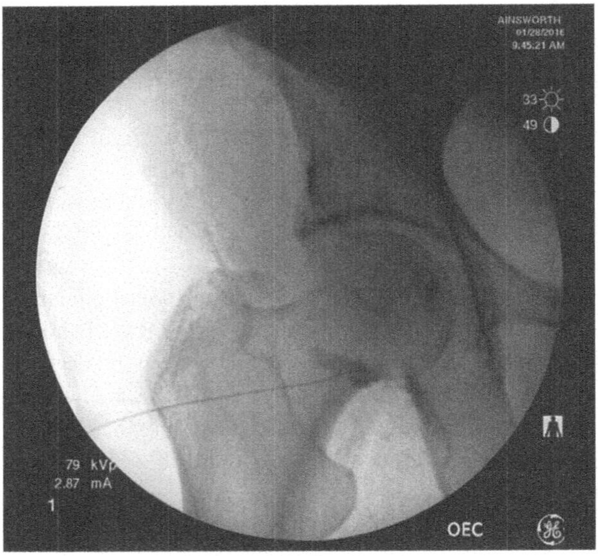

Fig. 45.9 Fluoroscopic image of intra-articular injection of PRP into the hip, with a positive arthrogram

- Once the needle is confirmed to be in the correct location, approximately 5–7.5 mL are administered in a fenestrating-fan technique, to fully surround the damaged area with the PRP.
- The needle is then withdrawn and a sterile bandage is applied.

45.6 Post-procedure Considerations

See Sect. 38.7.

45.7 Potential Complications and Pitfalls

See Sect. 38.7.2.

45.8 Clinical Pearls

See Sect. 38.8.

References

1. Halpern BC, Chaudhury S, Rodeo SA. The role of platelet-rich plasma in inducing musculoskeletal tissue healing. HSS J. 2012;8:137–45.
2. Monto RR. Platelet rich plasma treatment for chronic Achilles tendinosis. Foot Ankle Int. 2012;33:379–85.
3. Cheatham SW, Kolber MJ, Salamh PA, Hanney WJ. Rehabilitation of a partially torn distal triceps tendon after platelet rich plasma injection: a case report. Int J Sports Phys Ther. 2013;8:290–9.
4. Raeissadat SA, Rayegani SM, Hassanabadi H, Fathi M, Ghorbani E, Babaee M, Azma K. Knee osteoarthritis injection choices: platelet-rich plasma (PRP) versus hyaluronic acid (a one-year randomized clinical trial). Clin Med Insights Arthritis Musculoskelet Disord. 2015;8:1–8.
5. Hamilton B, Tol JL, Knez W, Chalabi H. Exercise and the platelet activator calcium chloride both influence the growth factor content of platelet-rich plasma (PRP): overlooked biochemical factors that could influence PRP treatment. Br J Sports Med. 2015;49:957–60.
6. Schilephake H. Bone growth factors in maxillofacial skeletal reconstruction. Int J Oral Maxillofac Surg. 2002;31:469–84.
7. Dhurat R, Sukesh M. Principles and methods of preparation of platelet-rich plasma: a review and author's perspective. J Cutan Aesthet Surg. 2014;7:189–97.
8. Zandim BM, Souza MV, Magalhães PC, Benjamin LA, Maia L, Oliveira AC, et al. Platelet activation: ultrastructure and morphometry in platelet-rich plasma of horses. Pesq Vet Bras. 2012;32:83–92.

9. Marlovits S, Mousavi M, Gäbler C, Erdös J, Vécsei V. A new simplified technique for producing platelet-rich plasma: a short technical note. Eur Spine J. 2004;13:S102–6.
10. Mishra A, Pavelko T. Treatment of chronic elbow tendinosis with buffered platelet-rich plasma. Am J Sports Med. 2006;34:1774–8.
11. Rabago D, Best TM, Zgierska AE, Zeisig E, Ryan M, Crane D. A systematic review of four injection therapies for lateral epicondylosis: prolotherapy, polidocanol, whole blood and platelet-rich plasma. Br J Sports Med. 2009;43:471–81.
12. McShane JM, Shah VN, Nazarian LN. Sonographically guided percutaneous needle tenotomy for treatment of common extensor tendinosis in the elbow: is a corticosteroid necessary? J Ultrasound Med. 2008;27:1137–44.
13. Fullerton BD, Reeves KD. Ultrasonography in regenerative injection (prolotherapy) using dextrose, platelet-rich plasma, and other injectants. Phys Med Rehabil Clin N Am. 2010;21:585–605.
14. Peerbooms JC, Sluimer J, Bruijn DJ, Gosens T. Positive effect of an autologous platelet concentrate in lateral epicondylitis in a double-blind randomized controlled trial: platelet-rich plasma versus corticosteroid injection with a 1-year follow-up. Am J Sports Med. 2010;38:255–62.
15. Merolla G, Paladini P, Saporito M, Porcellini G. Conservative management of rotator cuff tears: literature review and proposal for a prognostic. Prediction Score. Muscles Ligaments Tendons J. 2011;1:12–9.
16. Sallay PI, Hunker PJ, Lim JK. Frequency of various tear patterns in full-thickness tears of the rotator cuff. Arthroscopy. 2007;23:1052–9.
17. Azar FM. Evaluation and treatment of chronic medial collateral ligament injuries of the knee. Sports Med Arthrosc. 2006;14:84–90.
18. Paoloni J, De Vos RJ, Hamilton B, Murrell GA, Orchard J. Platelet-rich plasma treatment for ligament and tendon injuries. Clin J Sport Med. 2011;21:37–45.
19. Saiga K, Furumatsu T, Yoshida A, Masuda S, Takihira S, Abe N, Ozaki T. Combined use of bFGF and GDF-5 enhances the healing of medial collateral ligament injury. Biochem Biophys Res Commun. 2010;402:329–34.
20. Eirale C, Mauri E, Hamilton B. Use of platelet rich plasma in an isolated complete medial collateral ligament lesion in a professional football (soccer) player: a case report. Asian J Sports Med. 2013;4:158–62.
21. Schorfhaar AJ, Mair JJ, Fetzer GB, Wolters BW, LaPrade RF. Lateral and posterolateral injuries of the knee. In: DeLee JC, Drez Jr D, Miller MD, editors. DeLee and Drez's orthopaedic sports medicine. 3rd ed. Philadelphia, Pa: Saunders Elsevier; 2009. p. 1718–46.
22. Hauser RA, Orlofsky A. regenerative injection therapy (prolotherapy) for hip labrum lesions: rationale and retrospective study. Open Rehabil J. 2013;6:59–68.
23. Redmond JM, Gupta A, Stake CE, Hammarstedt JE, Finch NA, Domb BG. Clinical results of hip arthroscopy for labral tears: a comparison between intraoperative platelet-rich plasma and bupivacaine injection. Arthroscopy. 2015;31:445–53.
24. Sánchez M, Guadilla J, Fiz N, Andia I. Ultrasound-guided platelet-rich plasma injections for the treatment of osteoarthritis of the hip. Rheumatology (Oxford). 2012;51:144–50.
25. Petersen W, Petersen F, Tillmann B. Structure and vascularization of the acetabular labrum with regard to the pathogenesis and healing of labral lesions. Arch Orthop Trauma Surg. 2003;123:283–8.

Chapter 46
Technical Aspects of Regenerative Injection Therapy

Nyla Azam, Corey W. Hunter, and Sudhir Diwan

A number of regenerative treatment options are becoming more widely available to the pain management physician, but the field is still in its infant stage (Table 46.1). We are still learning when to use which therapy and for whom it is best indicated. The therapies have been shown to be safe, but potential complications may become apparent as their use becomes more prevalent.

46.1 Patient Selection

Patient selection for regenerative injections should be done carefully. As the purpose of regenerative treatments is to reverse an underlying degenerative disorder, the physician should use clinical and radiographic data to confirm that presenting symptoms are related to tissue damage [1]. Once there is a confirmed diagnosis, current standard treatment should be trialed first, including physical therapy, weight loss, bracing, and oral or topical analgesics [2]. Timing of treatment is another

N. Azam
Division of Pain Medicine, Weill Cornell Medical College, New York, NY, USA
e-mail: nyla.azam@gmail.com

C.W. Hunter
Ainsworth Institute of Pain Management, New York, NY, USA

Department of Physical Medicine and Rehabilitation, Mount Sinai Hospital, New York, NY, USA
e-mail: esponline@me.com

S. Diwan (✉)
Lenox Hill Hospital, New York, NY, USA

Manhattan Spine and Pain Medicine, New York, NY, USA
e-mail: sudhir.diwan63@gmail.com

S. Diwan, T.R. Deer (eds.), *Advanced Procedures for Pain Management*,
https://doi.org/10.1007/978-3-319-68841-1_46

Table 46.1 Comparison of the various categories of regenerative products currently available

Regenerative product	Growth factor concentrate	Stem cell concentrate	Commercial availability	Invasiveness of harvest	Degree of difficulty to harvest	Amount of processing	Evidence to support
Platelet-rich plasma (PRP)	Moderate	None	High	Low	Low	Minimal	Moderate
Amniotics	High	Very low/none	High	None	None	None	Sparse
Bone marrow aspirate concentrate (BMAC)	Moderate/high	High	High	Moderate	Low	Minimal	Minimal
Adipose-derived stromal stem cells	Moderate/high	Very high	None	High	High	High	Minimal
Allogeneic stem cells	Very low/none	Very high	In clinical trials	None	None	None	In clinical trials
Fibrin sealant	None	None	Limited	None	None	None	Minimal (intradiscal only)

important consideration. Patients who are being considered for regenerative treatments generally fall into one of three groups [1]:

- Asymptomatic patients who are at high risk for degeneration
- Symptomatic patients with early-stage disease
- Symptomatic patients with advanced-stage disease

Decreased effect and earlier return of pain have been shown in those with advanced stages of degeneration. In general, younger patients with lower body mass indices and less severe cases of disease have shown better results for a longer duration [3]. Offering treatment to patients with earlier-stage disease must be balanced, however, with the risk of undergoing treatment [1].

Ultimately, when deciding whether to consider a patient for this treatment modality, a few factors must be considered:

- Underlying pathology
- Severity of underlying disease
- Failure of response to standard treatment

Regenerative injections have been used to treat a number of pathologies [4]:

- Cartilage degeneration, such as knee osteoarthritis
- Tendon/ligament injuries
  - Epicondylitis
  - Rotator cuff injury
  - Patellar tendinopathy
  - Achilles tendinopathy
  - Plantar fasciopathy
- Muscle injuries
- Intervertebral disc degeneration

Other conditions should be ruled out or should be a reason for exclusion from regenerative treatment [3]:

- Underlying inflammatory arthritis, such as rheumatoid arthritis or ankylosing spondylitis
- Gout
- Infectious joint disease
- Radiculopathy from spinal disease
- Acute injury
- Neoplasm

46.2 Concerns, Contraindications and Precautions

Concerns surrounding regenerative injections include those one would have for any interventional procedure, such as bleeding or infection. The nature of the substance being injected brings with it its own set of precautions, however, and the following list of contraindications [5, 6]:

- Current localized or systemic infection
- Compromised immune system
- Use of NSAIDs within 5 days prior to the injection
- Hemoglobin level < 11 g/dL
- Platelet count <150,000 × 10^3/mL or platelet dysfunction
- Hypofibrinogenemia
- Inability to comply with post-procedure instructions

Precautions should be used in patients with a number of conditions:

- Coagulopathy
- Cancer history, particularly for stem cell use
- Prior arthroplasty
- Systemic disorder
- Smoking
- Pregnancy

Injections can be considered if the patient's INR is less than 2.5 if needle size is no larger than 25 G and the injection is not performed near spinal or noncompressible structures [5]. There have been no incidents of in vivo tumor growth or in vitro transformation of stem cells into tumor cells, but there is a theoretical potential that systemically administered cultured stem cells may be drawn to sites of latent tumor cells and support their growth [7]. For patients with prior arthroplasty, injecting into extra-articular tissues can be considered, as long as the clinician recognizes the catastrophic risk of infection [5]. A survey found that physicians are most hesitant about using regenerative injections for intervertebral disc pathologies, as the risk of doing harm near spine-related structures may be greater [1].

46.3 Choosing Between Various Therapies

The choice of which regenerative product or category is better for treating any particular pathology has not yet been determined. Going a step further, if one were to simply look at just one category, such as platelet-rich plasma (PRP), it remains to be seen whether even one particular platform is better than another. Proponents of a certain product will claim that their method is better because of higher cells counts, more growth factors, two spins instead of one, no buffy coat, and so forth, but there has never been a single study to prove that any one of these attributes is more beneficial or is even advantageous at all in treating injuries. At face value, stem cell therapy would seem to be better than PRP, for instance, but there is no evidence to support this idea, merely conjecture (*see* Table 46.1).

Until standardized studies are presented showing that a certain attribute has been proven to lead to increased healing, one should proceed with caution and choose the therapy that best fits their particular practice, patient population, and skill set. A number of questions should be considered when contemplating any regenerative injection [8]:

- What is the cost to the patient?
- How invasive of a procedure is the patient willing to endure?
- What kind to equipment is available *versus* what is needed?
- If stem cell therapy is chosen, what would be a sufficient number of cells?
- Will a combination with growth factors or genetic modification be needed?
- Will scaffolds or vehicles be used? Which type?
- What is the recovery time?
- When should the cells be delivered?

The answers to these questions will depend on various factors:

- Type of patient
- Location of the defect
- Size and type of defect
- Cell type being used
- The lineage desired

For the process of obtaining product/cells, one also must consider the hospitalization or office time, the time required to harvest the tissue and process it, and the time required to utilize scaffolds/vehicles, if desired (Table 46.2).

Finally, one must choose between autologous *versus* allogeneic cells. For an autologous donation, donor site morbidity should be determined, as it can affect the age and quality of stem cells and their ability to proliferate and differentiate. In some cases, an autologous donation may be unrealistic because it may be difficult to obtain a sufficient sample owing to the patient's body habitus or underlying disease. Allogeneic cells would present a better option because of their availability, and they may even be of better quality. Any underlying disease in the donor must be

Table 46.2 Comparison of Time and Equipment Needed to Prepare Each Regenerative Product

Regenerative product	Time to harvest and/or prepare	Equipment needed
Platelet-rich Plasma (PRP)	10–30 min	• Kit • Centrifuge
Amniotics	1–2 min	• Pre-packaged, ready-to-use product
Bone marrow aspirate concentrate (BMAC)	30–45 min	• Kit • Centrifuge
Adipose-derived-stromal stem cells	4–6 h	• Surgical tools to perform tumescent liposuction • Laminar flow hood • Tissue culture supplies and stem cell isolation kit • Incubator shaker • Centrifuge
Allogeneic stem cells	1–2 min	• Pre-expanded cell line, ready-to-use product
Fibrin sealant	1–2 min*	• Commercially available product[a]

[a]Fibrin sealant can be used by itself or in tandem with either BMAC or adipose-derived stromal stem cells as a scaffold. The time noted is for the application of fibrin sealant alone

considered, however, and may require prolonged cell storage, which can lead to deterioration [8]. Figure 46.1 presents a flow chart to aid in deciding between various regenerative treatments and products.

46.3.1 Platelet-Rich Plasma and Variants

Platelet-rich plasma (PRP) is relatively easy to procure and takes just minutes to prepare. A number of commercially available platforms are available, all claiming to have some aspect that makes their product superior to others, such as two spins instead of one, less buffy coat, or more platelets. Every manufacturer claims to have the highest platelet counts and/or concentration of growth factors in their final product. Physicians should keep in mind that the Food & Drug Administration (FDA) does not regulate PRP, so any claims made are not monitored. Under 21 CFR 1271 of the FDA's Code of Regulations, PRP is exempt from the traditional regulatory pathway, which includes animal studies and clinical trials. Moreover, there is not a single study that proves that one platform is superior to another, or even that more platelets are actually advantageous. Though it seems intuitive that a higher cell count would yield a better result, it has yet to proven what aspect of PRP—growth factors, volume, buffy count—is actually the most important, or whether cell count matters at all.

Those interested in utilizing PRP in their practice should consider cost and ease of use first, ignoring claims by the manufacturer as to which platform is best. For an independent review of the currently available platforms for harvesting and processing PRP.

46.3.1.1 Advantages

PRP has several advantages over other regenerative therapies [3]:

- Easiest cell type to acquire, as the cells are derived from peripheral blood obtained by venipuncture [9], which can be done in an outpatient setting and does not require additional procedures. The only required equipment is for performing venipuncture, cell collection, and spinning.
- Performed in an outpatient setting
- Typically cheaper than traditional stem cell therapy, but still effective
- Significantly decreased chance of blood-transmitted diseases and/or allergic reaction to treatment because the autologous transplant is derived from the patient's own blood

46.3.1.2 Disadvantages

The technique also has several disadvantages:

- Injection can be extremely painful
- Creates painful inflammatory reaction

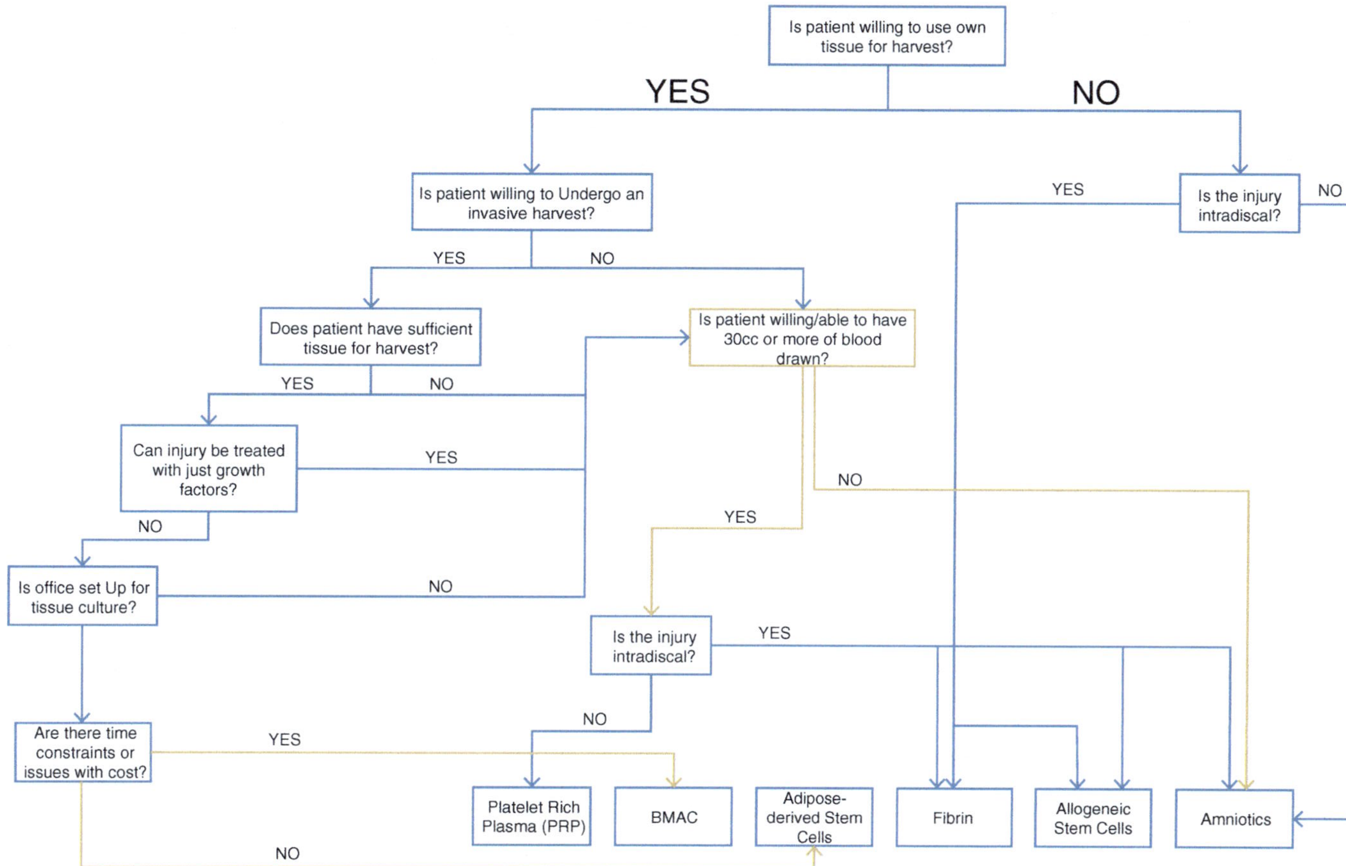

Fig. 46.1 Flowchart for deciding between various regenerative treatments/products. *BMAC* bone marrow aspirate concentrate

- Patient must avoid anti-inflammatory medication before the procedure and for several weeks afterward, so most non-narcotic pain medications (e.g., celecoxib, diclofenac) are restricted
- Not recommended for intradiscal use because of increased likelihood of discitis and inflammation

46.3.2 Autologous Stem Cells

Many consider stem cells to be the pinnacle of regenerative therapy. Scientists have studied stem cells for decades, owing to the sheer potential they hold for a variety of conditions. Much of the early research was focused on embryo-derived stem cells, but this cell line proved to be uncooperative: The cells were fragile and difficult to manipulate insofar as trying to "encourage" them to differentiate into whatever cell strain was needed, and there have been ethical debates surrounding their origin. Eventually, scientists turned to autologous mesenchymal stem cells (MSCs), also known as stromal stem cells [10].

MSCs are commonly derived from bone marrow or adipose, although results can vary depending on site of origin [11, 12]. MSCs are immunomodulatory, inhibiting the proliferation of local B and T lymphocytes and inflammatory cytokines. This makes them particularly useful for post-traumatic or inflammatory pain [13].

Ease of harvesting is an important factor to consider. Obtaining bone marrow-derived MSCs (BM-MSCs) entails a painful procedure, harvesting cells from the iliac crest in a procedure room, possibly requiring some form of anesthesia. Adipose-derived MSCs (AD-MSCs) can be just as painful to obtain, as liposuction is required. On the other hand, it is easier to obtain large numbers of cells without the morbidity associated with obtaining BM-MSCs. The stem cell isolate of adipose tissue left after the tissue is processed is known as the stromal vascular fraction (SVF). AD-MSCs can be obtained in large quantities, with MSCs being 500 times more prevalent in adipose tissue than in bone marrow, so the SVF will be richer in MSCs than the isolate from BM-MSC [14].

AD-MSCs are similar morphologically to BM-MSCs and can also differentiate into various lines (Table 46.3). They are less efficient at differentiating into osteogenic and chondrogenic lineages, however, and have greater adipogenetic capability than BM-MSCs. The difficulty in using AD-MSCs is in restricting their differentiation to the desired cell line, as they preferentially form adipocytes [8].

46.3.2.1 Bone Marrow-Derived MSCs

Advantages

BM-MSCs have several advantages:

- Harvest is easy to perform
- Minimal processing is required

Table 46.3 Differences between bone marrow and adipose tissue[a]

	SVF	BM-NC	AD-MSC	BM-MSC
CD34	+	±	±	–
CD45	+	++	–	–
CD13	±	++	++	++
CD73	±	±	++	++
CD90	±	±	++	++
CD105	±	±	++	++
CD10			++	±
CD36			+	–
CD106			±	+
CFU-F	>1%	>0.001%	>5%	>5%

From Bourin et al. [25]

BM-NC bone marrow nucleated cells, *CFU* colony forming units

[a]CD#: surface antigen markers illustrating the commonality of both cell lines: ++: >70%; +: >30–70%; ±: >2–30%; −: <2%

- Greater potential than AD-MSCs to differentiate into different lineages, including osteoblasts, chondrocytes, and adipocytes, with appropriate stimulation [8]

Disadvantages

They also have some disadvantages:

- Lower cell counts and need for expansion to increase.
- Cell numbers **cannot** be expanded in the United States, per guidelines set forth by the FDA. Should the harvested cells be expanded or manipulated in any way beyond simple concentration processing and purification, they cannot be injected back into the donor.
- May differentiate uncontrollably into an undesired lineage, such as fibroblasts.
- May decrease in quality with age of the donor.
- Yield a smaller number of MSCs, about 5×10^4 cells per 20 mL of aspiration [15]. The number decreases with age of the donor, but can be rapidly multiplied *ex vivo*, and can double to 50 times over 10 weeks [16].
- Because of the smaller cell count, BM-MSCs may need to be combined with bioengineered vehicles/scaffolds for transplantation to large sites [17].

46.3.2.2 Adipose-Derived MSCs

Advantages

AD-MSCs have several advantages:

- Higher cell counts; SVF richer in MSCs. One milliliter of adipose tissue contains 300–500 times more MSCs than bone marrow aspirate [19]

- Expansion not required to be effective
- May need to be combined with vehicles such as PRP for combined effect

Disadvantages

They also have some disadvantages:

- Harvest is invasive and more difficult to perform, as it requires tumescent liposuction
- Requires enzymatic processing, which typically includes lipase. To safely remove all enzyme, several washes are required
- Requires a great of equipment to process, as well as a dedicated room for culturing
- Takes more time to process
- As the cells are harvested from fat, the amount of tissue that can be harvested and the number of times a harvest can be performed are limited by the size of the person and body fat content
- Less prone to differentiating into osteogenic and chondrogenic lineages; preferentially differentiate into adipocytes [8]

46.3.3 Allogeneic Stem Cells

The ideal stem cell product would be one that possessed all the hypoimmunogenic properties of autologous MSC yet was readily available for purchase in a pre-expanded cell line, thus negating the need for harvest and processing. By nature, MSCs are hypoimmunogenic, because of their early, undifferentiated state, meaning they can be allogenically transplanted in a host without the fear of an immune response. MSCs expanded in vitro in the presence of growth factors typically will not express enough HLA/MHC surface antigens to elicit an immune response from the recipient.

46.3.3.1 Advantages

Allogeneic stem cells have several advantages:

- No need for harvest
- Pre-processed, pre-expanded cell line
- Hypoimmunogenic so an allogenic transplant may not require immunosuppression [8]
- "Off-the-shelf" cell lines, readily available and in constant supply
- No predilection for particular lineages (unlike AD-MSCs, which tend to differentiate into adipocytes)
- Lower risk of infection due to decreased need for processing
- One line of mesenchymal precursor cells, MPC-06-ID (Mesoblast Ltd., Melbourne) has shown initial promise in clinical trials for intradiscal use

46.3.3.2 Disadvantages

At the time of this publication, expanded cell lines are not FDA-approved in the United States and are still in clinical trials.

46.3.4 Amniotics

Cryopreserved amniotic tissue is purported to offer all the regenerative and restorative properties of the human embryonic tissue in a pre-packaged, ready-to-use product. These products are rich in growth factors, key proteins, and cytokines (occasionally containing umbilical tissue) meant to modulate inflammation and promote healing. A variety of products are commercially available; like PRP, they operate outside the regulation of the FDA.

46.3.4.1 Advantages

These products have some advantages over PRP:

- Comparable concentrations of the relevant growth factors present in PRP
- Ready for use without the need for harvest or processing
- No need to abstain from NSAIDs during treatment

46.3.4.2 Disadvantages

They also have some disadvantages:

- Supporting evidence is sparse, and most available publications are industry-sponsored
- Cell counts (platelets or stem cells) are extremely low, if present at all
- Not regulated by FDA

46.3.5 Fibrin Sealant

Fibrin sealant is a therapy aimed at repairing damaged intervertebral discs. The fibrin (comprised of thrombin and fibrinogen) is injected into the disc, acting like glue that will fill crevices and tears. Once the fibrin is in place, a natural inflammatory response takes place within the disc, causing collagen to reform within the disc, eventually being replaced with natural disc tissue. Thus the disc's natural architecture is restored. Fibrin has also been studied as a scaffold for MSCs, to increase their viability and survival [20].

46.3.5.1 Advantages

Fibrin sealant offers several advantages:

- Pre-packaged biologic product
- No need for tissue harvest or processing
- Easy to perform via a traditional discogram-type needle approach
- Can be used as a scaffold for MSCs

46.3.5.2 Disadvantages

It also has some disadvantages:

- Supporting evidence is sparse
- As a solo treatment, fibrin is limited to intradiscal use
- At the time of this publication, still in clinical trials
- Not regulated by FDA

46.4 Special Consent

Figure 46.2 shows an example of a consent form for regenerative medicine. Consent for these procedures should include some specific cautions:

- Risks associated with any articular or peri-articular injection, including bleeding, infection, bruising, nerve injury, allergic reaction to local anesthetic, and temporary irritation or worsening of pain [5].
- The fact that regenerative injections are still considered experimental treatment. Although numerous studies have been performed on the safety of these techniques, there may still be unknown adverse events [1].
- The possibility for stem cells to convert into malignant cells (perhaps the greatest concern regarding MSC therapy). The reasons why this treatment is efficacious—the cells' long life span, resistance to apoptosis, and ability to proliferate—are features shared by cancer cells [21], but no such occurrences have been reported in clinical studies so far [7].
- The cost for treatment, as it may not be covered by insurance. Cost varies amongst practices, based on the type of equipment being used. It can range from a few hundred dollars to tens of thousands [18].
- Procedural and anesthesia considerations for obtaining cell samples, such as for BM-MSCs and AD-MSCs. Drawing PRP requires equipment to draw samples and the ability to perform venipuncture, process the sample, and match the sample to the correct patient [5].

STANDARD PAIN MANAGEMENT PRACTICE
1234 Maple Street, Suite AB, Anywhere , USA 12345

DISCLOSURE & CONSENT FORM
FOR REGENERATIVE MEDICINE TREATMENT(S)

Patient Name: ______________________ Date of Birth: ______________

The purpose of this form is to allow the physician to obtain the required consent to perform the suggested procedure. If the procedure is to be performed on a minor or an individual that is not of sound mind or able to provide written consent, a legal guardian or representative must consent on the patient's behalf. My signature below provides written confirmation that I understand and agree to the following statements:

I, ______________________ (patient), do hereby authorize Dr. ______________ and any such assistants as may be selected by him to perform the following procedure(s) on me:

____

____

I affirm that I have been given appropriate information about my condition and the recommended medical, surgical, and/or diagnostic procedure(s) to be performed. I further affirm that the risk, benefits and potential complications have been explained to me regarding the procedure(s) I am consenting to.

I am aware that the practice of regenerative medicine, which includes but is not limited to: platelet rich plasma or PRP, stem cell therapy, bone marrow aspirate concentrate, amniotic tissue grafts, etc, is considered experimental and, in some cases, not regulated by the Food & Drug Administration (FDA). I attest that this has been explained to me that no guarantees have been made to me concerning the result of the procedure(s) nor the safety/efficacy of the therapy I am to receive today. I understand the risks of regenerative medicine as they have been explained to me by the Doctor and that not all possible complications can be predicted as this treatment is considered experimental. I further attest that other therapeutic alternatives that are not considered experimental have been offered to me and I have chosen to pursue this experimental therapy of my own volition. It has been explained to me that during the course of the procedure(s), unforeseen conditions may be revealed that necessitate additional or different procedures than those set forth in paragraph (2). I, therefore, authorize and request that the Doctor, his assistants, or his designees perform such procedures as are necessary and desirable in the exercise of professional judgement. The authority granted under this paragraph (5) shall extend to treating all conditions that are not known at the time of the procedure is undertaken.

I have been informed of the risks that are generally associated with the performance of any procedure and the administration of anesthesia. I further understand that there may be serious consequences such as headaches, neurological or sensory disturbances, bowel/bladder dysfunction, infection, soreness, permanent pain, delayed healing, numbness, tingling, non-healing, need for future procedures or other calamitous occurrence. I understand that there may be certain risks especially associated with the procedure(s) described in paragraph (2). I further acknowledge there may be an increased risk of complications due to the experimental nature of the procedure(s) I am to receive today; furthermore, I understand and acknowledge the complications which may arise may also carry an increased level of severity due to the experimental nature as well as the limited research surrounding its application in conventional medicine. I have asked and am satisfied that I know the extent that I wish to know what those risks may be. I accept those risks.

I consent, authorize and request the administration and management of such anesthesia as is deemed suitable by the anesthesiologist assigned to my procedure. It is my understanding that the anesthesiologist will have full charge of the administration and management of the anesthesia.

I acknowledge that the foregoing information does not cover all of the specific information that has been provided by the Doctor. But, the information set forth above was provided to me and I have had full opportunity to ask questions and to have received additional information.

______________________________ ______________________________
Signature of Patient or Authorized Representative Witness/Interpreter Signature

______________________________ ______________________________
Physician Signature Date Time

Fig. 46.2 Sample consent form when performing a regenerative medicine procedure. *This form should in no way be considered a legally binding document that will provide unlimited protection to the user. Each state has different requirements for informed consent, and different regulations for the application of regenerative medicine. Anyone considering adding regenerative medicine to his or her practice should first consult with legal counsel in his or her area*

46.5 Choosing Regenerative Therapies Over Approved and Nonexperimental Therapies

When deciding on whether to use regenerative treatments, one must keep in mind that they are still considered experimental, and their use must meet the guidelines put forth by the FDA. In Title 21, part 1271 of the Code of Federal Regulation, the FDA states that all clinics that participate in the manufacture of human cell and tissue products must meet criteria to comply with registration, donor-eligibility, good-manufacturing, and quality assurance requirements [22]. Human cell and tissue products are defined as any articles "containing or consisting of human cells and tissues that are intended for implantation, transplantation, infusion, or transfer into a human recipient" [23, 24]. Cell and tissue products that meet that definition require pre-marketing approval unless they are exempt as a "361 product" [20]. Exemptions as a 361 product are allowed if all of the following criteria are met:

- Minimally manipulated
- Intended for homologous use
- Not combined with other articles, with the exception of water or sterilizing, preservation, or storage agents
- Have no systemic or metabolic effect, or are for autologous use or allogeneic use in first- or second-degree blood relatives, or for reproductive use [20]

Cell and tissue products that are not classified as 361 products are considered to be drug treatments, subject to Section 351 and the Code of Federal Regulations for Food and Drug. If a Section 351 therapy does not already have market approval, it can be administered only with an Investigational New Drug application [20].

Based on the above criteria, stem cells would have to be used within a short period and only at the point of care, not allowing for extended *ex vivo* culturing and treatment with growth factors [22]. The FDA has brought suit against a clinic that it determined was more than "minimally manipulating" cells [19, 20]. Because the FDA has classified stem cell therapies as drug products, they are subject to the same rigorous standards applied to other drugs [18]. Any component of the manufacturing, distribution, or sale that occurs across state boundaries would be subject to the interstate commerce clause and FDA approval [19]. MSCs cannot be used for therapeutic purposes unless the facility shows that it follows Good Manufacturing Practice guidelines [18].

46.6 Complications

With careful patient selection and proper sterile technique, one should be able to minimize the risks of procedural complications such as bleeding or infection. A few complications are most commonly seen:

- Increased swelling and pain may follow the procedure, related to expansion of the joint space. This should resolve over the course of 1–2 weeks. To minimize swelling, the volume of injectate should be carefully considered.

- Warmth may be felt in the affected area, possibly as a result of the underlying inflammatory process. This should also resolve over the course of about a week.
- For bone marrow–derived stem cells, there may be some discomfort at the aspiration site over the iliac crest. Patients should be careful not to overexert themselves, to avoid development of bone spurs.
- Patients undergoing adipose tissue aspiration also may have soreness at the collection site.

46.7 Follow-Up and Post-procedure Considerations

- These are often same-day procedures, and patients can expect to go home.
- Post-procedural pain can be managed with simple analgesics such as acetaminophen, or tramadol if stronger medication is needed.
- Anti-inflammatories are avoided for 7–10 days before a PRP treatment, and for 3–4 weeks afterward, as they can hinder the inflammatory process that is necessary to facilitate healing.
- Regular daily activity level can be resumed as tolerated, and it is recommended to continue gentle range of motion exercises.
- Impact exercises should be avoided. The patient can be started with isometric exercises without range of motion for the first 2 weeks, and advanced to isotonic exercises with low-level resistance for a week. After 6 weeks, eccentric exercises can be added as tolerated. Full physical activity can be resumed at 8–10 weeks [5].
- The frequency of treatments varies. PRP is often performed with a 1- to 2-month interval between procedures. Injections may be repeated until there is about 80% relief of symptoms, or until there is a lack of response to treatment, in which case alternative therapies should be considered. Alternatives should also be considered if there is no response after two treatments [5].

46.8 Clinical Pearls

- Potential cost to the patient, the patient's tolerance for invasive harvesting, and processing time are all factors that should be taken into account when choosing between various regenerative therapies.
- Most therapies, if not all, are not regulated by the FDA, so claims made by manufacturers of commercially available products for regenerative treatments are not regulated.
- PRP and autologous stem cells require tissue to be harvested and processed, whereas allogeneic stem cells, amniotics,and fibrin sealant are commercially available (Figs. 46.3 and 46.4).
- Harvested MSCs **cannot** be expanded in the United States. If an MSC line is expanded, it cannot be transplanted back into the host or any other recipient.

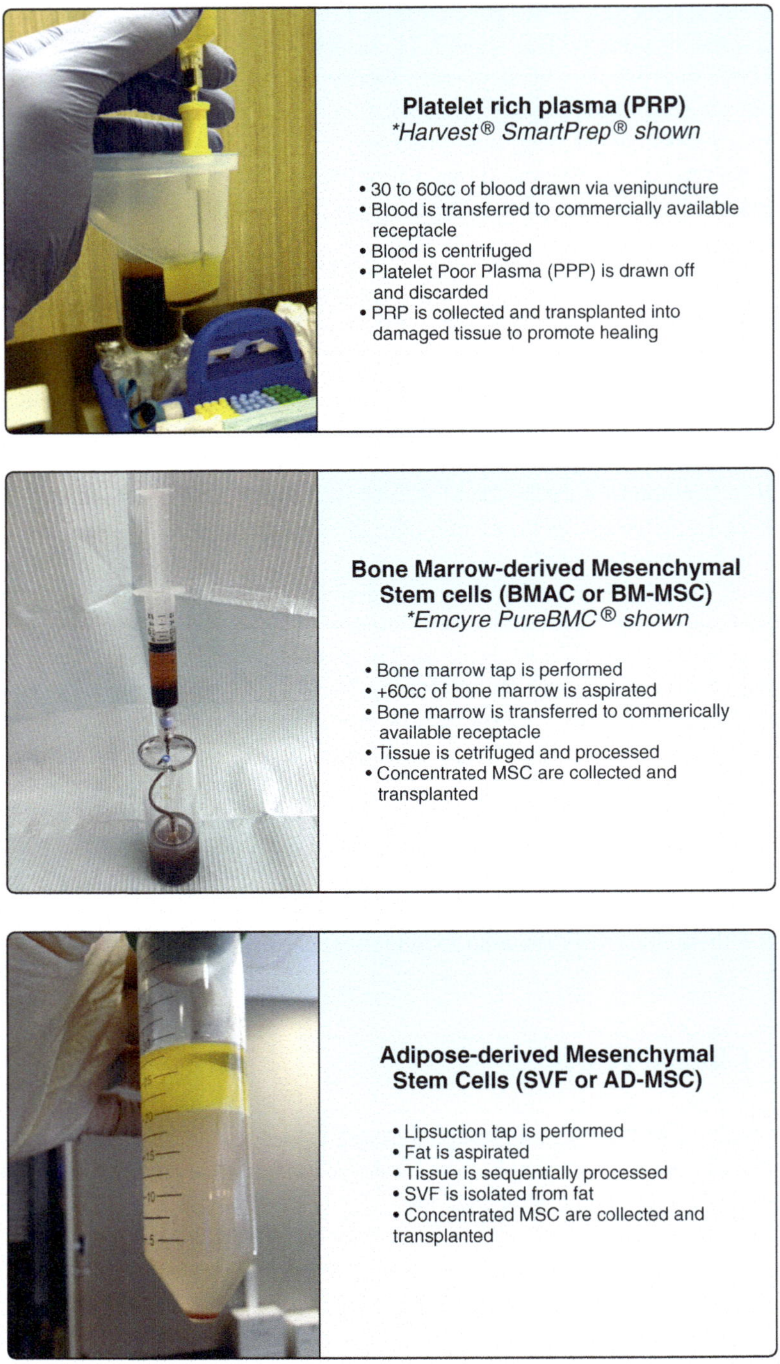

Fig. 46.3 Regenerative treatments requiring harvest and processing. *SVF* stromal vascular fraction

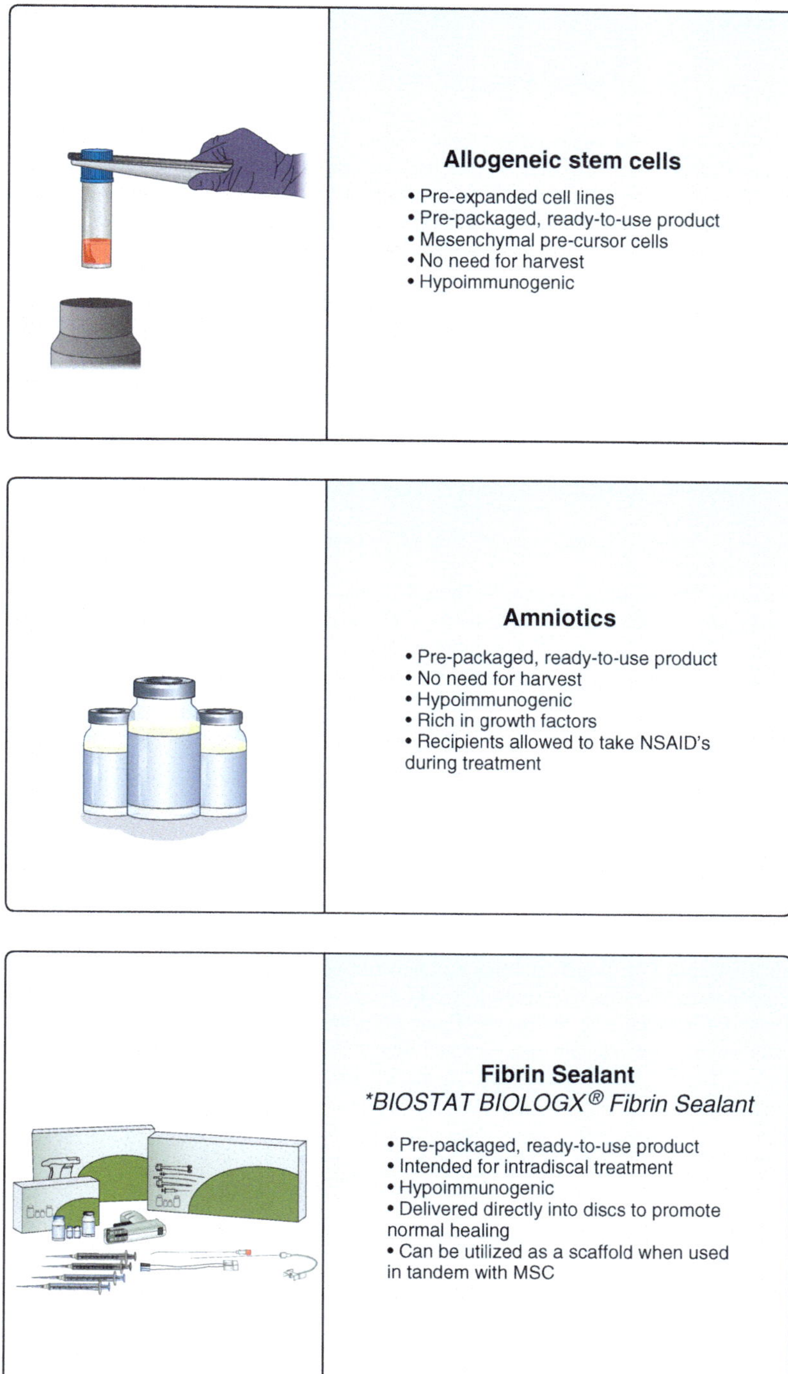

Fig. 46.4 Pre-packaged, ready-to-use regenerative products

References

1. Niemansburg SL, van Delden JJ, Oner FC, Dhert WJ, Bredenoord AL. Ethical implications of regenerative medicine in orthopedics: an empirical study with surgeons and scientists in the field. Spine J. 2014;14:1029–35.
2. Bertrand H, Reeves KD, Bennett CJ, Bicknell S, Cheng AL. Dextrose prolotherapy versus control injections in painful rotator cuff tendinopathy. Arch Phys Med Rehabil. 2016;97:17–25.
3. Jang SJ, Kim JD, Cha SS. Platelet-rich plasma (PRP) injections as an effective treatment for early osteoarthritis. Eur J Orthop Surg Traumatol. 2013;23:573–80.
4. Andia I, Maffulli N. Muscle and tendon injuries: the role of biological interventions to promote and assist healing and recovery. Arthroscopy. 2015;31:999–1015.
5. Vora A, Borg-Stein J, Nguyen RT. Regenerative injection therapy for osteoarthritis: fundamental concepts and evidence-based review. PM R. 2012;4:S104–9.
6. Cavallo C, Filardo G, Mariani E, Kon E, Marcacci M, Pereira Ruiz MT, et al. Comparison of platelet-rich plasma formulations for cartilage healing: an in vitro study. J Bone Joint Surg Am. 2014;96:423–9.
7. Dawson JI, Kanczler J, Tare R, Kassem M, Oreffo RO. Concise review: bridging the gap: bone regeneration using skeletal stem cell-based strategies – where are we now? Stem Cells. 2014;32:35–44.
8. Docheva D, Müller SA, Majewski M, Evans CH. Biologics for tendon repair. Adv Drug Deliv Rev. 2015;84:222–39.
9. Dragoo JL, Wasterlain AS, Braun HJ, Nead KT. Platelet-rich plasma as a treatment for patellar tendinopathy: a double-blind, randomized controlled trial. Am J Sports Med. 2014;42:610–8.
10. Bakshi A, Hunter C, Swanger S, Lepore A, Fischer I. Minimally invasive delivery of stem cells for spinal cord injury: advantages of the lumbar puncture technique. J Neurosurg Spine. 2004;1:330–7.
11. Keyser KA, Beagles KE, Kiem HP. Comparison of mesenchymal stem cells from different tissues to suppress T-cell activation. Cell Transplant. 2007;16:555–62.
12. Melief SM, Zwaginga JJ, Fibbe WE, Roelofs H. Adipose tissue-derivedmultipotent stromal cells have a higher immunomodulatory capacity than their bone marrow-derived counterparts. Stem Cells Transl Med. 2013;2:455–63.
13. Labusca L, Zugun-Eloae F, Mashayekhi K. Stem cells for the treatment of musculoskeletal pain. World J Stem Cells. 2015;7:96–105.
14. Baghaban Eslaminejad M, Malakooty Poor E. Mesenchymal stem cells as a potent cell source for articular cartilage regeneration. World J Stem Cells. 2014;6:344–54.
15. Majd H, Quinn TM, Wipff PJ, Hinz B. Dynamic expansion culture for mesenchymal stem cells. Methods Mol Biol. 2011;698:175–88.
16. Giordano A, Galderisi U, Marino IR. From the laboratory bench to the patient's bedside: an update on clinical trials with mesenchymal stem cells. J Cell Physiol. 2007;211:27–35.
17. Guan X, Furth ME, Childers MK. Stem cell use in musculoskeletal disorders. PM R. 2011;3:S95–9.
18. Aggarwal S, Pittenger MF. Human mesenchymal stem cells modulate allogeneic immune cell responses. Blood. 2005;105:1815–22.
19. Gimble JM, Katz AJ, Bunnell BA. Adipose-derived stem cells for regenerative medicine. Circ Res. 2007;100:1249–60.
20. Gasparotto VP, Landim-Alvarenga FC, Oliveira AL, Simões GF, Lima-Neto JF, Barraviera B, Ferreira RS. A new fibrin sealant as a three-dimensional scaffold candidate for mesenchymal stem cells. Stem Cell Res Ther. 2014;5:78.
21. Bashir J, Sherman A, Lee H, Kaplan L, Hare JM. Mesenchymal stem cell therapies in the treatment of musculoskeletal diseases. PM R. 2014;6:61–9.
22. Sipp D, Turner L. Stem cells. U.S. regulation of stem cells as medical products. Science. 2012;338:1296–7.

23. Lysaght T, Campbell AV. Regulating autologous adult stem cells: the FDA steps up. Cell Stem Cell. 2011;9:393–6.
24. U.S. Dept. of Health and Human Services. Minimal manipulation of human cells, tissues, and cellular and tissue-based products. Food and Drug Administration. 2014. http://www.fda.gov/downloads/BiologicsBloodVaccines/GuidanceComplianceRegulatoryInformation/Guidances/CellularandGeneTherapy/UCM427746.pdf. Accessed 15 Oct 2015.
25. Bourin P, Bunnell BA, Casteilla L, Dominici M, Katz AJ, March KL, et al. Stromal cells from the adipose tissue-derived stromal vascular fraction and culture expanded adipose tissue-derived stromal/stem cells: a joint statement of the International Federation for Adipose Therapeutics and Science (IFATS) and the International Society for Cellular Therapy (ISCT). Cytotherapy. 2013;15:641–8.

Chapter 47
Platelet-Rich Plasma Therapy: An Overview

Eric T. Lee and Steven M. Falowski

Given the multitude of potential sites of PRP treatment, it is important to understand the biological mechanism of its action, its indications, and its potential complications. The availability of commercial kits (each with its own instructions) makes harvesting easier for the physician, but it is still the physician's responsibility to understand the benefits of different harvesting, preparation, and activation techniques to maximize the therapeutic effect. The basic equipment and protocol (if one chooses not to use a commercial kit) is also integral to the application of PRP therapy.

47.1 Introduction

In the simplest terms, PRP is an autologous plasma serum with platelets concentrated above normal in vivo levels. The potential advantages of using a self-derived product to heal are reductions in complications and adverse effects from immune response. PRP has even been proposed as a more effective healing method than various other treatments. Essentially, in harvesting PRP we are taking the platelets found naturally in one's blood plasma, extracting them and concentrating them in plasma, and then injecting them directly into the injured body site.

To best understand the benefits of PRP, a brief overview of the process of tissue healing is important. When acute injury occurs, platelets aggregate, forming a plug

E.T. Lee (✉)
Musculoskeletal Care and Regenerative Medicine, Summit Pain Alliance, Santa Rosa, CA, USA
e-mail: eric.lee@summitpainalliance.com

S.M. Falowski
Department of Neurosurgery, St. Luke's University Health Network, Bethlehem, PA, USA
e-mail: sfalowski@gmail.com

S. Diwan, T.R. Deer (eds.), *Advanced Procedures for Pain Management*,
https://doi.org/10.1007/978-3-319-68841-1_47

at the site of injury, followed by fibrin clot. Once the platelets aggregate, they activate the secretion of various growth factors and induce inflammatory responses from other cells, such as monocytes, neutrophils, and lymphocytes [1]. The clotting process of blood begins, typically within 10–15 min, and is 95% complete within the first hour [2]. Cells such as fibroblasts are stimulated, creating collagen, which supplants the fibrin clot. Next, endothelial cells promote angiogenesis, the creation of a new vascular supply, which then bring nutrients to support the healing region.

It is this supply of nutrients and healing factors that is critical to soft tissue healing. A lack of blood supply to any injury site will limit the amount of healing cells, growth factors, and nutrients to the area, preventing the tissues from maximally healing. Thus, poorly vascularized structures such as cartilage, ligaments, and the entheses of muscles could benefit from direct injection of these factors with substances such as PRP.

47.1.1 Growth Factors

Platelets themselves play an important role in natural tissue healing as both producers and stimulators of a wide variety of healing factors:

- Platelet-derived growth factor AB (PDGF-AB)
- Transforming growth factor β1 (TGF β1)
- Fibroblast growth factor (FGF)
- Vascular endothelial growth factor (VEGF)
- Connective tissue growth factor (CTGF)
- Epithelial growth factor (EGF)
- Insulin-like growth factor 1&2 (ILGF)
- Keratinocyte growth factor (KGF)

47.2 Applications

Given what is found in PRP, it has been used for many applications, from cosmetics to wound healing to treating pain conditions. Theoretically, PRP should work well on any soft tissue structure (such as ligaments, tendons, or cartilage) that needs help in healing. It has been reported that musculoskeletal injuries are the most common cause of long-term pain and physical disability [3], and in terms of treating painful conditions, chronic tendon injuries, acute muscle and ligament injuries, and degenerative joint diseases are all potential targets.

47.2.1 Indications

Though there are many potential targets for PRP therapy, we have selected the most common areas that may benefit from treatment. Perhaps the most robust literature support exists for PRP injections for these conditions [4–7]:

- Lateral epicondylitis
- Medial epicondylitis
- Rotator cuff pathology
- Medial collateral ligament injury
- Lateral collateral ligament injury
- Shoulder labrum tear
- Hip labrum tear
- Wrist injuries (multiple ligaments and tendons)
- Biceps tendon partial tear
- Costochondritis
- Greater trochanter injury
- Meniscus injury
- Patella and quadriceps tendon injuries
- Achilles tendon (partial tear)
- Plantar fasciitis
- Triangular ligament sprains

Where PRP treatment fits in the algorithm is up to the treating physician, but it is most often used for those injuries that would not or have not responded well to conservative therapies [8]. We use PRP liberally to treat soft tissue injuries, to promote faster and better healing in synergy with conservative therapies. The number of injections administered has not been clearly established, but some suggest that one to three injections maximize the benefit of the procedure [9].

47.3 PRP Preparation

When considering the best preparation and use of PRP, several areas are often contested. Most often discussed are whether to include a buffy coat and whether it is important to activate the PRP prior to injection.

47.3.1 The Buffy Coat

The buffy coat is a layer of predominantly white blood cells that appears as a thin line on a post-centrifuged sample of fractionated blood. In addition to the white blood cells, there is a concentration of platelets, as well as the associated cytokines.

White blood cells play a role in tissue healing through the inflammatory cascade they evoke [10], but it is also thought that an increased inflammatory response can lead to increased pain and possibly more damage to the area without well-controlled healing. Given these two counterpoints, it is left to the treating physician as to whether to include leukocyte-rich *versus* leukocyte-poor buffy coat in the PRP preparation.

47.3.2 Activation

In choosing a preparation kit or a format for preparing the PRP, the physician must decide whether to activate the platelets prior to injection. Activation means pharmacologically adding a substance (typically calcium chloride) to the PRP to stimulate the release of growth factors such as platelet-derived growth factors (PDGF)-AB and insulin-like growth factor (IGF-1) from the platelets [11]. These factors will promote the healing cascade of events, resulting in the recruitment of other cells such as osteoblasts, stem cells, and epidermal cells [12]. The theory is that a high concentration of activated platelets will lead to better tissue repair. Once they are activated, the fibrin network begins to form a fibrin membrane, further invoking cell proliferation and leading toward tissue repair [13]. Activation is still considered controversial, however, as there is some evidence that a mix of active and resting platelets may perform tissue repair better [14], and that activation by substances already found in situ, such as collagen at the soft tissue, would be more effective [15]. Photo activation for PRP has been advocated for reduction in post-procedure immune response and pain. We will leave it to the discretion of the practicing physician as to whether activation is beneficial to their use of PRP.

A wide variety of PRP harvesting and preparation products are commercially available [16] (Table 47.1). The various kits employ activated as well as inactivated mediums and produce a variety of cell counts. The purpose of this book is to describe general principles behind using PRP and its application in treating musculoskeletal injuries with PRP injectate. The source and preparation of the final PRP product used is left to the discretion of the treating physician. For all procedures described here, the advantages of using ultrasound are readily apparent, as it allows for visualization of target areas, maximizing the delivery of the injectate to the areas of damage. Familiarity with ultrasound use, probes, and equipment is recommended for all physicians planning to use PRP as an effective treatment.

47.4 PRP Harvesting Technique

For those not using a commercial kit, it is worth describing a PRP harvesting technique. The goal when harvesting PRP is to fractionate the whole blood into separate components and extract the desired volume. Centrifuging allows one to do this.

Table 47.1 Commercial kit platelet concentrations

Commercially available kits	Manufacturer	Platelet concentration, cells in millions	WBC concentration, cells in millions
Arteriocyte MagellanPRP™	Arteriocyte Medical Systems; Hopkinton, MA	4.4	3.1
Arthrex ACP®	Arthrex; Naples, FL	1.6	1
Biomet GPS®III	Zimmer Biomet; Warsaw, IN	4.5	2.9
Cytomedix Angel® PRP	Cytomedix; Gaithersburg, MD	4.9	3.2
Cytonics APIC® PRP	Cytonics; West Palm Beach, FL	5.6	0.3
EmCyte Pure PRP® II	EmCyte; Fort Myers, FL	5.1	3.27
Harvest® SmartPreP®	Harvest Terumo BCT; Lakewood, CO	5.3	3.33
MTF CASCADE® PRP	MTF; Edison, NJ	2.9	1.88

WBC white blood cell

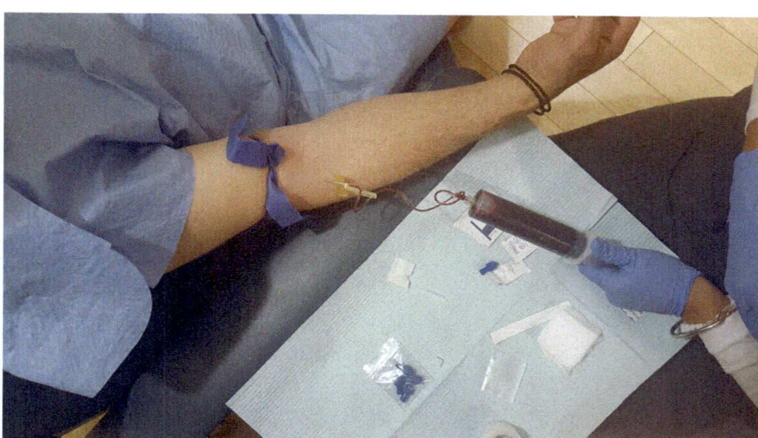

Fig. 47.1 Whole blood draw in 60 mL syringe

There are data describes single-spin and double-spin techniques. In theory, as a higher concentration of platelets potentially leads to better preparations [14], we advocate the double-spin method. One of the more validated protocols available is the Landesberg et al. [17] (double-spin) protocol, which is described briefly here:

- Using sterile technique, obtain venous access with a butterfly needle and withdraw 30 mL of blood into a blood collection vial (Fig. 47.1)
- Tubes are then placed in the centrifuge and spun at 200 × *g* for 15 min (Fig. 47.2).

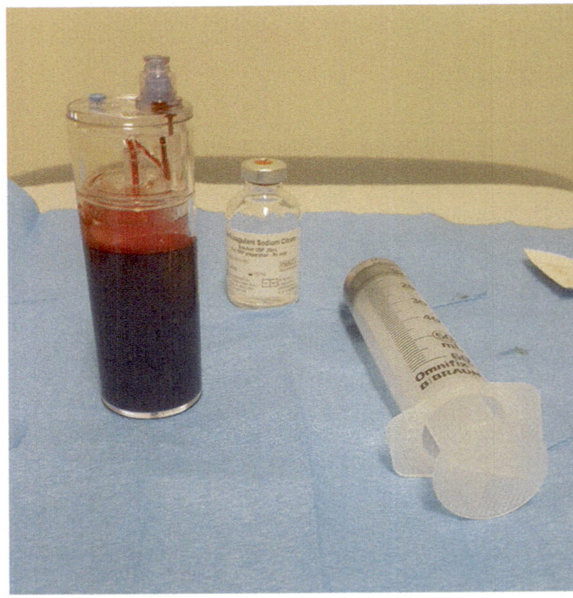

Fig. 47.2 Whole blood draw in centrifuging vial

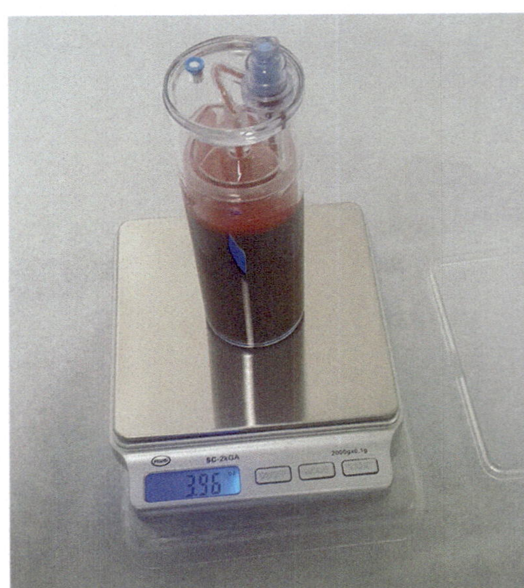

Fig. 47.3 Whole blood mass obtained

- Using the 20-mL syringe with an 18-G blunt-tip needle attached, the plasma and buffy coat are then drawn from the vials and transferred to a conical vial (Fig. 47.3).
- The conical vial with the plasma and the buffy coat is then placed back into the centrifuge.

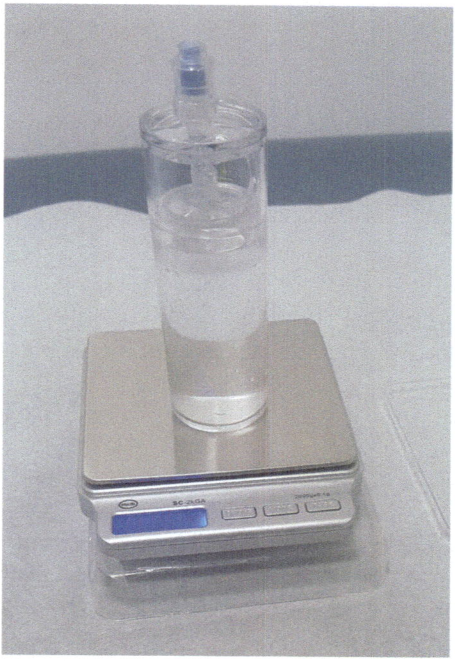

Fig. 47.4 Counterbalance mass obtained

- A second conical vial is filled with water to match the volume with plasma and the buffy coat to serve as a counterweight (Fig. 47.4).
- The centrifuge is then run a second time at 200 × *g* for 10 min (Fig. 47.5).
- The conical vial with sample is removed from the centrifuge (Fig. 47.6).
- Using a 10-mL syringe with a second blunt-tip needle attached, the upper half of the plasma is drawn up; this is the platelet-poor plasma (PPP).
- The PPP is discarded.
- The remaining volume in the conical vial is PRP; the yield should be 3–6 mL.

47.5 Basic Concerns

As with all patients undergoing a procedure, some medical concerns should be addressed. Any immunocompromised patients are potentially at high risk for infection, so it is important to make sure these patients are medically optimized, which may involve coordinating with other physicians who are managing their care. In several autoimmune degenerative joint conditions, some patients are receiving immunomodulating medications, and these should be evaluated prior to any PRP treatment.

Patients also may have thrombocytopenia or bleeding disorders, which must be considered. A decreased number of platelets may result in a bleeding disorder that increases the risk of procedural complications. A decreased number of platelets also

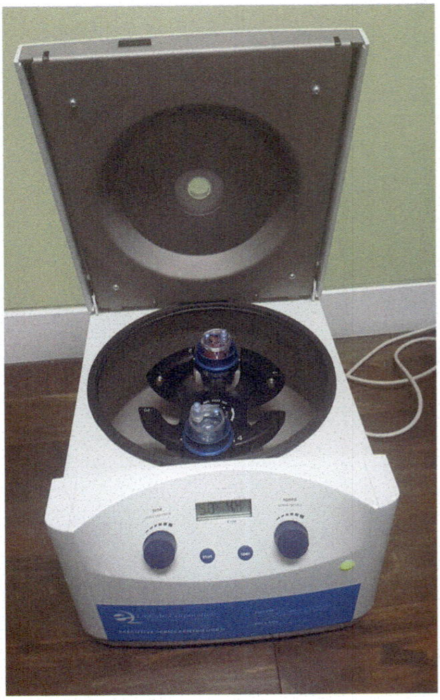

Fig. 47.5 Whole blood and counterbalance in centrifuge

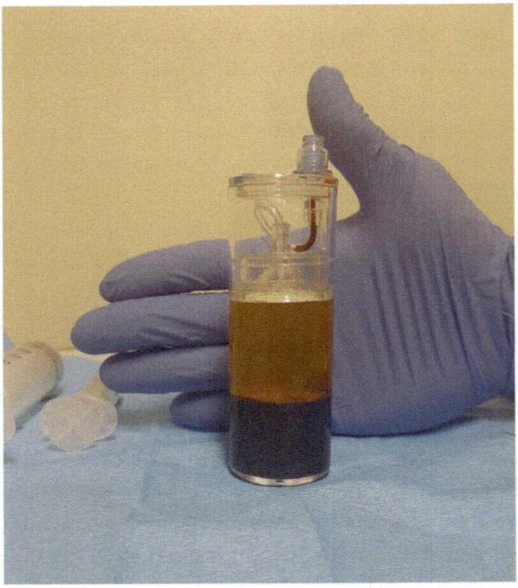

Fig. 47.6 Red blood cells (*left*), platelet-poor plasma (*center*), platelet-rich plasma (*right*)

may lead to a decrease in the final concentration of PRP, affecting the therapeutic value of the product.

Patients with active cancer, a history of cancer, or suspected oncologic disease should consult with an oncologist and receive medical clearance prior to treatment.

47.5.1 Basic Concerns and Contraindications for PRP

Immunocompromised patients are potentially at high risk for infection, and concern about patients with thrombocytopenia or bleeding disorders may be warranted. Patients with active cancer, history of cancer, or suspected oncological disease should consult with an oncologist and receive medical clearance prior to treatment with PRP.

- Infection, systemic or localized
- Coagulopathy, platelet dysfunction syndrome
- Complicated and irregular anatomy
- Chronic or continuous NSAID or steroid therapy
- Patient refusal or inability to provide informed consent

47.6 Preoperative Considerations

Each treatment should be carefully planned to determine the approximate volume of PRP required. This planning should take into account the particular injury and body part being treated, which will influence the amount of blood to be drawn. Strict sterile technique should be used throughout, as PRP is an optimal medium for transmission of infection.

47.6.1 Equipment Needed

- 18 G 1.5-in. needle
- 27 G 1.5-in. needle
- 3.5-in. spinal needle, 20 G/22 G/25 G, for shoulder labrum and shoulder rotator cuff tendons
- 1.5-in. needle, 20 G/22 G/25 G, for lateral and medial epicondyles and medial and lateral collateral ligaments
- 3- or 5-mL syringe, for local anesthetic
- 10-mL syringe, for collecting PRP from concentrating receptacle (if not included in the kit)

- 1% or 2% lidocaine
- Sterile fenestrated drape or utility drapes
- Chlorhexidine gluconate 2% or povidone-iodine
- PRP harvesting/processing kit
- Surgical marker
- Ultrasound
- Sterile sheath for ultrasound probe

After the harvesting of the PRP, the administration of the injectate will depend on the area being treated. Specific details regarding techniques to perform the injections are described in detail in Chap. 46.

47.7 Post-procedure Considerations

The post-procedure protocol is at the sole discretion of the physician, as there is evidence for both precautionary immobilization for several days to weeks [18], or for immediate mobilization [19]. Immobilization is controversial; in some cases it may be necessary, but sequential movement of the treated areas along the desired healing stress lines can be advantageous. Therefore, it is recommended that each patient be evaluated as to whether the effects of motion on the treated area will be beneficial in terms of stability and future healing, so as to make a determination on immobilization and bracing.

47.7.1 Potential Complications and Adverse Effects

All surgical procedures have a risk of complications and unwanted effects, which the performing physician should be aware of:

- Increased pain at the injection site.
- Increased inflammatory response at the treatment site from the injectate. The PRP goal in healing involves the signaling and promotion of healing factors and cell activation. These phases of healing can create increased inflammation.
- Infection is always a primary concern in performing any interventional technique. With the use of an autologous blood product, adherence to sterile technique is imperative to minimize infection risk.
- Proper labeling for samples and proper disposal should be used to prevent cross-contamination, especially if multiple patients are being treated.

47.8 Clinical Pearls

- PRP can be used for many potential applications to either induce or accelerate healing, especially in soft tissues.
- The goal—to bathe the injured tissue with the PRP—can be aided with good procedural technique and imaging such as ultrasound and fluoroscopy.
- A larger-gauge needle may aid in more rapid blood draw and minimized degradation of the cells.
- Activation of the platelets may be considered, per physician preference.
- Medications that interfere with the inflammatory cascades, such as NSAIDs, should be avoided for 7 days prior to PRP treatment (10 days for steroids) and for 1 month following treatment.

References

1. Golebiewska EM, Poole AW. Platelet secretion: from haemostasis to wound healing and beyond. Blood Rev. 2015;29:153–62.
2. Kevy SV, Jacobson MS. Preparation of growth factor enriched autologous platelet gel. Presented at the 27th annual meeting of the society for biomaterials, St. Paul, MN 26 Apr 2001.
3. Woolf AD, Pfleger B. Burden of major musculoskeletal conditions. Bull World Health Organ. 2003;81:646–56.
4. Mishra A, Pavelko T. Treatment of chronic elbow tendinosis with buffered platelet-rich plasma. Am J Sports Med. 2006;34:1774–8.
5. Rabago D, Best TM, Zgierska AE, Zeisig E, Ryan M, Crane D. A systematic review of four injection therapies for lateral epicondylosis: prolotherapy, polidocanol, whole blood and platelet-rich plasma. Br J Sports Med. 2009;43:471–81.
6. McShane JM, Shah VN, Nazarian LN. Sonographically guided percutaneous needle tenotomy for treatment of common extensor tendinosis in the elbow: is a corticosteroid necessary? J Ultrasound Med. 2008;27:1137–44.
7. Fullerton BD, Reeves KD. Ultrasonography in regenerative injection (prolotherapy) using dextrose, platelet-rich plasma, and other injectants. Phys Med Rehabil Clin N Am. 2010;21:585–605.
8. Peerbooms JC, Sluimer J, Bruijn DJ, Gosens T. Positive effect of an autologous platelet concentrate in lateral epicondylitis in a double-blind randomized controlled trial: platelet-rich plasma versus corticosteroid injection with a 1-year follow-up. Am J Sports Med. 2010;38:255–62.
9. Halpern BC, Chaudhury S, Rodeo SA. The role of platelet-rich plasma in inducing musculoskeletal tissue healing. HSS J. 2012;8:137–45.
10. Raeissadat SA, Rayegani SM, Hassanabadi H, Fathi M, Ghorbani E, Babaee M, Azma K. Knee osteoarthritis injection choices: platelet-rich plasma (PRP) versus hyaluronic acid (a one-year randomized clinical trial). Clin Med Insights Arthritis Musculoskelet Disord. 2015;8:1–8.
11. Fontenot RL, Sink CA, Werre SR, Weinstein NM, Dahlgren LA. Simple tube centrifugation for processing platelet-rich plasma in the horse. Can Vet J. 2012;53:1266–72.
12. Hamilton B, Tol JL, Knez W, Chalabi H. Exercise and the platelet activator calcium chloride both influence the growth factor content of platelet-rich plasma (PRP): overlooked biochemical factors that could influence PRP treatment. Br J Sports Med. 2015;49:957–60.
13. Schilephake H. Bone growth factors in maxillofacial skeletal reconstruction. Int J Oral Maxillofac Surg. 2002;31:469–84.

14. Dhurat R, Sukesh M. Principles and methods of preparation of platelet-rich plasma: a review and author's perspective. J Cutan Aesthet Surg. 2014;7:189–97.
15. Zandin BM, de Souza MV, Magalhães PC, Benjamin L, Maia L, de Oliveira AC, et al. Platelet activation: ultrastructure and morphometry in platelet-rich plasma of horses. Pesq Vet Bras. 2012;32:83–92.
16. Marlovits S, Mousavi M, Gäbler C, Erdös J, Vécsei VA. new simplified technique for producing platelet-rich plasma: a short technical note. Eur. Spine J. 2004;13(Suppl 1):S102–6.
17. Landesberg R, Roy M, Glickman RS. Quantification of growth factor levels using a simplified method of platelet-rich plasma gel preparation. J Oral Maxillofac Surg. 2000;58:297–301.
18. Monto RR. Platelet rich plasma treatment for chronic Achilles tendinosis. Foot Ankle Int. 2012;33:379–85.
19. Cheatham SW, Kolber MJ, Salamh PA, Hanney WJ. Rehabilitation of a partially torn distal triceps tendon after platelet rich plasma injection: a case report. Int J Sports Phys Ther. 2013;8:290–9.

Index

S. Diwan, T.R. Deer (eds.), *Advanced Procedures for Pain Management*,
https://doi.org/10.1007/978-3-319-68841-1

The manufacturer's authorised representative in the EU is Springer Nature Customer Service Centre GmbH, Europaplatz 3, 69115 Heidelberg, Germany. If you have any concerns regarding our products, please contact ProductSafety@springernature.com

Printed and bound by CPI Group (UK) Ltd, Croydon, CR0 4YY

30/09/2026

02225232-0012